Handbook of PEDIATRIC OBESITY

Etiology,

Pathophysiology,

and Prevention

Edited by

Michael I. Goran • Melinda S. Sothern

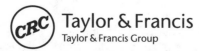

Taylor & Francis
Taylor & Francis Group

Boca Raton London New York

A CRC title, part of the Taylor & Francis imprint, a member of the
Taylor & Francis Group, the academic division of T&F Informa plc.

Published in 2006 by
CRC Press
Taylor & Francis Group
6000 Broken Sound Parkway NW, Suite 300
Boca Raton, FL 33487-2742

International Standard Book Number-10: 1-57444-912-5 (Hardcover)
International Standard Book Number-13: 978-1-57444-912-9 (Hardcover)
Library of Congress Card Number 2005050108

Library of Congress Cataloging-in-Publication Data

Handbook of pediatric obesity : etiology, pathophysiology, and prevention / edited by Michael I. Goran, Melinda Sothern.
    p. cm.
    Includes bibliographical references and index.
    ISBN 1-57444-912-5 (alk. paper)
    1. Obesity in adolescence--Handbooks, manuals, etc. 2. Obesity in children--Prevention--Handbooks, manuals, etc. 3. Overweight children--Nutrition--Handbooks, manuals, etc. 4. Obesity--Etiology--Handbooks, manuals, etc. 5. Obesity--Pathophysiology--Handbooks, manuals, etc. I. Goran, Michael I. II. Sothern, Melinda. III. Title.

RJ399.C6H363 2005
618.92'398--dc22
                                                    2005050108

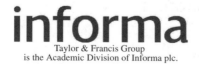
Taylor & Francis Group
is the Academic Division of Informa plc.

Visit the Taylor & Francis Web site at
http://www.taylorandfrancis.com

and the CRC Press Web site at
http://www.crcpress.com

Preface

We are delighted to introduce this timely and significant collection of papers on the topic of childhood obesity. Over the past 20 years the percentage of overweight adolescents in the United States has increased more than threefold from 5 to 16%, and the percentage of overweight children aged 6 to 11 years increased from 5 to 15%. The prevalence of overweight is even more striking among certain ethnic groups. In the United States, for example, recent data show that 44% of Latino and 40% of African American adolescents (ages 12 to 19) are considered overweight (above the 85th percentile for age and gender), which is approximately double the prevalence in Caucasians.

The general significance and scope of the pediatric obesity health problem was summarized in the 2004 report from the Institute of Medicine:

> Children's health has made tremendous strides over the past century. In general, life expectancy has increased by more than thirty years since 1900 and much of this improvement is due to the reduction of infant and early childhood mortality. Given this trajectory toward a healthier childhood, we begin the 21st century with a shocking development — an epidemic of obesity in children and youth. The increased number of obese children throughout the US during the past 25 years has led policymakers to rank it as one of the most critical public health threats of the 21st century.

When we first started working in this field 15 years ago, there was probably a handful of pediatric obesity experts. As the prevalence of childhood obesity continues to increase, and with the emergence of obesity-related diseases earlier in life, the number of investigators and studies in this area has proliferated, and the quality and sophistication of research in this area has evolved tremendously. We are extremely pleased to be able to present important summaries from some of the national leaders in this field of research. These investigators include a diverse group from multiple and complementary areas of expertise. This diversity reflects the nature and scope of the approaches that are required to understand and fix this societal problem at the level of social, behavioral, environmental, metabolic, and genetic factors. The chapters themselves are diverse, and within each chapter we purposefully attempted to assemble experts from many areas to provide a more comprehensive and balanced overview of the specific topic covered within each chapter.

In the first five chapters, we cover various topics related to the overall epidemiology of childhood obesity. In Chapter 1, Dr. Alison Field summarizes the epidemiology of obesity as well as its health and economic consequences. This chapter sets the stage by summarizing the overall scope of the problem at hand. In Chapter 2, Dr. Shumei Sun summarizes biological aspects of growth and development from birth through puberty. In Chapter 3, Dr. Dympna Gallagher and colleagues summarize current information related to ethnic differences in obesity and related outcomes. This is an important area of study because of the dramatic ethnic disparities, not only in the predisposition to obesity, but in the predisposition to obesity-related diseases. In Chapter 4, Dr. Barry Popkin and Dr. Penny Gordon-Larsen extend the epidemiological analysis to a more global perspective, with a focus on the complex interplay between economic and social factors, demonstrating that the burden of global obesity is shifting toward the poor and underserved. In Chapter 5, Dr. Stephen Daniels discusses the fascinating topic of critical periods for obesity during growth and development, covering aspects from before conception and *in utero* development, through early infancy and adolescence.

The second part of the book (Chapters 6 to 12) focuses on the etiology of childhood obesity, especially as it relates to the regulation of body weight and energy balance during growth and development. In Chapter 6, Dr. Nancy Butte and colleagues present an overview of genetic aspects of obesity and how they may be expressed at different stages of the life cycle. Genetic studies using various methodological approaches (twin studies, family studies, pedigree studies, candidate genes, genomic scans) are summarized, and there is a discussion on the various forms of monogenic obesity. Chapter 7, by Dr. Angelo Pietrobelli and Dr. David Fields, discusses methodological applications for the measurement of energy expenditure and body composition. This chapter is especially useful because it covers a wide range of applications and tools that are useful under different types of situations. Chapter 8, by Dr. Margarita Treuth and Dr. Linda Bandini, discusses the role of energy expenditure and physical activity in the regulation of body weight. This topic is relevant to the identification of factors that might predict the development of obesity, which has important implications for designing effective interventions. In Chapter 9, Dr. Cong Ning and Dr. Jack Yanovski cover endocrine factors and disorders associated with pediatric obesity. This discussion is especially relevant because the complex and dynamic changes in endocrine factors that occur during growth need to be accounted for when treating overweight and obesity. In Chapter 10, Dr. Paule Barbeau and colleagues provide a detailed overview of the interplay between physical activity and obesity in children, extending the discussion in Chapter 8 to incorporate obesity-related diseases and exercise-intervention studies.

Chapters 11 and 12 focus on obesity-related diseases in children. In particular, the incidence of pediatric type 2 diabetes has increased dramatically in the last 20 years, and in Chapter 11, Dr. Barbara Gower and Dr. Sonia Caprio discuss this finding, especially because this might relate to the observed changes in insulin dynamics that occur during puberty. In Chapter 12, Dr. Martha Cruz extends this discussion to cardiovascular disease risk factors and the metabolic syndrome, seen with increased frequency among obese children. Evidence from this chapter suggests that a state of insulin resistance associated with obesity during childhood may be responsible for the increased risk factors for type 2 diabetes and cardiovascular disease, as has been hypothesized in adults. Thus, preventive action should begin early in life and should perhaps focus on improving insulin resistance.

Chapters 13 to 15 focus in more detail on behavioral and environmental aspects. In Chapter 13, Dr. Tanja Kral and colleagues discuss behavioral aspects of food intake and how this may affect potential targets for preventing weight gain during growth and development. This chapter emphasizes modifiable factors that could serve as therapeutic targets. The discussion is presented at various levels of factors, including strategies related to food presentation (portion size, frequency of food exposure), food properties (energy density, sugar content, glycemic index), and familial patterns (family meals, TV dinners, snacking practices). In Chapter 14, Dr. Donna Spruijt-Metz and Dr. Brian Saelens present a similar discussion, this time based on an analysis of behavioral factors related to physical activity, and move toward considerations for the development of effective physical activity interventions that need to be based on sound theories of health behavior. In Chapter 15, Dr, Penny Gordon-Larsen and Dr. Kim Reynolds summarize the rapidly evolving area of research related to the influence of the built environment on obesity, especially those related to physical activity. The built environment incorporates factors in urban design and general land use (roadways, paths, access to parks and recreation, public transport). It has become clear that our environments can influence our physical activity levels in positive and negative ways, and therefore those developing strategies to increase physical activity and reduce obesity need to consider broader contexts in the environment and potentially reach a larger audience at the population level.

In the final four chapters (Chapters 16 to 19), we provide overviews on interventions for treatment and prevention. Chapter 16, by Dr. Leslie Lytle and Dr. Katie Schmitz, addresses community level influences and interventions. This chapter defines community and discusses ecological models and approaches for obesity prevention. Chapter 17, by Dr. Simone French and Dr. Mary Story, reviews school-based research and interventions, with a specific focus on obesity prevention based studies. Chapter 18, by Dr. Cara Ebbeling and Dr. David Ludwig, covers the broad topic of dietary approaches for obesity treatment and prevention. This chapter includes a fascinating review of how children's diets have changed over the past few decades and then summarizes various dietary intervention studies using conventional and popular approaches, ending with the suggestion that diets geared toward controlling postprandial glucose levels may be more effective than previous diets that used low calorie, low fat, and low carbohydrate approaches. In the final chapter, Dr. Elsie Taveras and Dr. Matthew Gillman review the link between breast-feeding and later risk of obesity, covering the epidemiological studies in this area and potential mechanisms, and ending with clinical and public health implications that may be useful for long-term obesity prevention.

In these chapters we can see why the topic of childhood obesity has become on the one hand so specialized and on the other so multidisciplinary. Trying to understand the numerous factors involved with body weight regulation and identifying interventions to prevent or treat the problem is an enormous task in and of itself. Addressing this issue in growing children is further complicated by numerous challenges specific to children, as discussed in these chapters.

For example, obesity is a moving target in growing children in that the growth process is associated with underlying increases in fat and fat free mass (i.e., growth itself requires energy imbalance to occur). This has implications for the definition and interpretation of data. Considering obesity as a dynamic condition provides a good model for studying it in children (i.e., growth is associated with a continual increase in body fatness, as opposed to adults, where obesity is generally a static model). The difficulty comes in trying to separate the changes in fat mass that are due to obesity (or obesity reduction) from those associated with growth itself.

The general philosophy underlying intervention approaches in children is also different for a number of reasons. First, pharmacological intervention is less of an option because of ethical concerns related to long-term drug use in children and because of unknown effects of pharmacological interventions on growth and development. Obesity treatment and prevention in children requires consideration of the specific social and environmental factors, such as family and school.

Despite these challenges, we have made considerable progress, and our goal was to summarize this progress. Because this is a rapidly evolving area of research, we are sure that we will need to modify this body of work in the not-too-distant future. We hope that you find this work as useful and as inspiring as we have in putting it together.

As a final note we would like to thank all of the authors and coauthors for their dedication and enthusiasm to the cause. None of the authors received an honorarium for this work. They contributed their chapters on the basis of an absolute commitment and enthusiasm for their research. To exemplify this outlook, the editors and authors have agreed to donate a portion of any royalties to the pediatric interest group of NAASO: The Obesity Society, a group that is committed to education and professional networking among pediatric obesity researchers and practitioners. It has been a wonderful and inspiring experience to have been able to collaborate with such a wonderful group who share a collective vision of a healthier and brighter outlook for future generations.

Michael I. Goran, Ph.D.
Professor of Preventive Medicine and Associate Director
USC Institute for Prevention Research
Keck School of Medicine
University of Southern California

Melinda S. Sothern, Ph.D.
Associate Professor and Director
Section of Health Promotion
School of Public Health
Louisiana State University Health Sciences Center

About the Editors

Michael I. Goran, Ph.D. is professor of preventive medicine and physiology and biophysics and associate director of the Institute for Prevention Research at the University of Southern California, Keck School of Medicine. He has been involved with studies related to childhood obesity since 1990. His earlier research focused on the regulation of energy balance and body composition, and the role of energy expenditure in the development of obesity in children. More recently, he has studied the relationship between body fat, especially visceral fat, and increased disease risk in children and adolescents. Dr. Goran's current studies include a natural history study of the development of type 2 diabetes in obese Hispanic adolescents, and a longitudinal cohort study of changes in insulin resistance across puberty in Caucasian and African American children. He is especially interested in ethnic differences in obesity, insulin resistance and associated complications during growth and development. Currently he is involved with several initiatives to design optimal interventions for the prevention and treatment of obesity and type 2 diabetes in children of various ethnic groups. Since 1991his research has been funded by the National Institutes of Health, the United States Department of Agriculture, and the American Diabetes Association.

He has published 170 peer-reviewed papers and reviews on topics related to the regulation of energy metabolism and body composition and the health effects of obesity, especially in children. He has received a variety of national and international awards for his research including The Nutrition Society Medal for Research (1999), the Kretchmer Award for research in childhood nutrition from the American Society for Clinical Nutrition (2000) and the Lilly Scientific Achievement Award from the North American Association for the Study of Obesity (2001).

Melinda S. Sothern, Ph.D. is an Associate Professor of Research and directs the Section of Health Promotion in the Division of Behavioral and Community Health in the Louisiana State University (LSU) Health Sciences Center, School of Public Health and the Prevention of Childhood Obesity Laboratory at the LSU Pennington Biomedical Research Center. Her research has been widely published in scientific journals and recently in a book for parents and pediatricians entitled *Trim Kids* (2001, Harper Resource, New York, NY). She is currently serving as Principal Investigator on two National Institute of Health (NIH)-sponsored studies entitled, *Insulin Sensitivity in Children with Low Birth Weight* and *Exploring Mechanisms of the Metabolic Syndrome in African American and Caucasian Youth*. She is also currently a co-investigator in the NIH sponsored, 6-year study entitled, *Increasing Physical Activity Patterns in Adolescent Girls: the TAAG Study*, with seven other sites nationwide, and directs the physical activity intervention of the NIH-sponsored study, *Environmental Approaches for the Prevention of Weight Gain: The Wise Mind Study*, and is Co-PI and mentor of the NIH-funded study, *Environmental Determinants of Physical Activity in Parks*.

Dr. Sothern recently co-authored a position paper and serves as faculty for the American Dietetic Association pediatric weight management certification program. She is considered a national spokesperson for overweight youth and has been featured extensively in national and international television, radio, and print media including *Good Morning America*, the *Today* show, *Fox News*, *48 Hours*, Nickelodeon TV, *The Oprah Winfrey Show*, Discovery Channel, CNN International, Yorkshire TV, British Broadcasting Co., *USA Today*, *Associated Press – World News*, *The Washington Post*, *Wall Street Journal*, *National Geographic*, *Parents Magazine*, *Parenting*, *Better Homes and Gardens*, *Prevention Magazine* and many others.

Dr. Sothern has led her field in establishing standardized guidelines for prescribing exercise for children with increasing levels of obesity and is best known for her work in promoting active play as a means of preventing and treating childhood obesity. She has been a member of the American College of Sports Medicine (ACSM) and the North American Association for the Study of Obesity (NAASO) for more than 15 years, is a fellow and council member of NAASO, and currently serves as Past Chairman of the Pediatric Obesity Interest Group. She is also past member of the NAASO Public Affairs Committee and current member of the Publication Committee and is a scientific presenter for the NAASO Distinguished Lecture Series. She has provided over 100 invited scientific lectures to universities and medical centers, is a reviewer for the National Institutes of Health and numerous pediatric, obesity and exercise scientific journals, and provides scientific advice to several major national and international corporations.

List of Contributors

Carlos A. Bacino
Department of Molecular and Human Genetics
Baylor College of Medicine
Houston, Texas

Linda G. Bandini, Ph.D., R.D.
Eunice Kennedy Shriver Center
University of Massachusetts Medical School
Waltham, Massachusetts
and
Boston University
Department of Health Sciences
Boston, Massachusetts

Paule Barbeau, Ph.D.
Georgia Prevention Institute
Department of Pediatrics
Medical College of Georgia
Augusta, Georgia

Nancy F. Butte
USDA/ARS Children's Nutrition Research
   Center
Department of Pediatrics
Baylor College of Medicine
Houston, Texas

Sonia Caprio, M.D.
Yale University School of Medicine
New Haven, Connecticut

Shelley A. Cole
Department of Genetics
Southwest Foundation for Biomedical Research
San Antonio, Texas

Anthony G. Comuzzie
Department of Genetics
Southwest Foundation for Biomedical Research
San Antonio, Texas

Martha L. Cruz, D.V.M., D.Phil.
Department of Preventive Medicine
Keck School of Medicine
University of Southern California
Los Angeles, California

Stephen R. Daniels, M.D., Ph.D.
Division of Cardiology, Department of
   Pediatrics
Cincinnati Children's Hospital Medical Center
Cincinnati, Ohio

Meredith S. Dolan, M.S., R.D.
Weight and Eating Disorders Program
University of Pennsylvania School of Medicine
Philadelphia, Pennsylvania

Cara B. Ebbeling, Ph.D.
Division of Endocrinology
Department of Medicine
Children's Hospital
Boston, Massachusetts

Myles S. Faith, Ph.D.
Weight and Eating Disorders Program
University of Pennsylvania School of Medicine
   and Children's Hospital of Philadelphia
Philadelphia, Pennsylvania

José R. Fernández, Ph.D.
Division of Physiology and Metabolism
Department of Nutrition Sciences
and
Statistical Genetics
Department of Biostatistics
University of Alabama at Birmingham
Birmingham, Alabama

Alison E. Field, Sc.D.
Children's Hospital Boston
Division of Adolescent/Young Adult Medicine
Boston, Massachusetts

David A. Fields, Ph.D.
Endocrinology and Diabetes
Department of Pediatrics
University of Oklahoma Health Science Center
Oklahoma City, Oklahoma

Simone A. French, Ph.D.
Division of Epidemiology and Community
  Health
University of Minnesota
Minneapolis, Minnesota

Dympna Gallagher, Ed.D.
Body Composition Unit–Obesity Research
  Center
St. Luke's–Roosevelt Hospital and Columbia
  University
New York, New York

Matthew W. Gillman, M.D., S.M.
Center for Child Health Care Studies
Department of Ambulatory Care and Prevention
Harvard Pilgrim Health Care and Harvard
  Medical School
and
Department of Nutrition
Harvard School of Public Health
Boston, Massachusetts

Penny Gordon-Larsen, Ph.D.
Department of Nutrition
Schools of Public Health & Medicine
University of North Carolina at Chapel Hill
Chapel Hill, North Carolina

Barbara A. Gower, Ph.D.
Department of Nutrition Sciences
University of Alabama at Birmingham
Birmingham, Alabama

Bernard Gutin, Ph.D.
Georgia Prevention Institute
Department of Pediatrics
Medical College of Georgia
Augusta, Georgia

Qing He, Ph.D.
New York Obesity Research Center
St. Luke's-Roosevelt Hospital
New York, New York

Paul B. Higgins, B.S.
Division of Physiology and Metabolism
Department of Nutrition Sciences
University of Alabama at Birmingham
Birmingham, Alabama

Julia Kerns, B.A.
Weight and Eating Disorders Program
University of Pennsylvania School of Medicine
Philadelphia, Pennsylvania

Tanja V.E. Kral, Ph.D.
Weight and Eating Disorders Program
University of Pennsylvania School of Medicine
Philadelphia, Pennsylvania

David S. Ludwig, M.D., Ph.D.
Division of Endocrinology
Department of Medicine
Children's Hospital
Boston, Massachusetts

Leslie A. Lytle, Ph.D., R.D.
Division of Epidemiology & Community
  Health
School of Public Health
University of Minnesota
Minneapolis, Minnesota

Cong Ning, M.D., Ph.D.
Unit on Growth and Obesity, Developmental
  Endocrinology Branch
National Institute of Child Health and Human
  Development
National Institutes of Health
Bethesda, Maryland

Angelo Pietrobelli, M.D.
Pediatric Unit
Verona University Medical School
Policlinic GB Rossi
Verona, Italy

Barry M. Popkin, Ph.D.
Department of Nutrition
Schools of Public Health & Medicine
University of North Carolina at Chapel Hill
Chapel Hill, North Carolina

Kim D. Reynolds, Ph.D.
Institute for Health Promotion & Disease
  Prevention Research
University of Southern California
Alhambra, California

Brian E. Saelens, Ph.D.
Cincinnati Children's Hospital Medical Center
Division of Behavioral Medicine and Clinical
  Psychology
University of Cincinnati College of Medicine
Department of Pediatrics
Cincinnati, Ohio

Kathryn Schmitz, Ph.D.
Assistant Professor
Center for Clinical Epidemiology and
  Biostatistics
University of Pennsylvania
Philadelphia, Pennsylvania

Melinda S. Sothern, Ph.D.
School of Public Health
Louisiana State University Health Sciences
  Center
New Orleans, Louisiana

Donna Spruijt-Metz, M.F.A., Ph.D.
Institute for Health Promotion and Disease
  Prevention
University of Southern California
Alhambra, California

Mary Story, Ph.D., R.D.
Division of Epidemiology and Community
  Health
University of Minnesota
Minneapolis, Minnesota

Shumei S. Sun, Ph.D.
Department of Community Health
Wright State University School of Medicine
Dayton, Ohio

Elsie M. Taveras, M.D., M.P.H.
Center for Child Health Care Studies
Department of Ambulatory Care and Prevention
Harvard Pilgrim Health Care and Harvard
  Medical School
Boston, Massachusetts

Margarita S. Treuth, Ph.D.
Center for Human Nutrition
Johns Hopkins Bloomberg School of Public
  Health
Baltimore, Maryland

Jack A. Yanovski, M.D., Ph.D.
Unit on Growth and Obesity, Developmental
  Endocrinology Branch
National Institute of Child Health and Human
  Development
National Institutes of Health
Bethesda, Maryland

Contents

1 Epidemiology of the Health and Economic Consequences of Pediatric Obesity

Alison E. Field

CONTENTS

INTRODUCTION: THE SCOPE OF THE PROBLEM

Pediatric obesity is a serious public health problem in the United States. During the past two decades, the prevalence of overweight has more than doubled among children and adolescents.[1]

According to the 1999 to 2002 National Health and Nutrition Examination Survey, approximately 31% of children and adolescents are overweight or at risk for overweight (i.e., body mass index [BMI] *greater than* or equal to the national 85th percentile for age and sex).[2] The prevalence of overweight is particularly high among African Americans and Hispanics. Among adolescents approximately 37% of African Americans and 41% of Mexican Americans are overweight or at risk for overweight, compared with 28% of white adolescents.[2] Pediatric and adolescent overweight are public health problems not only in the United States, but also in other developed and affluent countries, and now they are spreading to less affluent countries, such as Brazil and China.[3] (See Chapter 4, "An International Perspective on Pediatric Obesity.") Although genes may predispose certain individuals more than others to obesity, the increasing prevalence of obesity among pediatric and adolescent populations in recent decades suggests that important nongenetic factors are responsible for the magnitude of the current problem.

DEFINITIONS OF OVERWEIGHT

In the United States the terminology frequently used to describe excessive weight in childhood and adolescence is slightly different from the terminology used to describe it in adults. Among pediatric obesity researchers in the United States, the term *obesity* is infrequently used; instead the terms *at risk of overweight* and *overweight* are frequently used to define high weight status in childhood and adolescence.[4] In other countries these two groups are referred to as *overweight* and *obese*, respectively.[5] In the United States and elsewhere, among adults the terms *overweight* and *obesity* are used to define degrees of excessive weight. *Overweight* refers to weighing more than a standard level for height and age. Overweight individuals may have excessive stores of body fat; however, highly active people who have substantial muscle mass may weigh slightly more than the standard for their height despite low body fat. Thus people may be overweight, but not over-fat. *Obesity* traditionally has been classified based on body fat stores, but now is frequently defined as weighing much more than a standard level for age and height.

Body mass index, a formula that combines weight and height and is often used in epidemiologic studies assessing the relationship between weight and disease, is commonly used to determine if someone weighs much more than the standard or ideal level for his or her age and height. In addition, the public health recommendations on body weight for children are based on age- and gender-specific percentiles of BMI. The advantage of using BMI (kg/m^2) instead of weight in pounds or kilograms is that it accounts for height, an essential piece of information when evaluating weight. Because children and adolescents are growing, the age and gender of the child are needed to evaluate whether an individual child or adolescent is a healthy weight or overweight. One can use the same BMI percentile cutoff, such as being above the age- and gender-specific 85th percentile, at all ages, but the absolute BMI value will vary by age. For example, a 10-year-old boy with a BMI of 23 kg/m^2 has a BMI above the 95th percentile so he is overweight, whereas, a 15-year-old boy with a BMI of 23 kg/m^2 is within the normal weight range for height. The issue of the age cutoff for evaluating young people against the adult U.S. Dietary Guidelines,[6] as opposed to the pediatric standards from the Centers for Disease Control and Prevention,[7] has not received adequate attention. The adult guidelines classify BMI as follows: less than 18.5 kg/m^2 is underweight, 18.5 to 24.9 kg/m^2 is the healthy weight range, 25 to 29.9 kg/m^2 is overweight, and greater than 30 kg/m^2 is obese. The international pediatric standards developed by Cole and colleagues,[5] which are based on data from six countries, were created to map to the adult standards at age 18, and therefore, it is clear when the transition should be made. Moreover, they have age- and gender-specific BMI cutoff values to pass through a BMI of 25 kg/m^2 (overweight) and 30 kg/m^2 (obesity) at age 18. In the United States there is a strong bias toward using the CDC standards, based on several large U.S. datasets. Although the cutoff values are not extremely different from Cole's international standards, there is a problem with adolescents being considered overweight (BMI ≥ 25 kg/m^2) according to the adult standards, but not the pediatric standards (BMI 95th percentile for age and gender). This misclassification begins to occur before age 18; it starts at age 13.5 years for boys and age 12 for girls. The problem is much less of an issue when a BMI 85th percentile for age and gender is used to define the excessive weight outcome. In that case, the inconsistent classification does not occur until 17.5 years for the boys and 17 years for girls.

Categorizing people based on BMI or BMI percentiles for age and gender works fairly well on a population level, but on the individual level it has the disadvantage that someone with low body fat but very high muscle mass may be misclassified as obese (or overweight, if using the pediatric terminology). The use of direct measures of body fatness (alone or in combination with BMI) will lead to better classification of weight status, particularly among physically active individuals because BMI does not take into account lean body mass, but this may not be feasible in large cohort studies. Although the correlation between BMI, BMI percentiles, and body fat is very high,[8–10] BMI is not a direct measure of body fatness; therefore, there will be some misclassification when weight status is based on BMI alone. The gold standard for measuring body fat is underwater weighing or radiographic techniques (such as dual-energy x-ray absorptiometry, computed tomography [CT] scans, and magnetic resonance imaging[MRI]), but these methods are labor intensive, are expensive to collect, and require skilled collection personnel. Therefore, it is not feasible to collect these types of data in general clinical settings or large epidemiologic studies. As a result, many research studies classify children's weight status based on their BMI, age, and gender. Moreover, in the United States, clinicians are being urged to use the CDC pediatric BMI growth charts to monitor the weight status of their patients. Among adults, overweight is defined as having a BMI greater than or equal to 25 kg/m^2,[6] but in children and adolescents one cannot use one cutoff value because both weight and height should be changing as part of normal development. Therefore, instead of a uniform cutoff value that applies to children and adolescents of all ages and both genders, weight status is defined in terms of age- and gender-specific percentiles of BMI. In the United States, *at risk of overweight* is defined as having a BMI at or above the 85th percentile for age- and gender and *overweight* is defined as having a BMI above the 95th percentile. In other countries these two groups are referred to as *overweight* and *obese*, respectively.

TRACKING OF OVERWEIGHT FROM CHILDHOOD AND ADOLESCENCE INTO ADULTHOOD

One of the reasons for concern about the rising prevalence of childhood and adolescent overweight is that overweight children and adolescents are likely to become overweight or obese adults. Weight status tracks with age, and the risk of an overweight child becoming an obese adult rises with age.[11–14] In one study among preschool children, an obese child was about twice as likely as a nonobese child to become an obese adult.[15] Adolescents who were overweight, however, were almost 18 times more likely than their leaner peers to be obese in early adulthood.[16] Moreover, the risk of adult obesity is not limited to children who are overweight. Among 2617 participants in the Bogalusa Heart Study, Freedman et al.[17] observed that children in the 50th to 74th percentile were more likely than those with a BMI below the 50th percentile in childhood to become overweight or obese adults and that the percentage of children who were overweight or obese in adulthood increased with increasing BMI percentile in childhood.

CONSEQUENCES OF OBESITY IN CHILDHOOD AND ADOLESCENCE

Among adults obesity and higher relative weights are risk factors for cardiovascular disease (CVD),[18] certain cancers,[19,20] diabetes,[21] and mortality.[22] The health outcomes of pediatric obesity have been less studied.

ELEVATED BLOOD PRESSURE

Among children and adolescents, BMI has been observed to be positively associated with elevated blood pressure. Freedman et al.[23] assessed the relationship between overweight and cardiovascular risk factors among 9167 children, 5 to 17 years of age, in the Bogalusa Heart Study. They observed that children who were overweight were significantly more likely to have elevated diastolic blood pressure (odds ratio [OR] = 2.4, 95% confidence interval [CI] 1.8 to 3.0), systolic blood pressure (OR = 4.5, 95% CI 3.6 to 5.8), insulin levels (OR = 12.6, 95% CI 10 to 16), and triglycerides (OR = 7.1, 95% CI 5.8 to 8.6). Similar results were seen in the National Growth and Health Study. Morrison et al.[24] observed that among the 1166 white and 1213 black girls, 20% of the white girls and 30% of the black girls were overweight (BMI 85th percentile). The overweight girls in both races had significantly higher triglycerides, and systolic and diastolic blood pressure, and significantly lower HDL than nonoverweight girls.

IMPAIRED GLUCOSE TOLERANCE, INSULIN RESISTANCE, AND TYPE 2 DIABETES

Although there are minimal data on the relationship between early childhood obesity and the development of type 2 diabetes, there is ample evidence that childhood weight status is associated with impaired glucose tolerance and insulin resistance. For example, among the 679 children in the Minneapolis Children's Blood Pressure Study, BMI in childhood was positively related to fasting insulin levels in young adulthood (Pearson correlation = .3, $p < .001$).[25] Similarly, in the Bogalusa Heart Study, both BMI and percentage of body fat were associated with fasting insulin levels in childhood[23] and adulthood.[17] During childhood, overweight children were 12 times more likely than their leaner peers to have high fasting insulin levels, and the risk was greater for whites than blacks.[23] The race difference may reflect the finding that independent of body fatness, African Americans have lower insulin sensitivity than whites.[26,27] Less is known about insulin secretion and sensitivity among Hispanics; however, Goran et al.[28] observed that insulin sensitivity was significantly lower in Hispanics and African Americans compared with white children. In addition, in a study 55 obese children and 112 obese adolescents who had been referred to a pediatric obesity clinic, Sinha et al.[29] observed that 25% of the children and 21% of the adolescents had impaired glucose tolerance and 4 (4%) of the adolescents had asymptomatic type 2 diabetes. All the cases were either African American or Hispanic. Because the sample was clinic based, it is impossible to extrapolate the population prevalence of type 2 diabetes from this study; however, the study suggests that race disparities in the prevalence of type 2 diabetes begin in childhood and adolescence.

ASTHMA

Most,[30,31] but not all,[32] cross-sectional analyses have observed an association between childhood overweight and asthma; however, the results have been difficult to interpret because the temporal order of the association was unclear. Some have argued that the cross-sectional associations are due to asthmatic children becoming overweight because their asthma limits their activity and thus they gain more weight than their peers. However, recent prospective studies support the hypothesis that overweight children are more likely than their peers to develop asthma.[33,34] Among 3792 participants in the Children's Health Study in Southern California who were assessed annually between 1993 and 1998, overweight and obese children were significantly more likely than their leaner peers to develop asthma.[34] The association was stronger among the boys than the girls. Among 9828 children examined annually over 5 years in six U.S. cities, the risk of developing asthma was associated with BMI at baseline and BMI change during the study, but the association was stronger among the girls than the boys.[33] In addition, one study on the relationship between birth weight and emergency room visits for asthma during a 10-year period among 83,595 infants found that the risk of an emergency room visit related to asthma increased linearly with birth weight over 4.5 kg.[35] Taken together the results suggest that the most common chronic disease in childhood, obesity, is a risk factor for one of the other most common chronic diseases of childhood, asthma.

OTHER HEALTH CONSEQUENCES

Results from primarily cross-sectional and clinic-based studies suggest that overweight children may be at increased risk for certain orthopedic conditions, neurological conditions, and gallstones.[36] The orthopedic conditions most consistently linked to pediatric obesity are slipped capital epiphysis[37-40] and Blount's disease,[41] a growth disorder of the tibia that causes bowing of the lower legs. Another morbidity associated with pediatric obesity is idiopathic intracranial hypertension (pseudotumor cerebri), which can lead to blindness. Pseudotumor cerebri has been observed to be more common among overweight as compared with lean children.[42,43] Many of these studies have been conducted with children and adolescents with gallbladder disease from specialized clinics, thus the generalizability of the results to the general population is not well known.

Among adults, gallstones are a fairly common, often quite painful, condition that is most common among overweight individuals.[44] Gallstones are believed to form when the bile contains too much cholesterol or bilirubin or not enough bile salts, or when the gallbladder does not empty properly. Stones can range in size, and many of them are asymptomatic. Gallstones that are symptomatic can be very painful. The most common course of treatment is laparoscopic surgery to remove the gallbladder (laparoscopic cholecystectomy). Among adults the relationship among weight, weight change, and gallstone formation is very strong.[21,45] The association has been less studied among children and adolescents; however, several clinic-based studies have observed that overweight was more common among cases.[46-48]

SOCIAL AND PSYCHOSOCIAL CONSEQUENCES

Unlike many of the physical health consequences of childhood and adolescent overweight that may not become manifest until adulthood, the social and psychosocial consequences are immediate. Despite the rapid increase in the prevalence of overweight, there are considerable social consequences of being overweight in a Westernized society that values thinness and fitness. Although Phillips and Hill[49] observed that among 313 9-year-old girls, those who were overweight were not less popular than their leaner peers, Davison and Birch[50] observed that negative stereotypes of overweight people were common among 178 9-year-old girls and their mothers and fathers. Moreover, in a study of 5-year-old girls, higher weight status was associated with lower perceived cognitive ability,[51] suggesting that negative values associated with overweight are transmitted to young children. Other studies of older children have suggested that parents may play a role in the transmission of cultural values about desirable body weight and shape.[52-57]

Large studies among adolescents have observed that overweight youth are more likely than lean adolescents to be socially isolated.[58,59] There are numerous other adverse social consequences for overweight adolescents. Adolescent females who are overweight are less likely to be accepted to college[60] and less likely to marry.[61] Gortmaker et al.[61] followed a nationally representative sample of 10,039 young people, 16 to 24 years of age, over 8 years. They observed that compared with women who had not been overweight as adolescents, those who had been overweight completed fewer years of school (0.3 years less), were less likely to marry (20% less likely), and had lower household incomes ($6710 less). There were fewer consequences for males, but males who had been overweight were 11% less likely than their peers to be married at the follow-up visit.

Eating Disorders

Children and adolescents, particularly girls, who are overweight are more likely than their leaner peers to be extremely concerned with their weight and to engage in bulimic behaviors.[62-65] Clinical studies have found that bulimics frequently report having been overweight prior to the onset of the disorder.[66,67] Because bulimic patients have usually been ill for at least several years before seeking treatment,[68] it is possible that the reports of having been overweight are a distorted self-perception rather than accurate recall. In a series of case control studies, Fairburn and colleagues observed that a recalled history of childhood obesity was associated with having anorexia nervosa or bulimia nervosa in adulthood.[69,70] However, only univariate associations were presented, thus it is unclear whether the association with BMI was a true association or the result of confounding. We are aware of only one prospective study on the topic. In a 3-year prospective study, Patton et al.[71] did not observe an independent association between weight status and risk of developing eating disorders of at least subthreshold severity. In the Growing Up Today Study, over a 3-year period, Field et al. observed that boys who engaged in binge eating gained significantly more weight that their peers.[72] Moreover, binge eating severity has been observed to lessen with weight loss;[73] thus, it is possible that binge eating leads to, as opposed to results from, weight gain and overweight. More longitudinal studies are needed to better understand the relationship between weight status and the development of eating disorders.

Teasing and Bullying

Other adverse social consequences to overweight include teasing and bullying. In a cross-sectional study of 4746 adolescents in Minnesota, Neumark-Sztainer et al.[74] observed that both underweight and overweight adolescents were more likely than their average-weight peers to be teased about their weight. Among the overweight adolescents, a higher percentage of those who were teased engaged in binge eating and unhealthy weight regulation practices. Janssen et al.[75] assessed the relationship of weight status to being bullied and bullying others among a sample of 5749 Canadian 11- to 16-year-old boys and girls. Compared with normal-weight children of the same age, obese girls and boys were significantly more likely to be the victim of peer aggression, whereas neither overweight nor obese girls or boys were more likely than their normal weight peers to bully others.

Self-Esteem

The relationship of overweight to self-esteem is not well understood. Many cross-sectional studies report that self-esteem is lower in overweight or obese children compared with leaner children;[76,77] however, other studies have not observed this association.[78] There are limited prospective data on the relationship between obesity, weight change, and self-esteem. Strauss observed that there was no cross-sectional association at baseline between obesity and global self-esteem among 1520 children, 9 to 10 years of age, in the National Longitudinal Study of Youth.[76] However over a 4-year period, compared with nonobese white and Hispanic girls, the self-esteem levels of obese white and Hispanic girls decreased significantly. The decrease among black girls was not significant. As a result of the decreases in self-esteem, at ages 13 to 14 there was a cross-sectional difference in levels of self-esteem between obese and nonobese white and Hispanic girls. The decrease in self-esteem among the boys was significant, but less striking than among the girls.

Quality of Life

Among children and adults, obesity has an impact on many aspects of quality of life. One study of 371 children, 8 to 11 years of age, observed that overweight children scored significantly lower than normal weight children on physical functioning and a psychosocial health summary.[79] More striking is that in a study of 106 children and adolescents, Schwimmer et al.[80] observed that obese children and adolescents had a health-related quality of life that was lower than their peers who were not overweight and similar to that of children and adolescents diagnosed with cancer.

LONG-TERM HEALTH CONSEQUENCES OF PEDIATRIC OBESITY

MORTALITY

Excessive weight in adulthood increases the risk of death, particularly death due to cardiovascular disease. There are limited data on the relationship between childhood or adolescent BMI and risk of death in adulthood. Must et al.[81] studied 508 men and women who as 13 to 18 years olds had participated in the Harvard Growth Study in the 1920s and 1930s. Among the males, those who had been overweight as adolescents were 80% more likely to than their peers to have died from any cause and were 230% more likely to have died from cardiovascular disease. However, women who had been overweight as adolescents were no more likely than their peers to have died. Similar results were observed by Gunnell et al.[82] in a 57-year follow-up of the Boyd Orr cohort. Among the males, but not the females, Gunnell and colleagues observed that a high BMI in childhood was predictive of death during the follow-up. Compared with males who had a BMI between the 25th and 49th percentile in childhood, those who had a BMI above the 75th percentile were 90% more likely to have died during the follow-up (relative risk [RR] = 1.9, 95% CI 1.0 to 3.6) and 270% more likely to have died from ischemic heart disease (RR = 2.7, 95% CI 1.2 to 6.0).

Hoffmans et al.[83] assessed the relationship between BMI at age 18 (late adolescence) and mortality during 32 years of follow-up among a cohort of middle-aged Dutch men. They observed that men who had been overweight (BMI $\geq$ 25 kg/m^2) were 50% more likely to die during the follow-up than were their peers who had a BMI < 19 kg/m^2 at age 18. The elevation in risk was strongest for coronary deaths (RR = 2.5). Although Hoffmans did not observe an association between childhood BMI and mortality from cancer, that lack of an association may have been due to not separating out the cancers that are largely attributable to smoking. The inclusion of smoking-related cancers could dilute or obscure any associations between BMI and cancer mortality. Okasha et al.[84] observed that adolescent weight status was predictive of mortality from cancers not known to be related to smoking. Compared with women with a BMI < 20.14 in adolescence, women with a BMI between 21.5 and 22.9 were 240% (RR = 2.4, 95% CI 1.0 to 5.6) and women with a BMI greater than or equal to 22.9 were 260% (RR = 2.6, 95% CI 1.1 to 6.0) more likely to die from cancers not related to smoking. Among the men the elevation in risk was only seen among those in the highest quartile of adolescent BMI (RR = 1.3), but among the females the risk was more linear and the increase in risk was larger than seen among the males.

Although mortality is a clearly defined outcome, the results of mortality analyses can be difficult to interpret. Except for diseases that are almost always fatal regardless of treatment, mortality is a function of incidence of disease, stage of illness at diagnosis, and the effectiveness of treatment. Many forms of cardiovascular disease are treatable by either pharmacotherapy or intervention (i.e., angioplasty or surgery), thus the relationship between excess weight and death from cardiovascular disease does not necessarily translate to same relationship with the development of cardiovascular disease.

CARDIOVASCULAR DISEASE

Heart Disease

Although a high birth weight decreases risk, both weight and weight status in adolescence are positively related to the risk of developing heart disease in adulthood. Several studies have observed that males and females with an elevated BMI in late adolescence are more likely than their leaner peers to develop cardiovascular disease. In the Caerphilly Prospective Study, Yarnell et al.[85] studied 2335 middle-aged men who provided recalled information on weight and height at age 18. Men who had been obese (BMI > 30 kg/m^2) at age 18 were two times more likely (OR = 2.2, 95% CI 1.1 to 4.3) than their leaner male counterparts to have a coronary event within 14 years of joining the prospective study. Moreover, among the 508 men and women in the Harvard Growth Study, those who had been overweight as adolescents were more likely than their peers to have a coronary event in adulthood.[81]

Although high BMI in childhood and adulthood increases the risk of cardiovascular events, birth weight has an inverse association with risk. The risk is particularly elevated for people who are born small and grow rapidly during childhood. Barker and colleagues[86] observed that in a cohort study of 13,517 adults, those born weighing more than 4 kg were at the lowest risk of coronary heart disease (CHD), but within the leanest strata of birth weight, the risk of CHD increased with each higher category of BMI at age 11. The association between birth weight and later risk of disease is thought to be due to the effects of programming *in utero*.[87-89] Based on animal models, it is believed that perinatal nutrition might have a lasting effect on physiology and metabolism.[88] Thus, the increase in risk of developing CVD is believed to be at least partially due to the consequences of suboptimal nutrition during pregnancy. In addition, there are several mechanisms through which obesity and weight gain during later childhood and adolescence might increase the risk of coronary heart disease. Hyperlipidemia is one mechanism. BMI is positively correlated with triglyceride levels and inversely correlated with HDL levels. Low HDL levels are more predictive than high total cholesterol of developing heart disease. Thus, pediatric and adolescent obesity increases risk of heart disease in part by increasing total triglycerides, decreasing HDL levels, and making the HDL/LDL ratio less favorable.[90]

Hypertension

Although high blood pressure (i.e., hypertension) is a highly treatable condition, if left untreated its consequences are severe, and hypertension is a strong predictor of more severe CVD. The combination of obesity and hypertension is associated with an increased risk of cardiac failure due to thickening of the ventricular wall and increased heart volume.[91]

There is a linear relation between body weight and blood pressure among children, adolescents, and adults. The relationship between BMI and the risk of developing hypertension has been extensively researched among adults. Studies have observed that both weight[21,92,93] and weight gain[92,93] are positively associated with the development of hypertension in adulthood. Although not as extensively researched, it appears that BMI in childhood and adolescents is also predictive of the development of hypertension in adulthood. Among 82,473 female nurses in the Nurses' Health Study, Huang et al.[93] observed that women who were overweight (BMI > 25 kg/m^2) in late adolescence (age 18) were two times more likely (RR = 2.28, 95% CI 2.12 to 2.45) than women with a BMI less than 18.2 kg/m^2 to develop hypertension in middle age. Moreover, the increase in risk was linear. For every 1-kg/m^2 increase in BMI at 18 years of age, the risk for hypertension increased 8%. Srinivasan et al.[94] observed that in a biracial sample of 783 people, initially 13 to 17 years and then followed up when they were 27 to 31 years of age, those who had been overweight as adolescents were 8.5 times more likely than their leaner peers to have hypertension and high cholesterol as young adults.[94] They observed that males were more likely than females to develop elevated systolic blood pressure and that overweight youth were approximately four times more likely than children with a BMI between the 25th and 50th percentile to develop elevated systolic blood pressure.[94] In addition, they observed a significant, but weaker, association between overweight and elevated diastolic blood pressure.

There are several mechanisms through which obesity causes hypertension. Hyperinsulinemia, which is common among overweight and obese individuals, can cause activation of the sympathetic nervous system, as well as cause sodium retention, thus increasing the risk of developing hypertension.[95]

Diabetes

Type II diabetes is characterized by peripheral insulin resistance, impaired regulation of hepatic glucose production, and compromised β-cell function. Diabetics are at substantially elevated risk for blindness, kidney disease, heart disease, stroke, and death; thus, it represents a major public health problem. It is believed that the incidence of type II diabetes has risen steadily over the past 30 years and is becoming increasingly prevalent among adolescents and young adults;[96] however, the exact prevalence is not known among children and adolescents. One study was based on reviewing medical records from 1982 to 1995 at a regional, university-affiliated pediatric diabetes referral center. The authors attempted to ascertain whether there had been an increase in noninsulin dependent diabetes that paralleled the rise in the prevalence of obesity;[97] they observed that the incidence of noninsulin dependent diabetes among adolescent increased tenfold during the 12-year period, from 0.7/100,000 per year in 1982 to 7.2/100,000 per year in 1994. Because the study is based on record reviews at one referral center, it is unclear whether the results are generalizable to the greater U.S. population.

The relationship between body weight and risk of diabetes among adults is strong and well established.[98,99] Fewer studies have been conducted assessing the association of diabetes to weight status early in life, but it is believed that excessive weight in preadolescence, adolescence, and adulthood increases the risk of type II diabetes through insulin resistance.[100] In contrast, low birth weight increases the risk of developing diabetes in adulthood.

Weight at Birth and in Childhood as Risk Factors for Diabetes

There is ample evidence that birth weight and weight in early infancy have an inverse association,[101 103] whereas childhood and adolescent BMIs have a positive association with risk of developing diabetes. Among women in the Nurses' Health Study, those who weighed less than 7 lb at birth were significantly more likely than women who weighed between 7.1 and 8.5 lb at birth to develop diabetes.[101] Moreover, The association between birth weight and type 2 diabetes was strongest for the women who reported no family history of diabetes. In a longitudinal study of 13,517 men and women in Finland, Barker and colleagues observed that that the risk for developing diabetes decreased with increasing birth weight categories and increased with higher BMI at age 11. Thus the participants at the highest risk (RR = 2.5, 95% CI 1.2 to 5.5) were those who weighed less than 3 kg at birth, but had a BMI greater than 17.6 kg/m² at age 11. The association with birth weight is thought to reflect that inadequate nutrition *in utero* programs "the fetus to develop resistance to insulin-stimulated uptake of glucose later in life — a 'thrifty phenotype.'"[103]

Barker et al.[86] observed that BMI at age 11 was positively related to risk of developing diabetes among the 13,517 Finnish men and women in his study. In each strata of birth weight, the highest risk was seen among the participants who had a BMI > 17.6 kg/m² at age 11; however, the elevation in risk was only significant among the participants who had been in the leanest strata of birth weight. Similar results were seen by Bhargava et al.[104] who observed that among 1492 young adults who had been measured in infancy, childhood, and adolescence, those who were low weight at age 2 but made large increases in their BMI between age 2 and 12 were at increased risk of developing impaired glucose tolerance or diabetes. In addition, the risk of developing impaired glucose tolerance or diabetes was inversely associated with age at adiposity rebound.

Weight in Late Adolescence as a Risk Factor for Diabetes

Weight in later adolescence is strongly related to the risk of developing type 2 diabetes in adulthood. Colditz et al.[105] observed that among 114,281 females nurses, 30 to 55 years of age, BMI at age 18 (late adolescence) had a strong association with the development of type 2 diabetes in adulthood. Women with a BMI between 25 and 27 kg/m² were three times (RR = 3.3) and women with a BMI greater than or equal to 35 kg/m² were 13 times more likely (RR = 13.5) than women with a BMI

22 kg/m^2 at age 18 to develop diabetes. Moreover, independent of attained weight, weight gain since age 18 was predictive of developing diabetes. The effect of weight gain was greatest among those women with a family history of diabetes, but even among women without a family history, those who gained 5 to 9 kg since age 18 were two times more likely to develop diabetes mellitus (RR = 2.3; 95% CI 1.7 to 3.1). Although Holbrook et al.[106] in a study of 886 men and 1114 women found that adolescent overweight had a nonsignificant increase in risk (RR = 1.3) of developing noninsulin-dependent diabetes in adulthood, they did observe a strong association between weight gain since age 18 and the risk of developing diabetes.

CANCERS

Excessive weight in adulthood is associated with the development of numerous types of cancer, including postmenopausal breast cancer,[20] endometrial,[19] gastric,[107] and colon cancer.[21] Obesity in adulthood is thought to increase risk of developing cancer primarily through its effect on hormones. However, there are very limited data on the relationship between childhood or young adult weight status and the long-term risk of cancer.

Breast Cancer

Excessive weight in adulthood lowers the risk for premenopausal breast cancer but increases the risk for postmenopausal breast cancer. The relationship between childhood and adolescent BMI to risk of breast cancer is not as clear.[108] In a large population–based case control study in Sweden, recalled somatotype at age 7 was inversely related to postmenopausal breast cancer.[109] In both the Swedish case control study[109] and a large case control study in the United States,[110] BMI at age 18 was a weak inverse predictor of postmenopausal breast cancer. In a prospective analysis of 95,256 women in the Nurses' Health Study, Huang et al.[20] observed a stronger inverse association between BMI at age 18 and risk of either pre- or postmenopausal breast cancer than was observed in the Swedish or American case control studies.[109,110] However, Wenten et al.,[111] in a modest-sized case control study in the United States, did not observe any evidence of an association between BMI at age 18 and pre- or postmenopausal breast cancer. Nevertheless, the overall evidence supports a modest inverse association between BMI and risk of breast cancer. The decrease in risk may be due to a higher prevalence of menstrual irregularities and their associated low estrogen levels in overweight women.

In addition to the association with adolescent weight status, birth weight has also been observed to be related to the risk of developing breast cancer.[112–115] Michels et al.[114] conducted a nested case control study in the Nurses' Health Study and found that compared with women whose birth weight was at least 4000 g, those with birth weights below 3500 g were significantly less likely to have developed breast cancer (*p* for trend = .004). The majority of the cases were premenopausal, and the association was strongest in the younger women. Similar results were observed in a population-based case control study in Denmark comprising 881 women with breast cancer diagnosed before the age of 40 and 3423 age-matched controls. Mellemkjaer et al.[115] observed that compared with women with a birth weight between 3000 and 3499 g, those with a birth weight above 4000 g were 25% more likely (95% CI 1.00 to 2.51) to develop early-onset breast cancer. In a cohort of 106,504 Danish women, Ahlgren et al.[116] observed that birth weight was a significant predictor of both pre- and postmenopausal breast cancer. For every 1000 g increase in birth weight, the risk of breast cancer increased approximately 9% (95% CI 2 to 17). It is believed that exposure to estrogens and other hormones *in utero* is likely to be responsible for the relationship between birth weight and development of breast cancer.[114]

Ovarian Cancer

Although the data are limited, the results suggest that the risk of ovarian cancer increases with BMI at age 18.[117,118] In a case control study of 1269 cases of epithelial ovarian cancer and 2111 matched controls, Lubin et al.[117] observed that women who had been in the highest quartile of BMI at age 18 (BMI 22.9 to 35.2 kg/m^2) were 40% more likely than their peers with a BMI < 19 kg/m^2 at age 18 to have developed ovarian cancer. However, in an analyses of 109,445 women in the Nurses' Health Study who were followed for 20 years, women who had a BMI at age 18 years ≥ 25 kg/m^2 were two times more likely than women who had a BMI < 20 kg/m^2 at age 18 to develop premenopausal ovarian cancer.[118] However, there was no association between BMI at age 18 and risk of postmenopausal ovarian cancer.

Other Cancers

The relationship between childhood and adolescent BMI and other cancers has not been thoroughly researched. One large case control study based on the Swedish cancer registry observed a suggestion that birth weight, but not BMI at age 18, was associated with risk of developing testicular cancer.[119] Men with high birth weights were 35% (OR = 1.35, 95% CI 0.99 to 1.85) more likely than their peers to develop testicular cancer. The association has not been observed in other studies; thus, it is premature to conclude that birth weight is risk factor for testicular cancer.

Although adult BMI is a known risk factor for endometrial cancer, little is known about the relationship between pediatric BMI and endometrial cancer. In a large case control study of 709 cases and 3368 controls, Weiderpass et al.[120] observed that there was a modest association between BMI at age 18 and risk of endometrial cancer; however, the association was apparently due to BMI at age 18 being strongly related to BMI later in adulthood. When both BMI at age 18 and current BMI were included in the model, only the latter was significantly related to the risk of developing cancer. More research is needed to give a definitive answer about the relationship, or lack thereof, between BMI in childhood and adolescence and the risk of developing endometrial cancer.

Polycystic Ovarian Syndrome

Polycystic ovarian syndrome (PCOS) is one of the more common causes of female infertility, and it affects approximately 5 to 10% of premenopausal women.[121] In cross-sectional studies, a strong association between PCOS and obesity has been observed, but there are limited prospective data on the association between weight in childhood and development of PCOS. Cresswell et al.[122] observed that among women whose mothers were relatively heavy (weights above the median weight in the study), there was a positive association between birth weight and the prevalence of polycystic ovaries in adulthood (p for trend = 0.002); however, when women whose mothers were lean were included in the analysis, the association was no longer significant. Laitinen et al.[123] did not observe an association between birth weight and PCOS symptoms among 2007 Finish women in a longitudinal cohort. However, they did observe an association between obesity at age 14 and PCOS symptoms in adulthood (RR = 1.6, 95% CI 1.2 to 2.1). In addition, women who were overweight or obese at both ages 14 and 31 years had a slightly higher risk of PCOS symptoms than women who were normal weight at age 14 and become overweight or obese in adulthood. In addition, in the Nurses' Health Study, Rich-Edwards and colleagues[124] observed that compared with women with a BMI between 20 and 21.9 kg/m^2 at age 18 years, those with a BMI greater than 23.9 kg/m^2 were significantly more likely to have developed ovulatory infertility, which is common among women with PCOS. Although in cross-sectional and retrospective studies PCOS has been observed to be associated with insulin resistance, type 2 diabetes, and cardiovascular risks,[125] few studies have controlled for weight status; thus, confounding is likely. More research is needed on the independent association of PCOS with the development of other morbidities.

ECONOMIC COSTS OF PEDIATRIC OBESITY

Disease burden is commonly measured by mortality; however, it is an inadequate measure because it does not account for the morbidity associated with chronic conditions, nor does it capture the impact of lifestyle on health-related quality of life. This is particularly true for diseases, such as obesity, with an early age of onset that do not rapidly cause death. Economic measures, on the other hand, can summarize this broad range of health effects and account for both nonfatal and fatal conditions. Thus, they may provide a more comprehensive summary of the public health impact of conditions such as obesity.

Economic costs can be compartmentalized into direct and indirect costs. The direct costs of illness include the costs of diagnosis and treatment related to any disease (hospital stay, nursing home, medications, physician visits). Indirect costs include the value of lost productivity, including wages lost by people unable to work because of disease and years lost due to premature mortality.[126]

Most of the research on the costs of obesity has focused on adults.[126,127] Colditz estimated that the direct costs for obesity (BMI $\geq$ 30 kg/m^2), in 1995 dollars, was $70 billion.[126] However, he noted that because there are adverse health effects associated with overweight below a BMI of 30,[21] his estimate is the lower bound of the health care cost because there are substantial additional costs incurred among those who are overweight (i.e., have a BMI of 25 to 29.9 kg/m^2), but not obese.

In a recent study based on the 1998 Medical Expenditure Panel Survey and the 1996 and 1997 National Health Interview Surveys, Finkelstein et al.[128] estimated that at least 9.1% of the total medical expenditures in 1998 were related to adult overweight or obesity. In terms of dollars, the costs were estimated to be between $51.5 billion and $78.5 billion (if nursing home care is included in the estimate) and approximately half of the costs were paid by Medicaid and Medicare. More recently they estimated that the annual U.S. medical expenditures attributable to obesity were approximately $75 billion in 2003 dollars, but varied widely between the states.[129]

Only one paper has evaluated the health care costs of childhood obesity. Wang and Dietz used information from the 1979–1999 National Hospital Discharge Survey, a dataset based on a national sample of hospitals, to estimate trends in the obesity-related hospital utilization costs.[130] They estimated that the annual hospital cost was $110 million during 1997 to 1999, a large increase from $12.6 million during 1979 to 1981. In terms of 2001 dollars, the annual hospital costs were about $35 million during 1979 to 1981 and increased more than threefold to about $127 million during 1997 to 1999.

CONCLUSION AND SUMMARY

Obesity is a serious public health problem in the United States and other developed countries, and it is becoming a problem in developing countries as well. The prevalence of overweight in children and adolescents in the United States, as well as other westernized countries, is rising rapidly, so that we can expect the rates of CVD, diabetes, asthma, and certain cancers to rise over the next several decades.

The prevalence of pediatric obesity and other cardiovascular risk factors is greater among African Americans and Hispanics than whites,[2,131,132] but data are lacking on whether there are racial differences in the long-term health impact of pediatric obesity. Few of the large cohort studies have had sufficient numbers of African Americans, Hispanics, and Asian to investigate whether race or ethnicity modifies the association between weight status and long-term health risk. The studies that have been large enough to assess racial differences on the impact of adult BMI on morbidity and mortality have not been consistent across outcomes.[133–135] Thus, it is unknown how well the results from the cohort studies generalize to nonwhite populations; in some case the magnitude or risk may be underestimated and in others it may be overestimated. Moreover, it has been suggested that the use of relative measures of association (i.e., relative risk) rather than absolute measures (i.e., risk differences) may result in an underestimation of the true impact of obesity on morbidity and mortality among African Americans because of the higher morbidity and mortality rates among African Americans in all weight categories, including the reference group.[136]

Despite the health risks of obesity and the societal pressures to be thin, particularly for girls, the prevalence of pediatric overweight continues to rise. With rare exceptions, obesity is a preventable disease. Few adults are able to lose weight and maintain their weight loss,[137,138] thus highlighting the need for the prevention of the development of overweight. Although treatments for CVD and cancer have improved, prevention should be the goal. By preventing the development of obesity, a substantial proportion of the burden of CVD, cancer, and diabetes could be avoided. Children and adolescents should be encouraged to engage in physical activity. Activity is helpful for maintaining weight losses and preventing excessive weight gain; thus, children and adolescents should be encouraged to be active regardless of their weight.

REFERENCES

1. Flegal KM, Carroll MD, Kuczmarski RJ, Johnson CL. Overweight and obesity in the United States: prevalence and trends, 1960-1994. *Int J Obes Relat Metab Disord.* 1998;22(1): 39–47.
2. Hedley AA, Ogden CL, Johnson CL, Carroll MD, Curtin LR, Flegal KM. Prevalence of overweight and obesity among US children, adolescents, and adults, 1999-2002. *JAMA.* 2004;291(23): 2847–2850.
3. Wang Y, Monteiro C, Popkin BM. Trends of obesity and underweight in older children and adolescents in the United States, Brazil, China, and Russia. *Am J Clin Nutr.* 2002;75(6): 971–977.
4. Himes JH, Dietz WH. Guidelines for overweight in adolescent preventive services: recommendations from an expert committee. The Expert Committee on Clinical Guidelines for Overweight in Adolescent Preventive Services. *Am J Clin Nutr.* 1994;59(2): 307–316.
5. Cole TJ, Bellizzi MC, Flegal KM, Dietz WH. Establishing a standard definition for child overweight and obesity worldwide: international survey. *BMJ.* 2000;320(7244): 1240–1243.
6. Dietary Guideline Advisory Committee. Report of the Dietary Advisory Committee on the Dietary Guidelines for Americans: Secretary of Health and Human Services and the Secretary of Agriculture; 1995.
7. 2000 CDC Growth Charts: United States. http: //www.cdc.gov/growthcharts/.
8. Field AE, Laird N, Steinberg E, Fallon E, Semega Janneh M, Yanovski JA. Which metric of relative weight best captures body fatness in children? *Obes Res.* 2003;11(11): 1345–1352.
9. Daniels SR, Khoury PR, Morrison JA. The utility of body mass index as a measure of body fatness in children and adolescents: differences by race and gender. *Pediatrics.* 1997;99(6): 804–807.
10. Goulding A, Gold E, Cannan R, Taylor RW, Williams S, Lewis-Barned NJ. DEXA supports the use of BMI as a measure of fatness in young girls. *Int J Obes Relat Metab Disord.* 1996;20(11): 1014–1021.
11. Guo SS, Roche AF, Chumlea WC, Gardner JD, Siervogel RM. The predictive value of childhood body mass index values for overweight at age 35 y. *Am J Clin Nutr.* 1994;59(4): 810–819.
12. Williams S. Overweight at age 21: the association with body mass index in childhood and adolescence and parents' body mass index. A cohort study of New Zealanders born in 1972-1973. *Int J Obes Relat Metab Disord.* 2001;25(2): 158–163.
13. Lauer RM, Clarke WR. Childhood risk factors for high adult blood pressure: the Muscatine Study. *Pediatrics.* 1989;84(4): 633–641.
14. Magarey AM, Daniels LA, Boulton TJ, Cockington RA. Predicting obesity in early adulthood from childhood and parental obesity. *Int J Obes Relat Metab Disord.* 2003;27(4): 505–513.
15. Serdula MK, Ivery D, Coates RJ, Freedman DS, Williamson DF, Byers T. Do obese children become obese adults? A review of the literature. *Prev Med.* 1993;22(2): 167–177.
16. Whitaker RC, Wright JA, Pepe MS, Seidel KD, Dietz WH. Predicting obesity in young adulthood from childhood and parental obesity. *N Engl J Med.* 1997;337(13): 869–873.
17. Freedman DS, Khan LK, Dietz WH, Srinivasan SR, Berenson GS. Relationship of childhood obesity to coronary heart disease risk factors in adulthood: the Bogalusa Heart Study. *Pediatrics.* 2001;108(3): 712–718.
18. Manson JE, Colditz GA, Stampfer MJ, Willett WC, Rosner B, Monson RR, et al. A prospective study of obesity and risk of coronary heart disease in women. *N Engl J Med.* 1990;322(13): 882–889.

19. Shoff SM, Newcomb PA. Diabetes, body size, and risk of endometrial cancer. *Am J Epidemiol.* 1998;148(3): 234–240.

20. Huang Z, Hankinson SE, Colditz GA, Stampfer MJ, Hunter DJ, Manson JE, et al. Dual effects of weight and weight gain on breast cancer risk. *JAMA.* 1997;278(17): 1407–1411.

21. Field AE, Coakley EH, Must A, Spadano JL, Laird N, Dietz WH, et al. Impact of overweight on the risk of developing common chronic diseases during a 10-year period. *Arch Intern Med.* 2001;161(13): 1581–1586.

22. Manson JE, Willett WC, Stampfer MJ, Colditz GA, Hunter DJ, Hankinson SE, et al. Body weight and mortality among women. *N Engl J Med.* 1995;333(11): 677–685.

23. Freedman DS, Dietz WH, Srinivasan SR, Berenson GS. The relation of overweight to cardiovascular risk factors among children and adolescents: the Bogalusa Heart Study. *Pediatrics.* 1999;103(6 Pt 1): 1175–1182.

24. Morrison JA, Sprecher DL, Barton BA, Waclawiw MA, Daniels SR. Overweight, fat patterning, and cardiovascular disease risk factors in black and white girls: The National Heart, Lung, and Blood Institute Growth and Health Study. *J Pediatr.* 1999;135(4): 458–464.

25. Sinaiko AR, Donahue RP, Jacobs DR, Jr., Prineas RJ. Relation of weight and rate of increase in weight during childhood and adolescence to body size, blood pressure, fasting insulin, and lipids in young adults. The Minneapolis Children's Blood Pressure Study. *Circulation.* 1999;99(11): 1471–1476.

26. Gower BA, Nagy TR, Goran MI. Visceral fat, insulin sensitivity, and lipids in prepubertal children. *Diabetes.* 1999;48(8): 1515–1521.

27. Arslanian S, Suprasongsin C, Janosky JE. Insulin secretion and sensitivity in black versus white prepubertal healthy children. *J Clin Endocrinol Metab.* 1997;82(6): 1923–1927.

28. Goran MI, Ball GD, Cruz ML. Obesity and risk of type 2 diabetes and cardiovascular disease in children and adolescents. *J Clin Endocrinol Metab.* 2003;88(4): 1417–1427.

29. Sinha R, Fisch G, Teague B, Tamborlane WV, Banyas B, Allen K, et al. Prevalence of impaired glucose tolerance among children and adolescents with marked obesity. *N Engl J Med.* 2002;346(11): 802–810.

30. von Kries R, Hermann M, Grunert VP, von Mutius E. Is obesity a risk factor for childhood asthma? *Allergy.* 2001;56(4): 318–322.

31. von Mutius E, Schwartz J, Neas LM, Dockery D, Weiss ST. Relation of body mass index to asthma and atopy in children: the National Health and Nutrition Examination Study III. *Thorax.* 2001;56(11): 835–838.

32. To T, Vydykhan TN, Dell S, Tassoudji M, Harris JK. Is obesity associated with asthma in young children? *J Pediatr.* 2004;144(2): 162–168.

33. Gold DR, Damokosh AI, Dockery DW, Berkey CS. Body-mass index as a predictor of incident asthma in a prospective cohort of children. *Pediatr Pulmonol.* 2003;36(6): 514–521.

34. Gilliland FD, Berhane K, Islam T, McConnell R, Gauderman WJ, Gilliland SS, et al. Obesity and the risk of newly diagnosed asthma in school-age children. *Am J Epidemiol.* 2003;158(5): 406–415.

35. Sin DD, Spier S, Svenson LW, Schopflocher DP, Senthilselvan A, Cowie RL, et al. The relationship between birth weight and childhood asthma: a population-based cohort study. *Arch Pediatr Adolesc Med.* 2004;158(1): 60–64.

36. Must A, Strauss RS. Risks and consequences of childhood and adolescent obesity. *Int J Obes Relat Metab Disord.* 1999;23(Suppl 2): S2–S11.

37. Poussa M, Schlenzka D, Yrjonen T. Body mass index and slipped capital femoral epiphysis. *J Pediatr Orthop B.* 2003;12(6): 369–371.

38. Nicolai RD, Grasemann H, Oberste-Berghaus C, Hovel M, Hauffa BP. Serum insulin-like growth factors IGF-I and IGFBP-3 in children with slipped capital femoral epiphysis. *J Pediatr Orthop B.* 1999;8(2): 103–106.

39. Wilcox PG, Weiner DS, Leighley B. Maturation factors in slipped capital femoral epiphysis. *J Pediatr Orthop.* 1988;8(2): 196–200.

40. Loder RT, Aronson DD, Greenfield ML. The epidemiology of bilateral slipped capital femoral epiphysis. A study of children in Michigan. *J Bone Joint Surg Am.* 1993;75(8): 1141–1147.

41. Dietz WH, Jr., Gross WL, Kirkpatrick JA, Jr. Blount disease (tibia vara): another skeletal disorder associated with childhood obesity. *J Pediatr.* 1982;101(5): 735–737.

42. Carta A, Bertuzzi F, Cologno D, Giorgi C, Montanari E, Tedesco S. Idiopathic intracranial hypertension (pseudotumor cerebri): descriptive epidemiology, clinical features, and visual outcome in Parma, Italy, 1990 to 1999. *Eur J Ophthalmol.* 2004;14(1): 48–54.

43. Radhakrishnan K, Thacker AK, Bohlaga NH, Maloo JC, Gerryo SE. Epidemiology of idiopathic intracranial hypertension: a prospective and case-control study. *J Neurol Sci.* 1993;116(1): 18–28.

44. Maclure KM, Hayes KC, Colditz GA, Stampfer MJ, Speizer FE, Willett WC. Weight, diet, and the risk of symptomatic gallstones in middle-aged women. *N Engl J Med.* 1989;321(9): 563–569.

45. Must A, Spadano J, Coakley EH, Field AE, Colditz G, Dietz WH. The disease burden associated with overweight and obesity. *JAMA.* 1999;282(16): 1523–1529.

46. Honore LH. Cholesterol cholelithiasis in adolescent females: its connection with obestiy, parity, and oral contraceptive use — a retrospective study of 31 cases. *Arch Surg.* 1980;115(1): 62–64.

47. Fisher M, Rosenstein J, Schussheim A, Shenker IR, Nussbaum M. Gallbladder disease in children and adolescents. *J Adolesc Health Care.* 1981;1(4): 309–312.

48. Takiff H, Fonkalsrud EW. Gallbladder disease in childhood. *Am J Dis Child.* 1984;138(6): 565–568.

49. Phillips RG, Hill AJ. Fat, plain, but not friendless: self-esteem and peer acceptance of obese pre-adolescent girls. *Int J Obes Relat Metab Disord.* 1998;22(4): 287–293.

50. Davison KK, Birch LL. Predictors of fat stereotypes among 9-year-old girls and their parents. *Obes Res.* 2004;12(1): 86–94.

51. Davison KK, Birch LL. Weight status, parent reaction, and self-concept in five-year-old girls. *Pediatrics* 2001;107(1): 46–53.

52. Hill AJ, Franklin JA. Mothers, daughters and dieting: investigating the transmission of weight control. *Br J Clin Psychol.* 1998;37(Pt 1): 3-13.

53. Pike KM, Rodin J. Mothers, daughters, and disordered eating. *J Abnorm Psychol.* 1991;100(2): 198–204.

54. Smolak L, Levine MP, Schermer F. Parental input and weight concerns among elementary school children. *Int J Eat Disord* 1999;25(3): 263–271.

55. Levine MP, Smolak L, Moodey AF, Shuman MD, Hessen LD. Normative developmental challenges and dieting and eating disturbances in middle school girls. *Int J Eat Disord.* 1994;15(1): 11–20.

56. Abramovitz BA, Birch LL. Five-year-old girls' ideas about dieting are predicted by their mothers' dieting. *J Am Diet Assoc.* 2000;100(10): 1157–1163.

57. Lowes J, Tiggemann M. Body dissatisfaction, dieting awareness and the impact of parental influence in young children. *Br J Health Psychol* 2003;8(Pt 2): 135–147.

58. Falkner NH, Neumark-Sztainer D, Story M, Jeffery RW, Beuhring T, Resnick MD. Social, educational, and psychological correlates of weight status in adolescents. *Obes Res.* 2001;9(1): 32–42.

59. Strauss RS, Pollack HA. Social marginalization of overweight children. *Arch Pediatr Adolesc Med.* 2003;157(8): 746–752.

60. Canning H, Mayer J. Obesity — its possible effect on college acceptance. *N Eng J Med.* 1966;275: 1172–1174.

61. Gortmaker SL, Must A, Perrin JM, Sobol AM, Dietz WH. Social and economic consequences of overweight in adolescence and young adulthood. *N Engl J Med.* 1993;329(14): 1008–1012.

62. Field AE, Camargo CA, Jr., Taylor CB, Berkey CS, Frazier AL, Gillman MW, et al. Overweight, weight concerns, and bulimic behaviors among girls and boys. *J Am Acad Child Adolesc Psychiatry* 1999;38(6): 754–760.

63. Ackard DM, Neumark-Sztainer D, Story M, Perry C. Overeating among adolescents: prevalence and associations with weight-related characteristics and psychological health. *Pediatrics.* 2003;111(1): 67–74.

64. Boutelle K, Neumark-Sztainer D, Story M, Resnick M. Weight control behaviors among obese, overweight, and nonoverweight adolescents. *J Pediatr Psychol.* 2002;27(6): 531–540.

65. Neumark-Sztainer D, Story M, Hannan PJ, Perry CL, Irving LM. Weight-related concerns and behaviors among overweight and nonoverweight adolescents: implications for preventing weight-related disorders. *Arch Pediatr Adolesc Med.* 2002;156(2): 171–178.

66. Beumont PJ, George GC, Smart DE. "Dieters" and "vomiters" and "purgers" in anorexia nervosa. *Psychol Med.* 1976;6(4): 617–622.

67. Garner DM, Garfinkel PE, O'Shaughnessy M. The validity of the distinction between bulimia with and without anorexia nervosa. *Am J Psychiatry.* 1985;142(5): 581–587.

68. Herzog DB, Keller MB, Lavori PW, Ott IL. Short-term prospective study of recovery in bulimia nervosa. *Psychiatry Res.* 1988;23(1): 45–55.
69. Fairburn CG, Welch SL, Doll HA, Davies BA, O'Connor ME. Risk factors for bulimia nervosa. A community-based case-control study. *Arch Gen Psychiatry.* 1997;54(6): 509–517.
70. Fairburn CG, Cooper Z, Doll HA, Welch SL. Risk factors for anorexia nervosa: three integrated case-control comparisons. *Arch Gen Psychiatry.* 1999;56(5): 468–476.
71. Patton GC, Selzer R, Coffey C, Carlin JB, Wolfe R. Onset of adolescent eating disorders: population based cohort study over 3 years. *BMJ.* 1999;318(7186): 765–768.
72. Field A, Austin S, Taylor C, Malspeis S, Rosner B, Rockett H, et al. The relation between dieting and weight change among preadolescents and adolescents. *Pediatrics.* 2003;112: 900–990.
73. Stunkard AJ, Allison KC. Two forms of disordered eating in obesity: binge eating and night eating. *Int J Obes Relat Metab Disord.* 2003;27(1): 1–12.
74. Neumark-Sztainer D, Falkner N, Story M, Perry C, Hannan PJ, Mulert S. Weight-teasing among adolescents: correlations with weight status and disordered eating behaviors. *Int J Obes Relat Metab Disord.* 2002;26(1): 123–131.
75. Janssen I, Craig WM, Boyce WF, Pickett W. Associations between overweight and obesity with bullying behaviors in school-aged children. *Pediatrics.* 2004;113(5): 1187–1194.
76. Strauss RS. Childhood obesity and self-esteem. *Pediatrics.* 2000;105(1): e15.
77. Kimm SY, Barton BA, Berhane K, Ross JW, Payne GH, Schreiber GB. Self-esteem and adiposity in black and white girls: the NHLBI Growth and Health Study. *Ann Epidemiol.* 1997;7(8): 550–560.
78. French SA, Story M, Perry CL. Self-esteem and obesity in children and adolescents: a literature review. *Obes Res.* 1995;3(5): 479–490.
79. Friedlander SL, Larkin EK, Rosen CL, Palermo TM, Redline S. Decreased quality of life associated with obesity in school-aged children. *Arch Pediatr Adolesc Med.* 2003;157(12): 1206–1211.
80. Schwimmer JB, Burwinkle TM, Varni JW. Health-related quality of life of severely obese children and adolescents. *JAMA.* 2003;289(14): 1813–1819.
81. Must A, Jacques PF, Dallal GE, Bajema CJ, Dietz WH. Long-term morbidity and mortality of overweight adolescents. A follow-up of the Harvard Growth Study of 1922 to 1935. *N Engl J Med.* 1992;327(19): 1350–1355.
82. Gunnell DJ, Frankel SJ, Nanchahal K, Peters TJ, Davey Smith G. Childhood obesity and adult cardiovascular mortality: a 57-y follow-up study based on the Boyd Orr cohort. *Am J Clin Nutr.* 1998;67(6): 1111–1118.
83. Hoffmans MD, Kromhout D, Coulander CD. Body Mass Index at the age of 18 and its effects on 32-year-mortality from coronary heart disease and cancer. A nested case-control study among the entire 1932 Dutch male birth cohort. *J Clin Epidemiol.* 1989;42(6): 513–520.
84. Okasha M, McCarron P, McEwen J, Smith GD. Body mass index in young adulthood and cancer mortality: a retrospective cohort study. *J Epidemiol Community Health.* 2002;56(10): 780–784.
85. Yarnell JW, Patterson CC, Thomas HF, Sweetnam PM. Comparison of weight in middle age, weight at 18 years, and weight change between, in predicting subsequent 14 year mortality and coronary events: Caerphilly Prospective Study. *J Epidemiol Community Health.* 2000;54(5): 344–348.
86. Barker DJ, Eriksson JG, Forsen T, Osmond C. Fetal origins of adult disease: strength of effects and biological basis. *Int J Epidemiol.* 2002;31(6): 1235–1239.
87. Desai M, Hales CN. Role of fetal and infant growth in programming metabolism in later life. *Biol Rev Camb Philos Soc.* 1997;72(2): 329–348.
88. Kwong WY, Wild AE, Roberts P, Willis AC, Fleming TP. Maternal undernutrition during the preimplantation period of rat development causes blastocyst abnormalities and programming of postnatal hypertension. *Development.* 2000;127(19): 4195–4202.
89. Oken E, Gillman MW. Fetal origins of obesity. *Obes Res.* 2003;11(4): 496–506.
90. Bray GA. Health hazards of obesity. *Endocrinol Metab Clin North Am.* 1996;25(4): 907–919.
91. Alpert MA, Hashimi MW. Obesity and the heart. *Am J Med Sci.* 1993;306(2): 117–123.
92. Field AE, Byers T, Hunter DJ, Laird NM, Manson JE, Williamson DF, et al. Weight cycling, weight gain, and risk of hypertension in women. *Am J Epidemiol.* 1999;150(6): 573–579.
93. Huang Z, Willett WC, Manson JE, Rosner B, Stampfer MJ, Speizer FE, et al. Body weight, weight change, and risk for hypertension in women. *Ann Intern Med.* 1998;128(2): 81–88.

94. Srinivasan SR, Bao W, Wattigney WA, Berenson GS. Adolescent overweight is associated with adult overweight and related multiple cardiovascular risk factors: the Bogalusa Heart Study. *Metabolism.* 1996;45(2): 235–240.

95. Mikhail N, Golub MS, Tuck ML. Obesity and hypertension. *Prog Cardiovasc Dis.* 1999;42(1): 39–58.

96. Bloomgarden ZT. Type 2 diabetes in the young: the evolving epidemic. *Diabetes Care* 2004;27(4): 998–1010.

97. Pinhas-Hamiel O, Dolan LM, Daniels SR, Standiford D, Khoury PR, Zeitler P. Increased incidence of non-insulin-dependent diabetes mellitus among adolescents. *J Pediatr.* 1996;128(5 Pt 1): 608–615.

98. Colditz GA, Willett WC, Stampfer MJ, Manson JE, Hennekens CH, Arky RA, et al. Weight as a risk factor for clinical diabetes in women. *Am J Epidemiol.* 1990;132(3): 501–513.

99. Field AE, Manson JE, Laird N, Williamson DF, Willett WC, Colditz GA. Weight cycling and the risk of developing type 2 diabetes among adult women in the United States. *Obes Res.* 2004;12(2): 267–274.

100. Mahler RJ, Adler ML. Clinical review 102: Type 2 diabetes mellitus: update on diagnosis, pathophysiology, and treatment. *J Clin Endocrinol Metab.* 1999;84(4): 1165–1171.

101. Curhan GC, Willett WC, Rimm EB, Spiegelman D, Ascherio AL, Stampfer MJ. Birth weight and adult hypertension, diabetes mellitus, and obesity in US men. *Circulation.* 1996;94(12): 3246–3250.

102. Phipps K, Barker DJ, Hales CN, Fall CH, Osmond C, Clark PM. Fetal growth and impaired glucose tolerance in men and women. *Diabetologia.* 1993;36(3): 225–228.

103. Lithell HO, McKeigue PM, Berglund L, Mohsen R, Lithell UB, Leon DA. Relation of size at birth to non-insulin dependent diabetes and insulin concentrations in men aged 50-60 years. *BMJ.* 1996;312(7028): 406–410.

104. Bhargava SK, Sachdev HS, Fall CH, Osmond C, Lakshmy R, Barker DJ, et al. Relation of serial changes in childhood body-mass index to impaired glucose tolerance in young adulthood. *N Engl J Med.* 2004;350(9): 865–875.

105. Colditz GA, Willett WC, Rotnitzky A, Manson JE. Weight gain as a risk factor for clinical diabetes mellitus in women. *Ann Intern Med.* 1995;122(7): 481–486.

106. Holbrook TL, Barrett-Connor E, Wingard DL. The association of lifetime weight and weight control patterns with diabetes among men and women in an adult community. *Int J Obes.* 1989;13(5): 723–729.

107. Lagergren J, Bergstrom R, Nyren O. Association between body mass and adenocarcinoma of the esophagus and gastric cardia. *Ann Intern Med.* 1999;130(11): 883–890.

108. Okasha M, McCarron P, Gunnell D, Smith GD. Exposures in childhood, adolescence and early adulthood and breast cancer risk: a systematic review of the literature. *Breast Cancer Res Treat.* 2003;78(2): 223–276.

109. Magnusson C, Baron J, Persson I, Wolk A, Bergstrom R, Trichopoulos D, et al. Body size in different periods of life and breast cancer risk in post-menopausal women. *Int J Cancer.* 1998;76(1): 29–34.

110. Shoff SM, Newcomb PA, Trentham-Dietz A, Remington PL, Mittendorf R, Greenberg ER, et al. Early-life physical activity and postmenopausal breast cancer: effect of body size and weight change. *Cancer Epidemiol Biomarkers Prev.* 2000;9(6): 591–595.

111. Wenten M, Gilliland FD, Baumgartner K, Samet JM. Associations of weight, weight change, and body mass with breast cancer risk in Hispanic and non-Hispanic white women. *Ann Epidemiol.* 2002;12(6): 435–444.

112. Sanderson M, Williams MA, Malone KE, Stanford JL, Emanuel I, White E, et al. Perinatal factors and risk of breast cancer. *Epidemiology.* 1996;7(1): 34–37.

113. Vatten LJ, Maehle BO, Lund Nilsen TI, Tretli S, Hsieh CC, Trichopoulos D, et al. Birth weight as a predictor of breast cancer: a case-control study in Norway. *Br J Cancer.* 2002;86(1): 89–91.

114. Michels KB, Trichopoulos D, Robins JM, Rosner BA, Manson JE, Hunter DJ, et al. Birthweight as a risk factor for breast cancer. *Lancet.* 1996;348(9041): 1542–1546.

115. Mellemkjaer L, Olsen ML, Sorensen HT, Thulstrup AM, Olsen J, Olsen JH. Birth weight and risk of early-onset breast cancer (Denmark). *Cancer Causes Control.* 2003;14(1): 61–64.

116. Ahlgren M, Sorensen T, Wohlfahrt J, Haflidadottir A, Holst C, Melbye M. Birth weight and risk of breast cancer in a cohort of 106,504 women. *Int J Cancer.* 2003;107(6): 997–1000.

117. Lubin F, Chetrit A, Freedman LS, Alfandary E, Fishler Y, Nitzan H, et al. Body mass index at age 18 years and during adult life and ovarian cancer risk. *Am J Epidemiol.* 2003;157(2): 113–120.

118. Fairfield KM, Willett WC, Rosner BA, Manson JE, Speizer FE, Hankinson SE. Obesity, weight gain, and ovarian cancer. *Obstet Gynecol.* 2002;100(2): 288–296.

119. Richiardi L, Askling J, Granath F, Akre O. Body size at birth and adulthood and the risk for germ-cell testicular cancer. *Cancer Epidemiol Biomarkers Prev.* 2003;12(7): 669–673.

120. Weiderpass E, Persson I, Adami HO, Magnusson C, Lindgren A, Baron JA. Body size in different periods of life, diabetes mellitus, hypertension, and risk of postmenopausal endometrial cancer (Sweden). *Cancer Causes Control.* 2000;11(2): 185–192.

121. Dunaif A. Insulin resistance and the polycystic ovary syndrome: mechanism and implications for pathogenesis. *Endocr Rev.* 1997;18(6): 774–800.

122. Cresswell JL, Barker DJ, Osmond C, Egger P, Phillips DI, Fraser RB. Fetal growth, length of gestation, and polycystic ovaries in adult life. *Lancet.* 1997;350(9085): 1131–1135.

123. Laitinen J, Taponen S, Martikainen H, Pouta A, Millwood I, Hartikainen AL, et al. Body size from birth to adulthood as a predictor of self-reported polycystic ovary syndrome symptoms. *Int J Obes Relat Metab Disord.* 2003;27(6): 710–715.

124. Rich-Edwards JW, Goldman MB, Willett WC, Hunter DJ, Stampfer MJ, Colditz GA, et al. Adolescent body mass index and infertility caused by ovulatory disorder. *Am J Obstet Gynecol.* 1994;171(1): 171–177.

125. Gordon CM. Menstrual disorders in adolescents. Excess androgens and the polycystic ovary syndrome. *Pediatr Clin North Am.* 1999;46(3): 519–543.

126. Colditz GA. Economic costs of obesity and inactivity. *Med Sci Sports Exerc.* 1999;31(11 Suppl): S663–5667.

127. Katzmarzyk PT, Janssen I. The economic costs associated with physical inactivity and obesity in Canada: an update. *Can J Appl Physiol.* 2004;29(1): 90–115.

128. Finkelstein EA, Fiebelkorn IC, Wang G. National medical spending attributable to overweight and obesity: how much, and who's paying? *Health Aff.* (Millwood) 2003;Suppl: W3-219–W3-226.

129. Finkelstein EA, Fiebelkorn IC, Wang G. State-level estimates of annual medical expenditures attributable to obesity. *Obes Res.* 2004;12(1): 18–24.

130. Wang G, Dietz WH. Economic burden of obesity in youths aged 6 to 17 years: 1979–1999. *Pediatrics.* 2002;109(5): e81.

131. Winkleby MA, Kraemer HC, Ahn DK, Varady AN. Ethnic and socioeconomic differences in cardiovascular disease risk factors: findings for women from the Third National Health and Nutrition Examination Survey, 1988-1994. *JAMA.* 1998;280(4): 356–362.

132. Winkleby MA, Robinson TN, Sundquist J, Kraemer HC. Ethnic variation in cardiovascular disease risk factors among children and young adults: findings from the Third National Health and Nutrition Examination Survey, 1988-1994. *JAMA* 1999;281(11): 1006–1013.

133. Stevens J, Plankey MW, Williamson DF, Thun MJ, Rust PF, Palesch Y, et al. The body mass index-mortality relationship in white and African American women. *Obes Res* 1998;6(4): 268–277.

134. Calle EE, Thun MJ, Petrelli JM, Rodriguez C, Heath CW, Jr. Body-mass index and mortality in a prospective cohort of U.S. adults. *N Engl J Med* 1999;341(15): 1097–1105.

135. Bernstein L, Teal CR, Joslyn S, Wilson J. Ethnicity-related variation in breast cancer risk factors. *Cancer* 2003;97(1 Suppl): 222–229.

136. Stevens J, Juhaeri, Cai J, Jones DW. The effect of decision rules on the choice of a body mass index cutoff for obesity: examples from African American and white women. *Am J Clin Nutr* 2002;75(6): 986–992.

137. Field AE, Wing RR, Manson JE, Spiegelman DL, Willett WC. Relationship of a large weight loss to long-term weight change among young and middle-aged US women. *Int J Obes Relat Metab Disord* 2001;25(8): 1113–1121.

138. Anderson JW, Konz EC, Frederich RC, Wood CL. Long-term weight-loss maintenance: a meta-analysis of US studies. *Am J Clin Nutr* 2001;74(5): 579–584.

2 Growth and Development

Shumei S. Sun

CONTENTS

This chapter focuses on biological aspects of human growth and development. The first section describes measurements and the assessment of growth using growth charts. The second section reviews patterns of growth for individuals from birth through infancy, early and middle childhood, and puberty and sexual maturation. The third section concerns the use of growth curve models to quantify growth landmarks. The last section describes the significance of growth and development in relation to future size, function, and disease.

GROWTH MEASUREMENT AND ASSESSMENT

During the first three years of life, the three most clinically important growth measurements are weight, recumbent length, and head circumference. Weight-for-age and recumbent-length-for-age are primary indicators for monitoring growth, health, and nutritional status of infants. An infant's body weight, recumbent length, and head circumference not only provide information about current growth and health but also predict future health status. Infants with abnormal values for weight-for-age and recumbent-length-for-age may be receiving inadequate nutrition or may be suffering from a medical condition that affects their nutrition and growth. Weight is commonly assessed in relation to body length because length and weight differ among infants of the same age. Head circumference allows for an indirect evaluation of the status of brain size and development because of the close relationship between brain development and head circumference.[1]

Growth in length and weight reach maximal values in fetal life. During the first year of life, the rates decelerate; therefore, growth proceeds at a relatively steady pace until adolescence. At the onset of puberty, the adolescent growth spurt commences and secondary sexual characteristics appear. After puberty, a final acceleration of growth brings most children close to their final adult body size.

To monitor growth in weight, recumbent length (referred to subsequently as length), and head circumference during infancy, health professionals use growth charts to assess an infant in relation to the size of his or her peers and to identify growth retardation and obesity. A separate set of growth charts is needed to provide a reference for children because growth in childhood and adolescence differs from growth in infancy. There are documented differences in the growth of boys and girls during infancy, childhood, and adolescence. Girls, on average, pass through the adolescent growth spurt 1 to 2 years earlier than boys. Boys experience a greater velocity of growth during this period than girls, and the adolescent growth period lasts longer in boys than in girls. These differences call for separate growth charts for boys and girls at all ages.

The U.S. Center for Disease Control (CDC) growth charts include infant growth charts from birth to 3 years and child and adolescent growth charts from 2 to 20 years of age; there are separate charts for boys and girls. These charts were derived almost entirely from a series of cross-sectional nationally representative samples of the U.S. population from 1963 to 1994 that included subjects aged 2 months to 20 years.[2–4] The infant growth charts include gender-specific curves for the 3rd, 5th, 10th, 25th, 50th, 75th, 90th, 95th, and 97th percentiles for weight-for-age, length-for-age, head-circumference-for-age, and weight-for-length for infants with birth weights greater than 1500 g. In the child and adolescent growth charts, height is used in place of length, and body mass index (BMI; kg/m^2) is used in place of weight-for-length. Gender-specific percentiles are similar to those of the infant growth charts, but the ages run from 2 to 20 years at 6-month intervals for weight, height, and BMI.

To assess growth, nurses and clinicians should be trained to measure weight, length, and head circumference accurately and consistently following the *Anthropometric Standardization Reference Manual*.[5] These measurements should be plotted on the weight-for-age, length-for-age, weight-for-length, and head-circumference-for-age growth charts. The accepted normal ranges for these measurements lie within the 5th and 95th percentiles inclusive. The CDC defines overweight infants 2 years and younger as having a weight-for-length greater than the 95th percentile. For children 2 years and older, the measurements should be plotted on the weight-for-age, height-for-age, and BMI-for-age growth charts. Just as in the infant growth charts, the 5th and 95th percentiles are used to define normal ranges in children's growth charts. BMI-for-age is recommended to screen children aged 2 to 20 years for "at risk of overweight" and "overweight." A BMI below the 5th percentile of the U.S. BMI growth charts is considered as "underweight." A BMI between the 85th and 95th percentiles of the BMI growth charts is considered "at risk of overweight" and a BMI at or above the 95th percentile inclusive is considered "overweight."

If the measurements are unusually high or low, further examinations are necessary. Serial measurements should be plotted on the CDC growth charts. The use of incremental growth charts is recommended when measurements fall outside the normal range.[6] These allow more rapid detection of unusual growth rates than is possible when serial data are plotted on the CDC growth charts for status.[7] Growth charts for weight and length increments have been developed for 1-, 2-, and 3-month intervals from birth to 3 years and for 6-month intervals from birth to 18 years using data from the Iowa Longitudinal Study and the Fels Longitudinal Study, respectively.[6] One-month increments for head circumferencse from 1 to 12 months of age have also been developed using serial data from the Fels Longitudinal Study.[8] If a child grows at an unusual rate, the possible influences of acute or chronic illness, parental stature, rate of maturation, ethnicity, and maternal substance abuse should be considered.

PATTERNS OF GROWTH

The patterns of growth of a child or a group of children can be described mathematically through models that summarize the overall pattern of growth across an age range. Knowledge of these patterns is necessary to interpret previous changes in individuals. The patterns of growth are the basis of informed expectations of future changes. Patterns of growth in body size are shown in Figure 2.1 for weight, length/height, head circumference, and BMI using serial data from the participants in the Fels Longitudinal Study. The following sections describe the patterns of growth in a child during infancy (birth to 2 years of age), early childhood (2 through 6 years of age), middle childhood (7 through 10 years of age), and adolescence (11 through 18 years of age).

INFANCY

During infancy, body size increases at a faster rate than at any other time in postnatal life. Most normal infants double their birth weight by 5 months of age and triple it by 1 year. In the first year of life, weight increases about 200%, body length 55%, and head circumference 40%. Between 1 and 2 years of age, an average child grows about 12 cm in length and gains about 3.5 kg in weight. Compared with the size of its body, an infant's head is disproportionately large at birth. At birth, head circumference is about 35 cm and increases to about 47 cm during the first year.

EARLY CHILDHOOD

After infancy, the rate of growth slows to nearly a constant rate that begins at 4 to 5 years of age when the average annual increments are about 2 kg for weight and 6 cm for height. Sex differences in height and weight during the preschool years are slight.

MIDDLE CHILDHOOD

Middle childhood is a period of continued steady growth. On average, children increase in weight by about 3 kg/yr at 7 years and by about 4 kg/yr at 10 years, and they increase in height by about 5 cm/yr from 7 to 10 years. At 7 years, boys are, on average, about 2 cm taller than girls, but there is only a small sex difference in weight. By 10 years, the average girl is about 1 cm taller than the average boy and about 1 kg heavier. The sex difference in growth rate during middle childhood contributes to the earlier appearance of significant sex difference in size at the start of puberty.

BMI decreases from 1 year and reaches a nadir at 5 or 6 years and then begins to increase (see Figures 2.1 and 2.2). The timing of the nadir and the rebound that follows it are estimated from curve-fitting procedures in research studies. Clinically, the BMI nadir and rebound may be recognized from plots of three or more successive BMI values during the relevant age range. The timing of the nadir does not differ between the sexes.[4,9,10] The earlier the nadir occurs, the greater the child's ultimate BMI. In some children, the BMI nadir may occur as early as 2 years.[11] Figure 2.2 illustrates the mean value of the BMI rebound for 460 subjects in the Fels Longitudinal Study as well as values for two individuals. The nadir of the BMI has been called the adiposity rebound but is more accurately called the BMI rebound. An early BMI rebound is a risk factor for future obesity.[11]

PUBERTY AND SEXUAL MATURATION

Sexual maturity can be assessed from the development of secondary sex characteristics: pubic hair in boys and girls, genitalia in boys, breast development and menarche in girls. Standardized stages of secondary sex characteristics were popularized by Tanner and can be assigned from stage 1 (immaturity) to stage 5 (full maturity).[12] The onset of secondary sex characteristics in U.S. children is shown in Figure 2.3.[13]

The median age for the onset of breast development is about 9.5 years for non-Hispanic black girls, about 10 years for Mexican-American girls, and about 10.4 years for non-Hispanic white girls. Age at menarche is an important indicator of sexual maturation but is less useful than the grading of secondary sexual characteristics because it occurs late in puberty. Menarche is also not useful in determining whether a child is having a pubertal growth spurt because menarche occurs

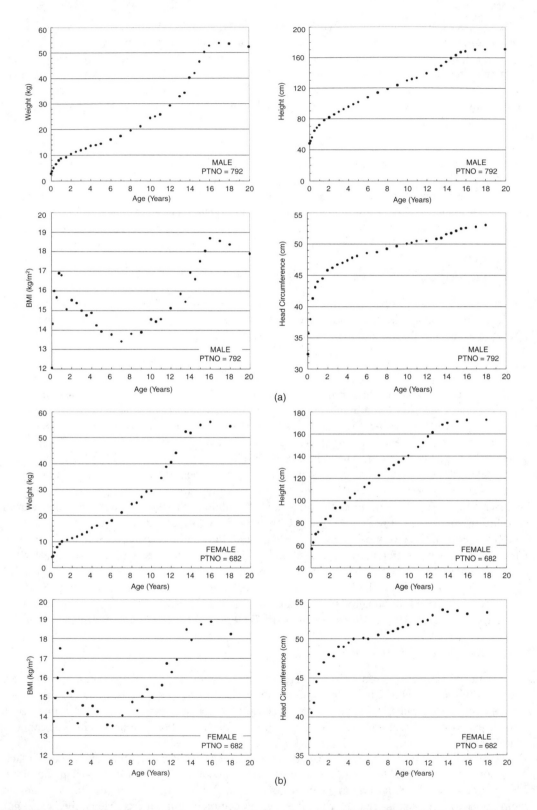

FIGURE 2.1 Individual serial data from birth to 20 years for weight, length/height, BMI, and head circumference for a representative boy (a) and an individual girl (b) from the Fels Longitudinal Study.

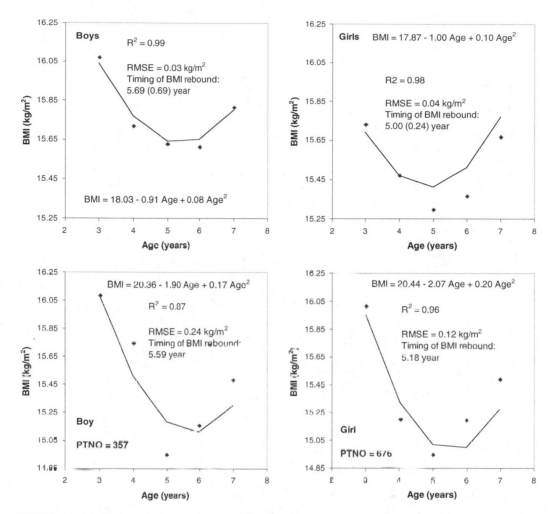

FIGURE 2.2 BMI rebound (data from The Fels Longitudinal Study).

about a year after peak height velocity (PHV). The median age at menarche for all U.S. girls is 12.43 years. Ten percent of all U.S. girls menstruate by 11.1 years of age, and 90% menstruate by 13.75 years of age.[14]

Estradiol is essential for the occurrence and timing of the normal pubertal growth spurt in girls, and testosterone is essential for the pubertal growth spurt in boys. Estradiol may also be responsible for pubertal increases in the body fat of girls, despite increases in growth hormone and IGF-1, which tend to reduce body fat. The reduction in the body fat of boys during puberty is due to testosterone, growth hormone, and IGF-1, which jointly increase fat-free mass and muscle mass. Estradiol is necessary in both sexes to cause a gradual cessation in linear growth by eradicating the growth plate and uniting the epiphyses and the metaphyses in long bones of the axial skeleton.[15]

The pubertal spurt in height (PHV) may be the best known feature of the human growth curve. PHV occurs at Tanner stages 2 to 4 of pubic hair development in each sex and at Tanner stages 3 to 5 of genital development in boys and Tanner stages 2 or 3 of breast development in girls.[7,16,17] The pubertal spurt begins in boys at about 11 years, and the PHV is reached at about 14 years.[18–21] These events occur about two years earlier in girls.

The patterns of growth in weight are similar to those in height, but peak velocities for weight occur about 6 months before PHV. Pubertal spurts can be recognized from serial data for height at 6-month intervals during a period of 18 months or at annual intervals during a period of 3 years.

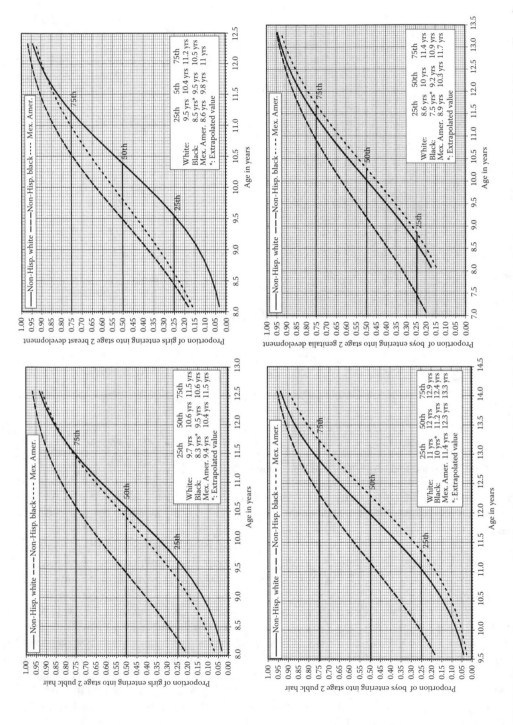

FIGURE 2.3 Timing of appearance of pubic hair in boys and girls, genitalia in boys, and breast development in girls in the United States. (From Sun et al., *Pediatrics*, 2002, 110(5).)

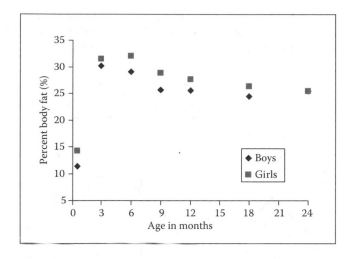

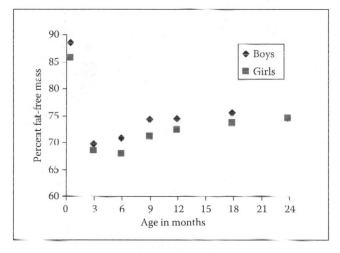

FIGURE 2.4 Percent of body fat and fat-free mass during first two years of life.

Data from only two examinations may show that growth is more rapid than usual, but evidence of a spurt requires a documented increase in rate of growth. Another method is to use growth curve models to fit serial data for height and identify the PHV from the fitted models. During puberty, BMI increases rapidly and reaches its maximum velocity at about 14 years in boys and 13 years in girls.[3] Small increases in BMI continue after puberty until at least 20 years in most studies,[3,22,23] but Luciano et al.[24] reported decreases in upper percentile levels for girls from 15 to 18 years that may be due to social pressures to lose weight.

The values for percent body fat are low at birth, but increase rapidly until 3 months in boys and 6 months in girls and then decrease slowly with larger values in girls than in boys.[25–27] Percent fat-free mass is high at birth, decreases to a nadir at 3 months in boys and at 6 months in girls, then increases thereafter.[26,27] The composition of fat-free mass changes during infancy, the percentage of water content decreases, and the percentages of mineral content and protein increase.[25] Figure 2.4 illustrates the age-related values for percent body fat from birth to 24 months.[25]

After infancy, values for percent body fat continue to decrease at slower rates throughout preschool years and middle childhood in each sex.[25] While sex differences in the relative composition of fat-free mass are negligible during infancy,[28] they become apparent in preschool years and middle childhood. Boys have less water and more protein and minerals than girls.[28] The pubertal growth spurt is not limited to height and weight but also occurs in body composition and bone mineral density.[12,29,30] The pubertal increases in BMI are mainly due to increases in fat-free mass in boys and in total body fat in girls, as shown in Figure 2.5.[31,32]

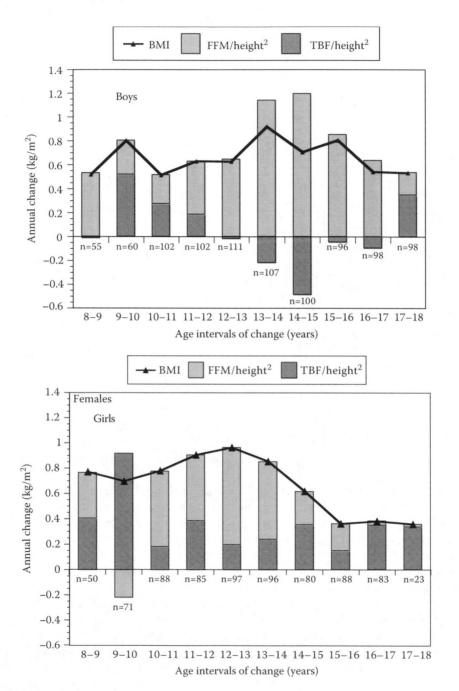

FIGURE 2.5 Annualized changes in BMI and total body fat/height^2 and fat-free mass/height^2 in the Fels Longitudinal Study.

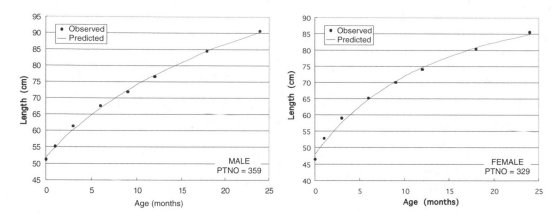

FIGURE 2.6 Observed (dots) and predicted (line) serial length data for two infants in the Fels Longitudinal Study.

MATHEMATICAL MODELS FOR DESCRIBING PATTERNS OF GROWTH

Childhood patterns of growth can be described by growth models. Several models of growth curves have been developed to fit a child's serial data for length, weight, and head circumference. For example, the model (Figure 2.6)

$$f(t) = a + b \log (t+1) + c(t+1)^{0.5} + e$$

was used to describe patterns of change in weight, length, and head circumference[6,8] and in the development of CDC growth charts.[2] In this model, $f(t)$ is the measurement at age t, a is the birth weight; b reflects the rates of change, c represents acceleration, and e is an error term.

Patterns of change in body weight have not been commonly described. This is partly due to the irregularity of body weight changes within children although, in general, body weight increases throughout the growth period. Using Fels data, change in BMI from 2 to 25 years is presented in Figure 2.7. The upper panel presents mean BMI, and the lower panel presents individual serial BMI data. The model

$$y = a + b \text{ age} + c \text{ age}^2 + d \text{ age}^3$$

was fitted to individual serial BMI values.[3] Three sets of BMI parameters were developed from the fitted data for each individual. BMI minimum and age at BMI minimum represent the early childhood period known as the BMI rebound. Maximum velocity of BMI, BMI value at maximum velocity, and age at maximum velocity of BMI represent puberty. BMI maximum and age at BMI maximum represent postpubescence.

Patterns of change in percent body fat and fat-free mass from 8 to 20 years of age are presented graphically in Figure 2.8.[31] The values for percent body fat and total body fat tend to be greater for girls than for boys at all ages throughout childhood. In girls, there is a steady increase in percent body fat. This pattern differs markedly from that in boys in whom percent body fat reaches a maximum at about age 12 years and decreases thereafter.[31,32] In both sexes, fat-free mass increases with age. There is little or no sex difference in fat-free mass before age 13, but the increase in fat-free mass is greater in boys after age 13. Between ages 14 to 20, the rates of increase in fat-free

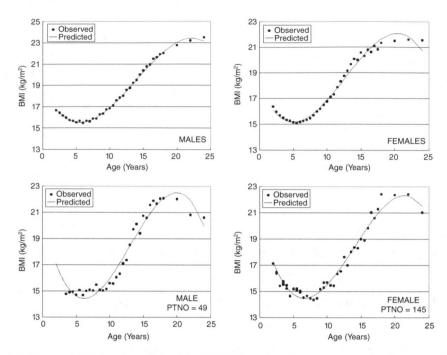

FIGURE 2.7 Observed (dots) and predicted (line) BMI. Upper panels are group means; lower panels are two individual participants; "PTNO" represents participant number.

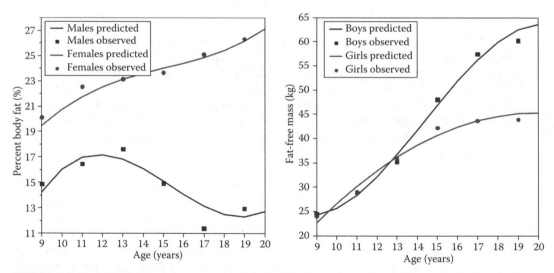

FIGURE 2.8 Patterns of growth in percent body fat and fat-free mass in the Fels Longitudinal Study. (From Guo et al., *Int. J. Obes.*, 1997, 21.)

mass show pronounced sexual dimorphism. The pubertal peak velocity of fat-free mass occurs at about the same age as PHV.

The sex differences in total body bone mineral content (BMC) are small up to 8 years. Between 9 and 13, girls have higher BMC than boys. The values for BMC are consistently higher in boys than in girls thereafter.[33] The higher BMC values in girls than in boys are due to differences in rates of maturation. At PHV, about 90% of adult stature has been reached, but only 60% of adult total body BMC.[34] The peak rate of increase in total body BMC occurs about 1 year after PHV.[34]

As a percentage of body weight, total body BMC increases from 4 to 18 years; this increase is rapid from 12 to 16 years, particularly in boys.[25,33]

SIGNIFICANCE OF GROWTH AND MATURATION

The timing and intensity of growth and maturation in body size and body composition determine the future risk of obesity, type 2 diabetes, and cardiovascular disease. Early growth is related to later growth. Body fat, fat distribution, fat-free mass, lipid profiles, blood pressure, and fasting plasma glucose concentration track, i.e., there is a positive correlation between repeated measurements taken in the same individuals at different points in time, from childhood into adulthood.[31,35–39] These studies indicate that the earliest onset of pathology begins during childhood.[40] The earlier the BMI rebound occurs, the greater the likelihood of later overweight.[9,41] High values for BMI peak velocity during puberty also pose risks for overweight in adulthood.[4,10,41,42] Girls of similar chronological ages who mature early sexually have significantly greater BMI values than those who mature later.[43] Both boys and girls who mature early have significantly greater total body fat, percent body fat, and fat-free mass than children who mature late.

TRACKING

Tracking refers to the prediction of future values from earlier values and the constancy of an individual relative to population percentiles.[44,45] Tracking is measured by correlations between values at pairs of ages for the same individual. Tracking also can be measured by canalization, the tendency of an individual's serial measurements to fall within the same channel of the population distribution. In the Fels Longitudinal Study, among children 8 to 13 years of age, one third of the boys and more than one half of the girls with BMI at or above the 95th percentile become overweight as adults. Furthermore, among children 13 to 18 years of age, more than one half of the boys and two thirds of the girls with BMI at or above the 95th percentile became overweight adults.[37,38]

Tracking in body composition is slight-to-moderate from birth and infancy through middle childhood to adolescence.[46] Tracking in total body fat, percent body fat, and fat-free mass is marked from the postpubertal period to adulthood.[4]

Tracking correlations ranged from 0.40 at 4-year intervals to 0.24 at a 20-year interval for systolic blood pressure, and from 0.37 (4 years) to 0.20 (20 years) for diastolic blood pressure in the Fels Longitudinal Study.[39] BMI deviations of +1 kg/m^2 from the population mean were associated with increases of 1.2 mm Hg in systolic blood pressure and increases of 0.6 mm Hg in diastolic blood pressure, and early elevations of blood pressure predicted significant risk for later hypertension.[43]

Significant tracking of lipids and lipoproteins from childhood into adolescence is well established.[36,47] Tracking was significant in total cholesterol, low density lipoprotein cholesterol, and high density lipoprotein cholesterol from childhood into young adulthood in the Fels Longitudinal Study.[36]

SIZE AT BIRTH AND INFANCY

There has been considerable interest in the possible relationships of low birth weight and length to hypertension, coronary heart disease, and insulin resistance in adulthood. Small weights-for-length may be related to later insulin resistance, and small head circumferences may predict poor cognitive performance and appear to correlate with the risk of Alzheimer's disease. The prevalence of coronary heart disease is inversely related to weight, length, and abdominal circumference at birth.[48–52] This relationship may be U-shaped because the prevalence of coronary heart disease is also related to large birth weights.[50] Data from the Fels Longitudinal Study show that birth weight is significantly and inversely related to plasma levels of triglycerides and significantly and positively

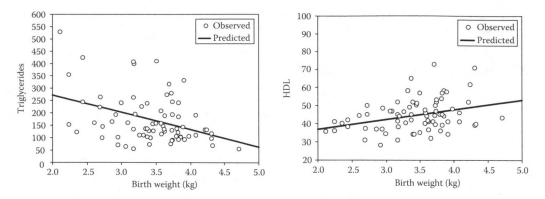

FIGURE 2.9 Significant correlations between birth weight and plasma triglycerides and high density lipo-protein cholesterol.

related to plasma levels of high-density lipoprotein cholesterol in adults 35 years and older (Figure 2.9).

The prevalence of the metabolic syndrome, a clustering of abdominal obesity, dyslipidemia, hypertension, and glucose intolerance is inversely related to birth weight.[53] There is considerable evidence that low birth weights and low ponderal indices at birth are related to the prevalence of type 2 diabetes mellitus later in life. Low birth weights are related to increased insulin resistance and elevated insulin levels in childhood and adulthood.[54,55] However, reports of the relationships between birth weights and glucose tolerance in adults are not in agreement.[56,57] Birth length is inversely related to the prevalence of coronary heart disease in men.[58] Forsen and colleagues[59] did not find such a relationship but noted a significant increase in the prevalence of coronary heart disease for those with small weights-for-length at birth. A faltering growth in head circumference can have serious implications for neural growth and maturation.

BMI REBOUND AND LATER OBESITY

An early BMI rebound is associated with a higher BMI in adolescence[10] and early adulthood.[3] Among the Fels boys, the average BMI value at the rebound was 15.33 kg/m², which occurred at a mean age of 5.4 years.[3] The corresponding mean values for Fels girls were 14.87 kg/m² at 5.3 years. There was a significant difference ($p < .05$) between boys and girls in their average BMI values at the rebound but not in their ages at the rebound. In the same study, age at the BMI rebound was significantly related to overweight at 35 to 45 years in girls but not in boys after adjustment for lifestyle variables and birth weight. A girl with an earlier BMI rebound by 1 year has two times the risk of having a BMI ≥25 as a woman compared with girls with later BMI rebounds.

ADOLESCENCE AND POSTADOLESCENCE

The maximum BMI velocity occurring during adolescence poses a risk for adulthood overweight that is related to cardiovascular diseases and type 2 diabetes. A boy with a higher peak velocity in BMI, V_{max}, by 1 kg/m²/yr during puberty has a risk of being overweight as a man nearly three times that of boys with mean V_{max}.[3] The corresponding risk of being overweight as a woman is 1.9. The maximum value for BMI at the postadolescent period was also predictive of the risk of being overweight in adulthood with an odds ratio of 1.8 and 2.2 for men and women, respectively.

RATES OF SEXUAL MATURATION

Early-maturing children tend to be taller and heavier than late-maturing children at the same chronological age, but the latter generally finish their growth as taller adults. Girls with an early menarche tend to be taller and heavier than those with a later menarche.[60] The timing of menarche appears to be related to adolescent weight gain. Girls who mature early have significantly greater BMIs than those of similar chronological ages who mature later.[43] Both boys and girls who mature early have significantly greater total body fat, percent body fat, and fat-free mass than children who mature late.

Accurate measurement and interpretation of human growth and maturation are essential to pediatric practice for early identification of aberrant values that may be associated with pathological conditions. Knowledge of growth patterns and the timing of the events during infancy, prepubertal and pubertal growth spurts, and sexual maturation is fundamental to the interpretation of growth. Tracking of growth measurements and body composition from childhood into adulthood is central to pediatric practice and public health policies and to epidemiological research in the prevention of childhood obesity and subsequent adverse outcomes in adulthood.

REFERENCES

1. Cooke RWI, Lucas A, Yudkin PLN, Pryse-Davies J. Head circumference as an index of brain weight in the fetus and newborn. *Early Hum Dev.* 1977;1/2: 145–149.
2. Kuczmarski RJ, Ogden CL, Grummer-Strawn LM, Flegal KM, Guo SS, Wei R, et al. CDC Growth Charts: United States. *Advance Data.* 2000; 314: 1–28.
3. Guo SS, Huang C, Maynard M, Demerath E, Towne B, Chumlea, WC, Siervogel RM. BMI during childhood, adolescence, and young adulthood in relation to adult overweight and adiposity. *Int J Obes.* 2000;24(12): 1628–1635.
4. Guo SS RA, Roche AF, Moore WM. The Revised U.S. National Growth Charts. *Nutrition and the M.D.* 1999;1–4.
5. Lohman T, Martorell R, Roche AF. *Anthropometric Standardization Reference Manual.* Champaign, IL: Human Kinetics, 1988.
6. Guo S, Roche A, Fomon S, Nelson S, Chumlea W, Rogers R, et al. Reference data on gains in weight and length during the first two years of life. *J. Pediatr.* 1991;119: 355–362.
7. Roche AF, Sun SS. *Human Growth: Assessment and Interpretation.* Cambridge: Cambridge University Press, 2004.
8. Guo S, Roche A, Moore W. Reference data for head circumference and 1-month increments from 1 to 12 months of age. *J Pediatr.* 1988;113: 490–494.
9. Dietz W. Critical periods in childhood for the development of obesity. *Am J Clin Nutr.* 1994;59: 955–959.
10. Rolland-Cachera MF, Deheeger M, Bellisle F, Sempe M, Guilloud-Bataille M, Patois E. Adiposity rebound in children: a simple indicator for predicting adiposity. *Am J Clin Nutr.* 1994;29: 129–135.
11. Bhargava, SK, Sachdev, HS, Fall, CHD, Osmond, C, Lakshmy, R, Barker, DJP, et al. Relation of serial changes in childhood body-mass index to impaired glucose tolerance in young adulthood. *New Engl J Med.* 2004;350: 865–875.
12. Roche A. Differential timing of maximum length increments among bones within individuals. *Human Biol.* 1974;46: 145–157.
13. Sun, SS, Schubert CM, Chumlea WC, Roche AF, Kulin HE, Lee PA, et al. National estimates of the timing of sexual maturation and racial differences among U.S. children. *Pediatrics.* 2002;110(5): 911–919.
14. Chumlea WC, Schubert CM, Roche AF, Kulin H, Lee PA, Himes JH, Sun SS. Age at menarche and racial comparisons in U.S. girls. *Pediatrics.* 2003;111: 110–113.
15. Grumbach M, Bilezikian JP, Monshima A, Bell, J. Increased bone mass as a result of estrogen therapy in a man with aromatase deficiency. *NE J Med.* 1998;339(9): 599–603.
16. Marshall WA, Tanner JM. Variations in pattern of pubertal changes in girls. *Arch Dis Child.* 1969;44: 291–303.
17. Marshall WA, Tanner JM. Variation in the pattern of pubertal changes in boys. *Arch Dis Child.* 1970;45: 13–23.
18. Buckler JMH. *A Longitudinal Study of Adolescent Growth.* London: Springer Verlag, 1990.

19. Gasser T, Kohler W, Muller H-G, Kneip A. Velocity and acceleration of height growth using kernel estimation. *Ann Human Biol.* 1984;11: 397–411.

20. Guo S, Siervogel R, Roche A, Chumlea W. Mathematical modelling of human growth: A comparative study. *Am J Human Biol.* 1992;4: 93–104.

21. Ramsay JO, Bock RD, Gasser T. Comparison of height acceleration curves in the Fels, Zurich, and Berkeley growth data. *Ann Human Biol.* 1995;22: 413–426.

22. Prokopec M, Bellisle F. Body mass index variations from birth to adulthood in Czech youths. *Acta Med Auxol.* 1992;24: 87–93.

23. Rolland-Cachera M, Cole T, Sepe M, Tichet J, Rossignol C, et al. Body mass index variations: centiles from birth to 87 years. *Eur J Clin Nutr.* 1991;45: 13–21.

24. Luciano A, Bressan F, Zoppi G. Body mass index reference curves for children aged 3-19 years from Verona, Italy. *Eur J Clin Nutr.* 1997;51: 6–10.

25. Fomon, SJ, Haschke, F, Ziegler, EE, Nelson, SE. Body composition of reference children from birth to age 10 years. *Am J Clin Nutr.* 1982;35: 1169–75.

26. Lapillonne A, Braillon P, Claris O, Chatelain PG, Delmas P, Salle B. Body composition in appropriate and in small for gestational age infants. *Acta Paediatri.* 1997;86: 196–200.

27. Butte NF, Hopkinson JM, Wong WW, O'Brian SF, Ellis KJ. Body composition during the first 2 years of life: an updated reference. *Pediatr Res.* 2000;47: 578–584.

28. Malina RM, Beunen G. Growth and physical performance relative to the timing of the adolescent spurt. *Exerc Sport Sci Rev.* 2004;16: 503–540.

29. Geithner CA, Satake T, Woynarowska B, Malina RM. Adolescent spurts in body dimensions: Average and modal sequences. *Am J Human Biol.* 1999;11: 287–295.

29. Parizkova J. Growth and growth velocity of lean body mass and fat in adolescent boys. *Pediatr Res.* 1976;10: 647–650.

30. Slemenda C, Reister T, Hui S, Miller J, Christian J, Johnston C. Influences on skeletal mineralization in children and adolescents: Evidence for varying effects of sexual maturation and physical activity. *J Pediat.* 1994;125: 201–207.

31. Guo SS, Chumlea WC, Roche AF, Siervogel RM. Age- and maturity-related changes in body composition during adolescence into adulthood: the Fels Longitudinal Study. *Int J Obes.* 1997;21: 1167–1175.

32. Maynard LM, Wisemandle W, Roche AF, Chumlea WC, Guo SS, Siervogel RM. Childhood body composition in relation to body mass index. *Pediatrics.* 2001;107: 344–350.

33. Maynard LM, Guo SS, Chumlea WmC, Roche AF, Wisemandle WA, Zeller CM, et al. Total-body and regional bone mineral content and areal bone mineral density in children aged 8 to 18 years: from the Fels Longitudinal Study. *Am. J Clin Nutr.* 1998;68: 1111–1117.

34. Bailey, DA. The Saskatchewan Pediatric Bone Mineral Accrual Study: Bone mineral acquisition during the growing years. *Int. J Sports Med.* 1997(Suppl);18: 191–194.

35. Porkka K, Viikari J, Taimela S, Dahl M, Akerblom H. Tracking and predictiveness of serum lipid and lipoprotein measurements in childhood: A 12-year follow-up — the cardiovascular risk in young Finns study. *Am J Epidemiol.* 1994;140: 1096–1110.

36. Guo SS, Beckett L, Chumlea WC, Roche AF, Siervogel RM. Serial analysis of plasma lipid and lipoproteins from 9 to 21 years. *Am J Clin Nutr.* 1993;58: 61–67.

37. Guo SS, Roche AF, Chumlea WC, Gardner JD, Siervogel RM. The predictive value of childhood body mass index values for overweight at age 35. *Am J Clin Nutr.* 1994; 59: 810–819.

38. Guo SS, Wu W, Chumlea WmC, Roche AF. Predicting overweight and obesity in adulthood from body mass index values in childhood and adolescence. *Am J Clin Nutr.* 2002;76(3): 653–658 (editorial p. 497).

39. Beckett LA, Rosner B, Roche AF, Guo SS. Serial changes in blood pressure from adolescence into adulthood. *Am J Epidemiol.* 1992;135: 1166–1177.

40. Berenson GS, Srinivasan SR. Emergence of obesity and cardiovascular risk for coronary artery diseases: The Bogalusa Heart Study. *Prev Cardiol.* 2001; 116–121.

41. Whitaker RC, Pepe MS, Wright JA, Seidel KD, Dietz WH. Early adiposity rebound and the risk of adult obesity. *Pediatrics.* 1998;101: E51–E56.

42. Wisemandle WA, Maynard LM, Guo SS, Siervogel RM. Childhood weight, stature and body mass index among never overweight, early-onset overweight and late-onset overweight groups. *Pediatrics.* 2000; U29–U36.

43. Guo S, Chi E, Wisemandle W, Chumlea WC, Roche AF, Siervogel RM. Serial changes in blood pressure from childhood into young adulthood for females in relation to body mass index and maturational age. *Am J Hum Biol.* 1998;10: 589–598.

44. Foulkes MA, Davis CE. An index of tracking for longitudinal data. *Biometrics.* 1981;37: 439–446.

45. Ware J, Wu M. Tracking: prediction of future values from serial measurements. *Biometrics.* 1981;37: 427–437.

46. Harsha DW, Smoak CG, Nicklas TA, Webber LS, Berenson GS. Cardiovascular risk factors from birth to 7 years of age: the Bogalusa Heart Study. Tracking of body composition variables. *Pediatrics.* 1987;80: 779–783.

47. Boulton TJC, Magarey AM, Cockington RA. Tracking of serum lipids and dietary energy, fat and calcium intake from 1 to 15 years. *Acta Paediatrica.* 1995;84: 1050–1055.

48. Barker DJP, Osmond C, Golding J, Kuch D, Wadsworkth MEJ. Growth in utero, blood pressure in childhood and adult life, and mortality from cardiovascular disease. *BMJ* 1989;298: 564–567.

49. Barker DJP, Winter PD, Osmaond C, Margetts B, Simmonds SJ. Weight in infancy and death from ischaemic heart disease. *Lancet.* 1989;ii: 577–580.

50. Barker DJP. Outcome of low birthweight. *Horm Res.* 1994;42: 223–230.

51. Barker DJP, Hales N, Fall CHD, Osmond C, Phipps K, Clark PMS. Type 2 (non-insulin-dependent) diabetes mellitus, hypertension and hyperlipidaemia (syndrome X) relation t reduced fetal growth. *Diabetologia.* 1993;36: 62–67.

52. Koupilova I, Leon DA, McKeigue PM, Lithell HO. Is the effect of low birth weight on cardiovascular mortality mediated through high blood pressure? *J Hypertens.* 1999;17: 19–25.

53. Yarbrough DE, Barrett-Connor E, Kritz-Silverstein D, Wingard DL. Birth weight, adult weight, and girth as predictors of the metabolic syndrome in postmenopausal women: The Rancho Bernardo Study. *Diabtetes Care.* 1998;21: 1652–1658.

54. Dabelea D, Petitt DJ, Hanson RL, Imperatore G, Bennett PH, Knowler WC. Birth weight, type 2 diabetes, and insulin resistance in Pima Indian children and young adults. *Diabetes Care.* 1999;22: 944–950.

55. Hofman PL, Cutfield WS, Robinson EM, Bergman RN, Menon RK, Sperling MA, Gluckman PD. Insulin resistance in short children with intrauterine growth retardation. *J Clin Endocrinol Metabol.* 1997;82: 402–406.

56. Lindsay RS, Dabelea D, Roumain J, Hanson RL, Bennett PH, Knowler WC. Type 2 diabetes and low birth weight: The role of paternal inheritance in the association of low birth weight and diabetes. *Diabetes.* 2000;49: 445–449.

57. McCance DR, Pettit DJ, Hanson RL, Jacobsson ITH, Knowler WC, Bennett PH. Birth weight and non-insulin dependent diabetes: thrifty genome, thrifty phenotype, or surviving small baby genotype? *BMJ.* 1994;308: 942–945.

58. Martyn CN, Barker DJP, Jespersen S, Greenwald S, Osmond C, Berry C. Growth in utero, adult blood pressure, and arterial compliance. *Br Heart J.* 1995;73: 116–121.

59. Forsen T, Eriksson JG, Tuomilehto J. Teramo K, Osmond C, Barker DJP. Mother's weight in pregnancy and coronary heart disease in a cohort of Finnish men: Follow-up study. *BMJ.* 1997;315: 837–840.

60. Yoneyama K, Nagata H, Sakamoto Y. A comparison of height growth curves among girls with different ages of menarche. *Human Biol.* 1988;60: 33–41.

3 Influence of Ethnicity on Obesity-Related Factors in Children and Adolescents

*Dympna Gallagher, José R. Fernández,
Paul B. Higgins, and Qing He*

CONTENTS

INTRODUCTION

The prevalence of obesity has increased significantly over the past 10 years across all populations and age groups. Twenty-five percent of U.S. children are overweight or at risk of becoming overweight, and this number has been increasing rapidly.[1] The incidence of overweight in children has nearly tripled over the past 30 years with approximately 11% of children and adolescents ages 6 to 19 years overweight and another 14% considered at risk for overweight. In children ages 2 to 19 years, overweight is defined as a body mass index (BMI kg/m^2) greater than the 95th percentile of the 2000 CDC growth charts for age and sex, and at risk for overweight is defined as a BMI greater than the 85th percentile and less than the 95th percentile. In addition, obesity disproportionately affects many minority populations and some lower income groups.[2] According to the third National Health and Nutrition Examination Survey (NHANES),[1] African-American girls are disproportionately affected. A recent study from the National Longitudinal Study[3] of Adolescent Health (n = 9795) examining the patterns of change in obesity among white, black, Hispanic, and Asian U.S. teens as they transitioned to young adulthood found that obesity incidence over the 5-year study period was 12.7%. Close to 10% of the population remained obese, 1.6% became nonobese, and the prevalence of obesity increased from 10.9 to 22.1%. Notably, obesity incidence was significantly higher in non-Hispanic black (18.4%) females compared with white females. Table 3.1 shows the incidence of overweight and obesity among different pediatric race groups based on consecutive NHANES reports.

Obesity is characterized as excess fat or adipose tissue mass. Total body adipose tissue and its distribution are known risk factors for metabolic abnormalities.[4] The risks associated with excess

TABLE 3.1
Age-Adjusted Prevalence of Overweight from National Surveys (1963 to 1994)

Population Group	Males	Females
Age 6 to 11		
All Races		
NHES II[a]	3.9	4.3
NHANES I	3.8	3.6
NHANES II	6.5	5.5
NHANES III	11.4	9.9
White		
NHES II[a]	4.2	4.1
NHANES I	3.8	3.7
NHANES II	6.5	4.9
NHANES III	11.2	9.1
Black		
NHES II[a]	1.5	5.0
NHANES I	3.8	3.4
NHANES II	6.0	9.5
NHANES III	11.9	15.6
Age 12 to 17		
All Races		
NHES III[b]	4.6	4.5
NHANES I	5.4	6.4
NHANES II	4.7	4.9
NHANES III	11.4	9.9
White		
NHES III[b]	4.8	4.3
NHANES I	5.5	5.8
NHANES II	4.6	4.2
NHANES III	12.2	9.4
Black		
NHES III[b]	3.1	5.8
NHANES I	5.2	10.3
NHANESI I	6.3	9.8
NHANES III	10.2	15.7

[a] National Health Examination Survey II.
[b] National Health Examination Survey III.

Source: Troiano RP, Flegal KM. *Pediatrics* 1998;101: 497–504.
With permission.

fatness result in part from where the fat is distributed.[4] Greater amounts of visceral adipose tissue are associated with increased insulin resistance and the metabolic syndrome[4,5] compared with subcutaneous adipose tissue. Race and ethnicity are known to affect fat and adipose tissue distribution,[6,7] and the association of fat distribution with insulin sensitivity varies by ethnicity.[7] Being African-American is an independent risk factor for type 2 diabetes mellitus and for insulin resistance. Bacha and colleagues[8] studied obese white and black adolescents, and observed that while differences in fat patterning may help explain the more atherogenic risk profile in whites, the cause of the more diabetogenic insulin sensitivity and secretion profile in blacks remains unknown.

HEALTH SIGNIFICANCE OF PEDIATRIC OBESITY

The higher prevalence of obesity in minority populations and individuals with lower income and education levels contributes to excess disease and mortality rates among these groups. Research has shown that obesity in childhood tracks into adulthood[9] and is associated with increased susceptibility to hypertension, dyslipidemia, and glucose intolerance.

Racial and ethnic differences in the prevalence of type 2 diabetes in adults in the United States are well established. The significant increase in the prevalence of childhood obesity over the past 30 years has coincided with a notable increase in the incidence of type 2 diabetes among adolescents. Substantial progress has been made toward identifying population-based risk factors for the development of type 2 diabetes that might lead to these racial–ethnic disparities including total body fatness or adiposity, central adiposity, duration of obesity, high caloric intake, physical inactivity, and genetic predisposition. While all racial and ethnic groups are at risk for type 2 diabetes, the way in which some groups respond to specific risk factors may predispose them to a greater risk of diabetes. Most available information on racial and ethnic disparities with regard to risk for diabetes and other cardiovascular risk factors has been derived from epidemiological studies and little is known about the metabolic and physiological effects of diabetes risk factors in specific racial and ethnic populations.

Detailed studies comparing ethnic differences in metabolic risk factors have been helpful in understanding why certain subgroups of the population may be at increased disease risk. Studies in children are of increased significance because they allow examination of potential underlying biological differences across subgroups of the population to be performed in the absence of potential confounding factors such as smoking, alcohol, aging, and menopausal status. Data from the Bogalusa Heart Study were the first to show evidence of increased insulin resistance based on measures of fasting insulin in African-American children compared with Caucasian children.[10] Subsequently, other studies have demonstrated greater insulin resistance and a greater acute insulin response in African-American than in Caucasian children,[11,12] and these differences were independent of body fat, visceral fat, dietary factors, and physical activity. Previous studies have shown that African-American children have a higher than expected acute insulin response to glucose than Caucasian children,[13] and the higher insulin levels in African-Americans are partly attributable to increased secretion and a lower hepatic extraction.[14,15]

The association between insulin sensitivity and obesity, hyperlipidemia, and hypertension in overweight and obese 5- to 10-year-old (Tanner stage 1 to 3) African-American children (n = 137) has been investigated.[16] In response to a glucose challenge, girls and older, heavier children produced significantly more insulin, and a statistically significant decrease in insulin sensitivity was found, particularly in girls, with increasing BMI. Insulin sensitivity was inversely related to increases in blood pressure, triglycerides, subcutaneous fat, percentage body fat, and Tanner stage. No relationship was observed with LDL and HDL. The authors concluded that reduced insulin sensitivity and the cluster of risk factors known as the insulin resistance syndrome are already apparent in the sample of overweight African-American children studied, while young African-American girls, in particular, were already showing signs of hyperinsulinemia in response to a glucose load, suggesting that the early stages of metabolic decompensation that lead to type 2 diabetes were already occurring.

Studies of obesity, insulin resistance, insulin secretion, and the β-cell response in the Latino population are limited, even in adults. Only a few studies have examined the relationship between obesity and insulin resistance among Latinos. Latino adults have greater fasting and postchallenge insulin,[17] and greater insulin resistance[18,19] than non-Latino whites. One study[20] assessed insulin action using the hyperglycemic clamp in healthy (glucose tolerant), nonobese, young adults including 16 Mexican-Americans. There was no ethnic difference in fasting insulin, but Mexican-Americans were more insulin resistant and had an appropriately higher second phase insulin response than Caucasians.

Goran and colleagues recently showed that Latino and African-American children are equally more insulin resistant than Caucasian children.[21] Interestingly, the compensatory response to the same degree of insulin resistance was different in Latino compared with African-American children. African-American children compensated with a higher acute insulin response to glucose, and this effect was in part due to a reduction in hepatic insulin extraction. Latino children compensated to the same degree of insulin resistance with greater second phase insulin secretion.[21] The well-documented ethnic differences in insulin action and secretion could be explained by either genetic or environmental factors. However, thus far, attempts at explaining the lower insulin sensitivity and higher acute insulin response in African-American compared with Caucasian children by factors such as diet, physical activity, and socioeconomic status[22,23] have proven unsuccessful. A genetic admixture determined from approximately 20 ancestry informative markers indicated that greater African-American genetic admixture was independently related to lower insulin sensitivity ($p < 0.001$) and higher fasting insulin ($p < 0.01$) and provides initial evidence that these ethnic differences may have a genetic basis.[24]

In adults, the effect of adiposity on stroke risk appears to vary by race and sex. What underlying phenomena mediate the relationship between excess adipose tissue and elevated cardiovascular disease risk? The biological implications of sex- and race-related differences in adipose tissue distribution are unclear. Epidemiological studies suggest that certain stages of life are associated with greater risk for the development of obesity in some individuals, including *in utero*, adiposity rebound, puberty, and adolescence stages during the preadult years.

Elevated blood pressure is a recognized component of the metabolic syndrome in adults. A school-based study[25] involving 5102 children (13.5 ± 1.7 years) where ethnicity distribution was 44% white, 25% Hispanic, 22% African-American, and 7% Asian revealed the prevalence of overweight to be 20%, which varied significantly by ethnicity (31% Hispanic, 20% African-American, 15% white, and 11% Asian). Elevated blood pressure was highest among Hispanics (25%) and lowest among Asians (14%); however, this ethnic effect disappeared after controlling for overweight. The prevalence of hypertension increased progressively as the BMI percentile increased from the 5th percentile or less (2%) to the 95th percentile or greater (11%). After adjustment for sex, ethnicity, overweight, and age, the relative risk of hypertension was significant (relative risk: 1.50) for sex and overweight (relative risk: 3.26). Because the prevalence of overweight was highest among Hispanic and African-American children, the risk of hypertension was greater in these groups.

An association between android fat and blood pressure was reported in an African-American and Caucasian pediatric population,[26] where significantly greater systolic and diastolic blood pressures (approximately 1.5 units) was found in African-American compared with Caucasian girls. However, this racial difference disappeared when the data were stratified by stage of sexual maturation. He and colleagues[27] reported in a large cross-sectional pediatric sample (n = 920, age 5 to 18 years) significant positive relationships between systolic and diastolic blood pressure and trunk fat adjusted for total fat in boys at all pubertal stages and in three racial groups (African-American, Asian, and Caucasian). Body fat and fat distribution were measured using two independent techniques, namely, dual energy x-ray absorptiometry (DXA) and anthropometric skinfolds. In girls, however, irrespective of racial group, trunk fat was not a significant predictor of blood pressure.

In summary, there is a disproportionate higher prevalence of obesity among African-Americans and Hispanic or Mexican-Americans. Obesity is a major contributor to the insulin resistant syndrome that often precedes type 2 diabetes. The prevalence of the insulin resistance syndrome is similarly greater in Mexican-Americans and African-Americans than in Caucasians and is identifiable in children, and these racial and ethnic differences manifest at a young age. Compared with Caucasians, obesity-related diseases such as diabetes and hypertension are more prevalent in minority racial and ethnic groups.

FATNESS/ADIPOSITY

The body consists of two compartments, fat and fat-free mass (FFM) (body weight = fat + FFM), and the relative contribution of fat in adults is age, race, and sex dependent.[28-30] Similar reference values do not exist at this time for pediatric populations. However, data exist showing age,[31,32] race,[33] and sex differences[34] in percent body fat as early as prepuberty. In a multiethnic, healthy male population (aged 3 to 18 years; n = 297), Hispanic (Mexican-American) males had higher body fat values than white males, and black males had lower values than white males. When adjusted for body size, the Hispanic males continued to have significantly higher body fat and percentage fat than the white or black males.[35] Among 313 females from a related cohort, Hispanic girls were found to have higher body fat and percentage body fat than their African-American and Caucasian counterparts.[36] Epidemiologic data from the NHANES and HHANES (The Hispanic Health and Nutrition Examination Survey) studies have shown higher skinfold thicknesses among Hispanic relative to African-American and Caucasian children.[37] Girgis et al.[38] have also reported greater percentage body fat in Mexican-American girls compared with Caucasian and African-American girls of similar age, body weight, and pubertal status. Typically, African-American and Caucasian prepubertal children of similar body size and age have not been found to differ by fat mass.[12,39,40] However, several studies have reported differences among older (adolescents) African-American and Caucasian children with regard to fat mass.[41,42] However, careful matching for stage of pubertal status is critical for comparisons among adolescents, and further study of ethnic differences in fat mass and change in fat mass are important in puberty.

Blacks were found to have had less total, visceral, and subcutaneous adipose tissue masses measured by abdominal magnetic resonance imaging (MRI) in a study of 20 black and 20 white normal-weight girls, aged 7 to 10 years, when matched for weight, BMI, bone age, chronological age, Tanner breast stage, and socioeconomic status.[39] Japanese premenarcheal girls had less fat and FFM (unadjusted for body size) than premenarcheal Caucasian girls measured by near-infrared interactance.[43]

Olhager et al.[44] used whole-body MRI in full-term healthy boys (n = 25) and girls (n = 21), 4 to 131 days old, to estimate adipose tissue volume (ATV) and the amounts of subcutaneous and nonsubcutaneous adipose tissue. Both sexes showed significant increases with increasing age in subcutaneous ATV (14.7 and 13.0 mL/d for boys and girls, respectively) and in nonsubcutaneous ATV (1.58 and 1.26 mL/d, respectively). Subcutaneous ATV was 90.5 ± 1.8% (boys) and 91.1 ± 1.9% (girls) of total ATV.

In a study of 73 neonates (26 white, 42 African-American, and 5 Hispanic) using DXA, an independent sex effect was demonstrated, with male infants having higher lean mass but lower fat mass. No significant race difference was found in fat mass or lean mass in this age group.[45] In a study of 76 children followed from 0.5 to 24 months of age, Butte et al.[46] reported percent fat mass as significantly higher in girls than in boys at 6 and 9 months of age ($p = 0.02$). The components of FFM on a percentage basis changed with age ($p = 0.001$) but not sex.

Johnson et al.[47] investigated whether insulin sensitivity was associated with longitudinal changes (3- to 6-year follow-up) in fatness in children (prepubertal at baseline) and found that low initial insulin sensitivity and a decrease in insulin sensitivity during the study were associated with increased fat gain over time. Greater baseline insulin sensitivity appeared to be associated with less gain in fat mass in Caucasians compared with African-Americans, suggesting that African-Americans may be more resistant to the apparent beneficial effect of increased insulin sensitivity. Of interest is that the increase in fat mass over the study period was not significantly different between Caucasian and African-American children, between boys and girls, or with increasing sexual maturation. Similarly Bray et al.[40] failed to find any differences in fat gain between African-American and Caucasian adolescents over a 2-year follow-up period.

In summary, differences in total body fat and percentage body fat, and fat accumulation with growth have been reported among some ethnic groups at very young ages, which could be contributors to the higher prevalence of certain diseases in those groups.

FAT-FREE MASS

Fat-free body mass is a widely studied "molecular level" body composition compartment that is highly correlated with resting energy expenditure (REE) and total energy expenditure in children[48] and adults.[49] During growth and development, skeletal muscle mass increases in proportion to body weight, accounting for ~6% of REE at 6 months of age, and increasing thereafter, reaching adults levels (~33% REE) likely in the late teenage years. Ellis[35] and Ellis et al.[36] reported racial differences in FFM between 5- to 7-year-old African-American and Caucasian children. Ellis[35] studied a young, multiethnic, healthy male population (aged 3 to 18 years; n = 297) consisting of three ethnic groups (European-American [white], n = 145; African-American [black], n = 78; and Mexican-American [Hispanic], n = 74]. Lean tissue mass by DXA was higher in black than in white males but not different between the white and Hispanic groups.

Sex differences in lean body mass[35,36,46] have been reported from birth throughout childhood with females having smaller amounts than males. Studies from our laboratory and others have reported that African-Americans have more appendicular skeletal muscle (ASM) than Caucasians in Tanner 1,[50,51] across Tanner stages,[50] and across the adult life span, even after controlling for weight, height, and age.[52,53] Song et al.[51] assessed ASM quantified by DXA in healthy prepubertal girls (n = 170) and boys (n = 166), using an analysis of variance and multiple regression analysis. The results showed (Figure 3.1) that after adjusting for age, height, and body weight: (1) African-American girls and boys had greater amounts of ASM than Asians ($p = 0.001$) and Caucasians ($p = 0.001$); (2) Caucasian girls had greater amounts of ASM than Asian girls ($p = 0.004$); (3) a trend toward greater ASM in Caucasian compared with Asian boys ($p = 0.06$); (4) irrespective of race, boys had significantly greater ASM than girls ($p = 0.001$); (5) the magnitude of the sex differences in ASM were not different across race; (6) within Asian and Caucasian girls, the race effect on ASM was dependent on height ($p = 0.023$). Age, height, and weight explained 90 to 95% of the variance in ASM in all races. These data suggest that prepubertal sex and racial differences in ASM are in the same direction and follow a similar pattern to that seen in adults, and these findings demonstrate that skeletal muscle mass as a fraction of body weight is smaller in Asian compared with African-American and Caucasian children.

African-American prepubertal children have relatively more bone mineral mass than Asian and Caucasian children. Bone mineral content (BMC) has been found to be lower in Caucasian than in African-American children at early ages (1 to 6 years).[54] Ellis[35] found that in healthy males (aged 3 to 18 years; n = 297) BMC (adjusted for age, weight, and height) was higher in black than in white males, but not different between the white and Hispanic groups. Horlick et al.[55] investigated total body BMC adjusted for total body bone area, age, height, and weight in prepubertal African-American and Caucasian females (n = 172) and males (n = 164). BMC was greater in males than in females ($p = 0.01$), and this sex difference was independent of race. African-American children had greater BMC than Asian and Caucasian children ($p = 0.001$). No differences were found between Asian and Caucasian children.

In a study of 232 healthy children, with about equal numbers of boys and girls and blacks and whites, aged 4 to 16 years, total body BMC was higher in blacks compared with whites of the same age and Tanner stage.[56] In a longitudinal study of 423 healthy Asian, black, Hispanic, and white males and females (aged 9 to 25 years), bone mass of the spine, femoral neck, total hip, and whole body were measured annually for up to 4 years by DXA. Age-adjusted mean bone mineral curves for areal and volumetric bone mineral density were compared for the four ethnic groups.

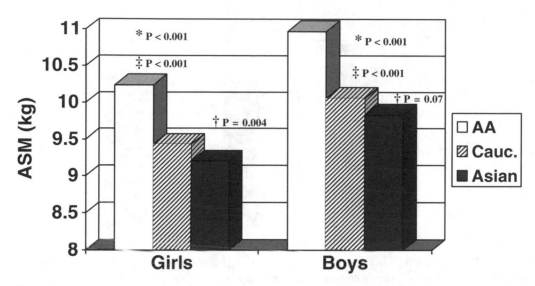

FIGURE 3.1 Appendicular skeletal muscle mass (ASM) in Asian, Caucasian (Cauc), and African-American (AA) girls and boys. Values are means adjusted for height, weight, and age. Significant differences: * Asian vs. African-American, $p < 0.001$; † Asian vs. Caucasian, $p = 0.004$ (girls) and $p = 0.07$ (boys); ‡ Caucasian vs. African-American, $p < 0.001$ (From Song, MY et al., *J Appl Physiol*. 2002; 92: 2285–2291. With permission.)

Consistent differences in areal and volumetric bone density were observed only between black and nonblack subjects. Among females, blacks had greater mean levels of areal and volumetric bone mineral density at all skeletal sites. Differences among Asians, Hispanics, and white females were significant for femoral neck and whole body bone mineral density, and whole body BMC to height ratio, for which Asians had significantly lower values; femoral neck volumetric density in Asian and white females was lower than that in Hispanics. Black males had consistently greater mean values than nonblacks for all areal and volumetric measurements. A few differences were also observed among nonblack male subjects. Whites had greater mean total hip areal, whole body areal, and whole body BMC to height ratio than Asian and Hispanic males; Hispanics had lower spine areal than white and Asian males. Overall, bone mineral density was on average 10% greater in African-Americans than in Caucasians.[57] Nelson et al.[58] in a longitudinal study of 561 African-American and white children and adolescents found that annual accrual of bone mineral was significantly higher in African-American boys and girls relative to their Caucasian counterparts. Furthermore, greater volumetric bone mineral density (as opposed to the DXA-derived areal BMD) of the spine was found in African-American males and females compared with Caucasians at the later stages of puberty.[59,60] Clear ethnic differences exist in skeletal mass and density, and are present in childhood and in adolescence. In particular, African-Americans have greater BMC and density than Caucasians.

In summary, racial and ethnic differences in FFM are already evident in the prepubertal years, including skeletal muscle mass and bone mineral. How early these differences manifest themselves has yet to be determined as insufficient data exist in the preschool and earlier ages. The implications of such differences in children are not known but could have consequences in the adult years when losses of these tissues have serious implications for functionality.

FAT/ADIPOSE TISSUE DISTRIBUTION

In Asians, despite a low prevalence of overweight and obesity (as defined by a BMI greater than 25 kg/m²), fat disproportionately accumulates in the abdominal cavity,[61,62] and this is thought to

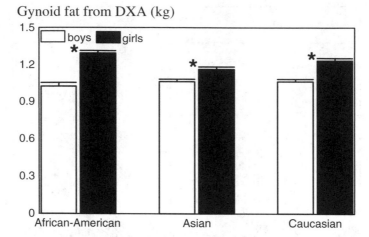

FIGURE 3.2 Adjusted means and standard error (SE) of log-transformed values for DXA-derived gynoid fat. *Sex difference in adjusted means within each race group from multiple *post-hoc* comparisons, $p < .01$. (From He et al., *J Clin Endocrinol Metab*. 2002;87: 2164–2170. With permission.)

increase insulin resistance. For African-Americans, however, the data have been contradictory. Despite African-Americans having less visceral adipose tissue (VAT) for a given BMI,[6,7] the prevalence of select risk factors for cardiovascular disease (e.g., lower peripheral insulin sensitivity) remains higher than that of other racial or ethnic groups.[8,17] Therefore, the question arises as to whether other adipose tissue depots in the body, independent of VAT and subcutaneous adipose tissue (SAT), might convey metabolic risk?

While the aforementioned findings relate to adults, prepubertal race and sex differences in fat distribution have also been reported. While sexual dimorphism of fat distribution was thought to emerge during puberty,[63–67] it is now known that sex differences exist well in advance of pubertal onset (Figure 3.2).[68] Race differences in fat distribution are clearly evident in adults but are less well characterized in prepubertal children. He et al.[68] investigated sex and race (African-American, Asian, and Caucasian) differences in body fat distribution using regression analysis in 358 children (176 girls and 182 boys) from a cross-sectional cohort, using anthropometry and DXA. In African-American and Caucasian children, sex differences in fat distribution were evident ($p < 0.01$), with girls having greater arm, leg and gynoid fat deposits compared with boys, after adjusting for trunk or android fat, and covariates including age, weight, height, race, and interactions. In Asians, significant sex differences ($p < 0.001$) were present in gynoid fat deposits only. Caucasian girls had greater total and subcutaneous limb fat than Asian girls ($p < 0.01$). Caucasian boys also had greater total limb fat than Asian boys ($p < 0.01$). These results demonstrate both sexual dimorphism and racial differences in fat distribution in prepubertal children, suggesting that the associated differences in cardiovascular and metabolic risk factors may begin before the onset of puberty. This comparison of African-American, Asian, and Caucasian prepubertal children suggests phenotypic differences in fat distribution. Because an android fat pattern is associated with greater visceral fat accumulation, a question is raised regarding the health risk attached.

Daniels et al.[26] reported racial differences in blood pressure in 9- and 10-year-old girls. Blood pressure was found to be associated with truncal fat during maturation (Tanner stages 1 to 5) in males but not in females[27] in a cross-sectional sample of females and males across Tanner stages 1 to 5. Subjects were 442 girls (145 African-American (AA), 161 Asian, 136 Caucasian) and 478 boys (128 AA, 184 Asian, 166 Caucasian), ages 5 to 18 years. The results demonstrated a sex difference in the relationship between blood pressure (BP) and trunk fat. After adjusting for height, weight, total fatness, and Tanner stage, a significant positive relationship was present between trunk fat and systolic BP and diastolic BP in boys only, across all three racial groups. In girls, trunk fat was not a significant predictor of BP.

Excess VAT is recognized as an important risk factor for the development of coronary heart disease and noninsulin dependent diabetes mellitus. Several studies have reported less VAT in African-American adults compared with Caucasian adults,[6,7] children, and adolescents.[8,13,39] Among women, whole-body VAT in Asian-Americans was compared with that of European-Americans.[61] VAT was measured using whole-body multislice MRI in 54 women (18 Asian-American, 36 European-American) and 53 men (19 Asian-American, 34 European-American) with a BMI (kg/m²) less than 30. Data were analyzed by multiple regression modeling. Asian-American women had higher log-transformed VAT compared with European-American women ($p < 0.05$), after adjusting for age and total body fat. There was a significant age by race interaction such that racial differences in VAT were most evident after the age of 30 years. No differences in VAT could be detected between Asian-American and European-American men, even after adjusting for potential covariates, including total adiposity. These data were the first to demonstrate higher amounts of VAT in healthy Asian-American adults, a finding that suggests normative VAT values or standards derived from Caucasians may not be applicable to Asians.

Yanovski et al.[39] found less VAT in normal-weight 7- to 10-year–old prepubertal African-American girls compared with Caucasians, despite no differences between groups in absolute waist circumference or waist-to-hip ratio. The groups were matched for weight, BMI, bone age, chronological age, Tanner breast stage, and socioeconomic status. Similarly, Goran et al.[13] found that African-American prepubertal children had significantly less VAT than Caucasian children.

Malina et al.[69] reported in their study of adolescent girls that the sequence from proportionally more to proportionally less trunk SAT was as follows: Asian > Mexican > White > Black by using skinfold measurements. Goran et al.[70] found body fat to be more centrally distributed in Mohawk compared with Caucasian children (4 to 7 years of age): chest skinfold thickness, the ratio of trunk skinfolds to extremity skinfolds, and the waist to hip ratio were all significantly higher in Mohawk children, and this effect was independent of sex and body fat content. Goran et al.[13] also reported that the relative distribution of adipose tissue measured by CT in the intra-abdominal compared with the subcutaneous abdominal region was significantly lower in prepubertal African-Americans compared with whites.

A less well studied fat–adipose tissue depot called intermuscular adipose tissue (IMAT), which is located below the subcutaneous adipose tissue fascial plane and between the muscle bundles, and quantified using whole body MRI, has recently been described.[71] In adults, the quantity of IMAT was assessed relative to other known fat depots within the body in relation to race (in African-American, Asian, and Caucasian).[72] IMAT deposits were not different in size in all racial groups at low levels of adiposity but accumulated as a greater proportion of total adipose tissue (TAT) in African-Americans compared with Caucasian and Asian subjects (58 g IMAT/kg TAT in African-Americans; 46 g IMAT/kg TAT in Caucasians; 44 g IMAT/kg TAT in Asians; interaction of slopes $p = 0.001$). VAT depots were not different in size at low levels of adiposity, but with increasing adiposity, VAT accumulation was greater in Asians and Caucasians compared with IMAT. Accumulation rates for IMAT and VAT did not differ in African-Americans.[72] Although the clinical significance of the IMAT depot has yet to be determined, two clinical investigations[73,74] quantified this depot in a single midthigh slice using computed tomography and found that insulin resistance was associated with increased subfacial adipose tissue in obese adults[73] and thinner older persons.[74] More specifically, Goodpaster et al.[73] found that adipose tissue located beneath the fascia lata, and therefore adjacent to skeletal muscle, was significantly negatively correlated with insulin resistance, whereas adipose tissue located above the fascia (i.e., SAT) and removed from skeletal muscle was not. Similar studies have yet to be conducted in children. Figure 3.3 shows the cross-sectional images from the midthigh in two 7-year-old prepubertal boys: obese (left) and lean (right). A greater amount of IMAT is evident in the obese boy.

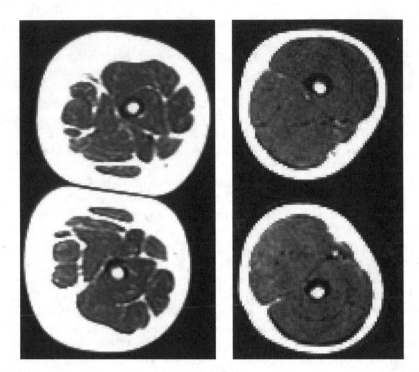

FIGURE 3.3 Cross-sectional images from midthigh in two 7-year-old prepubertal boys: obese (left) and lean (right) showing greater amounts of intermuscular adipose tissue (IMAT) in the obese boy.

Triglyceride or lipid stored within the myocyte of the muscle fiber (intramyocellular lipid, IMCL) and within adipocytes within muscle (extramyocellular lipid, EMCL) can be quantified using magnetic resonance spectroscopy. IMCL and EMCL have recently received attention as another component of body composition influenced by obesity and associated with insulin resistance.[75,76] These lipid stores have been found to be strongly associated with insulin resistance in obese[75,76] and nonobese adults,[77] and in nondiabetic offspring of type 2 diabetic subjects.[78,79] In obese adolescents,[80] both IMCL and EMCL contents of the soleus muscle were significantly greater than in lean control subjects. A strong inverse correlation was found between IMCL and insulin sensitivity, even after controlling for percent total body fat and abdominal subcutaneous fat mass (partial correlation $r = 0.73$, $p < 0.01$) but not when adjusting for visceral fat ($r = 0.54$, $p < 0.08$). In obese adolescents, increases in total body fat and central adiposity were accompanied by higher IMCL and EMCL lipid stores. Racial and ethnic differences in muscle IMCL and EMCL remain uninvestigated.

Fatty liver disease is another complication of obesity also seen in children. Nonalcoholic steatohepatitis (NASH) is associated with obesity, insulin resistance, diabetes, and hypertriglyceridemia. Children presenting with NASH tend to be prepubertal, male, more frequently of Hispanic origin, and with body weight above the 90th percentile.[81] However, there are no reports to date on racial and ethnic influences on liver fat and lipids in either adults or children.

In summary, fat and adipose tissue distribution is an independent risk factor for metabolic abnormalities. Several well-defined racial and ethnic differences in adipose tissue distribution have been described in both adults and children.

ETIOLOGY OF ETHNIC DIFFERENCES IN BODY COMPOSITION

The variables "ethnicity" or "race," typically encompass both genetic and environmental factors. Hence, when a trait differs by "ethnicity," this difference may be attributable to genetic and biologic

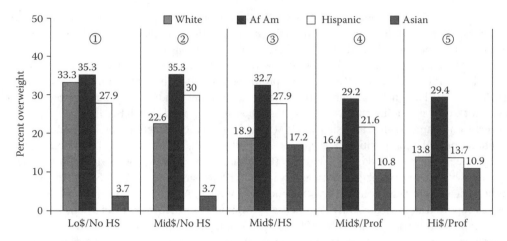

FIGURE 3.4 Predicted overweight prevalence among females by ethnicity and categories of family income and parental education. Low income (Lo$): $10,000 in continuous models; $0 to $20,000 in categorical models. Middle income (Mid$): $50,000 in continuous models; $40,000 to $60,000 in categorical models. High income (Hi$): $100,000 in continuous models; $80,000+ in categorical models. No HS, no high school; HS, high school (or GED) diploma; Prof, college or professional degree; Af Am, African-American. (From Gordon-Larsen P et al., *Obes Res.* 2003;11: 121–129. With permission.)

factors, environmental factors, or both. Recently, ancestral genetic admixture estimates have been used to explore ethnic differences in complex traits. Much of the current North American population was created by intermixing of European, West African, and Native American parental populations. Hence, alleles from these previously isolated populations have been combined to create a gene pool patchwork. The relative contribution of these parental populations to an individual's genome or ancestral genetic admixture can be determined from an array of DNA sequences that differ in frequency between the respective ancestral parental populations. These DNA sequences are known as ancestry informative markers. Estimates of ancestral genetic admixture, used in conjunction with measures of environmental influences such as socioeconomic status and habitual diet, can help to decompose the categorical variable "ethnicity" and to better understand the factors contributing to ethnic differences in complex traits.[82]

Several recent studies have used the ancestral genetic admixture approach to assess the contribution of genetic and environmental variables to ethnic differences in body composition variables. Bonilla et al. found that European admixture proportions among a group of Hispanic women living in New York City were negatively associated with bone mineral density.[83] In another study Fernandez et al.[84] found that West African admixture was positively associated with BMI and bone mineral density in African-American women. These data indicate that genetic factors may underlie ethnic differences in body composition phenotypes, a concept further supported by recent findings that African-American adolescents have a higher prevalence of overweight compared with Caucasian adolescents, after controlling for socioeconomic status (Figure 3.4).[85] West African genetic admixture was also associated with components of body composition in children.[86]

In summary, further work using ancestral genetic admixture and robust environmental measures will help yield a better understanding of the etiology of ethnic variation in body composition traits.

IMPLICATIONS OF RACIAL AND ETHNIC DIFFERENCES IN BODY COMPOSITION ON OBESITY

A larger skeletal muscle mass in African-Americans implies a smaller mass of organs for any given FFM. REE is lower in African-American girls and boys than in Caucasian girls and boys after controlling for body mass and FFM.[87–90] Skeletal muscle mass is significantly greater in African-American girls and boys, despite similar FFM, than in Caucasian girls and boys after controlling for body weight and age.[50,51] These two observations strongly suggest that FFM composition differs between racial groups and that African-Americans have a relative organ–tissue mass distribution that favors a lower REE. Over a prolonged period individuals with a relatively smaller organ mass will have a lower cumulative energy requirement and thus be susceptible to weight gain if intake is not adjusted.[91] A series of studies has reported that REE is lower in African-American compared with Caucasian adult women.[7,92–94] After adjusting for differences in body weight and/or body composition, Kushner et al.,[92] Albu et al.,[7] and Foster et al.[93] found REE to be 6% (160 kcal/d), 3% (120 kcal/d), and 6% (94 kcal/d), respectively, lower in African-American compared with Caucasian obese women. Similarly, REE was reported to be 7.5% lower in normal-weight African-American compared with Caucasian women. A 5 and 7% lower sleeping metabolic rate was reported in African-American men and women compared with Caucasians.[91] Total daily energy expenditure was found to be 10% lower in older (over 55 years) African-American men and women compared with Caucasians,[95] which was considered due to a 6% lower REE and 19% lower physical activity energy expenditure. Because REE comprises approximately 65% of daily energy expenditure in adults, the daily differences in REE observed in these studies (~100 to 150 kcal), over a prolonged period, may be one factor contributing to the greater incidence of obesity among African-American women. Regardless of the long-term effect on body weight, these observations suggest that racial differences in energy requirements may exist. It is noteworthy that similar ethnic patterns in REE have emerged in girls at all stages of pubertal maturation.[88] Sun et al.[50] published the results of a longitudinal investigation of how REE changes with pubertal maturation in relation to changes in body composition across race and sex. They reported that REE was significantly lower in African-American compared with Caucasian children (by ~250 kJ/d) and that REE declined with Tanner stage after adjusting for race, sex, fat mass, and FFM. These findings confirm earlier reports of lower daily REE in African-American girls compared with Caucasian girls, after adjusting for FFM: 212 kcal by Kaplan et al.,[87] 143 kcal by Morrison et al.,[88] 92 kcal by Yanovski et al.,[89] and 79 kcal by Wong et al.[90] Greater IMAT in African-Americans may confer greater metabolic risk although, at this time, the clinical significance of IMAT is unknown. Asians tend to have metabolic abnormalities at lower BMIs, which may be attributable to greater amounts of VAT. The strength of the associations between body composition and metabolic factors appears to be different among racial groups. For example, Yanovski et al.[39] reported that both basal ($r^2 = 0.46$, $p = 0.001$) and 2-h oral glucose tolerance test serum insulin levels ($r^2 = 0.31$, $p = 0.01$) were significantly correlated with SAT as assessed by MRI in black girls but not in white girls ($r^2 < 0.05$, for basal and 2-h insulin, not significant).

In summary, understanding body composition differences between racial and ethnic groups is important and should be taken into consideration when investigating and interpreting issues in obesity, disease, and biology, where racial and ethnic differences exist.

CONCLUSION

Striking racial and ethnic differences in the prevalence of obesity exist among children. Similarly, body composition varies by race and ethnicity (Table 3.2). There is a specific need to clearly understand the relationships between body fat and fat distribution, and the relation of these to cardiovascular and metabolic risk factors in different ethnic and racial groups. To do so, researchers need to conduct appropriate investigations involving the measurement of actual fat amount and fat distribution with less reliance on anthropometric indices such as body mass index and circumference measures. In pediatric populations, longitudinal studies with appropriate measures of environmental and cultural influences are required to better understand racial and ethnic differences in obesity and related comorbidities.

TABLE 3.2
Body Composition Differences by Race and Ethnicity in Children and Adolescents

Fat (%)	Greater in Ca compared with AA[33]
	Greater in AA compared with Ca[33]
	No differences between Ca and AA children[12,39]
	Greater in Hispanics (Mexican-American) compared with Ca boys and girls,[35–37] AA males and females,[35–37] and Ca and AA prepubertal females[38]
Visceral fat	Lower in AA compared with Ca[39]
Trunk fat	Greater in Asian compared with AA and Ca prepubertal males and females[68]
Total lean soft tissue	Greater in AA compared with Ca males and females[35,36]
	No differences between Ca and Hispanic (Mexican-American) males and females[35,36]
Limb soft tissue	Greater in AA compared with Asian and Ca males and females[51]
	Greater in Ca compared with Asian females[51]
Bone	Greater BMC in AA compared with Ca males and females,[35,36,54–57] and Asian males and females[55,57]
	No differences in BMC between Ca and Asian males and females[55]
	No differences in BMC between Ca and Hispanic (Mexican-American) males[35]
	Lower BMC in Asian and Ca compared with Hispanic females[57]
	Lower BMC in Asian and Hispanic compared with Ca males[57]

Note: AA = African-American; Ca = Caucasian; BMC = bone mineral content.

REFERENCES

1. Troiano RP, Flegal KM. Overweight children and adolescents: description, epidemiology, and demographics. *Pediatrics.* 1998;101: 497–504.
2. http://www.nhlbi.nih.gov/guidelines/obesity/ob_gdlns.pdf (accessed November 2004).
3. Gordon Larsen P, Adair LS, Nelson MC, Popkin BM. Five year obesity incidence in the transition period between adolescence and adulthood: the National Longitudinal Study of Adolescent Health. *Am J Clin Nutr.* 2004,80: 569–575.
4. Kissebah AH, Vydelingum N, Murray R, Evans DJ, Hartz AJ, Kalkhoff RK, Adams PW. Relation of body fat distribution to metabolic complications of obesity. *J Clin Endocrinol Metab.* 1982;54: 245–260.
5. Krotkiewski M, Bjorntorp P, Sjostrom L, Smith U. Impact of obesity on metabolism in men and women. Importance of regional adipose tissue distribution. *J Clin Invest.* 1983;72: 1150–1162.
6. Conway JM, Yanovski SZ, Avila NA, Hubbard VS. Visceral adipose tissue differences in black and white women. *Am J Clin Nutr.* 1995;61: 765–771.
7. Albu JB, Murphy L, Frager DH, Johnson JA, Pi-Sunyer FX. Visceral fat and race-dependent health risks in obese nondiabetic premenopausal women. *Diabetes.* 1997;46: 456–462.
8. Bacha F, Saad R, Gungor N, Janosky J, Arslanian SA. Obesity, regional fat distribution, and syndrome X in obese black versus white adolescents: race differential in diabetogenic and atherogenic risk factors. *J Clin Endocrinol Metab.* 2003;88: 2534–2540.
9. Dietz WH. Health consequences of obesity in youth: childhood predictors of adult disease. *Pediatrics.* 1998;101: 518–525.
10. Freedman DS, Srinivasan SR, Burke GL, Shear CL, Smoak CG, Harsha DW, et al. Relation of body fat distribution to hyperinsulinemia in children and adolescents: the Bogalusa Heart Study. *Am J Clin Nutr.* 1987;46: 403–410.
11. Arslanian S, Suprasongsin C, Janosky JE. Insulin secretion and sensitivity in black versus white prepubertal healthy children. *J Clin Endocrinol Metab.* 1997;82: 1923–1927.
12. Gower BA, Nagy TR, Goran MI. Visceral fat, insulin sensitivity, and lipids in prepubertal children. *Diabetes.* 1999;48: 1515–1521.

13. Goran MI, Nagy TR, Treuth MT, Trowbridge C, Dezenberg C, McGloin A, Gower BA. Visceral fat in Caucasian and African-American pre-pubertal children. *Am J Clin Nutr.* 1997;65: 1703–1709.

14. Gower BA, Granger WM, Franklin F, Shewchuk RM, Goran MI. Contribution of insulin secretion and clearance to glucose-induced insulin concentration in African-American and Caucasian children. *J Clin Endocrinol Metab.* 2002;87: 2218–2224.

15. Uwaifo GI, Nguyen TT, Keil MF, Russell DL, Nicholson JC, Bonat SH, et al. Differences in insulin secretion and sensitivity of Caucasian and African American prepubertal children. *J Pediatr.* 2002;140: 673–680.

16. Young-Hyman D, Schlundt DG, Herman L, De Luca F, Counts D. Evaluation of the insulin resistance syndrome in 5- to 10-year-old overweight/obese African-American children. *Diabetes Care.* 2001;24: 1359–1364.

17. Haffner SM, D'Agostino RJ, Saad MF, Rewers M, Mykkanen L, Selby J. Increased insulin resistance and insulin secretion in non-diabetic African-Americans, and Hispanics compared to non-Hispanic whites: the insulin resistance atherosclerosis study. *Diabetes.* 1996;45: 742–748.

18. Haffner SM, Stern MP, Mitchell BD, Hazuda HP, Patterson JK. Incidence of type II diabetes in Mexican Americans predicted by fasting insulin and glucose levels, obesity and body-fat distribution. *Diabetes.* 1990;39: 283–288.

19. Haffner SM, Miettinen H, Gaskill SP, Stern MP. Decreased insulin secretion and increased insulin resistance are independently related to the 7-year risk of NIDDM in Mexican-Americans. *Diabetes.* 1995;44: 1386–1391.

20. Chiu KC, Cohan P, Lee NP, Chuang LM. Insulin sensitivity differs among ethnic groups with a compensatory response in B-cell function. *Diabetes Care.* 2000;23: 1353–1358.

21. Goran MI, Bergman RN, Cruz ML, Watanabe R. Insulin resistance and associated compensatory response in African American and Hispanic children. *Diabetes Care.* 2002;25: 2184–2190.

22. Ku CY, Gower BA, Hunter GR, Goran MI. Racial differences in insulin secretion and sensitivity in prepubertal children: Role of physical fitness and physical activity. *Obes Res.* 2000;8: 506–515.

23. Lindquist C, Gower BA, Goran MI. Role of dietary factors in ethnic differences in early risk for cardiovascular disease and type 2 diabetes. *Am J Clin Nutr.* 2000;71: 725–732.

24. Gower BA, Fernandez JR, Beasley TM, Shriver MD, Goran MI. Using genetic admixture to explain racial differences in insulin-related phenotypes. *Diabetes.* 2003;52: 1047–1051.

25. Sorof JM, Lai D, Turner J, Poffenbarger T, Portman RJ. Overweight, ethnicity, and the prevalence of hypertension in school-aged children. *Pediatrics.* 2004;113: 475–482.

26. Daniels SR, Morrison JA, Sprecher DL, Khoury P, Kimball TR. Association of body fat distribution and cardiovascular risk factors in children and adolescents. *Circulation.* 1999;99: 541–545.

27. He Q, Horlick M, Fedun B, Wang J, Pierson RN, Jr., Heshka S, Gallagher D. Trunk fat and blood pressure in children through puberty. *Circulation,* 2002;105: 1093–1098.

28. Gallagher D, Visser M, Sepulveda D, Pierson RN, Harris T, Heymsfield SB. How useful is body mass index for comparison of body fatness across age, sex, and ethnic groups? *Am J Epidemiol.* 1996;143: 228–239.

29. Wang J, Thornton JC, Burastero S, Shen J, Tanenbaum S, Heymsfield SB, Pierson RN, Jr. Comparisons for body mass index and body fat percent among Puerto Ricans, blacks, whites and Asians living in the New York City area. *Obes Res.* 1996;4: 377–384.

30. Mott JW, Wang J, Thornton JC, Allison DB, Heymsfield SB, Pierson RN Jr. Relation between body fat and age in 4 ethnic groups. *Am J Clin Nutr.* 1999;69: 1007–1013.

31. Goulding A, Taylor RW, Jones IE, Lewis-Barned NJ, Williams SM. Body composition of 4- and 5-year-old New Zealand girls: a DXA study of initial adiposity and subsequent 4-year fat change. *Int J Obes Relat Metab Disord.* 2003;27: 410–415.

32. Taylor RW, Goulding A, Lewis-Barned NJ, Williams SM. Rate of fat gain is faster in girls undergoing early adiposity rebound. *Obes Res.* 2004;8: 1228–1230.

33. Morrison JA, Barton BA, Obarzanek E, Crawford PB, Guo SS, Schreiber GB, Waclawiw M. Racial differences in the sums of skinfolds and percentage of body fat estimated from impedance in black and white girls, 9 to 19 years of age: the National Heart, Lung, and Blood Institute Growth and Health Study. *Obes Res.* 2001;9: 297–305.

34. Zimmermann MB, Gubeli C, Puntener C, Molinari L. Detection of overweight and obesity in a national sample of 6–12-y-old Swiss children: accuracy and validity of reference values for body mass index from the US Centers for Disease Control and Prevention and the International Obesity Task Force. *Am J Clin Nutr.* 2004;79: 838–843.

35. Ellis KJ. Body composition of a young, multiethnic, male population. *Am J Clin Nutr.* 1997;66: 1323–1331.

36. Ellis KJ, Abrams SA, Wong WW. Body composition of a young, multiethnic, female population. *Am J Clin Nutr.* 1997;65: 724–731.

37. Greaves KA, Puhl J, Baranowski T, Gruben D, Seale D. Ethnic differences in anthropometric characteristics of young children and their parents. *Hum Biol.* 1989;61: 459–477.

38. Girgis R, Abrams SA, Castracane VD, Gunn SK, Ellis KJ, Copeland KC. Ethnic differences in androgens, IGF-1, and body fat in healthy prepubertal girls. *J Pediatr Endocrinol Metab.* 2000;13: 497–503.

39. Yanovski JA, Yanovski SZ, Filmer KM, Hubbard VS, Avila N, Lewis B, et al. Differences in body composition of black and white girls. *Am J Clin Nutr.* 1996;64: 833–839.

40. Bray GA, DeLany JP, Harsha DW, Volaufova J, Champagne CM. Body composition of African American and white children: a 2-year follow-up of the BAROC Study. *Obes Res.* 2001;9: 605–621.

41. Tershakovec AM, Kuppler KM, Zemel B, Stallings VA. Age, sex, ethnicity, body composition, and resting energy expenditure of obese African American and white children and adolescents. *Am J Clin Nutr.* 2002;75: 867–871.

42. He Q, Horlick M, Thornton J, Wang J, Pierson R, Jr., Heshka S, Gallagher D. Sex-specific fat distribution is not linear across pubertal groups in a multi-ethnic study. *Obes Res.* 2004;12: 725–733.

43. Sampei MA, Novo NF, Juliano Y, Colugnati FA, Sigulem DM. Anthropometry and body composition in ethnic Japanese and Caucasian adolescent girls: considerations on ethnicity and menarche. *Int J Obes Relat Metab Disord.* 2003;27: 1114–1120.

44. Olhager E, Flinke E, Hunnerstad U, Forsum E. Studies on human body composition during the first 4 months of life using magnetic resonance imaging and isotope dilution. *Pediatr Res.* 2003;54: 906–912.

45. Hammami M, Koo WW, Hockman EM. Body composition of neonates from fan beam dual energy X-ray absorptiometry measurement. *J Parenter Enteral Nutr.* 2003;27: 42–26.

46. Butte NF, Hopkinson JM, Wong WW, Smith EO, Ellis KJ. Body composition during the first 2 years of life: an updated reference. *Pediatr Res.* 2000;47: 578–585.

47. Johnson MS, Figueroa-Colon R, Huang TT, Dwyer JH, Goran MI. Longitudinal changes in body fat in African American and Caucasian children: influence of fasting insulin and insulin sensitivity. *J Clin Endocrinol Metab.* 2001;86: 3182–3187.

48. Elia M. Organ and tissue contribution to metabolic rate. In: Kinney JM, Ed. *Energy Metabolism: Tissue Determinants and Cellular Corollaries.* New York: Raven Press Ltd, 1992: 61–77.

49. Ravussin E, Lillioja S, Anderson TE, Christin L, Bogardus C. Determinants of 24-hour energy expenditure in man. Methods and results using a respiratory chamber. *J Clin Invest.* 1986;78: 1568–1578.

50. Sun M, Gower BA, Bartolucci AA, Hunter GR, Figueroa-Colon R, Goran MI. A longitudinal study of resting energy expenditure relative to body composition during puberty in African American and White children. *Am J Clin Nutr.* 2001;73: 308–315.

51. Song MY, Kim J, Horlick M, Wang J, Pierson RN, Jr., Heo M, Gallagher D. Prepubertal Asians have less limb skeletal muscle. *J Appl Physiol.* 2002;92: 2285–2291.

52. Gasperino JA, Wang J, Pierson RN, Jr., Heymsfield SB. Age-related changes in musculoskeletal mass between black and white women. *Metabolism.* 1995;44: 30–34.

53. Gallagher D, Visser M, De Meersman RE, Sepulveda D, Baumgartner RN, Pierson RN, et al. Appendicular skeletal muscle mass: effects of age, gender, and ethnicity. *J Appl Physiol.* 1997;83: 229–239.

54. Li JY, Specker BL, Ho ML, Tsang RC. Bone mineral content in black and white children aged 1 to 6 years of age. *Am J Dis Child.* 1989;143: 1346–1349.

55. Horlick M, Thornton J, Wang J, Levine LS, Fedun B, Pierson RN, Jr. Bone mineral in prepubertal children: gender and ethnicity. *J Bone Miner Res.* 2000;15: 1393–1397.

56. Hui SL, Dimeglio LA, Longcope C, Peacock M, McClintock R, Perkins AJ, Johnston CC, Jr. Difference in bone mass between black and white American children: attributable to body build, sex hormone levels, or bone turnover? *J Clin Endocrinol Metab.* 2003;88: 642–649.

57. Bachrach LK, Hastie T, Wang MC, Narasimhan B, Marcus R. Bone mineral acquisition in healthy Asian, Hispanic, black, and Caucasian youth: a longitudinal study. *J Clin Endocrinol Metab.* 1999;84: 4702–4712.

58. Nelson DA, Simpson PM, Johnson CC, Barondess DA, Kleerekoper M. The accumulation of whole body skeletal mass in third and fourth grade children: effects of age, gender, ethnicity, and body composition. *Bone* 1997;20: 73–78.

59. Gilsanz V, Roe TF, Mora S, Costin G, Goodman WG. Changes in vertebral bone density in black and white girls during childhood and puberty. *N Engl J Med.* 1991;325: 1597–1600.

60. Gilsanz V, Skaggs DL, Kovanlikaya A, Sayre J, Loro ML, Kaufman F, Korenman SG. Differential effects of race on the axial and appendicular skeletons of children. *J Clin Endocrinol Metab.* 1998;83: 1420–1427.

61. Park YW, Allison DB, Heymsfield SB, Gallagher D. Larger amounts of visceral adipose tissue in Asian Americans. *Obes Res.* 2001;9: 381–387.

62. Hayashi T, Boyle E, Leonetti D, McNeely M, Newell-Morris L, Kahn S, Fujimoto W. Visceral adiposity and the prevalence of hypertension in Japanese Americans. *Circulation.* 2003;108: 1718–1723.

63. Malina RM, Bouchard C. Subcutaneous fat distribution during growth. In: Bouchard C, Johnston FE, Eds. *Fat Distribution during Growth and Later Health Outcomes.* New York: Plenum, 1988: pp. 63–84.

64. Rolland-Cachera MF, Bellisle F, Deheeger M, Pequignot F, Sempe M. Influence of body fat distribution during childhood on body fat distribution in adulthood: a two-decade follow-up study. *Int J Obes.* 1990;4: 47–81.

65. Cowell CT, Briody J, Lloyd-Jones S, Smith C, Moore B, Howman-Giles R. Fat distribution in children and adolescents — the influence of sex and hormones *Horm Res.* 1997;48: 93–100.

66. Malina RM. Regional body composition: age, sex, and ethnic variation. In: Roche AF, Heymsfield SB, Lohman TG, Eds. *Human Body Composition.* Champaign IL: Human Kinetics, 1996: pp. 217–256.

67. Weststrate JA, Deurenberg P, van Tinteren H. Indices of body fat distribution and adiposity in Dutch children from birth to 18 years of age. *Int J Obes.* 1989;13: 465–477.

68. He Q, Horlick M, Thornton J, Wang J, Pierson RN, Jr., Heshka S, Gallagher D. Sex and race differences in fat distribution among Asian, African-American, and Caucasian prepubertal children. *J Clin Endocrinol Metab.* 2002;87: 2164–2170.

69. Malina RM, Huang YC, Brown KH. Subcutaneous adipose tissue distribution in adolescent girls of four ethnic groups. *Int J Obes Relat Metab Disord.* 1995;19: 793–797.

70. Goran MI, Kaskoun M, Johnson R, Martinez C, Kelly B, Hood V. Energy expenditure and body fat distribution in Mohawk children. *Pediatrics.* 1995;95: 89–95.

71. Song MY, Ruts E, Kim J, Janumala I, Heymsfield S, Gallagher D. Sarcopenia and increased adipose tissue infiltration of muscle in elderly African American women. *Am J Clin Nutr.* 2004;79: 874–880.

72. Gallagher D, Kuznia P, Heshka S, Albu J, Heymsfield S, Goodpaster B, et al. Adipose tissue in muscle: a novel depot similar in size to visceral adipose tissue. *Am J Clin Nutr.* 2005;81: 903–911.

73. Goodpaster BH, Thaete FL, Kelley DE. Thigh adipose tissue distribution is associated with insulin resistance in obesity and in type 2 diabetes mellitus. *Am J Clin Nutr.* 2000;71: 885–892.

74. Goodpaster BH, Krishnaswami S, Resnick H, Kelley DE, Haggerty C, Harris TB, et al. Association between regional adipose tissue distribution and both type 2 diabetes and impaired glucose tolerance in elderly men and women. *Diabetes Care.* 2003;26: 372–379.

75. Simoneau JA, Colberg SR, Thaete FL, Kelley DE. Skeletal muscle glycolytic and oxidative enzyme capacities are determinants of insulin sensitivity and muscle composition in obese women. *FASEB J.* 1995;9: 273–278.

76. Goodpaster BH, Thaete FZ, Simoneau JA, Kelley DE. Subcutaneous abdominal fat and tight muscle composition predict insulin sensitivity independently of visceral fat. *Diabetes.* 1997;46: 1579–1585.

77. Krssak M, Petersen KF, Dresner A, DiPietro L, Vogel SM, Rothman DL, et al. Intramyocellular lipid concentrations are correlated with insulin sensitivity in humans: a 1H-NMR spectroscopy study. *Diabetologia.* 1999;42: 113–116.

78. Perseghin G, Scifo P, DeCobelli F, Pagliato E, Battezzaeti A, Arcelloni C, et al. Intramyocellular triglyceride content is a determinant of in vivo insulin resistance in humans: a 1H-13C nuclear magnetic resonance spectroscopy assessment in offspring of type 2 diabetic parents. *Diabetes.* 1999;48: 1600–1606.

79. Jacob S, Machann J, Rett K, Bretchel K, Volk A, Renn W, et al. Association of increased intramyo-cellular lipid content with insulin resistance in lean non-diabetic offspring of type 2 diabetic subjects. *Diabetes.* 1999;48: 1113–1119.

80. Sinha R, Dufour S, Petersen KF, LeBon V, Enoksson S, Ma YZ, et al. Assessment of skeletal muscle triglyceride content by ^{1}H nuclear magnetic resonance spectroscopy in lean and obese adolescents: relationships to insulin sensitivity, total body fat, and central adiposity. *Diabetes.* 2002;51: 1022–1027.

81. Kerkar N. Non-alcoholic steatohepatitis in children. *Pediatr Transplantation.* 2004;8: 61–18.

82. Fernandez JR, Shriver MD. Using genetic admixture to study the biology of obesity traits and to map genes in admixed populations. *Nutr Rev.* 2004;62: S69–S74.

83. Bonilla C, Shriver MD, Parra EJ, Jones A, Fernandez JR. Ancestral proportions and their association with skin pigmentation and bone mineral density in Peurto Rican women from New York City. *Hum Genet.* 2004;115: 57–58.

84. Fernandez JR, Shriver MD, Beasley TM, Rafla Demetrious N, Parra E, Albu J, et al. Association of African genetic admixture with resting metabolic rate and obesity among women. *Obes Res.* 2003;11: 904–911.

85. Gordon-Larsen P, Adair LS, Popkin BM. The relationship of ethnicity, socioeconomic factors, and overweight in US adolescents. *Obes Res.* 2003;11: 121–129.

86. Fernandez J, Higgins P, Goran M, Gower B. Genetic admixture contributes to differences in body composition in children. *Obes Res.* 2004;12: A19.

87. Kaplan AS, Zemel BS, Stallings VA. Differences in resting energy expenditure in prepubertal black children and white children. *J Pediatr.* 1996;129: 643–647.

88. Morrison JA, Alfaro MP, Khoury P, Thornton BB, Daniels SR. Determinants of resting energy expenditure in young black girls and young white girls. *J Pediatr.* 1996;129: 637–642.

89. Yanovski SJ, Reynolds JC, Boyle AJ, Yanovski JA. Resting metabolic rate in African-American and Caucasian girls. *Obes Res.* 1997;5: 321–325.

90. Wong WW, Butte NF, Ellis KJ, Hergenroeder AC, Hill RB, Stuff JE, Smith EO. Pubertal African-American girls expend less energy at rest and during physical activity than Caucasian girls. *J Clin Endocrinol Metab.* 1999;84: 906 911.

91. Weyer C, Snitker S, Bogardus C, Ravussin E. Energy metabolism in African Americans: potential risk factors for obesity. *Am J Clin Nutr.* 1999;70: 13–20.

92. Kushner RF, Racette SB, Neil K, and Schoeller DA. Measurement of physical activity among black and white obese women. *Obes Res.* 1995;3: 261S 265S.

93. Foster GD, Wadden TA, Vogt RA. Resting energy expenditure in obese African American and Caucasian women. *Obes Res.* 1997;5: 1–6.

94. Hunter GR, Weinsier RL, Darnell BE, Zuckerman PA, Goran MI. Racial differences in energy expenditure and aerobic fitness in premenoapusal women. *Am J Clin Nutr.* 2000;71: 500–506.

95. Carpenter WH, Fonong T, Toth MJ, Ades PJ, Calles-Escandon J, Walston JD, Poehlman ET. Total daily energy expenditure in free-living older African-Americans and Caucasians. *Am J Physiol.* 1998;274: E96–E101.

4 An International Perspective on Pediatric Obesity

Barry M. Popkin and Penny Gordon-Larsen

CONTENTS

This chapter explores shifts in pediatric obesity around the world. The focus is on children and adolescents; however, data limitations force us to largely examine data on obesity trends in adults to provide a broader sense of changes in obesity over time. Specifically, this work provides a sense of change both in the United States and Europe, and the lower- and middle-income countries of Asia, Africa, the Middle East, and Latin America. The chapter shows that changes are occurring at great speed and at earlier stages of a country's economic and social development. The burden of obesity is shifting toward the pediatric poor. A case study of current U.S. adolescent obesity and shifts in the adolescent to young adult period is also provided. Dietary patterns and trends among children from four countries are used to highlight the great heterogeneity of these shifts.

INTRODUCTION

Over the past 15 years, there is increasing evidence that the structure of dietary intakes and the prevalence of obesity around the developing world have been changing at an increasingly rapid pace.[1-4] In many ways, these shifts are a continuation of large scale changes that have occurred repeatedly over time; however, we will assert and show that the changes facing low and moderate income countries appear to be very rapid. While initially these shifts were felt to be limited to higher income urban populations, it is increasingly clear that these are much broader trends affecting all segments of society.

On a global basis, there are several themes that we briefly explore. The first is the general shift toward obesity representing a global problem rather than one centered in a few high income countries. The second is the rapid increase in obesity found in lower- and middle-income developing countries — a rate of change that appears to be greater than that found in higher income countries. The third issue is the shift in the burden of obesity toward the poor on a worldwide basis. We then present the limited comparable data on trends in adolescent obesity across the globe, with specific attention to the link between obesity and economic and social development.

Fourth, we summarize some key patterns and trends in dietary behavior across children and adolescents in the United States, Russia, China, and the Philippines to provide some sense of the enormous shifts and also the heterogeneity of dietary changes among children and adolescents.

GLOBAL OBESITY

It is important to first present a few key issues related to adults to allow us to provide a full picture of obesity in youth because nationally representative data on children and adolescents are limited.[5]

THE NUTRITION TRANSITION

Two historic processes of change occur simultaneous with or preceding the nutrition transition. One is the demographic transition: the shift from a pattern of high fertility and high mortality to one of low fertility and low mortality (typical of modern industrialized countries). Even more directly relevant is the epidemiologic transition, first described by Omran:[6] the shift from a pattern of high prevalence of infectious diseases associated with malnutrition, periodic famine, and poor environmental sanitation to a pattern of high prevalence of chronic and degenerative diseases associated with urban–industrial life styles. A third pattern, that of delayed degenerative diseases, has been more recently formulated.[7] Accompanying this progression is a major shift in age-specific mortality patterns and a consequent increase in life expectancy. Interpretations of the demographic and epidemiologic transition share a focus with the nutrition transition on the ways in which populations move from one pattern to the next.

Similarly, large shifts have occurred in patterns of diet and physical activity and inactivity, and it is these shifts that delineate stages of the *nutrition transition*. These changes are reflected in nutritional outcomes, such as changes in average stature and body composition. Modern societies seem to be converging on a pattern of diets high in saturated fat, sugar, and refined foods, and low in fiber — often termed the "Western diet." Many see this dietary pattern to be associated with high levels of chronic and degenerative diseases and with reduced disability-free time.

Human diet, activity patterns, and nutritional status have undergone a sequence of major shifts, defined as broad patterns of food use and their corresponding nutrition-related diseases. Over the last three centuries, the pace of dietary and activity change appears to have accelerated, to varying degrees in different regions of the world. Further, dietary and activity changes are paralleled by major changes in health status, as well as by major demographic and socioeconomic changes. Obesity emerges early in these shifting conditions as does the age at death and the level and age of morbidity. One can think of five broad nutrition patterns. The two "earlier" patterns continue to characterize certain geographic and socioeconomic subpopulations, but much of the modern world is experiencing one or more of three latter patterns. The five stages or broad patterns are:

Stage 1. *Collecting food*, which characterizes hunter–gatherer populations;

Stage 2. *Famine*, characterized by periods of acute scarcity of food;

Stage 3. *Receding famine* as income rises;

Stage 4. *Degenerative disease*, where changes in diet and activity pattern lead to the emergence of new disease problems and increased disability;

Stage 5. *Behavioral change,* the negative tendencies begin to reverse and make possible a process of "successful aging."

These stages are not restricted to particular periods of human history. For convenience, the patterns are outlined as historical developments; however, "earlier" patterns are not restricted to the periods in which they first arose, but continue to characterize certain geographic and socioeconomic subpopulations.

Shifts in Adult Obesity Are Occurring across the Globe

The current levels of pediatric overweight in countries as diverse as Mexico, Egypt, and South Africa have been shown to be equal or greater than those in the United States.[3] Moreover, the rate of change in obesity in lower- and middle-income countries is shown to be much greater than in higher-income countries (see reference 3, for an overview). Figure 4.1 presents the level of obesity and overweight in several illustrative countries (Brazil, Mexico, Egypt, Morocco, South Africa, Thailand, and China). Most interesting is that many of these countries with high overweight levels are very low income. Moreover, it probably amazes many people that the levels of obesity of several countries — all with much lower income levels than the United States — are surprisingly high.

There is marked heterogeneity in the patterns, trends, and timing of obesity among developing countries. Many countries in Latin America began their transition earlier in the past century and certainly entered the nutrition-related noncommunicable disease (NR-NCD) stage of the transition far earlier than did other regions. However, other countries such as Haiti and subpopulations in Central America are still in the receding famine period, which means that there are still periodic famine and poor environmental sanitation. Moreover, some countries such as Mexico experienced an accelerated transition in the 1990s.[8] The Middle East, North Africa, and Asia appear to have begun their transition at a much later date as have most other countries in the developing world except for the western Pacific nations.

Changes in the Developing World Are Faster Than in Higher Income Countries!

Figure 4.1 shows how quickly overweight and obesity status have emerged as major public health concerns in some of these countries. Compared with the United States and European countries, where the annual increase in the prevalence of overweight and obesity among adult men and women is about 0.25 for each, the rates of change are very high in Asia, North Africa, and Latin America — two to five times greater than in the United States.

The Burden of Obesity Has Shifted to the Poor!

In a recent analysis, we have shown that a large number of low- and moderate-income countries already have a greater likelihood that adults residing in lower-income or lower-educated households are overweight and obese relative to adults in higher income or education households.[9,10] The Monteiro et al. study,[10] based on a multilevel analysis of 37 nationally representative data sets, shows that countries with a gross national product (GNP) per capita over about $2500 are likely to have a burden of obesity greater among the poor. We applied multilevel logistic regression analyses on the risk of obesity (body mass index [BMI] equal to or greater than 30 kg/m^2) to anthropometric and socioeconomic data collected by nationally representative cross-sectional

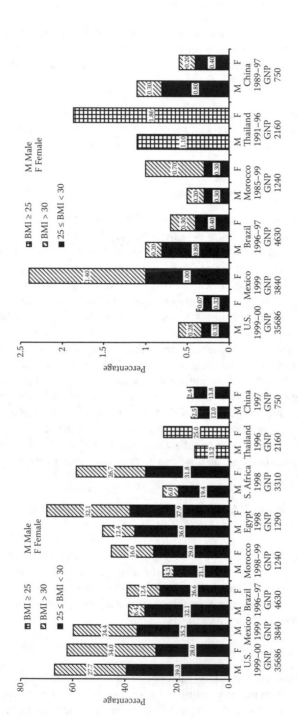

FIGURE 4.1 Obesity patterns and trends among adults in selected developing world countries (the annual percentage point increase in prevalence). (From Popkin BM. *Public Health Nutr.* 2002;5: 93–103.)

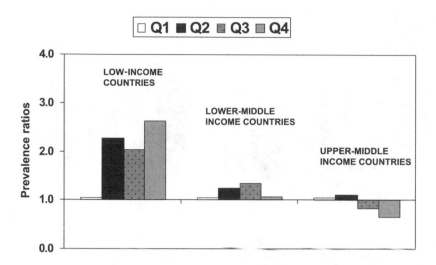

FIGURE 4.2 Prevalence ratios for women's obesity, for women aged 19 to 49 years, demographic and health surveys by quartiles of years of schooling in 37 developing countries (1992–2002). (From Monteiro, CA, Moura, EC, Conde, WL, Popkin, B, *Bull. WHO.* 2004, 82: 940 946. With permission.)

surveys on women aged 20 to 49 (n = 148,579) conducted from 1992 to 2000 in 37 developing countries within a wide range of world regions and stages of economic development (GNP from US$ 190 to 4440 per capita). Importantly, these analyses demonstrate the differential effect of individual level socioeconomic status (SES) factors within the level of the country's GNP.

Belonging to the lower SES group confers strong protection against obesity in low-income economies, can reduce or increase obesity in lower-middle income economies, and is a systematic risk factor for obesity in upper-middle income developing economies. The crude relationship between obesity and quartiles of education in lower-, middle-, and upper-income countries can be seen in Figure 4.2. A multilevel logistic model — including an interaction term between the country's GNP and each woman's SES — indicates that obesity starts to fuel health inequities in the developing world when the GNP reaches a value of about US$ 2500 per capita.[10] Examples of countries above the US$ 2500 per capita income level, those upper-middle income developing economies with higher obesity among the lower SES groups, include Mexico, Brazil, Turkey, and South Africa. Of course, the United States and all of Western Europe fits here. In all cases lower SES could be defined by household income or education levels and the same pattern would emerge.

CHILD AND YOUTH OBESITY PREVALENCE AND TRENDS

Globally there is no definitive set of nationally representative studies on children and adolescents available. The best overview and estimate of global prevalence of obesity and overweight among children and adolescents come from the review by Lobstein et al.[5] in which they provide an estimate of worldwide overweight and obesity (defined using the International Obesity Task Force [IOTF] cutoff points[12]) among school children at approximately 11% with rates over 30% in the Americans, about 20% in Europe, and the estimates are 17% in the Near and Middle East, 5% in Asia-Pacific, and 2% in sub-Saharan Africa.

Comparative Trends Research

A study of adolescent obesity dynamics was undertaken across four longitudinal studies.[13] Nationally representative data from Brazil (1975 and 1997), Russia (1992 and 1998), and the United States

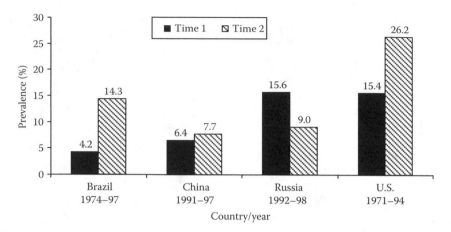

FIGURE 4.3 Child overweight prevalence has increased in Brazil, China, and the United States, but decreased in Russia. (From Wang Y, Monteiro C, Popkin BM. *Am J Clin Nutr.* 2002;75: 971–977.)

National Health and Nutrition Examination Survey (NHANES I [1971 to 1974] and NHANES III [1988 to 1994]) and nationwide survey data from China (1991 and 1997) were used. To define overweight, we used the sex- and age-specific BMI cutoffs recommended by the IOTF.[12]

Overweight prevalence measured by changes in the periods noted above (Figure 4.3) has increased in Brazil (4.2 to 14.3%), China (6.4 to 7.7%), and the United States (15.4 to 26.2%). In Russia, overweight decreased (15.6 to 9.0%). The annual increase rates of overweight prevalence (percentage points) are: 0.5 percentage points (Brazil), 0.2 percentage points (China), 1.1 percentage points (Russia), and 0.6 percentage points (United States). These are based on nationally representative weighted averages for Brazil, Russia, and the United States but do not adjust for any population composition changes.

The trends and current prevalence of overweight vary substantially across the four countries examined and seem to show a lag behind the changes experienced by adults in these countries. The burden of nutritional problems is shifting from energy imbalance deficiency to excess among older children and adolescents in Brazil and China. These changes and differences may relate to changes and differences in key environmental factors across countries. For example, the gross domestic product (GDP) tripled in the United States and Brazil and increased greater than 10-fold in China during this time (e.g., rise of living standards including an increase of food production and consumption, along with declines in physical activity and increases in inactivity and TV ownership). Conversely, Russia saw a worsening of the economy and a decline in living standards (including a decrease of food consumption and production). Over the past three decades, the percentage of older children and adolescents who were overweight tripled in Brazil and almost doubled in the United States.

The overweight prevalence was considerably higher in children than in adolescents in all three countries except for the United States. The far greater adolescent overweight prevalence in the United States stands out. It is possible that this relates partly to the use of the IOTF reference; however, these differences may be far too great to be explained by the use of this reference. Figure 4.4 presents these age–overweight patterns.

Similar to adults, the changes in youth obesity in these four countries varies across levels of household income. Over the past two decades, the increase in prevalence of overweight in Brazil was greatest in high-SES groups. Conversely, in the United States the increase was greatest in low-SES groups.[13] In addition, the prevalence of overweight was much higher in urban than rural areas in Russia and the United States.

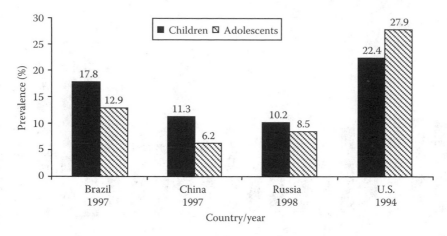

FIGURE 4.4 The age–overweight pattern is different in the United States than in other countries. (From Wang Y, Monteiro C, Popkin BM. *Am J Clin Nutr.* 2002;75: 971–977.)

Childhood and Adolescent Obesity Patterns across Europe

A recent comparative study conducted across Europe also utilizes the IOTF cutoff criteria for overweight.[12,14] These include measured (as opposed to self-reported) height and weight to derive BMI. All use representative samples of the general population of either the country or a region of the country. Four surveys (those for Belgium, Croatia, the Netherlands, and Switzerland) did not provide estimates of overweight using the IOTF criteria, and the authors used other methods to estimate the proportion of the sample that would exceed the IOTF cutoff points.

This study, as well as others, has shown that the prevalence of obesity has risen dramatically in many countries across Europe.[14,15] Among children (ages 7 to 11 years), overweight differs across Europe from France (19%), the United Kingdom (20%), Sweden (18%), and Denmark (15%) in western and northern Europe to Russia (10%) and Poland (18%) in the Eastern bloc to Spain (34%), Italy (36%), and Malta (35%) in southern Europe.[14] Adolescent (14 to 17 years) overweight is similar, with particularly high levels in the United Kingdom (21%) and southern Europe — Spain (21%), Greece (22%), and Cyprus (23%). Guillame and Lissau[15] postulate many reasons for these variations. For example, a north–south trend is clearly seen, with higher obesity in southern European countries. Further, the lower prevalence in central and eastern Europe occurs in countries whose economies suffered from recession during the economic and political transition of the 1990s (Figure 4.5 and Figure 4.6).

It seems across all regions of the world that the levels of adult obesity far exceed those of children. In addition it seems that rapid increases in child and adolescent obesity have emerged in recent years, but these increases still do not equal the rate of increase found among adults.

THE TRANSITION TO ADULTHOOD IN U.S. YOUTH

Gordon-Larsen et al.[16] sought to examine patterns of change in obesity among U.S. white, black, Hispanic, and Asian teens as they transition from adolescence to young adulthood. Using the IOTF cutoff points, obesity incidence over the 5-year study period was 12.7%, with 9.4% remaining obese, and 1.6% shifting from obese to nonobese. Obesity incidence was especially high among non-Hispanic black (18.4%) and Hispanic females (15.8%) relative to white females. Obesity prevalence increased from 10.9% in wave II to 22.1% in wave III, with 4.3% BMI ≥ 40 at wave III.

These results mirror many smaller studies that display a significant tendency for childhood and adolescent overweight to persist or track into adulthood.[17–19] The Gordon-Larsen et al.[16] findings indicate that the transition between adolescence and young adulthood appears to be a period of

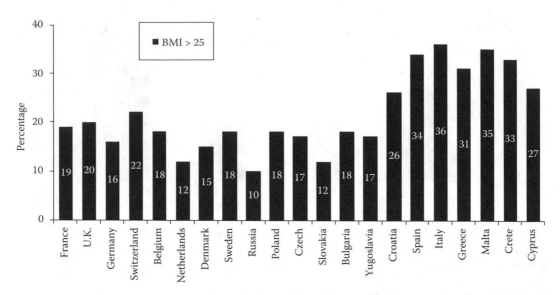

FIGURE 4.5 Overweight patterns across European children 7 to 11 years. (From Lobstein T, Frelut M-L. *Obes Rev.* 2003;4: 195–200.)

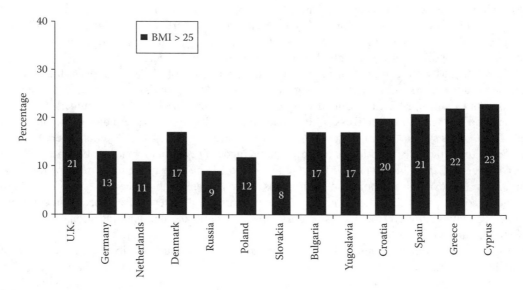

FIGURE 4.6 Overweight patterns across European adolescents 14 to 17 years. (From Lobstein T, Frelut M-L. *Obes Rev.* 2003;4: 195–200.)

increased risk for development of obesity. This upward trend is evident in both males and females, and in all major U.S. ethnic groups, particularly in non-Hispanic blacks. The trend foreshadows higher rates of diabetes and nutrition-related chronic degenerative diseases, emerging at younger ages[20,21] and underscores the major need for preventive strategies to curb this trajectory.

Shifts in Age-Specific Time Trends

There are few longitudinal mixed cohort studies that follow different age groups concurrently. Studies of both dietary and body composition trends seem to indicate an increase in rates of change across the world. This has been found in studies of income and price changes on the structure of

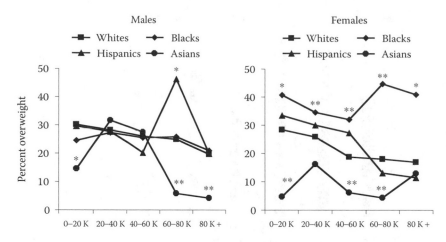

FIGURE 4.7 Overweight prevalence by category of income across sex and race/ethnic groups in U.S. adolescents. Whites vs. specified ethnic group: * = $p < 0.05$; ** = $p < 0.01$. (From Gordon-Larsen P, Adair LS, Popkin BM. *Obes Res.* 2003;11: 121–129.)

the Chinese diets as well as with obesity trends in the United States. In China, two studies have shown that shifts toward intake of higher fat foods and higher fat diets have accelerated changes in income.[22,23] In each case longitudinal analysis was used to show a significant increase in the impact of income on diet.

In the United States, McTigue et al.[24] conducted a longitudinal study of over 9000 U.S. young adults born between 1957 and 1964, and resurveyed 13 times over the span of two decades; they found that more than 25% were obese by age 35. Age of obesity onset was highest among black females, moderate in Hispanic females, and lowest in white females, while among males highest onset was seen for Hispanic males. In addition, McTigue et al.[24] found a large temporal weight trend: People born in later calendar years tended to have larger age-specific BMI. In every case in which the same age was sampled for both birth cohorts, the 1957-born group had a lower mean BMI than the 1964-born group. The intermediate birth cohorts had intermediate-range mean BMI values.

RELATIONSHIP BETWEEN INCOME AND OVERWEIGHT AMONG U.S. ADOLESCENTS

Gordon-Larsen et al.[25] examined the relationship between socioeconomic correlates of overweight and overweight (BMI ≥ 95th percentile[25]) in a nationally representative sample of over 20,000 U.S. adolescents from The National Longitudinal Study of Adolescent Health. The relationship between overweight prevalence and family income differed by ethnicity (Figure 4.7), with more pronounced differences among females. A clear inverse relationship between higher income and lower overweight was seen *only* among non-Hispanic white females. In females, overweight was highest for blacks across all SES levels and the black–white disparity in overweight actually increased at highest income levels. In males, there is less ethnic variation.

DIETARY CHANGES ACROSS THE GLOBE

Relative to what is known about changes over time in obesity, there is considerably less known about changes in the factors — dietary and physical activity patterns — responsible for these changes. There are limited systematic nationally representative or large representative studies of dietary change; however, we summarize a few key points here. There are even fewer such studies on physical activity. Aside from limited studies on leisure activities, little research on this topic for youth has been undertaken in the United States or Europe. We utilize nationally representative

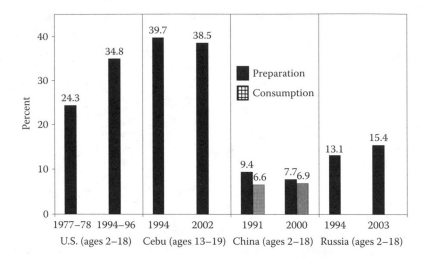

FIGURE 4.8 The proportion of energy consumed from foods prepared away from home.

dietary data from the United States (Continuing Survey of Individual Intakes[27]) and Russia (the Russia Longitudinal Dietary Survey[28]) along with a nine-province survey from China (the China Health and Nutrition Survey[29]) and a survey of a large metropolitan area in the Philippines (the Cebu Longitudinal Health and Nutrition Survey[30]) (for more detail see Adair and Popkin[31]).

ARE THERE SHIFTS IN AWAY-FROM-HOME DIETARY INTAKE?

There is great heterogeneity in this element of dietary change as seen in Figure 4.8. Interestingly, Filipino youth consumed higher percentages of their total food intake measured in calories away from home than American youth. Of course, there are age differences in the samples that might account for this discrepancy, but nonetheless the two countries with higher away-from-home patterns are the United States and the Cebuano region of the Philippines. Filipino youth consumed 39.7 (1994) and 38.5% (2002) of energy from foods purchased away from home, with food purchased from street vendors making up a significantly increasing proportion of away-from-home food purchases across the years. In the United States, 2 to 18 year olds consumed 24.3 and 34.8% of calories from foods eaten away from home in 1977 and 1994, respectively. The sharp increase in the United States indicates a trend that might lead to the higher levels found for U.S. children compared with those found in the Philippines. In contrast Russian children consumed about a third to half of these levels away from home, and Chinese children consumed less than 10% of their total energy away from home.

IS SNACKING BEHAVIOR CHANGING?

These results represent the composite of multiple snacking occasions, particularly in the Philippines and the United States. In the Philippines, snacking is very common, with an afternoon "merienda" part of the typical Filipino eating pattern. About 75% of sample youths reported consuming at least one food item as a snack in the 2002 survey, and on average, 17.2% of daily calories came from snacks, mostly in the form of traditional bakery products, candies, and soft drinks. There is no consistent trend in snacking behaviors in Cebu youth across time.

In the United States, snacks contributed about 21% of total calories in 1994 to 1996, and this represents a large increase since 1977 (Figure 4.9). The figures are much larger in Cebu for the 1994 survey and were still very high for the older group in 2002. While time trends are not evident in China and Russia (the latter owing to insufficient data to track snacking trends), about 1.2 and

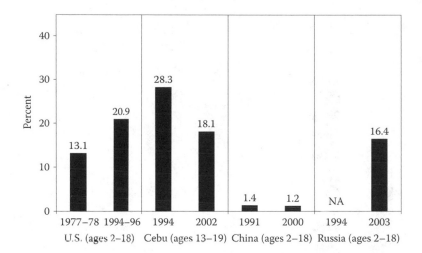

FIGURE 4.9 Snacking patterns: the proportion of daily energy from snacks.

16.4% of energy was derived from snacking in China, and Russia, respectively, in the most recent surveys in these countries.

ARE THE FOOD SHIFTS FOUND IN THE UNITED STATES COMMON ACROSS THE GLOBE AMONG CHILDREN?

The food pattern shifts in the United States among youth have been documented elsewhere in great detail.[32–34] Essentially they show marked increases in soft drinks combined with fruit drinks and also in fast foods (e.g., french fries, hamburgers, cheeseburgers, pizzas, and Mexican food) and salty snacks (Figure 4.10). Intake of these foods by children doubled from 8.3% of energy intake of the youth aged 2 to 18 to 16.1% over the 1977 to 1996 period. Soft drinks represent 8.5% of total energy intake in 1996 in the United States, only 3.0% in Cebu, and less than a half percentage point in China and Russia. The other items potentially categorized as fast foods in each country (e.g., traditional barbecued pork on skewers in the Philippines) also represent a smaller proportion of total energy. The total varies from 0.2 to 7.6% in the latest year of data for each country. Salty snacks are growing as a proportion of snacks in Russia and the United States, in particular. We present the comparison of the patterns and trends in Figure 4.10.

CONCLUSIONS

In this chapter we have shown a profound global shift in pediatric obesity. There are clear associations between global economies, recession, and economic factors and obesity in adults, adolescents, and children. The high obesity prevalence in adolescents is shown to be persistent into adulthood with high incidence in the transition to adulthood. The global obesity problem requires global obesity prevention and treatment solutions. Greater attention must be paid to research on economic, environmental, and social determinants of obesity in children and adolescents. It is evident from the U.S. case that the increase in obesity from adolescence to adulthood is tremendous. Other countries following this trajectory are likely to see substantial adult obesity and its associated comorbidities if this trajectory is not curbed.

The far greater proportion of adolescent overweight prevalence in the United States stands out. It is possible that this relates partly to the use of the IOTF reference,[12,35] but these differences may be far too great to solely be the result of the use of this reference. Differences in sexual

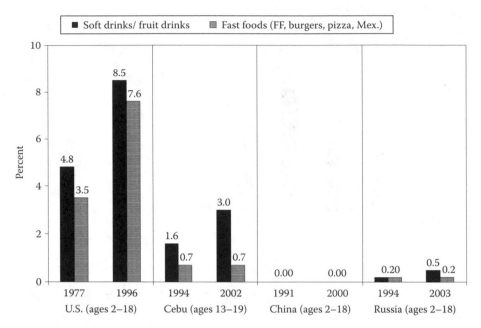

FIGURE 4.10 Food group shifts: Are modern fast foods and sweetened beverages the dominant shifts?

maturation patterns between the reference and study populations are one issue worthy of further consideration.[36,37]

In other research we have shown how the key relationships among global shifts in economic development, urbanization, income growth, and even declines in the real prices of food as key aspects driving these changes. Clearly globalization of mass media, the transfers of goods and services, and modern technology related to work, transportation, home production, and leisure are also important.[3,4,9,22,23]

The comparison of dietary results across the United States, Russia, China, and the Philippines provides some indication of the enormous heterogeneity of dietary patterns and trends across the world. While this comparison does not represent dietary change across the globe, it suggests that there are substantial variations in child dietary patterns across various countries. Further, it is difficult to extrapolate patterns of change from the United States (and possibly any other well-studied higher income developed country) to other regions of the world.

Given the universal shift to greater child obesity, it is clear that major population-based public health efforts to confront this trajectory are critically needed. This short review on obesity and diet trends demonstrates that programs and policies to encourage healthy eating must vary greatly in terms of focus to address global variation in diet trends.

References

1. Bell AC, Ge K, Popkin BM. The road to obesity or the path to prevention? Motorized transportation and obesity in China. *Obes Res*. 2002;10: 277–283.
2. Gordon-Larsen P, Adair LS, Popkin BM. Ethnic differences in physical activity and inactivity patterns and overweight status: The National Longitudinal Study of Adolescent Health. *Obes Res*. 2002;10: 141–149.
3. Popkin BM. An overview on the nutrition transition and its health implications: the Bellagio Meeting. *Public Health Nutr*. 2002;5: 93–103.

4. Popkin BM. The dynamics of the dietary transition in the developing world. In: Caballero B, Popkin BM, Eds. *The Nutrition Transition: Diet and Disease in the Developing World.* London: Academic Press, 2002: 111–128.

5. Lobstein T, Baur L, Uauy R. Obesity in children and young people: a crisis in public health. *Obes Rev.* 2004;5(Suppl 1): 4–97.

6. Omran AR. The epidemiologic transition: a theory of the epidemiology of population change. *Milbank Mem Fund Q.* 1971;49(4): 509–538.

7. Olshansky SJ, Ault AB. The fourth stage of the epidemiologic transition: the age of delayed degenerative diseases, *Milbank Mem Fund Q.* 1986;64: 355–390.

8. Rivera JA, Barquera S, Campirano F, Campos I, Safdie M, Tovar V. Epidemiological and nutritional transition in Mexico: rapid increase of non-communicable chronic diseases and obesity. *Public Health Nutr.* 2002;5(1A): 113–122.

9. Mendez MA, Monteiro CA, Popkin BM. Overweight now exceeds underweight among women in most developing countries! *Am J Clin Nutr.* 2005;81: 714–721.

10. Monteiro CA, Conde WL, Lu B, Popkin BM. Obesity and inequities in health in the developing world. *Int J Obes.* 2004;28: 1181–1186.

11. Monteiro, CA, Moura, EC, Conde WL, Popkin B. Socioeconomic status and obesity in developing countries: a review. *Bull. WHO.* 2004; 82: 940–946.

12. Cole TJ, Bellizzi MC, Flegal KM, Dietz WH. Establishing a standard definition for child overweight and obesity worldwide: international survey. *BMJ.* 2000;320: 1240–1243.

13. Wang Y, Monteiro C, Popkin BM. Trends of overweight and underweight in children and adolescents in the United States, Brazil, China, and Russia. *Am J Clin Nutr.* 2002;75: 971–977.

14. Lobstein T, Frelut M-L. Prevalence of overweight among children in Europe. *Obes Rev.* 2003;4: 195–200.

15. Guillame M, Lissau I. Epidemiology. In: Burniat W, Cole T, Lissau I, Poskitt EME, Eds. *Child and Adolescent Obesity: Causes and Consequences, Prevention and Management.* Cambridge: Cambridge University Press, 2002: 28–49.

16. Gordon-Larsen P, Adair LS, Nelson MC, Popkin BM. Five-year obesity incidence in the transition period between adolescence and adulthood: The National Longitudinal Study of Adolescent Health. *Am J Clin Nutr.* 2004;80: 569–575.

17. Power C, Lake JK, Cole TJ. Measurement and long-term health risks of child and adolescent fatness. *Int J Obes Relat Metab Disord.* 1997;21: 507–26.

18. Serdula MK, Ivery D, Coates JR, Freedman DS, Williamson DF, Byers T. Do obese children become obese adults? A review of the literature. *Prev Med.* 1993;22: 167–177.

19. Srinivisan SR, Bao W, Wattigney WA, Berenson GS. Adolescent overweight is associated with adult overweight and related multiple cardiovascular risk factors: the Bogalusa Heart Study. *Metabol Clin Exper.* 1996;45(2): 235–40.

20. Mokdad AH, Bowman BA, Ford ES, Vinicor F, Marks JS, Koplan JP. The continuing epidemics of obesity and diabetes in the United States. *JAMA.* 2001;286: 1195–1200.

21. Mokdad AH, Ford ES, Bowman BA, Dietz WH, Vinicor F, Bales VS, Marks JS. Prevalence of obesity, diabetes, and obesity-related health risk factors, 2001. *JAMA.* 2003;289: 76–79.

22. Du S, Mroz TA, Zhai F, Popkin BM. Rapid income growth adversely affects diet quality in China—particularly for the poor!? *Soc Sci Med.* 2004;59: 1505–1515.

23. Guo X, Mroz TA, Popkin BM, Zhai F. Structural changes in the impact of income on food consumption in China, 1989–93. *Econ Dev Cult Change.* 2000;48: 737–760.

24. McTigue KM, Garrett JM, Popkin BM. The natural history of obesity: Weight change in a large US longitudinal survey. *Ann Internal Med.* 2002;136: 857–864.

25. Gordon-Larsen P, Adair LS, Popkin BM. The relationship between ethnicity, socioeconomic factors and overweight: The National Longitudinal Study of Adolescent Health. *Obes Res.* 2003;11: 121–129.

26. 2000 CDC Growth Charts: United States. Centers for Disease Control and Prevention. National Center for Health Statistics. Available from http: //www.cdc.gov/growthcharts (accessed 21 April 2003).

27. Nielsen SJ, Popkin BM. Patterns and trends in portion sizes, 1977–1998. *JAMA.* 2003;289(4): 450–453.

28. Jahns L, Baturin A, Popkin BM. Obesity, diet, and poverty trends in the Russian transition to market economy. *Eur J Clin Nutr* 2003;57: 1295–1302.

29. Popkin BM, Du S. Dynamics of the nutrition transition toward the animal foods sector in China and its implications: a worried perspective. *J Nutr.* 2003;133: 3898S–3906S.

30. Adair LS, Cole TJ. Rapid child growth raises blood pressure in adolescent boys who were thin at birth. *Hypertension.* 2003;41: 451–456.

31. Adair LS, Popkin BM. Heterogeneity abounds in comparative child dietary trends. 2004. Unpublished manuscript.

32. Jahns L, Siega-Riz AM, Popkin BM. The increasing prevalence of snacking among U.S. children and adolescents from 1977 to 1996. *J Pediatr.* 2001;138: 493–498.

33. Nielsen SJ, Siega-Riz AM, Popkin BM. Trends in energy intake in the US between 1977 and 1996: Similar shifts seen across age groups. *Obes Res.* 2002;10: 370–378.

34. Nielsen S, Popkin BM. Changes in beverage intake between 1977–1998. *Am J Prev Med.* 2004;27: 205–10.

35. WHO Expert Committee. Physical status, the use and interpretation of anthropometry. WHO Technical Report Series No. 854. Geneva: WHO, 1995.

36. Wang Y, Wang JQ, Hesketh T, Ding QJ, Mulligan J, Kinra S. Standard definition of child overweight and obesity worldwide. [letters] *BMJ.* 2000;321: 1158–1159.

37. Wang Y, Adair L. How does maturity adjustment influence the estimates of obesity prevalence in adolescents from different countries using an international reference? *Int J Obes.* 2001;25: 550–558.

5 Critical Periods for Abnormal Weight Gain in Children and Adolescents

Stephen R. Daniels

CONTENTS

INTRODUCTION

Because overweight has become an epidemic pediatric health problem, substantial attention has turned to mechanisms of abnormal weight gain. At first glance, this appears very straightforward. Energy intake and energy expenditure operate under the first law of thermodynamics. In this schema, excess calories from the diet are stored for future use at a time when the need for calorie expenditure may be increased, or food availability decreased, or both. It is clear that the ability to accumulate, store, and maintain fat has been a survival advantage during the evolution of our species. For this reason, humans have evolved numerous and redundant biological mechanisms to defend fat, but few to limit the accumulation of fat. Therefore, it should be recognized that current medical approaches that consider obesity a disease may not recognize the importance of this physiology as an advantage for survival in environments where the availability of food is lower and a greater level of energy expenditure is required to obtain food. Nevertheless, the prevalence and severity of comorbid conditions associated with overweight make understanding abnormal weight gain and developing methods to prevent it of paramount importance.

It has been recognized that abnormal weight gain may occur throughout the life span. During fetal life, adipocytes begin to develop at around 15 weeks of gestation. There is an increase in both fat cell number and size that accelerates during the third trimester. This results in an increase in the percent of body fat from approximately 5 to 15%. During infancy, adipocytes appear to increase more in size than in number. In lean children, from age 2 to 14 years the fat cell size appears to remain stable. During this same developmental period, overweight children have an increase in fat cell size, which may then lead to a concomitant increase in fat cell number.[1]

Closer focus on the mechanisms of the development of obesity from both a research and a clinical perspective has raised the question of whether the risk of abnormal weight gain is uniform across development or whether there may be critical periods where the risk of abnormal weight gain is higher. It is important to understand this from a public health standpoint because such critical periods may offer windows of opportunity for identification of individuals at high risk for overweight and prevention of excess weight gain. The purpose of this chapter is to explore the level of current knowledge about critical periods for abnormal weight gain during childhood and adolescence.

DETERMINANTS OF CRITICAL PERIODS

Critical periods for abnormal weight gain may be defined by a variety of factors including genetic, biological, environmental, and behavioral. Table 5.1 presents potential determinants of such critical periods. A critical period refers to a specific developmental period or life stage when an abnormality may have an increased or enduring effect on the physiology of weight gain. The concept of critical periods has a very deterministic aspect to it. It may be more appropriate to consider these periods as sensitive rather than critical. It is also important to consider that an insult during a critical or sensitive period may have either an immediate effect on weight gain or a longer term, more remote effect. It is likely that there are multiple determinants for these periods that act together to increase weight gain. Finally, it is also likely that critical events may accumulate over time, and it is ultimately the aggregate effect of a number of factors that leads to abnormal weight gain. The potential for combined effects is presented in Figure 5.1.

TABLE 5.1
Potential Determinants of Critical Periods for Abnormal Weight Gain

1. Genetic
2. Biological
   - Development of adipocytes
   - Change in hormonal status
   - Change in resting energy expenditure
   - Change in appetite
   - Diet and activity
   - Pregnancy
3. Environmental
   - Availability of food
   - Availability of sedentary attractions
   - Barriers to physical activity
   - Home
   - School
   - Work
4. Behavioral
   - Breastfeeding
   - Developmental
   - Hunger cues
   - Peer influence
5. Other

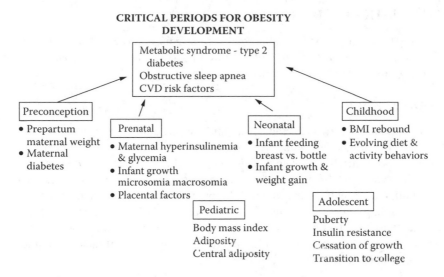

CRITICAL PERIODS FOR OBESITY DEVELOPMENT

FIGURE 5.1 Vulnerable periods for abnormal weight gain.

TABLE 5.2
Potential Critical Periods for Development of Overweight

1. Intrauterine life
    - Fetal growth & nutrition
    - Maternal diabetes
    - Adipocyte development
2. The first year of life
    - Infant feeding – breast vs. bottle
    - Weight gain in the first year
    - Changes in body composition
3. Preschool–school age
    - Body mass index rebound
    - Development of diet and activity behaviors
    - Solidification of diet and activity behaviors
    - School vs. home environment
    - Use of certain medications
4. Adolescence
    - Changes in insulin sensitivity
    - Changes in body composition
    - Use of certain medications
    - Pregnancy (females)
    - Family vs. peer influences
    - Transition to adulthood and independence

POTENTIAL CRITICAL PERIODS

A list of potential critical periods for abnormal weight gain is presented in Table 5.2. It is clear that a critical period can occur throughout the entire life course. Subsequent discussion focuses on those critical periods related to the pediatric population.

ADIPOCYTE DEVELOPMENT

There may be a number of periods during development where adipocytes may be adversely affected. This includes early feeding,[2] following the administration of steroids,[3] and with excess weight gain leading to peroxisome proliferator-activated receptor (PPAR)-mediated differentiation.[4] There remains much to be learned about the biology of the development of adipocytes and their responses to various stimuli. One might assume that weight loss that decreases the number of fat cells would provide a longstanding beneficial change in the adipocytes. However, it appears that the volume of adipocytes remains constant even after a liposuction procedure.[5] In addition, comorbidities may not improve after liposuction.[6] These results suggest that physiological factors continue to operate to maintain and restore fat mass once it has developed.

INTRAUTERINE FACTORS

Attention has been focused on intrauterine development as an important determinant of risk for future disease. As a general concept, these relationships have been referred to as the Barker hypothesis. In general, the hypothesis has related low birth weight to future adverse outcomes such as hypertension. There has been epidemiological research suggesting a direct relationship between intrauterine growth and birth weight, and body mass index (BMI) later in life.[7,8] Parsons et al. reviewed factors during childhood that are predictive of obesity later in life.[9] They found that birth weight was positively associated with the development of obesity in a number of large and reasonably long-term studies. However, when potential confounders such as gestational age, the fatness of the parents, and socioeconomic status were examined, the association was less consistent. In general, the relationship of birth weight to future obesity seems to be less certain than the relationship between birth weight and other cardiovascular risk factors such as blood pressure elevation.

A very important determinant of birth weight is gestational age. Unfortunately, many retrospective epidemiological studies have not had valid data on the gestational age. This means that it is not possible to evaluate whether the birth weight is appropriate, too low, or too high for the gestational age.

The mechanism by which birth weight might influence future weight gain is not clear. Possible mechanisms include alterations of body composition, central nervous system control of appetite, or regulation of glucose metabolism. To explain potential relationships between low birth weight and future obesity, it has been hypothesized that fetal undernutrition, whether due to poor maternal nutrition or placental insufficiency, sets up a thrifty metabolic program to be most efficient in energy storage and utilization. The program may prove to be maladaptive in later life as the child is exposed to greater availability of energy. Low birth weight has been associated with a future propensity to accumulate visceral adiposity.[7] The mechanism for this influence on fat distribution remains obscure. It may be mediated through changes in the hypothalamic–pituitary axis or in glucose metabolism.

A factor that may be operative in explaining the relationship of increased birth weight with future development of obesity is alterations of maternal–fetal glucose metabolism. This relationship may be underscored by the influence of gestational diabetes. Infants of diabetic mothers are usually macrosomic. Maternal hyperglycemia leads to excess fetal insulin production, which may act as a growth stimulator for the fetus. Animal studies have suggested that fetal hyperinsulinemia may lead to alterations in hypothalamic neurotransmitters, which can subsequently lead to later increased appetite and weight gain.[10] Epidemiological studies of the relationship of gestational diabetes to the risk of future obesity in offspring have produced mixed results. Some studies have shown a direct association,[11,12] while others have not found an association.[13] Gillman et al. found a direct relationship between gestational diabetes and risk of obesity in the offspring.[14] However, the relationship was explained in part by the mother's BMI and the baby's birth weight.

FIRST YEAR OF LIFE

Recent data suggest that weight gain during the first year of life may be an important determinant of obesity later in childhood and adolescence. Stettler et al. reported that the rate of weight gain during the first 4 months of life was associated with overweight at age 7 years after adjustment for confounding factors.[15] They found that the greatest risk of obesity was in the group with the highest birth weight and the greatest weight gain in early infancy. Early infancy is a period of rapid growth and weight gain. Birth weight usually doubles in the first 4 to 6 months of life. This means that mechanisms of energy balance may be quite important during this time. In addition, rapid weight gain during childhood after experiencing low birth weight has been associated with an increased risk of cardiovascular disease in adulthood.[16]

Another factor during the first year of life that may protect against the development of obesity is breastfeeding. Several studies have shown that breastfeeding is associated with lower risk of obesity in childhood and adolescence.[17,18] However, not all studies have shown this protective effect.[19,20] (See Chapter 19 for additional details.)

PRESCHOOL–SCHOOL AGE

The preschool years seem on the surface to be less important with respect to weight gain. However, these years are an important time when the physical activity and eating patterns become more adultlike and habits are developed. Thus, this may be a time when there is substantial opportunity to prevent short- and long-term abnormal weight gain.

Another occurrence during the preschool and early school age period has been called adiposity or BMI rebound. Normally the body mass index increases during the first 9 to 12 months of life. At that point it starts to decline over a period of years. The age when the body mass index begins to increase again after a reaching a nadir in childhood has been referred to as BMI rebound.[21] Epidemiological studies have shown that a younger age at BMI rebound is associated with a higher risk of future overweight.[22] Whitaker et al. demonstrated that this relationship was independent of BMI at the time of BMI rebound,[22] but this has not been clear in all studies. While this period has been called adiposity rebound, it has not yet been shown that changes in adiposity are responsible for the decrease and subsequent increase in BMI.

A younger age at BMI rebound has been associated with higher BMI in adolescence[23,24] and in early adulthood.[22,25] Whitaker et al. found that after adjustment for parental BMI and the child's BMI at the age of BMI rebound, the odds ratio for adult obesity when early rebound was compared with late rebound was 6.0 (95% confidence interval [CI] 1.3 to 26.6).[22] The average age at BMI rebound was 5.5 years in their study. Another question has been how the age at BMI rebound reflects the BMI at earlier ages. Rolland-Cachera et al. identified several paths of development in a cohort of French children.[25] They identified overweight infants who experienced a late BMI rebound and subsequently returned to normal weight. They also identified lean infants with BMI rebound at a younger age who then became overweight. Other groups of children remained in their original group, for example, overweight infants with an early BMI rebound who remained overweight in adolescence and adulthood.

The mechanism for BMI rebound and the determinants of its timing remain unknown. In addition, interventions to alter the age of BMI rebound have not been attempted. Further research is needed to examine the biological and behavioral determinants of BMI rebound and to understand how an earlier BMI rebound may influence the future development of obesity.

BMI rebound may also be associated with increased risk of diabetes mellitus. Bhargava and colleagues investigated a cohort from India.[26] They found that early BMI rebound was associated with increased risk of glucose intolerance and diabetes in adulthood. In addition they found that those with a younger age at BMI rebound had higher BMI at age 12 compared with those who had BMI rebound at an older age. This raises the question of whether early BMI rebound may also be related to differential deposition of fat. It may be that early BMI rebound is associated with greater fat deposition in the abdominal cavity, which may then predispose to insulin resistance, glucose intolerance, and type 2 diabetes mellitus.

Medications

There are medications that may be taken in the preschool and school age period that may predispose to weight gain. Included in this group of medications are corticosteroids, valproic acid, and atypical neuroleptic drugs such as olanzapine and risperidone.

The effects of endogenous corticosteroids have long been known. With excess steroid production, individuals develop Cushing's syndrome, which includes weight gain as a prominent manifestation. The effect of chronic administration of corticosteroids is also well known as patients who require these medications develop a typical round facial appearance (moon facies), obesity, and striae. Less certain is the role that short term or intermittent usage of steroids, such as might occur in patients with severe asthma, might have in obesity development. The use of oral dexamethasone for treatment of vitiligo was shown to be associated with weight gain even though suppression of endogenous cortisol production was not seen.[27] Eubanks et al. treated patients with cystic fibrosis with megestrol acetate and a significant increase in weight-for-age compared with placebo was seen.[28] The weight gain observed included increases in both fat mass and lean body mass. There is also some concern about the use of corticosteroids and the development of an eating disorder. Fornari et al. reported eight individuals who apparently developed an eating disorder after steroid administration for a medical condition.[29] These results suggest that the effect of corticosteroids on appetite and weight gain could be different for different individuals.

Valproic acid is used in the treatment of epilepsy. It may also be used in patients with mood disorders and other psychiatric illnesses. Weight gain is a common side effect of treatment with valproate. The age at which valproate is administered may be important. Caksen et al. found that long-term treatment with valproic acid was not associated with abnormal weight gain in prepubertal children.[30] Wirrell found that 14% of patients ages 10 to 17 years treated with valproic acid moved up to an overweight category after initiation of therapy.[31] The strongest predictor of weight gain was the weight category at the initiation of therapy. The mechanism by which valproic acid may lead to weight gain in some patients remains unknown. Possible mechanisms include stimulation of insulin secretion and impairment of beta oxidation of fatty acids. Demir and Aysun found that insulin concentration and the insulin to glucose ratio increased with treatment with valproic acid.[32] They speculated that these changes may lead to increased appetite and subsequent weight gain. Future research should focus on a better understanding of these mechanisms.

There have been a number of case studies documenting marked weight gain in patients treated with atypical antipsychotic agents.[33,34] Some reports have suggested that more than half of the children and adolescents treated with these agents have an excessive weight gain. Again, it is unknown why some patients seem to be prone to weight gain while others are not. Future research should elucidate the mechanisms involved in abnormal weight gain after administration of these medications.

ADOLESCENCE

Another sensitive or critical period for abnormal weight gain is adolescence. There are important changes in body composition that occur during pubertal development. There are also important differences between girls and boys in these body composition changes. In boys, fat-free mass tends to increase, while the percent of weight from fat decreases with advancing puberty.[21,35,36] In girls, both fat mass and fat-free mass increase while the percent of weight from fat also increases marginally.[21,35] The distribution of fat also changes during puberty. These changes are probably mediated by changes in hormone concentrations. Boys experience increased deposition of central fat, including both increased visceral fat and increased subcutaneous fat in this region. Girls tend to have increased fat deposition in the hips.[36]

The risk of becoming overweight in adolescence appears to be higher for girls compared with boys. However, in both boys and girls the amount of fat deposition and potentially the location of that fat deposition (central is worse than peripheral) during puberty appear to increase the risk of important obesity-related comorbidities later in life.

The presence of overweight in adolescence may be more important relative to future risk of obesity than at other ages during growth and development. For example, Whitaker et al. showed that the risk of obesity in adulthood was greater for an overweight adolescent compared with an overweight infant or young child.[37] It has been suggested that up to 80% of overweight adolescents will become overweight adults.[21] This increases the importance of weight gain during adolescence for both boys and girls.

There has also been concern that overweight developed during adolescence may be more likely to lead to adverse health effects later in life.[38,39] Better understanding of this potential relationship requires a comparison of obesity that is prevalent during adolescence, obesity that develops (incident) during adolescence, and obesity that develops in adulthood. Unfortunately, most epidemiological studies have not been able to make this comparison because data from one period or another are missing. Obesity that is present in adolescence (prevalent) has been associated with increased risk of morbidity from diabetes and cardiovascular disease and mortality in adulthood.[38,40] However, the extent to which these risks relate to mechanisms during childhood and adolescence, or are mediated solely through adult obesity remains unknown. The extent to which obesity present or incident during adolescence has increased effects on more central deposition of fat, greater insulin resistance, or increased effect on the heart, blood vessels, or other organ systems remains to be determined.

Adolescence is a time of rapid growth and developmental changes. Puberty is accompanied by a variety of hormonal changes and by transient insulin resistance.[41,42] The factors influencing the pubertal changes in insulin resistance are not completely understood. It is clear that insulin resistance during childhood is related to adiposity. However, the development of insulin resistance in puberty is not completely explained by differences in body mass index or adiposity.[43] Neither testosterone nor estrogen has been associated with insulin resistance.[44] Goran and Gower showed that the 30% drop in insulin sensitivity during puberty is similar across obesity status.[42] Moran et al. showed that growth hormone and insulinlike growth factor 1 were related to insulin resistance during puberty.[45] Insulinlike growth factor 1 rose and fell during puberty in parallel to the rise and fall of insulin resistance.

An important question is whether these changes in insulin resistance also create a sensitive period for abnormal weight gain. In adults, it has been proposed that insulin resistance is a physiological adaptation to obesity that limits fat accumulation and may help to stabilize weight.[46] This would suggest that increased insulin sensitivity may be a more permissive state for weight gain. Longitudinal studies in adults have been inconclusive. Some studies have shown that individuals with greater insulin sensitivity have greater weight gain than those who were more insulin resistant.[47,48] However, in two other studies the weight gain was greatest in the subjects who were most insulin resistant.[49,50] Further studies will be needed to resolve the mechanisms of these issues in adolescence. One study followed 111 healthy children over a 3-year period.[51] All subjects were Tanner stage 2 or 3 for pubertal development at baseline. They found that children who had greater insulin resistance had decreased gain in percent body fat estimated by skinfold thickness. This result appeared to be independent of the initial body weight. Odeleye et al. evaluated the relationship between insulin resistance and weight gain in prepubertal Pima Indian children.[52] Most of these children were overweight at baseline. They found that hyperinsulinemia was associated with higher rates of weight gain over a 10-year period that extended through adolescence. Steinberger et al. found that adiposity during childhood predicts insulin resistance and obesity in young adulthood.[53] However, it is not clear if increased insulin resistance was a causal factor for excess weight gain or occurred as a result of weight gain.

There are other factors that may influence insulin resistance during puberty. Murtaugh et al. found that low birth weight is associated with higher levels of insulin in adolescence suggesting insulin resistance.[54] This effect appeared to be independent of the weight in adolescence. Li et al. reported that low birth weight was a predictor of insulin resistance syndrome and its progression over age in childhood.[55] This effect was more pronounced among African-American children. The mechanism for this association between insulin resistance and low birth weight remains unknown.

There is clearly much to be learned about physiological changes in adolescence that may relate to abnormal weight gain. Future research should focus on methods that can disentangle a variety of longitudinal changes as they relate to acceleration of weight gain, growth, insulin resistance, and development of obesity.

Another factor that becomes important during adolescence for girls is the potential for pregnancy and childbirth. Childbearing has been shown to result in postpartum weight retention of greater than 5 kg in more than 20% of young women who become pregnant.[56–58] Pregnancy may also have adverse effects on other risk factors for type 2 diabetes mellitus and cardiovascular disease within 1 to 2 years postpartum.[59,60] Whether pregnancy in adolescence confers particular risks is not completely known.

Among adolescents in the United States who gave birth in 1996, 17% of those under age 16 and 25% of the 16 to 19 year olds were overweight prior to pregnancy.[61] In contrast to adult pregnant women who acquire fat with pregnancy during the first and second trimester and mobilize the fat in the third trimester, adolescents who are growing and become pregnant gain fat throughout gestation.[62] Adolescents may also retain more weight postpartum compared with adult women. Therefore, pregnancy during adolescence may alter normal growth processes and increase the risk of becoming overweight.[63]

The biological mechanisms for increased risk of overweight due to pregnancy in adolescence are unknown. Leptin levels are correlated with gestational weight gain but return to early pregnancy levels within 3 days of delivery. Gestational hormones have also been found to be related to leptin levels. Progesterone promotes changes in energy metabolism that have been associated with maternal weight gain.[64] Lactation has been reported to have at most a weak association with postpartum weight retention.[65] Other potential mechanisms have not been extensively studied.

Adolescence is also a time of changes in diet and physical activity. As children become adolescents, they may spend more time with friends and less time with their family. Time with friends may be spent in eating outside the home, which in turn may be related to increases in the intake of sodium and calories, particularly calories from fat.[66] Physical activity may change dramatically during adolescence. Kimm et al. found that substantial declines occurred for girls during adolescence.[67] The decline was even greater for African-American girls than white girls. Many girls declined to a level at which they had little or no leisure time physical activity. They also found that determinants of the decline in physical activity included greater BMI, previous pregnancy, and cigarette smoking. Clearly, with cessation of growth, decreased physical activity leads to changes in energy balance that are likely to lead to abnormal weight gain, even if dietary intake remains stable. Further research is needed to determine the biological and behavioral factors that determine these changes in diet and physical activity, which lead to problems with energy balance.

Medications

Adolescents may also use medication that can place them at risk for excess weight gain. For adolescent females, contraceptive use is a particular concern. Gallo et al. reviewed studies that included estrogen–progestin contraceptives for an association with weight gain.[68] They found that the three placebo controlled studies did not find evidence of weight gain related to oral or skin patch contraceptive use. They concluded that if there is an effect it is likely to be quite small. On the other hand, the use of Depo Provera® has been associated with excess weight gain. Bonny et al. evaluated weight gain related to use of Depo medroxyprogesterone for contraception in adolescents.[69] They found that both African-Americans and white females had an increase in weight and percent body fat after onset of medication use. However, the African-American girls had a significantly greater increase compared with the white girls. Baseline weight was a predictor for weight gain with Depo medroxyprogesterone in both African-American and white girls. Both white and African-American girls tended to gain weight in the first 3 months after initiation whereas the African-American girls also tended to gain weight in the next 2 months after beginning therapy. There are a number of issues to consider when prescribing contraceptives for adolescent females, and potential for weight gain should be included in the list.

There is also concern about abnormal weight gain in the period after high school. Individuals who go to college may have a substantial change in their environment leading to changes in energy balance. This may result in increased energy intake, decreased energy expenditure, or both. It should be emphasized that even as small a shift as 150 kcal/d could result in a weight gain of 15 lb that has been anecdotally reported for students during their freshman year (the freshman 15). Students who live at home may still have a substantial change in their schedule and have increased eating outside the home, leading to greater energy intake. Finally, those individuals entering the workforce for the first time and living independently of their parents also experience a substantial change in environment that could lead to a change in energy balance. These changes, which are occurring at a time when linear growth has stopped, may lead to abnormal weight gain and ultimately overweight.

CONCLUSION

It is clear that childhood and adolescence is an important developmental period for abnormal weight gain. It is likely that there are critical or sensitive periods where the risks and the consequences of weight gain are high. The pathophysiology of these critical periods is far from completely understood. It does appear that biological, environmental, behavioral, and other factors may be important and may combine to create a critical period. Future research should be directed at better understanding these critical periods during childhood and adolescence.

REFERENCES

1. Eckel, RH. Obesity: A disease or a physiologic adaptation for survival? In *Obesity Mechanisms and Clinical Management*, Eckel, RH (Ed.), Lippincott, Williams and Wilkins, Philadelphia, 2003.
2. Ivkovic-Lazar, T. Development and differentiation of adipose tissue. *Med Pregl.* 2003;56(3–4): 142–145.
3. Hauner H, Schmid P, Pfeiffer EF. Glucocorticoids and insulin promote the differentiation of human adipocyte precursor cells into fat cells. *J Clin Endocrinol Metab.* 1987;64(4): 832–835.
4. Vidal-Puig AJ, Considine RV, Jimenez-Linan M, Werman A, Pories WJ, Caro JF, Flier JS. Peroxisome proliferators-activated receptor gene expression in human tissues. Effects of obesity, weight loss, and regulation of insulin and glucocorticoids. *J Clin Invest.* 1997;99(10): 2416–2422.
5. Yost TJ, Rodgers CM, Eckel RH. Suction lipectomy: outcome relates to region-specific lipoprotein lipase activity and interval weight change. *Plast Reconstr Surg.* 1993;92(6): 1101–1108; Discussion 1109–1111.

6. Klein S, Fontana L, Young VL, Coggan AR, Kilo C, Patterson BW, Mohammed BS. Absence of an effect of liposuction on insulin action and risk factors for coronary heart disease. *N Engl J Med.* 2004;350: 2549–2557.

7. Barker M, Robinson S, Osmond C, Barker D. Birth weight and body fat distribution in adolescent girls. *Arch Dis Child.* 1997;77: 381–383.

8. Strauss RS, Dietz WH. Growth and development of term children born with low birth weight: effects of genetic and environmental factors. *J Pediatr.* 1998;133: 67–72.

9. Parsons TJ, Power C, Logan S, et al. Childhood predictors of adult obesity: a systematic review. *Int J Obes Relat Metab Disord.* 1999;23(Suppl 8): S1–S107.

10. Plagemann A, Harder T, Melchior K, Rake A, Rohde W, Dorner G. Elevation of hypothalamic neuropeptide Y-neurons in adult offspring of diabetic mother rats. *Neuroreport.* 1999;10: 3211–3216.

11. Dabelea D, Hanson RL, Lindsay RS, et al. Intrauterine exposure to diabetes conveys risks for type 2 diabetes and obesity: a study of discordant sibships. *Diabetes.* 2000;49: 2208–2211 [Abstract].

12. Silverman BL, Cho NH, Rizzo TA, Metzger BE. Long-term effects of the intrauterine environment. *Diabetes Care.* 1998;21: B142–B148.

13. Whitaker RC, Pepe MS, Seidel KD, Wright JA, Knopp RH. Gestational diabetes and the risk of offspring obesity. *Pediatrics.* 1998;101: E9.

14. Gillman MW, Rifas-Shiman S, Berkey CS, Field AE, Colditz GA. Maternal gestational diabetes, birth weight, and adolescent obesity. *Pediatrics* 2003;111(3): e221–e226.

15. Stettler N, Zemel B, Kumanyika S, Stallings VA. Infant weight gain and childhood overweight status in a multicenter, cohort study. *Pediatrics.* 2002;109: 194–199.

16. Eriksson JG, Forsen T, Tuomilehto J, Winter PD, Osmond C, Barker DJP. Catch-up growth in childhood and death from coronary heart disease: longitudinal study. *BMJ* 1999;318: 427–431.

17. Gillman MW, Rifas-Shiman SL, Camargo CA, Berkey CS, Frazier AL, Rockett HR, et al. Risk of overweight among adolescents who were breastfed as infants. *JAMA* 2001;285: 2461–2467.

18. Von Kries R, Koletzko B, Sauerwald T, et al. Breastfeeding and obesity: cross-sectional study. *BMJ* 1999;319: 147–150.

19. Hediger ML, Overpeck MD, Kuczmarski RJ, et al. Association between infant breastfeeding and overweight in young children. *JAMA* 2001;285: 2453–2460.

20. Li L, Parsons TJ, Power C. Breast feeding and obesity in childhood: cross sectional study. *British Medical Journal* 2003;327(7420): 904–905.

21. Dietz WH. Overweight in childhood and adolescence. *N Engl J Med.* 2004;350: 855–857.

22. Whitaker RC, Pepe MS, Wright JA, Seidel KD, Dietz WH. Early adiposity rebound and the risk of adult obesity. *Pediatrics* 1998;101(3): E5.

23. Rolland-Cachera MF, Deheeger M, Bellisle F, Sempe M, Guilloud-Bataille M, Patois E. Adiposity rebound in children: a simple indicator for predicting obesity. *Am J Clin Nutr* 1984;39: 129–135.

24. Siervogel RM, Roche AF, Guo S, Mukherjee D, Chumlea C. Patterns of change in weight^2/stature from 2 to 18 years: findings from long-term serial data for children in the Fels Longitudinal Growth Study. *Int J Obes Relat Metab Disord* 1991;15: 479–485.

25. Rolland-Cachera MF, Deheeger M, Guilloud-Bataille M, Avons P, Patois E, Sempe M. Tracking the development of adiposity from one month of age to adulthood. *Ann Hum Biol* 1987;14: 219–229.

26. Bhargava SK, Sachdev HS, Fall CH, Osmond C, Lakshmy R, Barker DJ, et al. Relation of serial changes in childhood body-mass index to impaired glucose tolerance in young adulthood. *N Engl J Med.* 2004;350(9): 865–875.

27. Radakovic-Fijan S, Furnsinn-Friedl AM, Honigsmann H, Tanew A. Oral dexamethasone pulse treatment for vitiligo. *J Am Acad Dermatol.* 2001;44(5): 814–817.

28. Eubanks V, Koppersmith N, Wooldridge N, Clancy JP, Lyrene R, Arani RB, et al. Effects of megestrol acetate on weight gain, body composition, and pulmonary function in patients with cystic fibrosis. *J Pediatr.* 2002;140(4): 439–444.

29. Fornari V, Dancyger I, La Monaca G, Budman C, Goodman B, Kabo L, Katz JL. Can steroid use be a precipitant in the development of an eating disorder? *Int J Eat Disord.* 2001;30(1): 118–122.

30. Caksen H, Deda G, Berberoglu M. Does long-term use of valproate cause weight gain in prepubertal epileptic children? *Int J Neurosci.* 2002;112(10): 1183–1189.

31. Wirrell EC. Valproic acid-associated weight gain in older children and teens with epilepsy. *Pediatr Neurol.* 2003;28(2): 126–129.

32. Demir E, Aysun S. Weight gain associated with valproate in childhood. *Pediatr Neurol.* 2000;22(5): 361–364.

33. Potenza MN, Holmes JP, Kanes SJ, McDougle CJ. Olanzapine treatment of children, adolescents, and adults with pervasive developmental disorders: an open-label study. *J Clin Psychopharmacol.* 1999;19: 37–44.

34. Kelly DL, Conley RR, Love RC, et al. Weight gain in adolescents treated with Risperidone and conventional antipsychotics over six months. *J Child Adolesc Psychopharmacol* 1998;8: 151–159.

35. Naumova EN, Must A, Laird NM. Tutorial in biostatistics: evaluating the impact of "critical periods" in longitudinal studies of growth using piecewise mixed effects models. *Int J Epidemiol.* 2001;30: 1332–1341.

36. Must A, Jacques PF, Dallal GE, Bajema CJ, Dietz WH. Long-term morbidity and mortality of overweight adolescents: a follow-up of the Harvard Growth Study of 1922 to 1935. *N Engl J Med.* 1992;327: 1350–1355.

37. Whitaker RC, Wright JA, Pepe MS, Seidel KD, Dietz WH. Predicting obesity in young adulthood from childhood and parental obesity. *N Engl J Med.* 1997;337(13): 869–873.

38. Hoffmans MD, Kromhout D, Coulander CD. Body mass index at the age of 18 and its effects on 32-year mortality from coronary heart disease and cancer. *J Clin Epidemiol.* 1989;42: 513–520.

39. Dietz WH. Critical periods in childhood for the development of obesity. *Am J Clin. Nutr.* 1994;59(5): 955–999.

40. Must A. Does overweight in childhood have an impact on adult health? *Nutr Rev.* 2003;61: 139–142.

41. Caprio S, Plewe G, Diamond MP, Simonson DC, Boulware SD, Sherwin RS, Tamborlane WV. Increased insulin secretion in puberty. *J Pediatr* 1989;114: 963–967.

42. Goran MI, Gower BA. Longitudinal study on pubertal insulin resistance. *Diabetes.* 2001;50(11): 2444–2450.

43. Moran A, Jacobs DR, Steinberger J, Hong C P, Prineas R, Luepker R, Sinaiko AR. Insulin resistance during puberty: results from clam studies in 357 children. *Diabetes* 1999;48: 2039–2044.

44. Travers SH, Jeffers BW, Bloch CA, Hill JO, Eckel RH. Gender and Tanner stage differences in body composition and insulin sensitivity in early pubertal children. *J Clin Endocrinol Metab* 1995;80: 172–178.

45. Moran A, Jacobs DR, Jr., Steinberger J, Cohen P, Hong CP, Prineas R, Sinaiko AR. Association between the insulin resistance of puberty and the insulin-like growth factor I/growth hormone axis. *J Clin Endocrinol Metab* 2002;87(10): 4817–4820.

46. Eckel RH. Insulin resistance: an adaptation for weight maintenance. *Lancet* 1992;340: 1452–1453.

47. Swinburn BA, Nyomba BL, Saad MF, Zurlo F, Raz I, Knowler WC, Lillioja S, Bogardus C, Ravussin E. Insulin resistance associated with lower rates of weight gain in Pima Indians. *J Clin Invest* 1991;88: 168–173.

48. Hoag S, Marshall JA, Jones RH, Hamman RF. High fasting insulin levels associated with lower rates of weight gain in persons with normal glucose tolerance: the San Luis Valley Diabetes Study. *Int J Obes* 1995;19: 175–180.

49. Hodge AM, Dowse GK, Alberti GMM, Tuomilehto J, Gareeboo H, Zimmet PZ. Relationship of insulin resistance to weight gain in nondiabetic Asian Indian, Creole, and Chinese Mauritians. *Metabolism* 1996;45: 627–633.

50. Folsom AR, Vitelli LL, Lewis CE, Schreiner PJ, Watson RL, Wagenknecht LE. Is fasting insulin inversely associated with rate of weight gain? Contrasting findings from the CARDIA and ARIC study cohorts. *Int J Obes* 1998;22: 48–54.

51. Travers SH, Jeffers BW, Eckel RH. Insulin resistance during puberty and future fat accumulation. *J Clin Endocrinol Metabol* 2002;87(8): 3814–3818.

52. Odeleye OE, de Courten M, Pettitt DJ, Ravussin E. Fasting hyperinsulinemia is a predictor of increased body weight gain and obesity in Pima Indian children. *Diabetes* 1997;46: 1341–1345.

53. Steinberger J, Moran A, Hong CP, Jacobs DR, Jr., Sinaiko AR. Adiposity in childhood predicts obesity and insulin resistance in young adulthood. *J Pediatr.* 2001;138(4): 469–473.

54. Murtaugh MA, Jacobs DR, Jr., Moran A, Steinberger J, Sinaiko AR. Relation of birth weight to fasting insulin, insulin resistance, and body size in adolescence. *Diabetes* 2003;26: 187–192.

55. Li C, Johnson MS, Goran MI. Effects of low birth weight on insulin resistance syndrome in Caucasian and African-American children. *Diabetes Care.* 2001;24(12): 2035–2042.

56. Gunderson EP, Abrams B. Epidemiology of gestational weight gain and body weight changes after pregnancy. *Epidemiol Rev.* 1992;21: 261–275.
57. Gunderson, EP, Abrams B, Selvin S. Does the pattern of postpartum weight change differ according to pregravid body size? *Int J Obes Relat Metab Disord.* 2001;25: 853–862.
58. Williamson DF, Madans J, Pamuk E, Flegal KM, Kendrick JS, Serdula MK. A prospective study of childbearing and 10-year weight gain in US white women 25 to 45 years of age. *Int J Obes Relat Metab Disord.* 1994;18: 561–569.
59. Lewis CE, Funkhouser E, Raczynski JM, Sidney S, Bild DE, Howard BV, Adverse effect of pregnancy on high density lipoprotein (HDL) cholesterol in young adult women. The CARDIA Study. Coronary Artery Risk Development in Young Adults. *Am J Epidemiol.* 1996;144: 247–254.
60. Haertel U, Heiss G, Filipiak B, Doering A. Cross-sectional and longitudinal associations between high density lipoprotein cholesterol and women's employment. *Am J Epidemiol.* 1992;135: 68–78.
61. US Department of Health and Human Services, Centers for Disease Control and Prevention. 1996. *Pregnancy Nutrition Surveillance 1996 Full Report.* Atlanta, GA: Author.
62. Scholl TO, Hediger ML, Schall JI, Khoo CS, Fischer RL. Maternal growth during pregnancy and the competition for nutrients. *Am J Clin Nutr.* 1994;60: 183–88.
63. Hediger ML, Scholl TO, Schall JI. Implications of the Camden Study of adolescent pregnancy: interactions among maternal growth, nutritional status, and body composition. *Ann NY Acad Sci.* 1997;817: 281–291.
64. Ledoux F, Genest J, Nowaczynski W, Kuchel O, Lebel M. Plasma progesterone and aldosterone in pregnancy. *Can Med Assoc J.* 1975;112: 943–947.
65. Ohlin A, Rossner S. Maternal body weight development after pregnancy. *Int J Obes Relat Metab Disord.* 1990;14: 159–173.
66. French SA, Story M, Neumark-Stzainer D, Fulkerson JA, Hannan P. Fast food restaurant use among adolescents: associations with nutrient intake, food choices, and behavioral and psychosocial variables. *Int. J Obes.* 2001;25: 1823–1833.
67. Kimm SY, Glynn NW, Kriska AM, Barton BA, Kronsberg SS, Daniels SR, et al. Decline in physical activity in black girls and white girls during adolescence. *N Engl J Med.* 2002;347(10): 709–715.
68. Gallo MF, Grimes DA, Schulz KF, Helmerhorst FM. Combination estrogen-progestin contraceptives and body weight: systematic review of randomized controlled trials. *Obstet Gynecol.* 2004;103(2): 359–373.
69. Bonny AE, Britto MT, Huang B, Succop P, Slap GB. Weight gain, adiposity, eating behaviors among adolescent females on depot medroxyprogesterone acetate (DMPA). *J Pediatr Adolesc Gynecol.* 2004;17(2): 109–115.

6 Genetics of Childhood Obesity

Nancy F. Butte, Carlos A. Bacino, Shelley A. Cole, and Anthony G. Comuzzie

CONTENTS

INTRODUCTION

Obesity is a complex disease influenced by multiple genetic and environmental factors.[1] Because of its complexity, obesity does not conform to simple Mendelian patterns of inheritance but displays variable expression. With the exception of rare single gene defects, obesity is an oligogenic disorder attributed to a few genes with relatively large measurable effects, whose expression is modulated by polygenic genes interacting with one another and with the environment. Classical genetic studies on twins, siblings, and nuclear families clearly have established the genetic influence on body weight and adiposity.

Teleologically, obesity genes may have been conserved in response to evolutionary pressures to promote weight gain in the face of food scarcity. This theory is put forth by the "thrifty" genotype hypothesis. Individuals genetically susceptible to overconsumption, efficient energy storage, and energy conservation would be more likely to survive famine and propagate the thrifty genes. These "thrifty" genes are maladaptive in present day environments with a plethora of highly palatable, energy-dense foods and sedentary lifestyles. The global epidemic of obesity in the past two decades cannot be attributed to a changing human gene pool, but more likely to susceptibility genes exerting their effects in highly permissive environments.

Body weight is regulated and defended by complex, highly redundant physiological systems.[2] The multiple pathways involved in adiposity development, regulation of food intake, and energy expenditure are subject to genetic modulation. Insulin, leptin, and ghrelin are key afferent signals involved in energy homeostasis. Central effector pathways that regulate body weight in response to the afferent signals are composed of catabolic and anabolic neuropeptides, which influence food intake and energy expenditure. The first-order neuronal targets of leptin and insulin are catabolic proopiomelanocortin (POMC) and anabolic neuropeptide-Y (NPY) and agouti-related protein (AgRP) neurons in the hypothalamic arcuate nucleus. Adaptive responses to perturbations in body fat involve reciprocal changes in the activity of these neuropeptides. Arcuate NPY/AgRP and POMC neurons project into the lateral hypothalamic area (LHA) and paraventricular nucleus (PVN) to connect with second-order neurons involved with fine control of appetite and energy expenditure. LHA releases anabolic neuropeptides such as melanin-concentrating hormone (MCH), and the PVN releases catabolic neuropeptides such as thyrotropin-releasing hormone (TRH), corticotropin-releasing hormone (CRH), and oxytocin. NPY/AgRP and POMC neurons also communicate with the brain stem, especially the nucleus of the solitary tract that is the target for enteric neurocrine peptides such as cholecystokinin, glucagon, glucagon-like peptide 1, amylin, and bombesin-related peptides.

INTRAUTERINE CRITICAL PERIOD FOR THE DEVELOPMENT OF OBESITY

The intrauterine period may play a role in the development of later obesity. In the early origins of adult diseases hypothesis, it is theorized that an environmental stimulus may occur at a critical period and have a lasting effect on the development of diabetes, cardiovascular diseases, and obesity.[3] A number of epidemiological studies have demonstrated a positive relationship between birth weight and body mass index (BMI) later in life.[4] Possible mechanisms underlying this relationship include alterations in fat cell number, structure and function of the appetite regulation centers of the brain, and pancreatic structure and function. Other studies have documented an association between low birth weight and later risk of central obesity, insulin resistance, and the metabolic syndrome, possibly mediated through hypothalamic pituitary axis, insulin regulation, and vascular responsiveness.

Genetic factors are likely to be major confounders of data supporting the early origins of obesity hypothesis. Genetic inheritance may entrain birth weight, insulin regulation and obesity, and components of the metabolic syndrome. Genetic imprinting also plays an important role in fetal growth and development. A handful of autosomal genes are inherited in a silent state from one of the two parents, and in a fully active state from the other.[5] Only a single copy is expressed, depending on the parent of origin. This imprint is established and erased in the germ line cells.

Early examples of genomic imprinting and its bearing on fetal growth is clearly exemplified by abnormal pregnancies that result in triploid fetuses.[6-8] In those instances, when two paternal and one maternal haploid component are present in the fetus, the placenta presents with large cystic and partial molar changes. A mole is an intrauterine mass formed by the degeneration of the partly developed products of conception. In this case fetal development is poor and will only show survival if there is mosaicism with normal diploid cells mixed with the triploid cell line. On the opposite end, if the triploid conception is the result of two paternal and one maternal haploid component, the fetus will develop but the placenta is very underdeveloped. In complete moles, the placenta develops cystic changes and not embryonic structures. Complete moles are androgeneic, in other words, they have solely paternal contribution and not maternal. This indicates that maternal genes are needed for embryo development and paternal genes are crucial for the development of placental and extra-embryonic tissues. The role of paternal and maternal genomes, similar to what is seen in humans, is also a well-known phenomenon in mouse development.[8]

Monozygotic twins discordant for birth weight could provide a unique approach for testing the influence of fetal environment on later adiposity that is independent of genetic and postnatal environmental factors. The Minnesota Twin Registry was used to implement this study design.[9] Adult height and weight were available for 4020 twin pairs. Birth weight was significantly correlated (all $P < 0.0005$) with adult height ($r = 0.236$), weight ($r = 0.188$), and BMI ($r = 0.078$). In monozygotic twins discordant for birth weight, the between-pair differences in birth weight correlated with between-pair differences in adult height and weight ($r = 0.316$ and 0.136, $P < 0.0005$), but not adult BMI ($r = 0.026$, $P = 0.331$), refuting the intrauterine environment as critical to programming later adiposity. The intrauterine period had a lasting effect on height, but not adiposity. There was no evidence of tracking of BMI independent of genetic effects. It should be noted, however, that most of the discordance in birth weight in monozygotic twins occurs in the third trimester. These results do not preclude long-term effects of environmental influences during the first two trimesters on later adiposity.

POSTNATAL CRITICAL PERIODS FOR THE DEVELOPMENT OF OBESITY

Substantial evidence supports the notion that adiposity tracks over the life span. Tracking refers to the prediction of future measures from earlier values and to the constancy of an individual's expected measures relative to population percentiles. Tracking of birth weight or early infant weight into adulthood was demonstrated in four studies.[10-13] Tracking may be genetic or environmental in origin. Two postnatal critical periods for the development of adiposity are the first year of life and puberty.[14] Infancy is characterized by an impressive hyperplasia and hypertrophy of adipose tissue. The rapid rate of fat deposition slows from weaning onward. BMI falls after the first year of life and begins to increase after age 4. Rapid maturation may predispose to the development of obesity. Markers of maturation, i.e., menarche, stage of puberty, or peak height velocity, are associated with subsequent fatness. Forbes[15] noted that obese children with onset in infancy have a greater proportion of fat-free mass (FFM) and bone mass than children who develop obesity later. Rolland-Cachera[16] found that the younger a child was at his or her lowest attained BMI, the greater the obesity in adulthood. Siervogel[17] also showed that the earlier children reach their nadir in BMI, the higher their BMI at age 18. The Amsterdam Growth and Health Study showed that individuals who matured rapidly in adolescence were generally more obese than slowly maturing adolescents between 13 and 27 years of age.[18] Obese children have accelerated linear growth, displaying advanced height and bone age. Because the growth spurt is less pronounced, final adult heights are not different from nonobese children. These age–sex dependent changes in body fat are driven by differences in preadipocyte proliferative activity, lipolysis, and lipogenesis, processes that all may be influenced by inheritance or gene–environment interactions.

GENETIC EPIDEMIOLOGY

HERITABILITY: INTERPRETATION FROM GENETIC EPIDEMIOLOGY STUDIES

Heritability (h^2) is defined as the relative proportion of the total phenotypic variance in a complex trait that is attributable to the additive effects of genes. Estimates of heritability apply only to the specific population studied and only to the environment at the time and place the population was studied. All the components of genetic variance are dependent on the gene frequencies so any estimates of them are valid only for the population from which they are estimated.[19]

Using quantitative genetic analysis, the total phenotypic variance (σ_P^2) is decomposed into its genetic (σ_G^2) and environmental (σ_E^2) components, such that $\sigma_P^2 = s_G^2 + \sigma_E^2$.[19,20] By extension, these components can be further decomposed, such that σ_G^2 can be separated into components representing the variance attributable to additive genetic effects (σ_A^2), dominance (σ_D^2), and epistasis (i.e., gene–gene interactions, σ_I^2), while σ_E^2 can be decomposed into components attributable to measured environmental factors and random, unmeasured factors. Nutritional and climatic factors are the commonest external causes of environmental variation. Maternal prenatal and postnatal effects are other sources of environmental variation. The proportion of phenotypic variation attributable to all genetic effects (i.e., additivity, dominance, epistasis) is referred to as the "broad sense" heritability ($h^2 = \sigma_G^2/\gamma_P^2$), while the "narrow sense" refers to the proportion of the variation attributed to the additive genetic effects only ($h^2 = \sigma_A^2/\sigma_P^2$).

Violations of the assumptions underlying the additive model will usually cause an upward bias of σ_A^2. The model assumes that the phenotypic variance is due to the additive effects of many genes (polygenes), not major dominant or recessive genes, and that there is no heterogeneity with regard to the mode of inheritance. Heritability estimates may be inflated when derived from siblings, particularly identical twins, because of shared environmental factors that are included under σ_A^2. Twins share a common environment from conception to birth and the period reared together. Therefore, the between-pair variance contains the variance due to common shared environment. To minimize this bias, researchers should derive heritability estimates from other relative sets.

TWINS, SIBLINGS, NUCLEAR FAMILIES, EXTENDED PEDIGREE STUDIES

Over the last several decades there has been much work substantiating a familial influence in the transmission of obesity. Observations on twins, siblings, nuclear families, and in extended pedigrees have all repeatedly shown that an individual's chances of being obese are increased when he or she has relatives who are also obese. Childhood-onset obesity has been associated with increased relative risk (RR = 2.14) for obesity in first-degree relatives, suggesting higher genetic loading and familial aggregation.[21] Although most obese adults were not obese as children, individuals with childhood-onset obesity may have a high genetic loading predisposing them to a highly familial form of adult obesity.

In fact, formalized quantitative genetic analyses of various measures of adipose tissue accumulation and distribution along with various metabolic parameters have consistently found significant heritabilities for these obesity-associated phenotypes, substantiating an additive or oligogenic component to obesity.[21-32]

Family and twin studies indicate that genes contribute substantially to variation in body fat accumulation and distribution. Estimates of the heritability of BMI generally range from 20 to 60%, as reviewed in Mitchell et al.[33] In several different studies, evidence for a major gene influencing BMI has been reported. For example, Burns et al.[34] found evidence for a single genetic locus that accounted for 37% of the total phenotypic variance in BMI. They also reported that this major locus had pleiotropic effects on blood pressure and high-density lipoprotein cholesterol (HDL)-C variability. Similar findings concerning a major gene effect for BMI have also been reported.[24,35-38] Rice et al.[27] and Comuzzie et al.[30] have also demonstrated a major gene effect for fat mass. In a sample of 176 French Canadian families, a major gene locus accounted for 45% of the variance in fat mass.[27] In a sample of Mexican-American families, a major gene accounted for 37 and 43% of the variance in fat mass in males and females, respectively.

Twin studies during late childhood and adolescence provide the most consistent and highest heritability estimates for BMI.[39] A study from Columbia University in monozygotic and dizygotic twins, 3 to 17 years of age, indicated that genes accounted for 75 to 80% of the phenotypic variation in percent body fat and 86% in BMI.[40] These results corroborate earlier reports of heritabilities for BMI in adolescents ranging from 0.67 for 8- to 10-year old twins, to 0.88 for 11- to 13-year-old twins, to 0.93 for 14- to 16-year-old twins.[41-44] In the Columbia University study, the remaining variation was attributed to nonshared environmental influences. The nonshared environment explains considerably more variance of the phenotype BMI than shared environment.[39]

The relationship between childhood stature growth parameters and adult overweight status was examined in the Fels Longitudinal Study.[45] Heritability estimates for stature parameters and overweight were between 52 to 92%. There is little evidence for shared genes influencing stature and adult overweight, although there were shared environmental factors that lead to an earlier age at peak height velocity and adult overweight.

The genetic contribution to the epidemic of childhood obesity may also involve an increase in assortative mating.[39] If this were occurring, children born to two obese parents would have a substantial chance of inheriting susceptibility gene variants from both parents and of developing severe obesity. High genetic loading may underlie the secular upward trend in the overweight and obese ranges.

ROLE OF ENVIRONMENTAL FACTORS IN THE ETIOLOGY OF CHILDHOOD OBESITY

The prevalence of obesity is increasing in most industrialized countries at a rate that is far too rapid to be attributed to evolutionary changes in the gene pool.[46,47] Modern environments have unmasked obesity in genetically susceptible individuals. Genetic predisposition to obesity has to be expressed by the induction of a positive energy balance due to changes in food intake and/or physical activity. Even though childhood and adult BMI are substantially heritable (70%), evidence is largely absent for shared family environmental factors.[46,48] The weight and fatness of adoptive siblings, who share their rearing environment but no genes, were not correlated. Monozygotic twins reared together showed no greater resemblance than did monozygotic twins reared apart. Adoptees do not resemble adoptive parents in weight or fatness. Offspring resemble their biological parents in weight equally, whether or not they were given up for adoption. Environmental experiences that are not shared between monozygotic twins were etiologically important for weight and obesity, accounting for approximately 20% of the variation.[46] The nature of these nonshared environmental factors is largely unknown, but they do not appear to be closely related with either age or sex.

The lack of evidence for shared environmental effects was apparent in 11-year-old twins[41] and adopted children studied from birth to 9 years of age.[49] Societal modernization has resulted in clear changes in lifestyle in the direction of decreased energy expenditure. Paradoxically, lifestyle changes apparently haven't influenced energy expenditure on a family basis, even though modern conveniences such as cars, TV, and computers are available to the household. A possible explanation is the near-universal ownership of modern conveniences. Individuals may respond differently to household environments, as suggested by different patterns of TV watching[50] and sports participation[51] found in twin family and adoption studies. It will be important to explore nonshared experiences, such as peer influences on diet and exercise, or within family differences in diet and exercise.

MONOGENIC OBESITY

Six single gene disorders involved in the leptin–melanocortin pathway cause early-onset morbid obesity. All give rise to voracious hyperphagia and profound childhood obesity.[14] Discovery of these mutations has provided insight into the biological pathways controlling body weight. Tertiary diagnostic and treatment facilities are needed for the care of these children. Health care workers require training to screen, refer, and treat these children appropriately. For instance, leptin deficiency is amenable to treatment[52] with replacement hormone therapy.

Leptin (LEP)

Congenital leptin deficiency has been described in six cases from two families.[53–55] Two cousins of Pakistani origin who had early onset severe obesity were homozygous for a guanine deletion that caused a frameshift mutation and lower circulating leptin levels.[53] Four members of a consanguineous Turkish family had a C to T substitution in codon 105 of the leptin gene that caused an Arg-Trp substitution in the protein.[54,55] Leptin treatment caused a dramatic decrease in body weight and a reversal of endocrine abnormalities.[52,56] Congenital leptin deficiency is characterized by severe hyperphagia, impaired T-cell mediated immunity, and hypogonadotropic hypogonadism.

Leptin Receptor (LEPR)

A mutation in the leptin receptor that resulted in a truncated receptor that lacked the intracellular and transmembrane portion was described in three sisters in a consanguineous family of Kabilian origin.[57] These women had hyperphagia, obesity, and sexual immaturity.

Pro-Opiomelanocortin (POMC)

Defects in the *POMC* gene result in a deficiency of some or all of the peptides derived from POMC, i.e., α-, β-, and γ-MSH (melanocyte stimulating hormone), ACTH (adrenocorticorticotrophin), N-terminal peptide, joining peptide, and β-lipotropin. *POMC* mutations were originally reported in three obesity cases, two of which were in children.[58] One child was a heterozygote for mutations in exon 3 and the other homozygous for a single mutation in exon 2 of the *POMC* gene. These children had red hair, corticotropin deficiency, and obesity. Three additional children have been identified with the same phenotype, with mutations in the *POMC* gene.[59] Disruption of central melanocortin signaling causes dysfunction of the hypothalamic–pituitary–thyroid axis. Some of the children with POMC deficiency also have elevated TSH (thyroid stimulating hormone) levels, reduced T4 values, and normal responses to TRH stimulation.

In a pooled data set, a missense R236G mutation in the coding region of the *POMC* gene was found in 0.9% of the subjects with early-onset obesity compared with 0.2% of the normal-weight controls.[60] This mutation disrupts the dibasic cleavage site between β-MSH and β-endorphin, and produces an aberrant fusion protein that binds to MC4R that interferes with central melanocortin signaling. Mutations at this site may make an appreciable contribution to the genetic predisposition to severe childhood obesity. Observations of haploinsufficiency of *POMC* causing an obesity phenotype are consistent with the findings of significant linkage detected on chromosome 2 containing the *POMC* gene as a susceptibility locus for common human obesity.[32]

Pro-Hormone Convertase (PC1)

Pro-hormone convertase 1 cleaves POMC into α-MSH and adrenocorticotropin (ACTH). There is one reported case of a mutation in the gene encoding PC1 (Gly593Arg), which causes failure of maturation of the inactive propeptide form of PC1. This woman was obese and had hypocortisolism, hypogonadatrophic hypogonadism, and increased POMC levels.[61] A second case of congenital PC1 deficiency was recently identified in a patient who had severe small intestinal absorptive dysfunction in addition to severe early-onset obesity, impaired prohormone processing, and hypocortisolemia.[62] PC1 also may be involved in the maturation of propeptides within the enteroendocrine cells and nerves that express PC1 throughout the gut.

Melanocortin 4 Receptor (MC4R)

MC4R mutations are by far the most common form of monogenic human obesity, accounting for 4 to 6% of common morbid obesity. Heterozygous mutations in the *MC4R* were first reported in individuals with early-onset severe obesity.[63–65] MC4R deficient individuals not only have increased fat mass and hyperphagia, but also increased lean mass, increased linear growth, hyperinsulinemia, and mild hypothalamic hypothyroidism.[66] Homozygotic mutations cause more severe obesity than heterozygotic ones. Mutations retaining residual signaling capacity manifest in a less severe phenotype.

MC4R mutations are usually autosomal codominant with variable penetrance, arising from haploinsufficiency in *MC4R* signaling rather than from dominant negative mechanisms.[63,67] MC4R is a member of the rhodopsin-like G protein-coupled receptor family. The binding of α-MSH to the MC4R leads to increased cAMP (cyclic adenosine monophosphate) production. Numerous mutations of *MC4R* have been found in children in early-onset severe obesity.[63,66] Experiments have been performed to determine which allelic variants result in impairment of the receptor's function.[63,68] Six mutants were found to have decreased (S58C, N62S, Y157S, C271Y) or no (P78L, G98R) ligand binding, with proportional impairments in α-MSH-stimulated cAMP production.[68] The most prevalent defect in loss-of-function *MC4R* mutants appears to be decreased cell surface expression due to intracellular retention of these mutants. MC4R is a superb target for pharmacological agonists to treat obesity.

Single-Minded Homologue 1 (SIM1)

A balanced translocation between chromosomes 1p22.1 and 6q16.2 was reported in one girl with morbid obesity. The translocation did not affect the transcription unit on 1p22.1, but it disrupted the transcription factor *SIM1* on 6q16.2.[69] The *SIM1* gene is essential for formation of the PVN, a principal site of MC4R expression. Haploinsufficiency of *SIM1*, possibly acting upstream or downstream of MC4R in PVN, could be responsible for the obesity seen in this child. Her early-onset obesity was characterized by hyperphagia, accelerated linear growth, and increased fat mass and bone mineral density. There was no evidence of developmental delay or precocious puberty. Her high weight gain was attributed to excessive food intake because her measured energy expenditure was normal. Larger chromosome 6 deletions containing *SIM1* have been reported with early-onset obesity in boys and girls who also may display developmental delay.[70]

SYNDROMIC OBESITY

Obesity syndromes refer to complex clinical syndromes in which obesity is only one of the physical and developmental anomalies.[71–73] Positional genetic analyses have led to the identification of causative genetic defects underlying these syndromes. In most cases, the defective gene product is an intracellular protein of unknown function expressed throughout the body. Both autosomal and X-linked "genes" have been seen associated with obesity conditions in children. In many cases, hyperphagia and/or other indications of hypothalamic dysfunction suggest a central origin of the obesity seen with these syndromes. Loss of function mutations often is the underlying cause of these syndromes, suggesting that less severe coding mutations or sequence variants may produce milder phenotypes in common obesities. Interestingly, several obesity syndromes involve imprinted genes.

Down Syndrome

Down syndrome is caused by trisomy 21, or three copies of chromosome 21 in 95% of the affected individuals instead of the usual two copies.[74] Prevalence is approximately 1 in 800 live-born infants. In most cases, the extra chromosome 21 is maternal in origin, and in almost 80% of these cases, nondisjunction occurred in maternal meiosis I. About 4 to 5% of cases are due to translocations that can be inherited or are *de novo*. Down syndrome is characterized by growth retardation, variable but often severe mental retardation, physical abnormalities including a flattened face and occiput, upward slanting eyes, large tongue, and small ears. Other defects include congenital heart disease (AV canal), gastrointestinal anomalies (duodenal atresia and Hirschprung's disease), leukemia, cataracts, thyroid dysfunction, and premature incidence of Alzheimer disease. Complications of autoimmune thyroiditis and congenital heart disease may compromise growth. Down syndrome individuals may develop obesity as they progress through a rather deficient pubertal development.[14]

Prader–Willi Syndrome

Prader–Willi syndrome is caused by a deletion or disruption of a paternally imprinted gene or genes on the proximal long arm of chromosome 15. Prader–Willi is an example of genomic imprinting, where the differential expression of alleles depends on the parent from which the gene originated. Approximately 70 to 75% of children with Prader–Willi syndrome have a microdeletion of paternal chromosome 15q11-q13. Another 20 to 25% has two copies of the maternal chromosome 15 and no copy of the paternal chromosome, also known as maternal uniparental disomy. There are 10 known paternally expressed loci potentially involved in the etiology of Prader–Willi syndrome, including intronless genes, complex polycistronic locus, and five classes of small nucleolar RNA. Multiple genes cluster in the genome.[73] Prevalence is about 1 in 10,000 live births.[74] Diminished fetal activity, hypotonia, and poor feeding are commonly seen in early infancy. Other clinical findings include hypogonadism, short stature, small hands and feet, mild to moderate mental retardation, and obsessive-compulsive behavior. Compulsive eating results in massive obesity, beginning after about age 2. Body composition is unusual with high fat mass and low muscle mass. Growth hormone therapy has been shown to lower fat mass, increase fat-free mass, growth velocity, and resting metabolic rate, and produce positive behavioral–cognitive effects.[14]

A Prader–Willi-like phenotype has been described in five children who share some features with Prader–Willi syndrome patients — obesity, hypotonia, short extremities, and developmental delay.[75] Normal cytogenetic and molecular studies of the 15q11-q13 region ruled out Prader–Willi syndrome, but an interstitial deletion of chromosome 6q16.2 of paternal origin was detected, which includes the *SIMI1* gene.

Angelman Syndrome with Obesity

Angelman syndrome is characterized by severe developmental delay with speech impairment, ataxic gait, and a happy disposition with inappropriate laughter.[76] Loss of maternal expression of *UBE3A*, located in the chromosome region 15q11-q13, results in Angelman syndrome. This can result from large deletions (70%), uniparental paternal disomy (2%), an imprinting defect (4%), or intragenic *UBE3A* mutations (5 to 10%). The remaining group may represent different etiologies. *UBE3A* encodes the E6-AP ubiqitin protein ligase, which marks proteins for degradation. A recent report describes an Angelman syndrome child with an imprinting defect associated with obesity and other clinical features seen in Prader–Willi syndrome patients.[77] Except for cases due to large deletions, one- to two-thirds of Angelman cases are associated with elevated BMI. The lack of an obese phenotype with large deletions might be due to severe underlying motor defects.

DUCHENNE MUSCULAR DYSTROPHY

Duchenne muscular dystrophy (DMD) is an X-linked recessive disease mostly affecting boys.[74] Prevalence is estimated at 1/4000 males.[78] The protein encoded by the *DMD* gene is called dystrophin, which is involved in the contractile apparatus of muscle cells. About 70% of DMD patients have a deletion of one or more exons of the *DMD* gene. Obesity frequently develops in these boys around age 7, resulting from deteriorating muscles being replaced by fat, inactivity, and poor control of dietary intake associated with low IQ. Later in adolescence, undernutrition often develops in greater than 50% of the boys.

ALBRIGHT HEREDITARY OSTEODYSTROPHY

Albright hereditary osteodystrophy is an autosomal dominant disorder due to gene mutations that decrease expression or function of G-alpha-S protein (*GNAS1*). Maternal transmission of the disease results in short stature, obesity, skeletal defects (short stature, brachydactyly), and impaired olfaction. The syndrome also entails resistance to several hormones including parathyroid hormone, which activates G-alpha-S in target tissues (pseudohypoparathyroidism type IA), whereas paternal transmission results only in the pseudohypoparathyroidism. Dysfunction of autonomic pathways in the central nervous system may cause the obesity associated with Albright's syndrome. Decreased β-adrenergic stimulation of adenylate cyclase, which requires Gs activity, is depressed in patients with this syndrome.[72]

FRAGILE X SYNDROME

Fragile X syndrome is caused by mutations in the *FMR1* gene at Xq27.3 and occurs in 1–2/2600 males and 1–2/4100 females.[78] Hypermethylation and silencing of transcription resulting in loss of function are recognized to be the mechanism by which triplet repeats cause this disease. Features include moderate to severe mental retardation, macroorchidism, and facial abnormalities including prominent forehead, square jaw, and large ears. Affected females usually have milder features. The fragile X syndrome is the most common inherited form of mental retardation.

BARDET–BIEDL SYNDROME

Bardet–Biedl syndrome is an autosomal recessive disorder, although approximately 10% of the cases are accounted for by a triallelic mode of inheritance.[79] There are eight known chromosome loci, and mutations have been identified in all of them — *BBS1, BBS2, BBS3, BBS4, BBS5, BBS6, BBS7,* and *BBS8*. However, approximately 50% of BBS patients are unaccounted for by the currently known mutations. There are no apparent differences in the phenotypes caused by mutations at each of the know *BBS* genes, suggesting that the BBS proteins participate in the same biochemical processes. The prevalence is 1/25,000. Bardet–Biedl syndrome is characterized by early-onset obesity, mental retardation, limb defects (syndactyly, brachydactyly, or polydactyly), retinal dystrophy or pigmentary retinopathy, hypogonadism or hypogenitalism, and structural abnormalities of the kidney. The cause of the obesity is unknown; although a hypothalamic deficiency has been suggested, abnormalities in energy metabolism have not been found.

COHEN SYNDROME

Cohen syndrome is characterized by modest obesity, microcephaly, severe mental retardation, short stature, ophthalmopathy, and facial abnormalities including prominent central incisors. Obesity is usually truncal, idiopathic, and nonubiquitous. Mutations in *COH1*, a novel gene on chromosome 8q22, whose function is unknown, cause Cohen syndrome.[80]

ALSTRÖM SYNDROME

Alström syndrome is a multisystem genetic disease manifested by childhood blindness related to retinal degeneration, infantile obesity, nerve deafness, diabetes mellitus with insulin resistance, acanthosis nigricans, chronic nephropathy, and hypogonadism in males but not females. Hyperphagia and obesity begin early in life. Endocrine abnormalities including growth hormone deficiency, hypothyroidism, and hypogonadism have been reported. Mental impairment is described in only a minority of patients. Alström syndrome is attributed to mutations in *ALMS1*, a ubiquitously expressed gene of unknown function.

BORJESON–FORSSMAN–LEHMANN SYNDROME

In addition to obesity, severe mental retardation, hypogonadism, epilepsy, short stature with relative microcephaly, and large fleshy ears characterize this X-linked recessive disorder.[72,73] Onset of obesity is at approximately 8 to 10 years of age. Hypopituitarism and optic nerve hypoplasia suggest a defect of midline development that could involve hypothalamic control of energy balance. Mutations in a gene, located in the Xq26 region coding for the PHF6 zinc-finger protein, cause the Borjeson–Forssman–Lehmann syndrome.[81]

SIMPSON–GOLABI–BEHMEL SYNDROME TYPE 1

Simpson–Golabi–Behmel syndrome (SGB) is an X-linked disorder characterized by generalized prenatal and postnatal overgrowth, macrosomia, mental retardation, coarse facial features, multiple congenital anomalies, and obesity.[82,83] Patients with SGB have macrocephaly, a coarse and stocky appearance with prominent jaw, wide nasal bridge, upturned nose tip, cleft palate, large tongue, lower lip groove, short and broad fingers with postaxial polydactyly, rib anomalies (cervical ribs, 13 pair of ribs, abnormal sternum), supernumerary nipples, congenital heart disease, and central nervous system anomalies (agenesis of the corpus callosum, hypoplasia of the cerebellar vermis, hydrocephalus).

The defect in SGB was mapped in two females with an X-autosomal translocation in which the glypican 3 gene (*GPC3*) was disrupted.[84] The *GPC3* gene encodes a putative extracellular proteoglycan believed to play an important role in growth control in embryonic mesodermal tissues. This protein forms insulinlike growth factor-2 (IGF-2) complex that appears to modulate IGF-2 action. IGF-2 is also implicated in the pathophysiology of other overgrowth conditions as in the case of Beckwith–Wiedemann Syndrome.

ENDOCRINE DISORDERS

Cushing's syndrome, hypothyroidism, hyperadrenocorticism, hypophosphatemic rickets, and growth hormone resistance may be associated with obesity. In contrast to the accelerated growth seen with common childhood obesity, these disorders are usually associated with short stature and growth retardation. The obesity seen with these disorders may be secondary to physical disabilities leading to inactivity or parental overindulgence leading to dietary overconsumption.

TABLE 6.1
Genome-Wide Linkage Studies for BMI in Children and Adolescents

Chromosome Location	LOD Score	Population	N	Candidate Gene	Reference
5q34-q35	2.8 (total)	American	n = 237		87
16p13	3.12 (total)	Caucasian			
16p11.2-p13.1	2.45 (total)				
20p12-p13	3.55 (total)				
20p11.2p	4.08 (total)				
10p	2.24	German	89 families	Glutamic acid	88
			76 families	decarboxylase	
2q33.2-q36.3	3.05, 2.33	French	115 families;	For chr 6:	89
6q22.31-q23.2	4.06, 3.77	Caucasian	n = 506	SIMI1, MCHR2,	
15q12-q15.1	2.53			PC-1	
16q22.1-q24.1	2.54				

GENOME-WIDE SCANS OF OBESITY IN CHILDREN

Genome-wide scans utilize polymorphic markers to identify chromosomal regions that are likely to harbor obesity-susceptibility genes. The technique involves genotyping 300 to 500 highly polymorphic short tandem repeat (STR) markers at regular intervals throughout the genome in sibling pairs or larger families. These markers are highly susceptible to mutations that increase or decrease the number of repeats, and therefore a population accumulates a large number of alleles at these loci that differ in the number of repeats present. Linkage analysis is performed to identify the chromosomal regions or alleles that affected obese family members share more commonly than would be expected by chance. The statistical probability of allele sharing is expressed as the log of the odds (LOD) score.

The genes that influence body weight in childhood may not be the same as those that are relevant in adults. Expression of genes influencing adiposity may be sex- and age-dependent. During periods of cell differentiation and proliferation, specific genes may interact with hormones and growth factors to promote excess fat mass.[85] Selected genes may play a role in the development of obesity and adipose cell differentiation such as PPAR-γ, C/EBP transcription factors, and HMG1-C DNA binding protein.[86]

Three genomic scans aimed at identifying obesity-related genes in children have been published (Table 6.1). A genomic scan was performed on 1909 individuals from 255 three-generation pedigrees participating in the Rochester Family Heart Study.[87] Linkage to BMI was detected on 1p36 in all sib pairs. Age-stratification identified a number of regions showing linkage with BMI in the younger children. In the 237 children aged 5 to 11 years, linkage to BMI was seen on 5q34-q35, 16p13, 16p11.2-p13.1, 20p12-p13, and 20p11.2p. Six regions displayed evidence for imprinting of BMI in children: 3p23-p24 (paternal expression), 4q31.1-q32 (maternal expression), 10p14-q11 (paternal expression), and 12p12-pter (paternal expression). Because imprinted genes are involved in many aspects of growth and development, imprinting may affect traits related to childhood obesity.

Another genomic scan was conducted in two sets of 89 and 76 German families with two or more obese children.[88] Three regions provided evidence for linkage with LOD scores of 1.65 to 2.24 on 10p11.23, 11q11-q13.1, and 19p13-q12. Peaks on chromosomes 10p and 11q coincide with linkage findings from genomic scans of obese European adults and harbor candidate genes for glutamic acid dehydrogenase 2, angiotensin receptor-like 1, ciliary neurotrophic factor, galanin, UCP2, and UCP3.

A genomic scan in 506 individuals from 115 French Caucasian families with at least one obese proband found significant linkage with obesity on 6q22.31-q23.2.[89] Within this region are the strong candidate obesity genes — *SIM1*, melanocortin concentrating hormone receptor 2 (*MCHR2*), and the plasma cell membrane glycoprotein (*PC-1*).

While the results from these studies appear modest, they do represent the first efforts to identify specific genes involved in the development of childhood obesity. It is encouraging that at least several of the regions identified appear to correspond to regions previously identified in genome scans for obesity-related traits in adults. However, additional work perhaps in larger and/or more complex samples of children will yet reveal genes with unique influence on the development of childhood obesity.

CANDIDATE GENE STUDIES IN CHILDREN

Based on known roles in energy homeostasis or sequence variations associated with human obesity, a number of putative susceptibility genes have been identified. Studies testing for associations between candidate genes and obesity-related phenotypes have been conducted in several pediatric studies.[71] While a role of these candidate genes in the development or expression of obesity-related phenotypes can be posited based on their known or suspected physiological role, the magnitude of their impact at the population level remains to be demonstrated.

3-ADRENERGIC RECEPTOR (*ADRB3*)

ADRB3 is located on chromosome 8p12-p11 and is expressed primarily in visceral adipose tissue. It is involved in regulation of lipid metabolism and thermogenesis. A common missense mutation is where tryptophan is substituted by arginine at codon 64 (Tryp64Arg) in the *ADRB3* gene. The BMI of obese Japanese children with the Trp/Arg or Arg/Arg (19.4 kg/m2) genotypes was significantly higher than that of those with the Trp/Trp genotype (18.9 kg/m^2).[90] Obese Finnish subjects carrying the Arg64 allele developed obesity more often before age 15 than those without it.[91] Trp64Arg mutation was not found to be a major factor affecting obesity in Chinese children.[92]

PEROXISOME PROLIFERATOR ACTIVATED RECEPTOR GAMMA (PPAR-γ)

PPAR-γ is a nuclear receptor located on chromosome 3p25, involved in adipogenesis and insulin signaling. A common variant, in which a proline is substituted for alanine at codon 12 of the γ2 isoform, results in decreased binding of the receptor to PPAR-γ responsive elements. The Pro12Ala mutation was associated with early-onset obesity.[93] The Pro12Ala mutation was observed more frequently in obese individuals with obesity onset in early adulthood than in normal weight individuals (29% vs. 15%; $P = .05$).

ADIPONECTIN (APM1)

Adiponectin is an adipocyte-derived protein with insulin-sensitizing and anti-inflammatory properties. Plasma adiponectin has been shown to be inversely correlated with BMI, body fat, fasting insulin, blood pressure, and plasma lipids. *APM1* is located on chromosome 3q27, a region in which linkage to BMI has been replicated. A silent substitution (T/G) at nucleotide 94 was associated with increased BMI in carriers of the G allele.[94]

Ghrelin (GHRL)

GHRL is an orexigenic hormone, which activates NPY/AgRP neurons in the ARC. GHRL increases short-term food intake in rodents and may decrease energy expenditure and fat catabolism.[2] Circulating GHRL levels are negatively correlated with BMI, implying a compensatory rather than a causal role in common obesity. Children with Prader–Willi syndrome have markedly elevated plasma ghrelin levels, possibly contributing to the associated hyperphagia and obesity.[95] In a study of 300 obese Italian children, two previously described polymorphisms were replicated; one (Leu72Met) was associated with earlier onset of childhood obesity.[96] This common polymorphism has been confirmed in obese French children,[97] but not obese German children.[96] This polymorphism also was associated with high BMI and lower insulin secretion in tall, obese French children.[97]

Uncoupling Proteins (UCP)

Uncoupling proteins (UCPs) are mitochondrial transporters that uncouple cellular respiration, releasing stored energy as heat. Genetic variants in the coding region of *UCP1* gene are not a common factor contributing to juvenile-onset obesity in the Danish population.[98] Neither were variants in the coding region of the *UCP3* gene, which is expressed primarily in skeletal muscle, found to contribute to obesity.[99] In 105 children aged 6 to 10 years, a polymorphism of *UCP2* (exon 8 ins/del) was found to be associated with higher BMI and body fat.[100]

Pro-Opiomelanocortin (POMC)

Mutations in the *POMC* coding region in Italian children with very early onset obesity were identified.[101] Mutations in codons 7 and 9 of the signal peptide may alter the translocation of pre-POMC into the endoplasmic reticulum.

CONCLUSION

In summary, obesity is a complex disease with multiple etiologies. The current surge in obesity in the United States is due to an interaction between a genetic predisposition toward efficient energy storage and a permissive environment of readily available food and sedentary behaviors. At different times of life, the relative influence of genes, development, and environment may vary. Genes that mediate susceptibility to obesity during development may affect energy intake, energy expenditure, and partitioning of energy to fat and lean tissues during development. The complex patterns of inheritance, the causative genes, and underlying mechanisms of childhood obesity are being unraveled through genomics, quantitative genetics, biochemistry, human physiology, and molecular epidemiology.

RESEARCH NEEDS

1. A greater understanding of the role of the intrauterine environment and gene-environment interactions on programming later obesity is needed.
2. Identification of the major genes regulating growth and maturation and gene-environment interactions affecting critical periods of adiposity development is needed.
3. Development of gene arrays is needed to identify monogenic and syndromic forms of early-onset obesity that could be used clinically in the classification and treatment of childhood obesity.
4. Genomic scans with sufficient sample size and appropriate sampling schemes are needed to identify major gene loci influencing childhood obesity.

5. Positional candidate gene research will be needed to identify the polymorphisms responsible for the heightened susceptibility to childhood obesity in human populations.

References

1. Comuzzie AG, Williams JT, Martin LJ, Blangero J. Searching for genes underlying normal variation in human adiposity. *J Mol Med.* 2001;79: 57–70.
2. Cummings DE, Schwartz MW. Genetics and pathophysiology of human obesity. *Annu Rev Med.* 2003;54: 453–471.
3. Oken E, Gillman MW. Fetal origins of obesity. *Obes Res.* 2003;11: 496–506.
4. Whitaker RC, Dietz WH. Role of the prenatal environment in the development of obesity. *J Pediatr.* 1998;132: 768–776.
5. Bartolomei MS, Tilghman SM. Genomic imprinting in mammals. *Annu Rev Genet.* 1997;31: 493–525.
6. Lawler SD, Povey S, Fisher RA, Pickthall VJ. Genetic studies on hydatidiform moles. II. The origin of complete moles. *Ann Hum Genet.* 1982;46: 209–222.
7. Jacobs PA, Szulman AE, Funkhouser J, Matsuura JS, Wilson CC. Human triploidy: relationship between parental origin of the additional haploid complement and development of partial hydatidiform mole. *Ann Hum Genet.* 1982;46: 223–231.
8. Barton SC, Surani MA, Norris ML. Role of paternal and maternal genomes in mouse development. *Nature.* 1984;311: 374–376.
9. Allison DB, Paultre F, Heymsfield SB, Pi-Sunyer FX. Is the intra-uterine period *really* a critical period for the development of adiposity? *Int J Obes.* 1995;19: 397–402.
10. Charney E, Goodman HC, McBride M, Lyon B, Pratt R. Childhood antecedents of adult obesity. Do chubby infants become obese adults? *N Engl J Med.* 1976;295: 6–9.
11. Braddon FEM, Rodgers B, Wadsworth MEJ, Davies JMC. Onset of obesity in a 36 year birth cohort study. *BMJ.* 1986;293: 299–303.
12. Rolland-Cachera MF, Deheeger M, Guilloud-Bataille M, Avons P, Sempe M. Tracking the devleopment of obesity from one month of age to adulthood. *Ann Hum Biol.* 1987;14: 219–29.
13. Garn SM, LaVelle M. Two-decade follow-up of fatness in early childhood. *Am J Dis Childhood.* 1995;139: 181–185.
14. Astrup A. Obesity in children and young people. A crisis in public health. *Obesity Rev.* 2004;5: 1–104.
15. Forbes GB. Lean body mass and fat in obese children. *Pediatrics.* 1964;308–314.
16. Rolland-Cachera MF, Deheeger M, Bellisle F, Sempé M, Guilloud-Bataille M, Patois E. Adiposity rebound in children: a simple indicator for predicting obesity. *Am J Clin Nutr.* 1984;39: 129–135.
17. Siervogel RM, Roche AF, Guo S, Mukherje ED, Chumlea WC. Patterns of change in weight/stature^2 from 2 to 18 years: findings from long-term serial data for children, in the Fels Longitudinal Growth Study. *Int J Obes.* 1991;15: 479–485.
18. van Lenthe FJ, Kemper HCG, van Mechelen W. Rapid maturation in adolescence results in greater obesity in adulthood: The Amsterdam Growth and Health Study. *Am J Clin Nutr.* 1996;64: 18–24.
19. Falconer DS, Mackay TFC. *Introduction to Quantitative Genetics,* 4th ed. Englewood Cliffs, NJ: Prentice-Hall, 1996.
20. Lynch M, Walsh B. *Genetics and Analysis of Quantitative Traits.* Sunderland, MA: Sinauer, 1998.
21. Price RA, Stunkard AJ, Ness R, Wadden T, Heshka S, Kanders B, Cormillot A. Childhood onset (age <10) obesity has high familial risk. *Int J Obes.* 1990;14: 185–195.
22. Fisler JS, Warden CH. Mapping of mouse obesity genes: a generic approach to a complex trait. *J Nutr.* 1997;127: 1909S–1916S.
23. Province MA, Arnqvist P, Keller J, Higgins M, Rao DC. Strong evidence for a major gene for obesity in the large, unselected, total Community Healthy Study of Tecumseh. *Am J Hum Genet.* 1990;47: A143.
24. Moll PP, Burns TL, Lauer RM. The genetic and environmental sources of body mass index variability: the Muscatine Family Ponderosity Study. *Am J Hum Genet.* 1991;49: 1243–1255.
25. Hasstedt SJ, Ramirez ME, Kuida H, Williams RR. Recessive inheritance of a relative fat pattern. *Am J Hum Genet.* 1989;45: 917–925.

26. Borecki IB, Rice T, Perusse L, Bouchard C, Rao DC. Major gene influence on the propensity to store fat in trunk versus extremity depots: evidence from the Quebec Family Study. *Obes Res*. 1995;3: 1–8.

27. Rice T, Borecki IB, Bouchard C, Rao DC. Segregation analysis of fat mass and other body composition measures derived from underwater weighing. *Am J Hum Genet*. 1993;52: 967–973.

28. Comuzzie AG, Blangero J, Mahaney MC, Mitchell BD, Stern MP, MacCluer JW. The quantitative genetics of sexual dimorphism in body fat measurements. *Am J Hum Biol*. 1993;5: 725–734.

29. Comuzzie AG, Blangero J, Mahaney MC, Mitchell BD, Stern MP, MacCluer JW. Genetic and environmental correlations among skinfold measures. *Int J Obes*. 1994;18: 413–418.

30. Comuzzie AG, Blangero J, Mahaney MC, Mitchell BD, Hixson JE, Samollow PB, et al. Major gene with sex-specific effects influences fat mass in Mexican Americans. *Genet Epidemiol*. 1995;12: 475–488.

31. Comuzzie AG, Blangero J, Mahaney MC. Genetic and environmental correlations among hormone levels and measures of body fat accumulation and topography. *J Clin Endocrinol Metab*. 1996;81: 597–600.

32. Comuzzie AG, Hixson JE, Almasy L, Mitchell BD, Mahaney MC, Dyer TD, et al. A major quantitative trait locus determining serum leptin levels and fat mass is located on human chromosome 2. *Nat Genet*. 1997;15: 273–276.

33. Mitchell BD, Kammerer CM, Blangero J, Mahaney MC, Rainwater DL, Dyke B, et al. Genetic and environmental contributions to cardiovascular risk factors in Mexican Americans: the San Antonio Family Heart Study. *Circulation*. 1996;94: 2159–2170.

34. Burns TL, Moll PP, Lauer RM. Cardiovascular risk factor levels and a gene for obesity: the Muscatine Ponderosity Family Study. *Circulation*. 1989;80(Suppl 2): II–82.

35. Price RA, Ness R, Laskarzewski P. Common major gene inheritance of extreme overweight. *Hum Biol*. 1990;62: 747–765.

36. Province MA, Keller J, Higgins M, Rao DC. A commingling analysis of obesity in the Tecumsch community health study. *Am J Hum Biol*. 1991;3: 435–445.

37. Kammerer CM, Mitchell BD, Stern MP. Preliminary evidence that major genes affect two-hour insulin levels and body mass index in Mexican Americans. *Am J Hum Genet*. 1992;51(Suppl): A152.

38. Gage TB, Blangero J, Mitchell BD, Stern MP, MacCluer JW. Segregation analysis of body mass index incorporating nutritional covariates and gentoype by sex interactions. *Am J Hum Genet*. 1993;53(Suppl); A1649.

39. Hebebrand J, Sommerlad C, Geller F, Görg T, Hinney A. The genetics of obesity: practical implications. *Int J Obes*. 2001;25: S10–S18.

40. Faith MS, Pietrobelli A, Nuñez C, Heo M, Heymsfield SB, Allison DB. Evidence for independent genetic influences on fat mass and body mass index in a pediatric twin sample. *Pediatrics*. 1999;104: 61–67.

41. Bodurtha JN, Mosteller M, Hewitt JK, Nance WE, Eaves LJ, Moskowitz WB, et al. Genetic analysis of anthropometric measures in 11-year-old twins: The Medical College of Virginia Twin Study. *Pediatr Res*. 1990;28: 1–4.

42. Allison DB, Heshka S, Neale MC, Heymsfield SB. Race effects in the genetics of adolescents' body mass index. *Int J Obes*. 1994;18: 363–368.

43. Beunen G, Maes HHM, Vlietinck R, Malina RM, Thomis M, Feyes E, et al. Univariate and multivariate genetic analysis of subcutaneous fat distribution in early adolescence. *Behav Genet*. 1998;28: 279–288.

44. Meyer JM, Silberg JL, Eaves LJ, Maes HH, Simonoff E, Pickles A, Rutter ML, Hewitt JK. Variable age of gene expression: Implications for developmental genetic models. In: LaBuda MC, Grigorenko EL, Eds. *On the Way to Individuality: Methodological Issues in Behavioral Genetics*. Commack, NY: Nova Science Publications, 1999.

45. Czerwinski SA, Towne B, Williams JT, Wisemandle WA, Demerath EW, Chumlea WC, et al. Childhood growth and adult overweight risk: a quantitative genetic analysis. In: Gilli G, Schell LM, Benso L, Eds. *Human Growth from Conception to Maturity*. London: Smith-Gordon, 2002: 125–131.

46. Grilo CM, Pogue-Geile MF. The nature of environmental influences on weight and obesity: a behavior genetic analysis. *Psychol Bull*. 1991;110: 520–537.

47. Hewitt JK. The genetics of obesity: What have genetic studies told us about the environment? *Behav Genet*. 1997;27: 353–358.

48. Guillaume M, Björntorp P. Obesity in children. Environmental and genetic aspects. *Horm Metab Res.* 1996;28: 573–581.

49. Cardon LR. Genetic influences on body mass index in early childhood. In: Turner JR, Cardon LR, Hewitt JK, Eds. *Behavioral Genetic Approaches in Behavioral Medicine.* New York: Plenum, 1995: 133–143.

50. Plomin R, Corley R, DeFries JC, Fulker DW. Individual differences in television viewing in early childhood: *Nature* as well as nurture. *Psychol Sci.* 1990;1: 371–377.

51. Boomsma DI, van den Bree MB, Orlebeke JF, Molenar PC. Resemblance of parents and twins in sports participation and heart rate. *Behav Genet.* 1989;19: 123–141.

52. Farooqi IS, Matarese G, Lord GM, Keogh JM, Lawrence E, Agwu C, et al. Beneficial effects of leptin on obesity, T cell hyporesponsiveness, and neuroendocrine/metabolic dysfunction of human congenital leptin deficiency. *J Clin Invest.* 2002;110: 1093–1103.

53. Montague CT, Farooql S, Whitehead JP, Soos MA, Rau H, Wareham NJ, et al. Congenital leptin deficiency is associated with severe early-onset obesity in humans. *Nature.* 1997;387: 903–908.

54. Strobel A, Issad T, Camoin L, Ozata M, Strosberg AD. A leptin missense mutation associated with hypogonadism and morbid obesity. *Nat Genet.* 1998;18: 213–215.

55. Ozata M, Ozdemir IC, Licinio J. Human leptin deficiency caused by a missense mutation: multiple endocrine defects, decreased sympathetic tone, and immune system dysfunction indicate new targets for leptin action, greater central than peripheral resistance to the effects of leptin, and spontaneous correction of leptin-mediated defects. *J Clin Endocrinol Metab.* 1999;84: 3686–3695.

56. Farooqi IS, Jebb SA, Langmack G, Lawrence E, Cheetham CH, Prentice AM, et al. Effects of recombinant leptin therapy in a child with congenital leptin deficiency. *N Engl J Med.* 1999;341: 879–884.

57. Clement K, Vaisse C, Lahlou N, Cabrol S, Pelloux V, Cassuto D, Gourmelen M, Dina C, Chambaz J, Lacorte JM, Basdevant A, Bougneres P, Lebouc Y, Froguel P, Guy-Grand B. A mutation in the human leptin receptor gene causes obesity and pituitary dysfunction. *Nature.* 1998;392: 398–401.

58. Krude H, Biebermann H, Luck W, Horn R, Brabant G, Gruters A. Severe early-onset obesity, adrenal insufficiency and red hair pigmentation caused by POMC mutations in humans. *Nat Genet.* 1998;19: 155–157.

59. Krude H, Biebermann H, Schnabel D, Tansek MZ, Theunissen P, Mullis PE, Gruters A. Obesity due to proopiomelanocortin deficiency: three new cases and treatment trials with thyroid hormone and ACTH4-10. *J Clin Endocrinol Metab.* 2003;88: 4633–4640.

60. Challis BG, Pritchard LE, Creemers JW, Delplanque J, Keogh JM, Luan J, et al. A missense mutation disrupting a dibasic prohormone processing site in pro-opimeolanocortin (POMC) increases susceptibility to early-onset obesity through a novel molecular mechanism. *Hum Mol Genet.* 2002;11: 1997–2004.

61. Jackson RS, Creemers JWM, Ohagi S, Raffin-Sanson M-L, Sanders L, Montague CT, et al. Obesity and impaired prohormone processing associated with mutations in the human prohormone convertase 1 gene. *Nat Genet.* 1997;16: 303–306.

62. Jackson RS, Creemers JW, Farooqi IS, Raffin-Sanson M-L, Varro A, Dockray GJ, et al. Small-intestinal dysfunction accompanies the complex endocrinopathy of human proprotein convertase 1 deficiency. *J Clin Invest.* 2003;112: 1550–1560.

63. Yeo GS, Lank EJ, Farooqi IS, Keogh J, Challis BG, O'Rahilly S. Mutations in the human melanocortin-4 receptor gene associated with severe familial obesity disrupts receptor function through multiple molecular mechanisms. *Hum Mol Genet.* 2003;12: 561–574.

64. Yeo GS, Farooqi IS, Aminian S, Halsall DJ, Stanhope RG, O'Rahilly S. A frameshift mutation in MC4R associated with dominantly inherited human obesity. *Nat Genet.* 1998;20: 111–112.

65. Vaisse C, Clement K, Guy-Grand B, Froguel P. A frameshift mutation in human Mc4R is associated with a dominant form of obesity. *Nat Genet.* 1998;20: 113–114.

66. Farooqi IS, Keogh JM, Yeo GSH, Lank EJ, Cheetham T, O'Rahilly S. Clinical spectrum of obesity and mutations in the melanocortin 4 receptor gene. *N Engl J Med.* 2003;348: 1085–1095.

67. Coll AP, Farooqi IS, Challis BG, Yeo GSH, O'Rahilly S. Proopiomelanocortin and energy balance: insights from human and murine genetics. *J Clin Endocrinol Metab.* 2004;89: 2557–2562.

68. Tao Y-X, Segaloff DL. Functional characterization of melanocortin-4 receptor mutations associated with childhood obesity. *Endocrinology.* 2003;144: 4544–4551.

69. Holder JL, Butte NF, Zinn AR. Profound obesity associated with a balanced translocation that disrupts the SIM1 gene. *Hum Mol Genet*. 2000;9: 101–108.

70. Holder JL, Jr., Zhang L, Kublaoui BM, DiLeone RJ, Oz OK, Bair CH, et al. *Sim 1* gene dosage modulates the homeostatic feeding response to increased dietary fat in mice. *Am J Physiol Endocrinol Metab*. 2004;287: E105–E113.

71. Snyder EE, Walts B, Perusse L, Chagnon YC, Weisnagel J, Rankinen T, Bouchard C. The human obesity gene map: the 2003 update. *Obes Res*. 2004;12: 369–439.

72. Deirue M-A, Michaud JL. Fat chance: genetic syndromes with obesity. *Clin Genet*. 2004;66: 83–93.

73. Stefan M, Nicholls RD. What have rare genetic syndromes taught us about the pathophysiology of the common forms of obesity? *Curr Diabetes Rep*. 2004;4: 143–150.

74. Gelehrter TD, Collins FS, Ginsburg D. *Principles in Medical Genetics*. Baltimore: Williams & Wilkins, 1998.

75. Faivre L, Cormier-Daire V, Lapierre JM, Colleaux L, Jacquemont S, Genevieve D, et al. Deletion of the SIM1gene (6q16.2) in a patient with a Prader–Willi-like phenotype. *J Med Genet*. 2004;39: 594–596.

76. Williams CA, Angelman H, Clayton-Smith J, Driscoll DJ, Hendrickson JE, Knoll JH, et al. Angelman syndrome: consensus for diagnostic criteria. Angelman Syndrome Foundation. *Am J Med Genet*. 1995;56: 237–238.

77. Gillessen-Kaesbach G, Demuth S, Theile J, Lich C, Horsthemke B. A previously unrecognised phenotype characterised by obesity, muscular hypotonia, and ability to speak in patients with Angelman syndrome caused by an imprinting defect. *Eur J Hum Genet*. 1999;7. 638 644.

78. Scriver CR, Beaudet AL, Sly WS, Valle D. *The Metabolic Basis of Inherited Disease*, 6th ed. New York: McGraw-Hill, 1989.

79. Katsanis N, Ansley SJ, Badano JL, Eichers ER, Lewis RA, Hoskins BE, et al. Triallelic inheritance in Bardet–Biedl syndrome, a Mendelian recessive disorder. *Science*. 2001;293: 2256–2259.

80. Kolehmainen J, Black GC, Saarinen A, Chandler K, Clayton-Smith J, Traskelin AL, et al. Cohen syndrome is caused by mutations in a novel gene, COH1, encoding a transmembrane protein with a presumed role in vesicle-mediated sorting and intracellular protein transport. *Am J Hum Genet*. 2003;72: 1359–1369.

81. Lower KM, Turner G, Kerr BA, Matthews KD, Shaw MA, Gedeon AK, et al. Mutations in PHF6 are associated with Borjeson–Forssman–Lehmann syndrome. *Am J Hum Genet*. 2002;32: 661–665.

82. Simpson JL, Landey S, New M, German J. A previously unrecognized X-linked syndrome of dysmorphia. *Birth Defects Original Article Series XI*. 1975;2: 18–24.

83. Garganta CL, Bodurtha JN. Report of another family with Simpson–Golabi–Behmel syndrome and a review of the literature. *Am J Med Genet*. 1992;44. 129 135.

84. Pilia G, Hughes-Benzie RM, MacKenzie A, Baybayan P, Chen EY, Huber R, et al. Mutations in GPC3, a glypican gene, cause the Simpson–Golabi–Behmel overgrowth syndrome. *Nat Genet*. 1996;12: 241–247.

85. Prins JB, O'Rahilly S. Regulation of adipose cell number in man. *Clin Sci*. 1997;92: 3–11.

86. Guerre-Millo M, Staels B, Auwerx J. New insights into obesity genes. *Diabetologia*. 1996;39: 1528–1531.

87. Gorlova OY, Amos CI, Wang NW, Sanjay S, Turner ST, Boerwinkle E. Genetic linkage and imprinting effects on body mass index in children and young adults. *Eur J Hum Genet*. 2003;11: 425–432.

88. Saar K, Geller F, Ruschendorf F, Reis A, Friedel S, Schauble N, et al. Genome scan for childhood and adolescent obesity in German families. *Pediatrics*. 2003;111: 321–327.

89. Meyre D, Lecoeur C, Delplanque J, Francke S, Vatin V, Durand E, et al. A genome-wide scan for childhood obesity — associated traits in French fmailies shows significant linkage on chromosome 6q22.31-q23.2. *Diabetes*. 2004;53: 803–811.

90. Endo K, Yanagi H, Hirano C, Hamaguchi H, Tsuchiya S, Tomura S. Association of Trp64Arg polymorphism of the beta3-adrenergic receptor gene and no association of Gln223Arg polymorphism of the leptin receptor gene in Japanese schoolchildren with obesity. *Int J Obes Relat Metab Disord*. 2000;24: 443–449.

91. Oksanen L, Mustajoki P, Kaprio J, Kainulainen K, Janne O, Peltonen L, Kontula K. Polymorphism of the beta 3-adrenergic receptor gene in morbid obesity. *Int J Obes Relat Metab Disord*. 1996;20: 1055–1061.

92. Xinli W, Xiaomei T, Meihua P, Song L. Association of a mutation in the beta3-adrenergic receptor gene with obesity and response to dietary intervention in Chinese children. *Acta Paediatr.* 2001;90: 1233–1237.

93. Vaccaro O, Mancini FP, Ruffa G, Sabatino L, Colantuoni V, Riccardi G. Pro12Ala mutation in the peroxisome proliferator-activated receptor gamma2 (PPARgamma2) and severe obesity: a case-control study. *Int J Obes Relat Metab Disord.* 2000;24: 1195–1199.

94. Stumvoll M, Tschritter O, Fritsche A, Staiger H, Renn W, Weisser M, et al. Association of the T-G polymorphism in adiponectin (Exon 2) with obesity and insulin sensitivity. Interaction with family history of type 2 diabetes. *Diabetes.* 2002;51: 37–41.

95. Cummings DE, Clement K, Purnell JQ, Vaisse C, Foster KE, Frayo RS, et al. Elevated plasma ghrelin levels in Prader Willi syndrome. *Nat Med.* 2002;8: 643–644.

96. Hinney A, Hoch A, Geller F, Schafer H, Siegfried W, Goldschmidt H, et al. Ghrelin gene: identification of missense variants and a frameshift mutation in extremely obese children and adolescents and healthy normal weight students. *J Clin Endocrinology Metab.* 2002;87: 2716.

97. Korbonits M, Gueorguiev M, O'Grady E, Lecoeur C, Swan DC, Mein CA, et al. A variation in the ghrelin gene increases weight and decreases insulin secretion in tall, obese children. *J Clin Endocrinol Metab.* 2002;87: 4005–4008.

98. Urhammer SA, Fridberg M, Sorensen TIA, Echwald SM, Andersen T, Tybjærg-Hansen A, et al. Studies of genetic variability of the uncoupling protein 1 gene in Caucasian subjects with juvenile-onset obesity. *J Clin Endocrinol Metab.* 1997;82: 4069–4074.

99. Urhammer SA, Dalgaard LT, Sorensen TIA, Tybjærg-Hansen A, Echwald SM, Andersen T, Clausen JO, Pedersen O. Organisation of the coding exons and mutational screening of the uncoupling protein 3 gene in subjects with juvenile-onset obesity. *Diabetologia.* 1998;41: 241–244.

100. Yanovski JA, Diament AL, Sovik KN, Nguyen TT, Hongzhe L, Sebring NG, Warden CH. Associations between uncoupling protein 2, body composition, and resting energy expenditure in lean and obese African American, white, and Asian children. *Am J Clin Nutr.* 2000;71: 1405–1420.

101. Miraglia del Giudice E, Cirillo G, Santoro N, D'Urso L, Carbone MT, Di Toro R, Perrone L. Molecular screening of the proopiomelanocortin (POMC) gene in Italian obese children: report of three new mutations. *Int J Obes Relat Metab Disord.* 2001;25: 61–67.

7 Energy Expenditure and Body Composition Techniques

Angelo Pietrobelli and David A. Fields

CONTENTS

INTRODUCTION

Physical changes that occur throughout childhood are generally related to growth and chemical maturation.[1] Growth and maturation are complex biological processes influenced by multiple factors including genetics, environment (e.g., life style), demography (age, gender, and race), hormones, and health status. All of these factors influence a child's height and body composition during the growth years. Clinical assessment of growth and maturation may be enhanced by accurate measurement of body composition. However, body composition measurement techniques used in adults are not always directly applicable to the pediatric population.

Body composition analysis in children provides a window into the complex changes that occur throughout childhood and provides the opportunity for metabolic and physiological correlations. Once body composition measurements are determined in a large population of healthy children, it will be possible to attain a greater understanding of the normal compartmental changes that occur during growth and development, and the effects of disease and medication on body composition. Additionally, longitudinal body composition and energy expenditure studies will help to clarify the relationship between childhood body composition and diseases that appear in adults. No matter the reasons for assessing body composition and the factors influencing energy expenditure, nutritionists and clinicians in health-related fields should have a general understanding of body composition and energy expenditure measurements methods as they apply to a pediatric population.

This chapter examines issues and techniques specifically related to a pediatric population in the field of body composition and energy expenditure. The chapter is broadly divided into two sections. The first section discusses body composition measurements — underlying principles, advantages, disadvantages, and consensus. The second section reviews energy expenditure measurements techniques. In conclusion, more fundamental theoretical issues for future research in the field of body composition and energy expenditure with children and adolescents are examined.

BODY COMPOSITION

Body composition studies include quantification and distribution of fat and fat-free mass (FFM), and their variation as a function of gender, race, and age. Quantifying the main components of the body is fundamental to describing deficiency or excess that has associations with the risk or onset of disease. Measurement of body mass in children is extremely challenging because we do not have direct measurements except *in vivo* neutron activation analysis and chemical analysis of the cadaver. There are, however, several indirect methods for measuring fat and fat-free mass, all of which have assumptions and age-specific considerations. In the following sections we review pertinent techniques that are considered appropriate for research and clinical application in children.

ANTHROPOMETRY

Anthropometry represents a group of inexpensive, noninvasive methods available to assess size, shape, limb lengths, circumferences, and breadths of the human body. These measurements could be used as markers of adiposity and fat distribution. However, these measurements in a pediatric population may be of limited utility.

Body Mass Index (BMI)

Among several weight for height indices reported in the pediatric literature, Quetelet's body mass index (BMI),[2] weight in kilogram divided height in meter squared (BMI = kg/m^2), may provide childhood fat estimates in large epidemiological studies.[3] BMI shows significant variations during childhood, which is why age and gender specific reference standards must be used. In adolescents, the pubertal status should also be evaluated. Pediatric population–based BMI reference curves are available for children from the United States,[4] Britain,[5] Sweden,[6] China,[7] the Netherlands,[8] and Italy[9] among others. Recently Cole and colleagues[10] proposed a definition using sex- and age-specific percentiles of the BMI pooled from several nationally representative data sets. In that paper, overweight equivalent in children corresponds to the cutoff in adults — a BMI at or above 25.0. A consensus has also been reached that the obesity equivalent corresponds to a BMI at or above 30.0 in adults.[10]

Weight and height reference charts are important for monitoring excess weight and, subsequently, fatness. However, BMI lacks adequate sensitivity and/or specificity in defining a single child as obese or normal weight.[11] It is important also to emphasize that the relation between BMI and adiposity is independently influenced by height, weight, gender, age, ethnicity, and fat distribution.[11,12] BMI reflects both fat and fat-free mass and is not a direct measure of adiposity; thus, it is not a qualitative measure (i.e., it does not reflect percent body fat) of overall body weight.

There is a good correlation between fat and BMI in groups, but the variation is large and BMI cannot predict fatness in individual subjects. BMI may be a surrogate measurement of adiposity, but it lacks adequate sensitivity and specificity, and a child could be misclassified as obese or nonobese.

Recently we validated the new growth charts from the Center for Disease Control and Prevention (CDC) and sex-specific BMI ranges-for-age and compared their performance (i.e., sensitivity and specificity) with that of the Rohrer index-for-age (RI: weight [kg]/height^3 [m^3]) and weight-for-height in screening both underweight and overweight in children aged 2 to 19 years. We found that the CDC's BMI-for-age is better than the Rohrer index-for-age in predicting both underweight and overweight but is similar to that of weight-for-height in the studied population.[13] In another study we tested the short-term stability of BMI, BMI z-scores, and BMI percentiles in a group of 135 preschool children. Across the three weight fluctuation metrics, BMI percentiles were more variable among nonobese than obese children and BMI z-scores were more variable among nonobese girls than obese girls. The stability of BMI was unrelated to child obesity status.[14] The principal finding of our study was that for certain BMI-based measures of adiposity, variability in adiposity depends on baseline adiposity status, while for other measures it did not. Specifically, variability in BMI was unrelated to baseline adiposity, whereas variability in BMI z-score and BMI percentile was highly significantly and inversely related to adiposity status. These results suggest that short-term changes in adiposity are best evaluated by changes in BMI units.[14]

Skinfolds

A long-standing method for determining body density, FFM, fat mass, and percent body fat (%BF) is skinfold measurement. This method is widely applied and can be used alone in evaluating nutritional status or incorporated into prediction equation formulas for body component estimation.[15] This technique uses special calipers to "pinch" and ascertain the thickness of skinfold at specific body sites.[16] The most useful skinfold thickness in pediatric populations is the triceps and subscapular sites. The anatomic reference for subscapular thickness is the inferior angle of the scapula and the fold is along the natural cleavage line of skin just inferior to the inferior angle of scapula, with the caliper placement approximately 1 cm below the fingers. The anatomical reference of triceps thickness is the acromial process of the scapula and olecranon process of the ulna. The distance between these two processes is measured using a tape measure on lateral aspect of arm with elbow flexed 90°; the midpoint is marked on lateral site of arm with the fold lifted 1 cm above the marked line on the posterior aspect of the arm with the caliper applied at the marked level.[16]

Age- and race-specific equations for estimating body fat were developed by Slaughter et al.,[17] using multicompartment model reference measures. These equations used the sum of two skinfolds (triceps + subscapular and triceps + calf) to predict body fatness with the prediction error ranging from 3.6 to 3.9% in boys and girls 8 to 17 years of age.[17] One must keep in mind that the skinfold thicknesses taken at different sites correlates differently with %BF and total fat;[17,18] triceps has a better correlation with %BF while subscapular skinfolds correlate better with total body fat mass. These measurements are useful indicators because of their relationships with risk factors. Centile charts for triceps and subscapular skinfolds have been published for several countries (e.g., United Kingdom, United States, and France) and are used to assess the body composition, specifically %BF in boys and girls.

Circumferences

Pediatric body composition can be estimated by measuring the size and proportion of the human body. For this reason circumferences and skeletal breadth measurements are used. This method is based on the principle that circumferences reflect fat mass (FM) and FFM, and skeletal size is related to lean body mass.[19] Circumferences at the waist, hip, and thigh are used to predict body fat distribution, and those of the waist and hip are good predictors of intraabdominal fat.[20] Waist circumference is associated with cardiovascular risk factors[21] and with metabolic syndrome.[22] Fernandez et al.[23] provided the distribution of waist circumferences among children aged 2 to 18 years in nationally representative samples of three major ethnic groups (African-American, Hispanic, and European-American) in term of percentile — 10, 25, 50, and 90. For a detailed report of the percentile distribution of waist circumferences, the reader is directed to Fernandez et al.[23]

Near-Infrared Interactance

The near-infrared interactance (NIR) method was originally developed for use in agriculture to measure the protein, fat, and water composition of grains and seeds[24] using a high-precision spectrophotometer. Investigators later discovered that the fat and water content of human tissues could be measured by using lower wavelengths than those used to assess agricultural products.[25] The degree of infrared light absorbed and reflected is related to the composition of the tissues through which the light is passing and to specific wavelength of the near-infrared light. Peak absorption wavelengths for pure fat and pure water are known, and the shape of the interactance curve is a function of the amount of fat and water present in the sample being measured.[25] The NIR instrument includes equations for children 5 to 12 years and adolescents 13 to 18 years. Manufacturer equations predict %BF from optical densities at the biceps skinfold site along with gender and body weight and height. The manufacturer's equations tend to overestimate %BF in children (2.5 to 4.1%) and have large prediction errors (standard error of estimate or SEE = 4.9%BF to 5.5%BF).[19,26,27]

Hydrostatic Weighing

The density of the human body (D_b) is equivalent to the ratio of its mass (M) and volume (V) where:[28]

$$D_b = M/V$$

Hydrostatic weighing (HW) has been commonly considered the "gold standard" and used as a criterion method in validation studies of new body composition assessment methods, nonetheless it has limitations when applied to pediatric age individuals; this is because of the changes that occur with growth and maturation and because of the maneuvers needed to perform the test (namely blowing out all the air from the lungs and submerging the body totally under the water).[29] The density of fat is accepted across all ages (0.9007 g/cm^3) and the FFM (1.100 g/cm^3) is considered to be the normal density in adults; however in children this is known to be incorrect.[29,30]

Hydrostatic weighing systems consist of a large tank of water with the water temperature about 37°C (this ensures adequate subject compliance). The system has a seat (i.e., chair) that is attached to a scale; this scale comes in many forms such as a cadaver scale or load cells (i.e., one up to four). The subject is asked to exhale maximally while his or her body is totally submerged; at this point body weight is recorded. This is an estimate of the subject's body weight under water; the subject's body weight is then measured outside the tank. Many researchers also measure residual lung volume during or following the underwater weighing procedures. The results are used to calculate body volume and D_b. Body density is then used to calculate the proportion of body weight as FM and FFM. The use of HW as a measurement tool to evaluate body composition in children is challenging, partly because subjects' compliance is poor.

Air-Displacement Plethysmography

Air displacement pleythysmography (ADP) is a relatively new application in pediatric body composition, thus a brief discussion is warranted. The basic underlying principles of plethysmography originated in Germany in the early 1900s,[31-34] with more recent work following.[35-38] It wasn't until the late 1980s that issues such as heat and moisture were resolved,[39–42] thus making way in 1995 for the BOD POD® (Life Measurement Incorporated, Concord, CA). The BOD POD represents an innovative and exciting technology in the field of pediatric body composition, partly because of the ease of the testing procedure, but also because of favorable results when compared with more established and customary body composition techniques.

The foundations of air displacement, and the BOD POD specifically, have been described in detail elsewhere.[43,44] In brief, the BOD POD is a single-unit, dual-chamber plethysmograph consisting of a testing chamber (front ~450 L) and a reference chamber (rear ~300 L). Body volume is determined by the ratio of the pressure amplitudes in the reference and testing chambers based upon Boyle's Law.[43] The manufacturer suggests wearing a compression swim cap and a tight fitting Lycra swimsuit to diminish hair and clothing issues. Interestingly, it has been reported that clothing, scalp hair, and facial hair, if not adequately controlled (i.e., wearing a tight fitting swimsuit and a compression swim cap), can result in percent fat being underestimated by ~6%.[45–47]

Since 1999 numerous studies have compared ADP with multicompartment models,[48–50] with dual energy x-ray absorptiometry (DXA),[48,49,51–54] and with HW[48,53–57] in children ranging in age from 4 to 18 years of age. Most of these studies have shown favorable agreement between the BOD POD and these more traditional body composition techniques; for a detailed review of these specific studies refer to Fields et al.[58]

An exciting development in the application of air-displacement plethysmography for the testing of infants (i.e., less than 1 year old) has recently emerged. Life Measurement Incorporated has developed an air-displacement plethysmograph specifically for infants called the Pea Pod. Though considered investigational, recent studies have shown the feasibility of using the Pea Pod, though more work needs to be done.[59–62]

In summary, the use of the BOD POD as an alternative method to more traditional body composition techniques has shown promise as indicated by generally positive results; however, at this time more studies that use a multicompartment approach are needed.

DILUTION METHODS

Total body water (TBW) can be measured using the dilution principle with the analogy of measuring the amount of water in a beaker by adding a know amount of dye.[63] The volume of water in the body can be measured by isotope dilution using tritium, deuterium (D_2O), or ^{18}O-labeled water. Adult human cadaver studies have been performed to determine the hydration constant (0.73) according with Fomon;[64] however, the hydration of the FFM changes during growth, with a maximum value at birth, and declines steadily until it reaches the adult value approximately during adolescence (Table 7.1). The TBW technique has a source of error because it relies on the assumption of a constant hydration status of FFM. Some investigators[48] attempted to reduce variable

TABLE 7.1
Percent Hydration of FFM in Children

Age (years)	Boys	Girls
Birth (full term)	80.6	80.6
3	77.0	77.4
5–6	75.9	77.0
7–8	75.4	76.8
9	74.9	76.6

Source: Modified from Fomon SJ, Haschke F, Ziegler EE, Nelson SE. *Am J Clin Nutr.* 1982;35:1169–1175. With permission.

hydration status resulting from growth by using gender and age constants developed by Lohman.[29,30] Even though this approach has been used, TBW showed a wide between-individual variation in the hydration of FFM, and this method may not be the optimum technique for the assessment of total body fat in children and adolescents, in particular newborns.[29,30]

Total Body Electrical Conductivity

As mentioned earlier, water and electrolytes have electric properties, and they can be measured to estimate TBW and FFM. Pediatric and adult devices that measure total body electric conductivity (TOBEC) can be used to provide accurate, rapid, noninvasive estimates of FFM and then define FM (weight less FFM) and %BF. The technique has been shown to be highly influenced by the geometry of the subjects.[65,66] The subjects pass through a low-energy electromagnetic coil, causing alterations in the conductance in the coil. The measured change in the electric signal is proportional to the total body electrolyte content (i.e., highly conductive FFM and a minimal component of the poorly conductive FM). This measurement then is converted to body composition estimates using prediction equations developed specifically for this method.[66,67] The only reference so far where this method has been applied in children uses the isotope dilution technique. Infant TOBEC has been calibrated for FFM and TBW using data from chemical analysis of infant miniature pigs[66,68] while De Bruin et al.[69] performed TOBEC in 435 infants (age 21 to 365 days) and the derived equation had a standard error for FFM of 77 g.

Bioimpedance Analysis

Bioimpedance analysis (BIA) uses the electric impedance of the body by introducing a small alternating electric current into the body and measuring the potential differences that result. The impedance magnitude (Z) is the ratio of the magnitude of the potential difference to the magnitude of the current. Alternating electric current flows through the body and has several different physical characteristics.[70] Tissues rich in water and electrolytes offer considerably less resistance to passage of an electric current than does lipid-rich adipose tissue. Conceptually, a human devoid of adipose tissue would have minimum impedance, which would increase to a maximum when all lean tissue was replaced by fat-filled adipose tissue.[71,72] A limitation of BIA is that it provides an estimate of TBW. Age or pubertal specific equations have been recommended because age related differences in electrolyte concentration in the extracellular space relative to the intracellular space may alter the relationship between bioelectric resistance and TBW.[70,73,74] Also, race-specific prediction equations for FFM have been developed.[75]

Until recently body composition measurements using BIA have employed a single frequency of 50 kHz. In accordance with the axioms of impedance plethysmography, the total resistance measurement (R) is combined with stature as length of the conductor (S) to compute stature squared derived by resistance (S^2/R) as an index of the total conductive volume of the body. The ability of this impedance index to describe the volume of FFM is related to the greater electrolyte content and measured conductivity of FFM compared with adipose tissue or bone. Fat mass can then be calculated as the difference between body weight and FFM.[70,72–74]

An important issue is that subject measurement conditions must be rigorously standardized in order to obtain accurate body composition estimates. Room and subject temperature, position of the patient, correct electrode placement, use of appropriate equations, and several other factors (e.g., eating or drinking) influence measured impedance and must be standardized to the extent possible during BIA measurements.[72] Table 7.2 presents some prediction equations for children using BIA.

TABLE 7.2
Prediction Equations for Children Using BIA

Ethnicity/Gender	Equation	Reference
White/boys and girls (6–10 years)	TBW (l) = 0.593 (Ht^2/R) + 0.065 (BW) + 0.04	73
White/boys and girls (10–19 years)	FFM (kg) = 0.61 (Ht^2/R) + 0.25 (BW) + 1.31	74
White/boys and girls (8–15 years)	FFM (kg) = 0.62(Ht^2/R) + 0.21 (BW) + 0.10(Xc) + 4.2	16
Japanese/boys (9–14 years)	FFM (kg) = 0.56(Ht^2/Z) + 0.20 (BW) + 1.66	27
Japanese/girls (9–15 years)	FFM (kg) = 0.42(Ht^2/Z) + 0.60 (BW) – 0.75 (arm C) + 7.72	27
Black children	FFM (kg) = 0.84 (Ht^2/R) + 1.10	75

Note. TDW = total body water, Ht = height (cm), R = resistance (Ω), BW = body weight (kg), FFM = fat free mass, Xc = reactance (Ω), Z = impedance (Ω), arm C = arm circumference (cm).

Dual Energy X-Ray Absorptiometry

Recent advances in techniques for measuring body composition have provided dual energy x-ray absorptiometry (DXA) for assessment of whole body as well as regional measurements of bone mass, lean mass, and fat mass.[76,77]

DXA is based on the exponential attenuation due to absorption by body tissues of photons emitted at two energy levels (40 and 70 keV). Subjects lie on their backs on a padded table wearing a hospital gown. The counter moves in a raster pattern above the subject's body from head to foot and counts attenuation rates of photons from the x-ray source within the table. The total dose for a scan is less than several hours of background exposure (0.02 mREM).[78] DXA is commonly used in the assessment of body composition in children because it is easy to perform and has advantages over other laboratory techniques that estimate whole body as well as regional composition. The greatest advantage of DXA may be its ability to assess regional body composition (e.g., arms, trunk, and legs). Nutritional status of diseases and growth disorders can be evaluated by analyzing the individual compartments of the body and could offer a new method for the study of skeletal maturation, mineral homeostasis, and environmental and nutritional factors involved in development.[79,80]

IMAGING METHODS

Computerized axial tomography (CT) and magnetic resonance imaging (MRI) allow investigators to evaluate pediatric and adult subjects at the tissue–system level, thus providing *in vivo* analysis.[81,82] CT and MRI can produce cross-sectional high-resolution images, and multiple cross-sectional images can be used to reconstruct tissue volumes including total, subcutaneous, and visceral adipose tissue; skeletal muscle; brain; heart; kidney; liver; skin; and bone.[83] Imaging techniques could explain the physiology of intraabdominal adipose tissue[84] and its relation to health and ultimately the associations between intraabdominal adipose tissue and metabolic factors.[79] None of the currently available methods can assess tissue–system level body composition components with the same accuracy as CT and MRI. The early accumulation of intraabdominal adipose tissue in childhood is clinically relevant because there are significant relationships with adverse health, including dyslipidemia and glucose intolerance, in obese children.[85] The accuracy of the measurements that we have with CT and MRI should help to explain ethnic differences in fat distribution as well as gender differences.[20]

CT and MRI are accurate imaging techniques for assessing body fat distribution, but the disadvantages are cost and radiation exposure (i.e., CT), and limited use in a research setting.

Multicompartment Body Composition

A two-compartment (2C) model, such as TBW and densitometry, is commonly used to estimate pediatric body composition. The 2C model can be derived from measurement of body weight combined with a body property of another component, such as body density or TBW. The 2C model, which partitions the body into FFM and FM, is influenced by age and maturation[86] and may not be the most accurate in children because of the potential changes in hydration and the density of FFM.[29]

According to previous studies in pediatric populations,[30,86] the four-compartment model (4C) is used to describe growth and estimate FM and the main component of FFM. This multicompartment approach involves assessment of body density, TBW, and bone. The 4C accounts for deviations in the quality of FFM because it measures the constituents of FFM (i.e., water, protein, and minerals) rather than assuming a constant density of 1.100 g/cm^3 and hydration of 73.2%.[48]

The 4C has advantages over 2C in children because it can take into account maturation, hydration status of the FFM, and bone in the estimation of body fat without relying upon assumptions that are incorrect in a pediatric population. This is important because it is known that hydration status decreases and bone increases with age (see Table 7.1).[29,48,87]

Body composition is exceptionally difficult to measure early in life for technical reasons and the concerns mentioned earlier. In fact accurate measurements require careful consideration of the selected methods. Butte and colleagues[86] provided reference body composition estimates in young children and extended earlier pediatric models reported by Fomon et al.[64] In this multicomponent model TBW was measured by deuterium dilution, total body potassium (TBK) by 40K,* and intra- and extracellular water calculated from TBW and TBK estimates. Finally bone mineral content was measured using DXA.

Conclusion

Given the literature review in this chapter, the following general clinical suggestions are offered regarding pediatric body composition measurements and assessment. More detailed discussions of the specific techniques can be found in the references.

1. Effects of growth, aging, nutrition, and physical activity in body composition:
   a. Overfeeding of normal and undernutrition individuals results in an increase in lean body mass and an increase of fat mass.
   b. Use of androgenic steroids and exercise could increase lean body mass but not body fat.
   c. Feeding a low energy diet to obese and nonobese subjects decreased both lean body mass and body fat.
   d. Feeding a high energy, low protein diet will increase both body fat with minor changes in lean body mass.
2. Taking into account the various factors (e.g., growth, diet, physical activity, hormones) that influence body composition and using an accurate and precise body composition method, health professions may be able to control growth development. It could be possible also to control several parameters in order to reduce risk factors of various diseases (e.g., high blood pressure, diabetes, obesity).

---

* Natural potassium (K) is distributed in three isotopic states (^{39}K, ^{41}K, ^{40}K). Only ^{40}K is radioactive.

3. There is no single body composition method that is the "best" for pediatric samples. The clinicians and the researcher need to know the practical considerations of body composition assessment with the limitations and strengths of the methods, e.g., a multicompartment method is best, but when taking into account the cost and equipment needed, this approach is impractical (Table 7.3).

4. Regardless of the method chosen to assess body composition, it is fundamental to rigorously follow the standard guidelines and protocols associated with each method to limit measurement error.[88]

TABLE 7.3
Comparison of Common Body Composition Techniques

Method	Cost per Test	Advantages	Disadvantages
BMI		Simple and inexpensive Good for health-risk stratification Suited for large studies	Does not provide qualitative body composition data (i.e., cannot give fat or fat-free mass nor provide visceral or subcutaneous fat)
Skinfolds	$10–$20	Quick and simple Suited for large studies	Operator must be skilled Regression equations must be used to calculate total body fat
HW	$20–$75	Measures whole body density Accurate	Difficult procedure for young children Some people cannot swim
ADP	$30–$75	Quick (5–8 minutes per test) Easier than HW	Requires a tight fitting swimsuit Breathing maneuver that must be performed is difficult for young children
TBW	$20–$75	Robust measure of total body water Easy to administer and collect sample	Not practical for large studies Requires collection of body fluid (e.g., blood, urine, saliva) Expensive if done in a large study
BIA	$10–$20	Simple and inexpensive Useful for large studies	Hydration status affects results Electrode placement is crucial for accurate results
DXA	$100–$150	Radiation (small dose) vs. CT Determines regional fat and fat free mass	Scanning bed cannot accommodate large subjects (>200 lb) Testing takes 30–50 minutes for large subjects
CT	$400–$700	Determines visceral and subcutaneous fat (considered the gold standard)	Radiation dose is large, equivalent to a chest x-ray Large subjects cannot fit in tube Claustrophobia may be a problem
MRI	$400–$700	No radiation Determines visceral and subcutaneous fat	Large subjects cannot fit in tube Claustrophobia may be a problem

Note: Body mass index = BMI; hydro-static weighing = HW; air-displacement plethysmography = ADP; total body water = TBW; bio-impedance analysis = BIA; dual energy x-ray absorptiometry = DXA; computed tomography = CT; magnetic resonance imaging = MRI.

MEASUREMENT OF ENERGY EXPENDITURE

Energy expenditure refers to anything that requires the body to expend energy such as body movement (e.g., organized sports, exercise, walking, fidgeting), muscular contraction (e.g., sitting), and bodily functions (e.g., respiration). There are three components that make up total energy expenditure (TEE). The largest component is resting metabolic rate (RMR) and this composes ~65% of the total energy consumed in a 24-h period.[89] RMR refers to the energy expended at rest to maintain basic physiological function (e.g., respiration, muscle tone, heart rate, brain function, and maintaining body temperature). The largest consumers of energy at rest are the organs (60 to 75%), with the liver and brain the largest consumers at 29 and 19%, respectively, with skeletal muscle consuming ~18%.[90] When performing RMR in children, it is important to carefully control the testing environment to reduce outside stimulation.[91] Typically, the subject arrives for testing between 5:30 and 6:00 A.M. after an overnight fast. Testing involves having the subject lie quietly on a bed for 15 min prior to a 30-min period of breath collection. The second, but most varied, source of TEE is physical activity–related energy expenditure and typically ranges from 15 to 30% of TEE. The last component of TEE is the thermic effect of feeding (TEF) or meal-induced thermogensis. After eating a meal, metabolism rises in part to digest, metabolize, and store food stuffs that were just consumed; this rise in metabolism makes up ~7 to 13% of TEE.[89] Interestingly, the nutritional makeup of the meal has a dramatic effect on TEF with a mixed diet creating a larger increase than simple sugars or carbohydrates.[92]

Energy expenditure is typically measured using indirect calorimetry, although it can be measured directly. In a clinical setting, energy expenditure is meaningful only when it is expressed as a calorie, i.e., the amount of heat necessary to raise the temperature of 1 L of water 1°C, from 14.5 to 15.5°C. Direct calorimetry involves the measurement of actual heat production; though highly accurate, the method is impractical for human metabolism studies and is rarely used today.

Indirect calorimetry typically involves the measurement of expiratory gases (O_2 and CO_2) at the mouth, specifically the amount of O_2 consumed and CO_2 produced when a food source is oxidized and is based on the caloric equivalent of 1 L of O_2 liberating ~5 calories.[93]

$$\text{Food source (fat, carbohydrate, protein, alcohol)} + O_2 \rightarrow CO_2 + H_2O$$

Indirect calorimetry can be used to measure activity related energy expenditure or aerobic fitness using a mask or mouthpiece from a variety of commercially available metabolic systems (V-Max Senor Medics, Yorba Linda, CA; TrueOne 2400 ParvoMedics, East Sandy, UT; K4b² COSMED, Chicago, IL; MOXUS Modular VO_2 System AEI Technologies, Naperville, IL; MAX II Cart Physio-Dyne, Quogue, NY; and Vacu Med VISTA Vacu Med, Ventura, CA), as well as resting energy expenditure with a canopy hood (Delta Trac II Senor Medics, Yorba Linda, CA) or lightweight, portable systems that use either a mask or mouthpiece (ReeVue KORR Medical Technologies, Salt Lake City, UT, and MedGem HealtheTech, Golden, CO).

Respiratory gas analysis by indirect calorimetry provides two invaluable pieces of information for exercise physiologists and clinical researchers: (1) it allows for the respiratory exchange ratio (RER) to be calculated (VCO_2 produced/VO_2 consumed), which provides crucial information on substrate utilization. For example, when 100% fat is oxidized (palmitic acid), the RER is 0.7:

$$C_{16}H_{32}O_2 + 23O_2 \rightarrow 16CO_2 + 16H_2O$$

$$\text{RER} = \frac{16CO_2}{23O_2} = 0.7$$

When 100% glucose is oxidized, the RER is 1.0:

$$C_6H_{12}O_6 + 6O_2 \rightarrow 6CO_2 + 6H_2O$$

$$RER = \frac{6CO_2}{6O_2} = 1.0$$

Thus, fat oxidation has an RER of 0.7 and glucose oxidation has an RER of 1.0 with protein oxidation and a mixed diet falling somewhere between 0.7 and 1.0 (~0.85). The second piece of information that indirect calorimetry provides is a gauge of the subject's physical exertion. By definition RER cannot be greater than 1.0 from fuel oxidation; however, in maximal exercise, RER levels typically are greater than 1.1, in part because the sodium bicarbonate system buffers lactic acid (a product of maximal exercise) to maintain the proper acid–base balance in the blood:

$$HLa + NaHCO_3 \leftrightarrow NaLa + H_2CO_3 \leftrightarrow H_2O + CO_2$$

This nonmetabolic CO_2 is blown off, thus elevating the RER above 1.0.

Another form of indirect calorimetry, though typically measured using urine, and less commonly blood and breath, is the double-labeled water technique that utilizes stable isotope techniques in the measurement of CO_2 and allows total energy expenditure to be measured.[94–96] An excellent source that explains the underlying principles, techniques, and unique issues with this technique is a consensus report by the IDECG[94] (International Dietary Energy Consultancy Group) in 1990. Briefly, deuterated hydrogen (^2H) and ^{18}O are given, usually orally after a baseline urine sample is taken to determine the natural baseline background of ^2H and ^{18}O. After 7 to 14 d, a second sample is obtained. The ^2H remains solely as body water, and it decreases and becomes diluted as unlabeled ^1H in the form of water enters the body (primarily as food and drink), where ^{18}O is also lost as water but some is lost as CO_2, which is the end product of metabolism.[94] Thus, the greater divergence between the slopes of the disappearance of each isotope reflects the amount of CO_2 produced.[94] The main advantage the double-labeled water technique has in the measurement of energy expenditure as compared with metabolic carts is that the subject is in a free-living situation unfettered by bulky hoses or masks, and the measurement is taken over an extended period, consequently reflecting a "true" real world energy expenditure. The double-labeled water technique has been validated with metabolic chambers and has produced results that are within 5 to 10% difference.[97] A major limitation is the cost of the isotope, with ^{18}O costing ~$200 to $350 per subject, and the analysis requires an isotope ratio mass spectrometer, thus limiting its use to only the most established laboratories.

MEASUREMENT OF PHYSICAL ACTIVITY

Physical activity is a rather ambiguous term loosely used to describe body movement or activity and is characterized by type (i.e., organized vs. recreational vs. occupational, aerobic vs. anaerobic), intensity, duration, and frequency.[98,99] There are a number of excellent reviews on physical activity assessment and issues related specifically to children.[100–103] It has become increasingly popular to measure physical activity instead of energy expenditure because the instruments used are markedly cheaper, unobtrusive, and allow investigators to categorize the intensity of the activities (low intensity vs. high intensity).[104,105] This has led to a new body of research that challenges long held beliefs that only "exercise and organized physical activity" can have a positive impact on health outcomes (e.g., diabetes, coronary heart disease, cancer, obesity). Data has begun to emerge that would suggest that exercise and physical activity are distinctly different and should not be used interchangeably, especially in children who engage in long periods of physical activity (e.g., play) but may never actually take part in a structured exercise regimen.

Unlike energy expenditure, physical activity does not measure energy expended (calories); rather it measures past activity, steps, frequencies, accelerations, counts, habits, and trends. This is because physical activity is measured with questionnaires, motion sensors (e.g., pedometers and accelerometers), observation booths, heart rate monitors, and diaries.

QUESTIONNAIRES

Most questionnaires (recalls, diaries, and history surveys) involve the subject, and many times the parent, to self-report the past week's activities. Typically self-report techniques, as compared with an objective measure (e.g., double-labeled water), have produced a modest correlation, with the child overestimating the amount and quantity of the actual physical activity performed.[106] To date little is known about why self-reports are so difficult to implement in this population, but typically children are able to recall only about 50% of their past week's activity, which is why the best self-report method is to have the child recall only what they did for that particular day or from the day before vs. recalling what they did for the past week.[107–109]

One must not forget that for qualitative instruments (questionnaires) to have real value and meaning, they must be converted into a quantifiable measure. For example, it is quite difficult to translate qualitative information (e.g., playing kickball in gym class for 20 min or playing hop scotch for 1 h) to a quantifiable outcome (e.g., calories burned for this period).[20] This conversion relies on the use of activity factors or intensity factors, which are interrelated to metabolic equivalents (MET).[20] One MET by definition is the amount of oxygen consumed per body weight at rest (3.5 ml $O_2 \cdot kg^{-1} \cdot min^{-1}$), thus a person playing at 5 METs would require 5 times as much oxygen as they would at rest. Once the MET level is determined, calories can be calculated because 1 MET $= \sim (1 \; kcal \cdot kg^{-1} \cdot h^{-1})$.

One of the first physical activity and behavior questionnaires used specifically in children was the Netherlands Health Education Questionnaire.[110] The questionnaire consisted of eight questions that concerned "behavior or patterns" related to physical activity and play, and were graded on a scale from 1 to 5. In the broadest sense it was a physical activity questionnaire that really evaluated the child's play habits and preferences. In another questionnaire developed with Pima Indians, the number of hours spent sleeping, napping, watching TV, and in specific physical activities is logged and used to determine the number of hours spent in physical activity.[111] The Amsterdam Growth Questionnaire is used in children and obtains the type, intensity, and duration of the physical activity at school in an unstructured environment.[112] As stated by others, though these questionnaires are extensively used and quite popular, their validity has not been scrupulously examined against true criterion measures of physical activity such as the double-labeled water technique or even movement based techniques (pedometers and accelerometers).[20]

Currently, there are two studies that have attempted to explore the validity of questionnaires vs. an objective measure of physical activity (double-labeled water and accelerometers) in children.[113,114] In the study by Goran et al. physical activity was obtained from questionnaires and compared with the actual energy expenditure from double-labeled water in 101 Caucasian children.[113] They concluded that physical activity was not related to energy expenditure from the double-labeled water technique. However, in a more recent study a 3-day physical activity recall was significantly related to the CSA activity accelerometer in 15-year-old girls.[114]

The apparent ease and low cost of using questionnaires are reasons they are so popular in studies that involve children; nonetheless prudence should be used because children simply do not have the cognitive ability to properly fill out the survey or recall their activities over the course of several days, especially if they are younger than 15 years old.[115,116] This is why it is imperative to adequately control the testing environment, ensuring as few distractions as possible, and to properly train staff in the use of these questionnaires and surveys.[117] Time-based and activity-based approaches have been employed to help children better recall past activity in filling out questionnaires. The Previous Day Physical Activity Recall (PDPAR) and the 3 Day Physical Activity Recall

(3DPAR) are examples of time-based approaches that ask the child to begin with the most recent day and working backward, reporting the dominate activity performed in half-hour blocks of time.[114,118] Another recall technique is an activity-based approach such as the Self-Administered Physical Activity Checklist (SAPAC).[114,118,119] This approach focuses on the kinds of activities the child performed with minimal cues about time of day; the child is then asked to give an estimate of the number of minutes he or she performed this particular activity over the last 3 d. In a recent study by McMurray et al., both recall approaches showed feasibility in adolescents in recalling activity over 1 d, but activity patterns over a 3-d period appeared to be too long even for these approaches to accurately determine activity.[120]

MOVEMENT-BASED TECHNIQUES

The gold standard for evaluating physical activity in children is to directly observe them at play through a one-way mirror.[121,122] Undoubtedly, this approach is time consuming and limits the number of children that can be studied while restricting the play area; thus, alternative approaches have been developed that are easier to implement while giving the children freedom to move about freely and unimpeded.

The two most commonly used movement based devices are pedometers and accelerometers. It is beyond the scope of this chapter to describe the actual mechanism and principle for each device, but they are explained very well by previous authors.[123,124] Principally, pedometers measure the number of steps taken and are generally worn on the hip but could be worn on the ankle and are inexpensive ($20 to $50). Accelerometers measure the change in acceleration; they too are typically worn at the hip and are modestly more expensive (e.g., $200 to $500). Pedometers and accelerometers measure vertical displacement only from ambulation, thus certain types of activities (e.g., bicycling, computer game playing, and swimming) are missed.

A limited number of studies have validated pedometers with a criterion method, with most studies to date using pedometers in a descriptive manner. One of the first studies examining the validity of pedometers in children was performed in kindergarten children (5 years old) using direct observation as the criterion method.[125] The pedometer was worn at the waist and was significantly correlated with the direct observation results; however, the authors reported that the pedometer tended to underestimate activity at higher intensities. Another study validated pedometers in 12- to 18-year-old boys using the actual step rate on a treadmill as the criterion method.[126] They reported that the pedometer vs. the actual step rate at both ends of the spectrum (i.e., walking at 1.3 mph and running at 4 mph) resulted in the estimation of caloric expenditure being off by -5 to 8%. The validity of pedometers vs. the Tritrac-R3D was performed in 34 children aged 8 to 10 years.[127] The correlation between activity counts from the pedometer and the Tritrac-R3D was 0.85. However another study reported that a pedometer was not reliable in the measurement of physical activity in African-American girls between 8 and 9 years old.[128] And in another study with 9-year-old Welsh children, a significant relationship existed between pedometers and VO_2 while walking on a treadmill.[129] A not so obvious issue when validating pedometers with a criterion method is that pedometers currently do not have the ability to store time; thus, (1) duration and intensity of a specific discrete activity at a specific time cannot be parsed from other discrete activities making it nearly impossible to extrapolate or convert steps into energy expenditure or even distance traveled, because 3000 steps for a child with legs 25 inches long would not cover the same distance if another child had legs 33 inches long; and (2) the researcher is dependent upon the subject to reset the pedometer counts from the previous day. However, in a practical sense, pedometers may be the easiest to employ in large epidemiological studies and from the subject's point of view may be the easiest to understand (i.e., the number of steps taken).

Accelerometers measure the body's acceleration and have the capability to differentiate between different intensities while being able to store and download data over a period of time (up to 7 d). Accelerometers can be either uniaxial, such as the Caltrac, MTI Actigraph, and the CAS, or triaxial, such as Tritrac and Tracmor, to name a few. Generally speaking, energy expenditure estimated by accelerometery correlates quite nicely ($r = .70$ to $.80$) with energy expenditure measured in a laboratory setting.[20,130,131] The first attempt to validate a uniaxial accelerometer (Caltrac) in a free living situation with double-labeled water proved unsuccessful.[132] Johnson et al. found the Caltrac in a sample of 31 children (8 years old) to have limited usefulness as a physical activity monitor when validated with the double-labeled water technique. However, another study directly refuted this by reporting a significant correlation ($r = .39$) between computer science and application (CSA) and double-labeled water in twenty-six 9-year-old boys and girls. It would be reasonable to suggest that a triaxial accelerometer may be able to capture more physical activity because it is three dimensional. In 2003 Hoos et al. reported that the Tracmor2, a triaxial accelerometer, was a valid tool in the assessment of energy expenditure ($r = .79$; $P < .01$) in 11 children whose average age was 7 years old vs. the double-labeled water technique.[133]

A problem when using pedometers or accelerometers is to convert the steps or activity counts into something more meaningful, such as calories or the appropriate MET level. A recently published paper by Treuth et al. involving 74 healthy 13- to 14-year-old girls reported a shared variance of $R^2 = .84$ between the predicted MET value from the activity counts using an Actigraph accelerometer (formerly the CAS) and O_2 consumed.[134] And in another study by Puyau et al., the predicted calories expended in a whole room calorimeter and free-living condition using the Actigraph in a group of 6- to 16-year-old boys and girls produced a $R^2 = .75$ (adjusted).[135]

In conclusion, pedometers and accelerometers have both strengths and weaknesses with both providing distinctively different types of information. Pedometers measure the number of steps taken without regard to distance traveled, whereas accelerometers provide intensity of movement and time; however, both lack the sensitivity to measure upper body movement. Because for many investigators a pedometer will be the only reasonable tool, more movement-based instrument studies are needed to improve the validity and reliability of current technologies while at the same time providing the creation of better and newer devices. Additionally, more studies are needed to produce conversion equations that can convert steps and activity counts to calories or METs.

HEART RATE MONITORS

Heart rate monitors provide an objective measure of physical activity due to the linear relationship between VO_2 (i.e., energy expenditure) and physical activity (i.e., movement), and have been used for quite some time in children, in part because they are inexpensive and subject compliance is generally high.[136–140] However, there are limitations using this approach because the heart rate–VO_2 relationship can be affected by such things as age, gender, training status, ambient temperature, and motivation, not to mention mental stresses (e.g., anxiety, excitement, and sadness).[141,142] Another weakness to consider when using the heart rate method is subject conformity. Oftentimes children will complain that the strap is pinching, hurting, or restricting their ability to breathe, thus reducing compliance.

A study by Welk et al. demonstrated how factors other than physical activity affect heart rate.[143] This study investigated heart rate vs. direct observation in children in active play (i.e., physical education class) and active rest (i.e., the classroom).[143] When heart rate was compared with direct observation while the children were actively engaged in physical education class, the correlation was $r = .79$; however, when the children were evaluated in the classroom (i.e., under resting conditions), the correlation between heart rate and physical activity was $r = .49$. Even so, Livingstone has reported good agreement between heart rate and the double-labeled water technique in children

(7 to 15 years old) when heart rate was measured over the course of 2 to 3 d and double-labeled water over 10 to 15 days, and states "heart-rate monitoring provides a close estimation in total energy expenditure in both boys and girls when compared to the double-labeled water technique."[136] Because the double-labeled water technique was used in this study as a true criterion method, one should seriously consider the feasibility of heart-rate monitoring as a viable and valid tool in the assessment of energy expenditure in children.

CONCLUSION

The following general recommendations and guidelines should be considered when evaluating energy expenditure and physical activity in children.

1. Physical activity questionnaires in children younger than 12 years old may be impractical and, worse, may give spurious results. The data obtained are difficult to interpret, mainly because of the child's cognitive ability to recall past activity patterns, Consequently in many instances the parent intervenes, thus restricting a "true" evaluation of activity the parent did not actually observe.
2. Though pedometers and accelerometers are objective measures of physical activity, one must keep in mind they measure distinctively different things.
3. Regardless of the method chosen to assess physical activity in children, one must first consider the subject's age and the type of information wanted. For a synopsis of each method's strengths and weaknesses, see Table 7.4.
4. Whenever possible, objective measures of physical activity (movement) should be employed as opposed to questionnaires.[117,120]

TABLE 7.4
Comparison of Common Physical Activity Techniques

Method	Advantages	Disadvantages
Questionnaires	Inexpensive	Relies upon memory to recall the past week's activity
	Easy to administer	Child's ability to understand question may be limited
	Suited for large studies	If parent helps child fill out questionnaire, the activity captured is limited only to activity the parent actually witnessed
		Modestly correlated to more objective measures
Movement-based techniques		
Pedometers	Inexpensive	Must be reset at the end of each day
	Measures steps taken	Cannot measure distance traveled or intensity
		Captures only steps taken
Accelerometers	Measures intensity of activity	Substantially more expensive than a pedometer
	Records time of activity	Does not capture certain types of activity (e.g., swimming, bike riding, many upper body movements)
	Has memory for up to 7 days	
Heart rate monitors	Objective measure of movement	Uncomfortable if worn for a long period
		Receiver must be "tamper" resistant
	Accurate	No way to convert heart beats into energy expended

REFERENCES

1. Forbes GB. Body composition in infancy, childhood, and adolescence. In: Forbes GB, Ed. *Human Body Composition: Growth, Aging, and Activity Level*. New York: Springer Verlag, 1987: 125–196.
2. Quetelet A. *Physique Sociale ou Essay Sur le Development des Facultes de L'homme*. Vol. 2. Muquardt, Brussels, 1869.
3. Must A, Jacques PF, Dallal GE, Bajema CJ, Dietz WH. Long-term morbidity and mortality of overweight adolescents. A follow-up of the Harvard Growth Study of 1922 to 1935. *N Engl J Med.* 1992;327: 1350–1355.
4. Kuczmarski RJ, Ogden CL, Grummer-Strawn LM, et al. CDC growth charts: United States. *Adv Data.* 2000: 1–27.
5. Cole TJ, Freeman JV, Preece MA. Body mass index reference curves for the UK, 1990. *Arch Dis Child.* 1995;73: 25–29.
6. He Q, Albertsson-Wikland K, Karlberg J. Population-based body mass index reference values from Goteborg, Sweden: birth to 18 years of age. *Acta Paediatr.*2000;89: 582–592.
7. Leung SS, Cole TJ, Tse LY, Lau JT. Body mass index reference curves for Chinese children. *Ann Hum Biol.* 1998;25: 169–174.
8. Cole TJ, Roede MJ. Centiles of body mass index for Dutch children aged 0–20 years in 1980—a baseline to assess recent trends in obesity. *Ann Hum Biol.* 1999;26: 303–308.
9. Cacciari E, Milani S, Balsamo A, et al. Italian cross-sectional growth charts for height, weight and BMI (6–20 y). *Eur J Clin Nutr.* 2002;56: 171–180.
10. Cole TJ, Bellizzi MC, Flegal KM, Dietz WH. Establishing a standard definition for child overweight and obesity worldwide: international survey. *BMJ.* 2000;320: 1–6.
11. Ellis KJ, Abrams SA, Wong WW. Monitoring childhood obesity: assessment of the weight/height index. *Am J Epidemiol.* 1999;150: 939–946.
12. Mast M, Langnase K, Labitzke K, Bruse U, Preuss U, Muller MJ. Use of BMI as a measure of overweight and obesity in a field study on 5–7 year old children. *Eur J Nutr.* 2002;41: 61–67.
13. Mei Z, Grummer-Strawn LM, Pietrobelli A, Goulding A, Goran MI, Dietz WH. Validity of body mass index compared with other body-composition screening indexes for the assessment of body fatness in children and adolescents. *Am J Clin Nutr.* 2002;75: 978–985.
14. Cole TJ, Faith MS, Pietrobelli A, Heo M. What is the best measure of adiposity change in growing children: BMI, BMI%, BMI z-score or BMI centile? *Eur J Clin Nutr.* 2005;59: 419–425.
15. Pietrobelli A, Wang Z, Heymsfield SB. Techniques used in measuring human body composition. *Curr Opin Clin Nutr Metab Care.* 1998;1: 439–448.
16. Lohman TG. *Advances in Body Composition Assessment. Current Issues in Exercise Science*. Monograph No 3. Champaign, IL: Human Kinetics, 1992.
17. Slaughter MH, Lohman TG, Boileau RA, et al. Skinfold equations for estimation of body fatness in children and youth. *Hum Biol.* 1988;60: 709–723.
18. Rolland-Cachera MF. Prediction of adult body composition from infant and child measurements. In: Davies PWD, Cole TJ, Eds. *Body Composition Techniques in Health and Disease*. Cambridge: Cambridge Press, 1995: 100–145.
19. Wagner DR, Heyward VH. Techniques of body composition assessment: a review of laboratory and field methods. *Res Q Exerc Sport.* 1999;70: 135–149.
20. Goran MI. Measurement issues related to studies of childhood obesity: assessment of body composition, body fat distribution, physical activity, and food intake. *Pediatrics.* 1998;101: 505–518.
21. Cruz ML, Weigensberg MJ, Huang TT, Ball G, Shaibi GQ, Goran MI. The metabolic syndrome in overweight Hispanic youth and the role of insulin sensitivity. *J Clin Endocrinol Metab.* 2004;89: 108–113.
22. Weiss R, Dziura J, Burgert TS, et al. Obesity and the metabolic syndrome in children and adolescents. *N Engl J Med.* 2004;350: 2362–2374.
23. Fernandez JR, Redden DT, Pietrobelli A, Allison DB. Waist circumference percentiles in nationally representative samples of African-American, European-American and Mexican-American children. *J Pediatr.* 2004;145: 439–444.
24. Norris AH. Instrumental techniques for measuring quality of agricultural crops. In: Lieberman M, Ed. *Post-harvest Physiology and Crop Preservation*. New York: Plenum Press, 1983: 471–484.

25. Conway JM, Norris KH, Bodwell CE. A new approach for the estimation of body composition: infrared interactance. *Am J Clin Nutr.* 1984;40: 1123–1130.

26. Cassady SL, Nielsen DH, Janz KF, Wu YT, Cook JS, Hansen JR. Validity of near infrared body composition analysis in children and adolescents. *Med Sci Sports Exerc.* 1993;25: 1185–1191.

27. Heyward VH, Stolarczyk LM. Body composition basics. In: Heyward VH, Stolarczyk LM, Eds. *Applied Body Composition Assessment.* Champaign, IL: Human Kinetics, 1996: 2–20.

28. Going SB. Densitometry. In: Roche AF, Heymsfield SB, Lohman TG, Eds. *Human Body Composition.* Champaign, IL: Human Kinetics, 1996: 3–23.

29. Lohman TG. Applicability of body composition techniques and constants for children and youths. *Exerc Sport Sci Rev.* 1986;14: 325–357.

30. Lohman TG. Assessment of body composition in children. *Pediatr Exerc Sci.* 1989;1:19–30.

31. Jongloed J, Noyons AKM. Die bestimmung des wahren bolumens und des spezifischen Gewichtes von Menshcen mittels Luftdruckveranderung. *Pflugers Archiv.* 1938;240: 197.

32. Kohlrausch W. Methodik zur Quantitativen Bestimmung der Korperstoffe *in vivo. Arbeitsphysiol.* 1929;2: 23.

33. Pfaundler M. Korpermass-studien an kindern. Von korpervolumen und der korperdichte. *Ztschr f Kinderheilk.* 1916;14: 123–137.

34. Murlin JR, Hoobler BR. The energy metabolism of normal and marasmic children with special reference to the specific gravity of the child's body. *Proc Soc Exp Biol Med.* 1913;11: 115–116.

35. Faulkner F. An air displacement method of measuring body volume in babies: a preliminary communication. *Ann NY Acad Sci.* 1963;110: 75–79.

36. Gnaedinger RH, Reineke EP, Pearson AM, Van Huss WD, Wessel JA, Montoye HJ. Determination of body density by air displacement, helium dilution, and underwater weighing. *Ann NY Acad Sci.* 1963;110: 96–108.

37. Friis-Hansen B. Body water compartments in children. Changes during growth and related changes in body composition. *Pediatrics.* 1961;28: 169.

38. Friis-Hansen B. The body density of newborn infants. *Acta Paediatrica.* 1963;52: 513–521.

39. Gundlach BL, Visscher GJW. The plethysmometric measurement of total body volume. *Hum Biol.* 1986;58: 783–799.

40. Gundlach BL, Nijkrake HGM, Hautvast JGAJ. A rapid and simplified plethysmometric method for measuring body volume. *Hum Biol.* 1980;52: 23–33.

41. Taylor A, Scopes JW, du Mont G, Taylor BA. Development of an air displacement method for whole body volume measurement of infants. *J Biomed Eng.* 1985;7: 9–17.

42. Sly PD, Lanteri C, Bates JHT. Effect of the thermodynamics of an infant plethysmograph on the measurement of thoracic gas volume. *Pediatr Pulmonol* 1990;8: 203–208.

43. Dempster P, Aitkens S. A new air displacement method for the determination of human body composition. *Med Sci Sports Exerc.* 1995;27: 1692–1697.

44. McCrory MA, Gomez TD, Bernauer EM, Molé PA. Evaluation of a new air displacement plethysmograph for measuring human body composition. *Med Sci Sports Exerc.* 1995;27: 1686–1691.

45. Vescovi JD, Zimmerman SL, Miller WC, Fernhall BO. Effects of clothing on accuracy and reliability of air displacement plethysmography. *Med Sci Sports Exerc.* 2002;34: 282–285.

46. Higgins PB, Fields DA, Gower BA, Hunter GR. The effect of scalp and facial hair on body fat estimates by the BOD POD. *Obes Res.* 2001;9: 326–330.

47. Fields DA, Hunter GR, Goran MI. Validation of the BOD POD with hydrostatic weighing: influence of body clothing. *Int J Obes.* 2000;24: 200–205.

48. Fields DA, Goran MI. Body composition techniques and the four-compartment model in children. *J Appl Physiol.* 2000;89: 613–620.

49. Gately PJ, Radley D, Cooke CB, et al. Comparison of body composition methods in overweight and obese children. *J Appl Physiol.* 2003;95: 2039–2046.

50. Wells JC, Fuller NJ, Wright A, Fewtrell MS, Cole TJ. Evaluation of air-displacement plethysmography in children aged 5–7 years using a three-component model of body composition. *Br J Nutr.* 2003;90: 699–707.

51. Buchholz AC, Majchrzak KM, Chen KY, Shankar SM, Buchowski MS. Use of air displacement plethysmography in the determination of percentage of fat mass in African American children. *Pediatr Res.* 2004;56: 47–54.

52. Nicholson JC, McDuffie JR, Bonat SH, et al. Estimation of body fatness by air displacement plethysmography in African American and white children. *Pediatr Res.* 2001;50: 467–473.

53. Lockner DW, Heyward VH, Baumgartner RN, Jenkins KA. Comparison of air-displacement plethysmography, hydrodensitometry, and dual X-ray absorptiometry for assessing body composition of children 10 to 18 years of age. *Ann NY Acad Sci.* 2000;904: 72–78.

54. Nuñez C, Kovera AJ, Pietrobelli A, et al. Body composition in children and adults by air displacement plethysmography. *Eur J Clin Nutr.* 1999;53: 382–387.

55. Dewit O, Fuller NJ, Fewtrell MS, Elia M, Wells JCK. Whole body air displacement plethymography compared with hydrodensitometry for body composition analysis. *Arch Dis Child.* 2000;82: 159–164.

56. Wells JCK, Douros I, Fuller NJ, Elia M, Dekker L. Assessment of body volume using three-dimensional photonic scanning. *Ann NY Acad Sci.* 2000;904: 247–254.

57. Demerath EW, Guo SS, Chumlea WC, Towne B, Roche AF, Siervogel RM. Comparison of percent body fat estimates using air displacement plethysmography and hydrodensitometry in adults and children. *Int J Obes.* 2002;26: 389–397.

58. Fields DA, Goran MI, McCory MA. Body-composition assessment via air-displacement plethysmography in adults and children: a review. *Am J Clin Nutr.* 2002;75: 453–467.

59. Yao M, Nommsen-Rivers L, Dewey K, Urlando A. Preliminary evaluation of a new pediatric air displacement plethysmograph for body composition assessment in infants. *Acta Diabetol.* 2003;40 Suppl 1: S55–S58.

60. Ma G, Yao M, Liu Y, et al. Validation of a new pediatric air-displacement plethysmograph for assessing body composition in infants. *Am J Clin Nutr.* 2004;79: 653–660.

61. Sainz RD, Urlando A. Evaluation of a new pediatric air-displacement plethysmograph for body-composition assessment by means of chemical analysis of bovine tissue phantoms. *Am J Clin Nutr.* 2003;77: 364–370.

62. Urlando A, Dempster P, Aitkens S. A new air displacement plethysmograph for the measurement of body composition in infants. *Pediatr Res.* 2003;53: 486–492.

63. Schoeller DA. Hydrometry. In: Roche AF, Hemsfield SB, Lohman TG, Eds. *Human Body Composition.* Champaign, IL: Human Kinetics, 1996: 25–43.

64. Fomon SJ, Haschke F, Ziegler EE, Nelson SE. Body composition of reference children from birth to age 10 years. *Am J Clin Nutr.* 1982;35: 1169–1175.

65. Sutcliffe JF, Smye SW, Smith MA. A further assessment of an electromagnetic method to measure body composition. *Phys Med Biol.* 1995;40: 659–670.

66. Fiorotto ML, Cochran WJ, Funk RC, Sheng HP, Klish WJ. Total body electrical conductivity measurements: effects of body composition and geometry. *Am J Physiol.* 1987;252: R794–R800.

67. Van Loan M. Assessment of fat-free mass in teen-agers: use of TOBEC methodology. *Am J Clin Nutr.* 1990;52: 586–590.

68. Boileau RA. Utilization of total body electrical conductivity in determining body composition. In: Boileau RA, (Ed.), *Designing Foods.* New York: Science Publisher, 1988: 251–327.

69. De Bruin NC, Luijenddijk IH, Visser HK, Degenhart HJ. The effect of alterations in physical and chemical characteristics on TOBEC-derived body composition estimates: validation with non human models. *Phys Med Biol.* 1994;39: 1143–1156.

70. Yanovski JA, Heymsfield SB, Lukaski HC. Bioelectrical impedance analysis. *Am J Clin Nutr.* 1996;64: 387–532.

71. Deurenberg P, Kusters CS, Smit HE. Assessment of body composition by bioelectrical impedance in children and young adults is strongly age-dependent. *Eur J Clin Nutr.* 1990;44: 261–268.

72. Pietrobelli A, Heymsfield SB, Wang ZM, Gallagher D. Multi-component body composition models: recent advances and future directions. *Eur J Clin Nutr.* 2001;55: 69–75.

73. Kushner RF, Schoeller DA, Fjeld CR, Danford L. Is the impedance index (ht2/R) significant in predicting total body water? *Am J Clin Nutr.* 1992;56: 835–839.

74. Houtkooper LB, Going SB, Lohman TG, Roche AF, Van Loan M. Bioelectrical impedance estimation of fat-free body mass in children and youth: a cross-validation study. *J Appl Physiol.* 1992;72: 366–373.

75. Lewy VD, Danadian K, Arslanian S. Determination of body composition in African-American children: validation of bioelectrical impedence with dual energy X-ray absorptiometry. *J Pediatr Endocrinol Metab.* 1999;12: 443–448.

76. Pietrobelli A, Formica C, Wang Z, Heymsfield SB. Dual-energy X-ray absorptiometry body composition model: review of physical concepts. *Am J Physiol*. 1996;271: E941–E951.

77. Mazess R, Chesnut CH, 3rd, McClung M, Genant H. Enhanced precision with dual-energy X-ray absorptiometry. *Calcif Tissue Int* 1992;51: 14–17.

78. Lohman TG. Dual energy X-ray absorptiometry. In: Roche AF, Heymsfield SB, Lohman TG, Eds. *Human Body Composition*. Champaign, IL: Human Kinetics, 1996: 63–78.

79. Goran MI, Figueroa R, McGloin A, Nguyen V, Treuth MS, Nagy TR. Obesity in children: recent advances in energy metabolism and body composition. *Obes Res*. 1995;3: 277–289.

80. Lapillonne A, Braillon PM, Delmas PD, Salle BL. Dual-energy X-ray absorptiometry in early life. *Horm Res*. 1997;48 Suppl 1: 43–49.

81. Heymsfield SB, Wang Z, Baumgartner RN, Ross R. Human body composition: advances in models and methods. *Annu Rev Nutr*. 1997;17: 527–558.

82. Sjostrom L. A computer-tomography based multicompartment body composition technique and anthropometric predictions of lean body mass, total and subcutaneous adipose tissue. *Int J Obes*. 1991;15(Suppl 2): 19–30.

83. Shen W, Wang Z, Punyanita M, et al. Adipose tissue quantification by imaging methods: a proposed classification. *Obes Res*. 2003,11: 5–16.

84. Fox KR, Peters DM, Sharpe P, Bell M. Assessment of abdominal fat development in young adolescents using magnetic resonance imaging *Int J Obes*. *Relat Metab Disord*. 2000;24: 1653–1659.

85. Caprio S, Hyman LD, McCarthy S, Lange R, Bronson M, Tamborlane WV. Fat distribution and cardiovascular risk factors in obese adolescent girls: importance of the intraabdominal fat depot. *Am J Clin Nutr*. 1996;64: 12–17.

86. Butte NF, Hopkinson JM, Wong WW, Smith EO, Ellis KJ. Body composition during the first 2 years of life: an updated reference. *Pediatr Res*. 2000;47: 578–585.

87. Pietrobelli A, Faith MS, Wang J, Brambilla P, Chiumello G, Heymsfield SB. Association of lean tissue and fat mass with bone mineral content in children and adolescents. *Obes Res*. 2002,10: 56–60.

88. Dietz W, Bellizzi MC. Assessment of childhood and adolescent obesity. *Am J Clin Nutr*. 1999;50: 117S–170S.

89. Elia M. Energy expenditure in the whole body. In: Kinney JM, Tucker HN, Eds. *Energy Metabolism. Tissue Determinats and Cellular Corollaries*. New York: Raven Press, Ltd., 1993: 19–47.

90. Grande F. Energy expenditure of organs and tissues. In: *Assessment of Energy Metabolism in Health and Disease*. Kinney JM, Ed. Columbus, OH: Ross Laboratories, 1989: 88–92.

91. Goran MI, Nagy TR. Effect of the pre-testing environment on measurement of metabolic rate in children. *Int J Obes*. 1996,20: 83–87.

92. St-Onge MP, Rubiano F, DeNino WF, et al. Added thermogenic and satiety effects of a mixed nutrient vs a sugar-only beverage. *Int J Obes*. *Relat Metab Disord*. 2004;28: 248–253.

93. Zuntz N. Ueber die Bedeutung der verschiedenen Nährstoffe als Erzeuger der Muskelkraft. *Pflugers Arch*. 1901;83: 557–571.

94. Prentice AM. *The Doubly-Labelled Water Method for Measuring Energy Expenditure: Technical Recommendations for Use in Humans. A Consensus Report by the IDECG Working Group*. Vienna, Austria: International Atomic Energy Agency, 1990.

95. Goran MI, Poehlman E, Johnson RK. Energy requirements across the life span: new findings based on measurement of total energy expenditure with doubly labeled water. *Nutr Res*. 1995;15: 115–150.

96. Schoeller DA, Fijeld CR. Human energy metabolism: what have we learned from the doubly labeled water method. *Annu Rev Nutr*. 1991;11: 355–373.

97. Goran MI. Application of the doubly labeled water technique for studying energy expenditure in young children: a review. *Pediatr Exerc Sci*. 1994;6: 11–30.

98. Caspersen CJ, Powell KE, Christenson GM. Physical activity, exercise, and physical fitness: definitions and distinctions for health-related research. *Public Health Rep*. 1985;100: 126–131.

99. Montoye HJ. Introduction: evaluation of some measurements of physical activity and energy expenditure. *Med Sci Sports Exerc*. 2000;32: S439–S441.

100. Riddoch CJ, Boreham CA. The health-related physical activity of children. *Sports Med*. 1995;19: 86–102.

101. Rowlands AV, Eston RG, Ingledew DK. Measurement of physical activity in children with particular reference to the use of heart rate and pedometry. *Sports Med*. 1997;24: 258–272.

102. Baranowski T, Bouchard C, Bar-Or O, et al. Assessment, prevalence, and cardiovascular benefits of physical activity and fitness in youth. *Med Sci Sports Exerc*. 1992;24: S237–S247.

103. Baranowski T, Simons-Morton BG. Dietary and physical activity assessment in school-aged children: measurement issues. *J Sch Health*. 1991;61: 195–197.

104. Lee IM, Rexrode KM, Cook NR, Manson JE, Buring JE. Physical activity and coronary heart disease in women. *JAMA*. 2001;285:1447–1454.

105. Wannamethee SG, Shaper AG. Physical activity in the prevention of cardiovascular disease: an epidemiological perspective. *Sports Med*. 2001;31: 101–114.

106. Sallis JF. Self-report measures of children's physical activity. *J Sch Health*. 1991;61: 215–219.

107. Baranowski T. Validity and reliability of self report measures on physical activity: an information processing perspective. *Res Q Exerc Sport*. 1988;59: 314–327.

108. Durant R, Ainsworth BE. The recall of physical activity: using a cognitive model of the question-answering process. *Med Sci Sports Exerc*. 1996;28: 1282–1291.

109. Pate RR. Physical activity assessment in children and adolescents. *Crit Rev Food Sci Nutr*. 1993;33: 321–326.

110. Saris WHM, The assessment and evaluation of daily physical activity in children. A review. *Acta Paediatr*. 1985;318(5): 37–48.

111. Kriska AM, Knowler WC, LaPorte RE, et al. Development of questionnaire to examine relationship of physical activity and diabetes in Pima Indians. *Diabetes Care*. 1990;13: 401–411.

112. Kemper HC. *The Amsterdam Growth Study: A Longitudinal Analysis of Health, Fitness, and Lifestyle*. Champaign, IL: Human Kinetics, 1997.

113. Goran MI, Hunter G, Nagy TR, Johnson R. Physical activity related energy expenditure and fat mass in young children. *Int J Obes Relat Metab Disord*. 1997;21: 171–178.

114. Pate RR, Ross R, Dowda M, Trost SG, Sirard JR. Validation of a 3-day physical activity recall instrument in female youth. *Pediatr Exer Sci*. 2003;15: 257–265.

115. Sallis JF, Strikmiller PK, Harsha DW, Feldman HA, Ehlinger S, Stone EJ, et al. Validation of interviewer- and self-adminstered physical activity checklists for fifth grade students. *Med Sci Sports Exerc*. 1996;28: 840–851.

116. Sallis JF, Buono MJ, Roby JJ, Carlson D, Nelson JA. the Caltrac accelerometer as a physical activity monitor for school-age children. *Med Sci Sports Exerc*. 1990;22: 698–703.

117. Welk GJ, Corbin CB, Dale D. Measurement issues in the assessment of physical activity in children. *Res Q Exerc Sport*. 2000;71: S59–S73.

118. Weston AT, Petosa R, Pate RR. Validation of an instrument for measurement of physical activity in youth. *Med Sci Sports Exerc*. 1997;29: 138–143.

119. Sallis JF, Condon SA, Goggin KJ, Roby JJ, Kolody B, Alcaraz JE. The development of self-administered physical activity surveys for 4th grade students. *Res Q Exerc Sport*. 1993;64: 25–31.

120. McMurray RG, Ring KB, Treuth MS, et al. Comparison of two approaches to structured physical activity surveys for adolescents. *Med Sci Sports Exerc*. 2004;36: 2135–2143.

121. Sleap M, Warburton P. Physical activity levels of 5–11-year-old children in England as determined by continuous observation. *Res Q Exerc Sport*. 1992;63: 238–245.

122. Bullen BA, Reed RB, Mayer J. Physical activity of obese and nonobese adolescent girls appraised by motion picture sampling. *Am J Clin Nutr*. 1964;14: 211–223.

123. Bassett DR, Jr., Strath SJ. Use of pedometers at assess physical activity. In: Welk GJ, Ed. *Physical Activity Assessments for Health-Related Research*. Champaign, IL: Human Kinetics, 2002: 163–177.

124. Welk GJ. Use of accelerometry-based activity monitors to assess physical activity. In: Welk GJ, Ed. *Physical Activity Assessments for Health-Related Research*. Champaign, IL: Human Kinetics, 2002: 125–142.

125. Saris WH, Binkhorst RA. The use of pedometer and actometer in studying daily physical activity in man. Part II: validity of pedometer and actometer measuring the daily physical activity. *Eur J Appl Physiol*. 1977;37: 229–235.

126. Kemper HC, Verschuur R. Validity and reliability of pedometers in habitual activity research. *Eur J Appl Physiol*. 1977;37: 71–82.

127. Rowlands AV, Eston RG, Ingledew DK. Relationship between activity levels, aerobic fitness, and body fat in 8- to 10-yr-old children. *J Appl Physiol*. 1999;86: 1428–1435.

128. Treuth MS, Sherwood NE, Butte NF, et al. Validity and reliability of activity measures in African-American girls for GEMS. *Med Sci Sports Exerc*. 2003;35: 532–539.

129. Eston RG, Rowlands AV, Ingledew DK. Validity of heart rate, pedometry, and accelerometry for predicting the energy cost of children's activities. *J Appl Physiol*. 1998;84: 362–371.

130. Melanson EL, Jr., Freedson PS. Validity of the Computer Science and Applications, Inc. (CSA) activity monitor. *Med Sci Sports Exerc*. 1995;27: 934–940.

131. Freedson PS. Electronic motion sensors and heart rate as measures of physical activity in children. *J Sch Health*. 1991;61: 220–223.

132. Johnson RK, Russ J, Goran MI. Physical activity related energy expenditure in children by doubly labeled water as compared with the Caltrac accelerometer. *Int J Obes*. Relat Metab Disord 1998;22: 1046–1052.

133. Hoos MB, Plasqui G, Gerver WJ, Westerterp KR. Physical activity level measured by doubly labeled water and accelerometry in children. *Eur J Appl Physiol*. 2003;89: 624–626.

134. Treuth MS, Schmitz K, Catellier DJ, et al. Defining accelerometer thresholds for activity intensities in adolescent girls. *Med Sci Sports Exerc*. 2004;36: 1259–1266.

135. Puyau MR, Adolph AL, Vohra FA, Butte NF. Validation and calibration of physical activity monitors in children. *Obes Res*. 2002;10: 150–157.

136. Livingstone MB, Coward WA, Prentice AM, et al. Daily energy expenditure in free-living children: comparison of heart rate monitoring with the doubly labeled water (2H$_2$(18)O) method. *Am J Clin Nutr*. 1992;56: 343–352.

137. Spady DW. Total daily energy expenditure of healthy, free ranging school children. *Am J Clin Nutr*. 1980;33: 766–775.

138. Treuth MS, Adolph AL, Butte NF. Energy expenditure in children predicted from heart rate and activity calibrated against respiration calorimetry. *Am J Physiol*. 1998;275: E12–E18.

139. Durant RH, Baranowski T, Davis H, et al. Reliability and variability of indicators of heart-rate monitoring in children. *Med Sci Sports Exerc*. 1993;25: 389–395.

140. Treiber FA, Musante L, Hartdagan S, Davis H, Levy M, Strong WB. Validation of a heart rate monitor with children in laboratory and field settings. *Med Sci Sports Exerc*. 1989;21: 338–342.

141. Strath SJ, Swartz AM, Bassett DR, O'Brien WL, King GA, Ainsworth BE. Evaluation of heart rate as a method for assessing moderate intensitity physical activity. *Med Sci Sports Exerc*. 2000;32: 465–470.

142. Li R, Deurenberg P, Hautvast J. A critical evaluation of heart rate monitoring to assess energy expenditure in individuals. *Am J Clin Nutr*. 1993;58: 602–607.

143. Welk GJ, Corbin CB, Kampert JB. The validity of the Tritrac-R3D activity monitor for the assessment of physical activity: II. Temporal relationships among objective assessments. *Res Q Exerc Sport*. 1998;69: 395–399.

8 Regulation of Body Weight: Energy Expenditure and Physical Activity

Margarita S. Treuth and Linda G. Bandini

CONTENTS

INTRODUCTION

The average healthy 5-year-old child consumes 500,000 kcal/yr and shows a remarkable ability to regulate the body by matching energy intake to energy expenditure and storage for growth. The regulation of body weight is dependent on multiple factors, but in general, weight gain occurs when there is an imbalance between energy intake and energy expenditure. This chapter focuses on the relationship of energy expenditure to body weight in children, in particular the components of energy expenditure (EE) and physical activity (PA). Measurement aspects are covered in Chapter 7. The effects of exercise on obesity are discussed in Chapter 10, and behavioral aspects of physical activity can be found in Chapter 14. Although energy intake is equally as important as expenditure or activity in energy balance, dietary intake will be covered elsewhere in terms of eating behaviors (Chapter 13) and dietary approaches for the prevention of childhood obesity (Chapter 18).

One area of particular research interest involves studies on the predictors of weight gain that focus on energy expenditure in infants, children, and adolescents.[1–9] Most studies suggest that lower energy expenditure does not influence weight gain,[2–5,8,9] except for the earliest study by Roberts et al.[1] and an even earlier study by Griffiths and Payne.[10] Energy expenditure related to physical activity is the most variable component among individuals. In adults, physical activity is associated with weight maintenance or weight loss. In children, it is more complicated because it is difficult to separate out the effects of the contribution of physical activity to energy expenditure from that due to normal growth and maturation.

ENERGY BALANCE

Energy balance is achieved when energy intake of food matches energy expenditure of the body. When intake exceeds expenditure and a positive energy balance has occurred, weight gain results. The converse is true for weight loss where energy expenditure exceeds intake and a negative energy balance has occurred. In infants, children, and adolescents who are in a rapid period of growth, additional energy is required for growth, and this amount is dependent on the age of the child (see section on Energy Requirements).

Total energy expenditure (TEE) is composed of basal metabolic rate (BMR; or resting metabolic rate, RMR, which is about 5% higher than BMR due to arousal), the thermic effect of food, and activity energy expenditure (activity EE). Resting metabolic rate accounts for about 60 to 70% of the TEE, whereas the thermic effect of food is much smaller (10%); the activity component constitutes the remainder. Physical activity EE, defined as the increase in metabolic rate that is caused by use of skeletal muscles for any type of movement, is the most variable component of daily EE.[11] Because RMR accounts for the largest portion of TEE, interindividual differences in RMR have been hypothesized to contribute to the development of obesity. Individuals with low RMR may be at risk for weight gain, whereas those with high activity EE may be less likely to become overweight.

Mayer et al.[12,13] first suggested that there was a threshold of inactivity that was associated with poor weight control. Persons with high levels of physical activity can maintain energy balance, whereas those with low physical activity cannot regulate this as precisely; therefore they become overweight. Physical activity level (PAL) is defined as TEE/RMR and can be quantified using a highly accurate technique, namely doubly labeled water, to measure TEE in conjunction with indirect calorimetry to measure RMR (see measurement aspects in Chapter 7). When examining existing data sets of TEE, fat mass (FM) and fat-free mass (FFM), Westerterp[14] reported that a higher PAL was associated with a lower fat mass in males. Schulz and Schoeller[15] found a highly significant negative relationship between PAL and body fatness, suggesting that a low PAL is a permissive factor for obesity. The threshold of physical activity that was found to protect against weight gain was 1.75, as supported by cross-sectional doubly labeled water data in adults.[16] These thresholds are likely different and more complicated for children because additional energy is required for growth, and PAL appears to be influenced by body weight.[17]

ENERGY REQUIREMENTS

The most recent report from the Institute of Medicine contains the Dietary Reference Intakes (DRI) for energy.[18] This is important in the context of childhood obesity in that these estimates are influenced by physical activity levels. The estimated energy requirement (EER) is defined as the dietary energy intake that is predicted to maintain energy balance in a healthy adult of a defined age, gender, weight, height, and level of physical activity consistent with good health.[18] Requirements for children and adolescents differ from adults in that energy requirements increase because of growth and developmental changes. Therefore, the committee developed prediction equations specific for infants, children, and adolescents based on a comprehensive review of the scientific data. The report[18] has equations for infants 0 to 2 years of age, children 3 to 8 years of age, and adolescent girls and boys 9 through 18 years of age. Infants require an additional 20 to 175 kcal/d for energy deposition, depending on the age of the infant. For children and adolescents, an extra

25 kcal/d was added for energy deposition to the EER. This was based on the rates of weight gain of children enrolled in the Fels Longitudinal Study[19] and rates of protein and fat deposition for adolescents.[20] During adolescence, fat deposition is higher in girls than in boys and that may influence the energy requirements.

The estimated energy requirement equations utilize age, weight, height, the extra requirement for energy deposition, and physical activity. There are four levels of activity — sedentary, low active, active, and very active — based on PALs derived from previous doubly labeled water studies. These four PALs were given different physical activity coefficients (PA coefficients) in the equations. Thus, to estimate the energy requirements, the activity coefficient must be chosen by estimating the child's activity level. Because of the differences between boys and girls in growth and fat deposition, gender-specific equations were developed. These equations were developed for each age group (infants, children, and adolescents) and can be found in the report.[18] These equations are useful to estimate the energy needs of individuals and are fairly straightforward as only age, weight, and height are needed.

Two equations are provided below for boys and girls age 9 to 18 years to understand how these equations are also useful when comparing individuals with different physical activity levels.

$$\text{Boys: EER} = 88.5 - [61.9 \times \text{age (yr)}] + \text{PA} \times [26.7 \times \text{weight (kg)}]$$
$$+ [903 \times \text{height (m)}] + 25 \text{ kcal/d for energy deposition}$$

$$\text{Girls: EER} = 135.3 - [30.8 \times \text{age (yr)}] + \text{PA} \times [10.0 \times \text{weight (kg)}]$$
$$+ 934 \times [\text{height (m)}] + 25 \text{ kcal/d for energy deposition}$$

For example, a male adolescent 14 years of age with a weight of 51.0 kg, height of 1.64 m, and a sedentary PAL would have an estimated energy requirement of 2090 kcal/d. The same adolescent who had a high active PAL would have an estimated energy requirement of 3283 kcal/d. An adolescent girl 14 years of age with a weight of 49.4 kg, height of 1.60 m, and a sedentary PAL would have an estimated energy requirement of 1718 kcal/d. If this female adolescent increased her activity level to high active, her estimated energy requirement would be 2831 kcal/d. These examples are useful to illustrate the marked differences in requirements between an adolescent classified as either sedentary or having a high physical activity level. These same comparisons are applicable to infants and children. If one wishes to accurately predict a child's energy requirements, it is clear that the physical activity level must be chosen correctly. Otherwise, a mismatch between intake and expenditure could lead to either under or overnutrition. Choosing the appropriate activity level (and therefore the activity coefficient) is one difficult challenge and a limitation of using these equations.

ENERGY EXPENDITURE

There have been several excellent review papers on EE in infants and children.[11,21–23] However, the focus in this chapter is on the relationship between energy expenditure and body weight.

In a cross-sectional study of infants that used doubly labeled water to measure TEE, no significant relationship was observed between body fat and total energy expenditure in infants 12 weeks of age.[24] In another cross-sectional study in older infants (9 to 12 months of age), FFM explained less than 20% of the variation in TEE.[25] The findings of these two studies suggest that other factors such as behavior contribute to the energy needs of infants.[25]

Cross-sectional studies of obese and nonobese children and adolescents have not shown differences in RMR and TEE after adjustment for body composition.[26–29] Other studies have compared EE in children grouped by parental adiposity.[30–33] Griffiths and Payne[10] found that total energy expenditure by heart rate monitoring and resting EE were lower in 4- to 5-year-old children with one obese parent than those with two normal-weight parents. Wurmser et al.[31] reported that overweight preadolescent girls with two obese parents had the lowest RMR. The normal-weight girls with overweight parents had a higher RMR than the overweight girls with two obese parents. In contrast, Goran et al.[32] reported no differences in TEE and activity EE measured by doubly labeled water in 73 normal-weight and overweight boys and girls with overweight parents. Treuth et al.[33] designed a study to determine whether energy expenditure, measured by 24-h calorimetry and doubly labeled water, differed among normal-weight-for-height, multiethnic, prepubertal girls. The children were grouped according to parental leanness or overweightness and/or obesity, classified by body mass index (BMI). Among familial groups, BMR, sleeping metabolic rate (SMR), 24-h EE, and activity counts were similar. No significant familial group differences in free-living TEE, activity EE, or PAL were observed. Bandini et al.[34] measured RMR and TEE in 196 premenarcheal nonobese girls with a mean age of 10.1 years. RMR was higher in girls with at least one overweight parent than those with two lean parents. There was no significant difference in nonresting EE, but TEE tended to be higher in the girls with an overweight parent, but the results were of borderline significance. Overall, these cross-sectional studies do not suggest that parental overweight is associated with reduced energy expenditure in children and adolescents.

Other investigators have looked cross-sectionally at the relationship between pubertal status, race and ethnicity, and energy expenditure. Morrison et al.[35] reported a lower RMR among girls who were postmenarcheal than in girls who were premenarcheal, while Molnar and Schutz[29] did not find any differences in RMR related to puberty in girls. In the MIT growth and development study,[34] nonresting EE was found to be significantly lower in pubertal girls (Tanner 2 and 3) than in prepubertal girls (Tanner 1). In a subcohort of 44 girls in the MIT growth and development study, RMR was measured at premenarche, menarche, and 4 years after menarche.[36] Absolute RMR measured around the time of menarche was significantly higher than RMR measured at premenarche or 4 years after menarche despite the fact that FFM was significantly higher at 4 years postmenarche. There was also a significant interaction between FFM, time, and parental overweight, indicating that RMR related to FFM over the period differed between the two parental weight status groups. In girls with overweight parents, RMR adjusted for FFM was lower 4 years postmenarche in comparison with premenarche and menarche. However there was no difference in adjusted RMR at the three time points for girls with normal-weight parents. These findings suggest that the energy required for RMR after controlling for FFM decreases over the adolescent period and that parental overweight may influence the change in RMR during this period.

It has been consistently reported that black children and adolescents have lower RMR than white children and adolescents,[34,37–39] although one study did not find a lower RMR in black girls compared with white girls.[40] Bandini et al.[34] report a lower TEE and nonresting EE in black girls compared with white girls. Treuth et al.[33] also reported a lower TEE in black girls than white girls; however, no difference was observed in activity EE between the two groups. These findings of lower energy expenditure in black children compared with white children suggest that they may be at increased risk for the development of obesity.

These studies illustrate the importance of consideration of variables such as parental weight status, race and ethnicity, and pubertal status in studies of energy expenditure in children and adolescents. Longitudinal studies designed to examine the relationship of energy expenditure with growth and development during childhood and adolescence must consider these factors.

Several well-designed studies[1,2,4,5,7–9] on children at risk of becoming obese by virtue of parental obesity, or reduced energy expenditures have yielded fairly consistent results as to whether energy expenditure plays a role in the development of obesity. The studies that have been conducted in infants, children, and adolescents are reviewed below.

INFANCY

To date, four studies have been conducted with infants to determine the relationship between energy expenditure and weight gain; they are summarized in Table 8.1. In the earliest study, Roberts et al.[1]

TABLE 8.1

Energy Expenditure and the Relationship to Weight Gain in Infants

N	Characteristics of Study Participants (Age, Gender, Race/Ethnicity	Length of Follow-up (months)	Component of Energy Expenditure Measured	Outcome Measure	Results	Ref.
18	Age: 3 months 9 F/9M Race/Eth N/A	9	RMR, TEE	BMI, skinfold thickness	TEE at 3 months of age lower in infants who became overweight	1
33	Age: 3 months 13 F/30 M Race/Eth: N/A	6–21	TEE	BMI, skinfold thickness	No relationship observed between TEE at 3 months and follow-up	2
30	Age: 9 months 16 F/14 M Race/Eth N/A	9	SMR, TEE	BMI, skinfold thickness, % body fat	No relationship observed between SMR and TEE at 9 months and follow-up	3
78	Age: 3 months 39 F/39 M Race/Eth: white	9	SMR, TEE	Weight, weight-for-length, FM, skinfold thickness	No relationship observed between SMR and TEE at 9 months and follow-up	4

Note: F = females; M = males; SMR = sleeping metabolic rate; RMR = resting metabolic rate; TEE = total energy expenditure; BMI = body mass index; FM = fat mass; % body fat = percent body fat by total body water

measured RMR and TEE in infants born to lean mothers and overweight mothers. At 3 months of age, TEE, but not RMR, was lower in the infants who became overweight. The authors concluded that reduced energy expenditure, particularly that which is associated with physical activity, contributed to the excess weight gain in the infants who gained weight. However, three large studies in infants subsequently failed to find evidence of a relationship between reduced RMR, SMR, or TEE and weight gain.[2-4] Davies et al.[2] studied 33 infants, Wells et al.[3] studied 30 infants, and Stunkard et al.[4] studied 78 infants. By comparison, a smaller sample size of only 18 infants was studied by Roberts et al.,[1] and only 6 became overweight. Furthermore, in the study by Stunkard et al.,[4] two groups of infants were studied: one group with obese mothers and one group with lean mothers. Neither mothers' weight status nor energy expenditure related to changes in body weight or fatness over a 9-month period. Thus, the preponderance of evidence does not suggest that a lower RMR or TEE during early infancy is predictive of weight gain.

CHILDHOOD

Several longitudinal studies conducted with children to evaluate the role of EE in the regulation of body weight have yielded consistent results.[5-9,41] Table 8.2 summarizes the main findings of these studies, which are briefly discussed here. In the first study,[5] body composition, and resting and total EE by calorimetry and doubly labeled water, respectively, were measured in Caucasian preadolescent boys and girls over a 4-year period. Using hierarchial linear modeling and analysis of variance, the influence of sex, EE, initial FM, and parental FM on the rate of change in FM was analyzed. The major determinants of the change in FM adjusted for FFM were sex, initial fatness, and parental fatness. A reduced EE (either RMR, TEE, or activity EE) was not a predictor of the change in FM. In another study, Figueroa-Colon et al.[7] studied 47 prepubertal girls using 24-h room respiration calorimetry. Two follow-up measures were taken, at 1.6 and 2.7 years, after the baseline measures. At the 1.6-year follow-up, sleeping EE was positively related to change in body fat and activity EE was inversely related to change in body fat. However, after 2.7 years of follow-up, neither SMR or activity EE were related to change in body fat. Salbe et al.[41] found no relationship

TABLE 8.2

Energy Expenditure and the Relation to Weight Gain in Children and Adolescents

N	Characteristics of Study Participants (Age, Gender, Race/Ethnicity)	Length of Follow-up (yr)	Component of Energy Expenditure Measured	Outcome Measure	Results	Ref.
75	4–7.2 yr M and F Caucasian	4	TEE, PAEE by DLW	Rate of change in FM adjusted for FFM	Strongest predictors of change in FM were fatness in fathers and mothers. After adjusting for parental fatness, EE was not related to change in FM.	5
115	4.6–11 yr M and F Caucasian, African American	3 to 5	TEE, PAEE by DLW	Rate of increasing FM relative to increasing FFM	Significant predictor of FM gain was aerobic fitness (negative relationship between aerobic fitness and FM).	6
47	4.8–8.9 yr F Race/Eth N/A	2.7	TEE, Activity EE, Sleep EE by calorimetry	Change in FM and % fat	No relationship of EE with change in body fat at 2.7 yr	7
138	5 yr M and F Native American	5	RMR, TEE, PAEE by DLW	% fat	No significant predictors of the change in % body fat	41
101	8–9 yr F Caucasian, African American, Hispanic	2	TEE, PAEE by DLW TEE, BMR, Activity EE, Sleep EE by calorimetry	FM, % fat Change in FM and % fat	Predictors of change in % fat were free-living total EE (negative) and muscle oxidative capacity (positive).	8
196	8–12 yr F Caucasian, African American, Hispanic, Asian	7.2 ± 2.6 (mean ± SD)	RMR, TEE by DLW, activity EE	Change in BMI z score; change in % fat by bioimpedance	No relationship between RMR, activity EE, TEE, and % fat activity EE positively associated with change in BMI-z score	9

Note: F = females; M = males; TEE = total energy expenditure; PAEE = physical activity energy expenditure; EE = energy expenditure; DLW = doubly labeled water; RMR = resting metabolic rate; BMR = basal metabolic rate; FM = fat mass; FFM = fat-free mass

of EE and body fat in 5-year-old overweight Native American boys and girls who were followed for 5 years. Treuth et al.[8] studied 101 prepubertal, multiethnic, normal-weight girls over a 2-year period. Measures of fitness, baseline EE by 24-h calorimetry, TEE by doubly labeled water, and muscle oxidative capacity by nuclear magnetic resonance imaging, were used to examine the predictors of weight or fat gain in these girls. Free-living TEE was negatively predictive of the change in percent fat. Muscle oxidative capacity, an indicator of fitness, was positively predictive of the change in percent fat. Johnson et al.[6] studied 115 boys and girls over a 3- to 5-year period. Measures of TEE and activity EE were examined as predictors of the rate of increasing FM relative to the increase in FFM. Neither of these variables was found to be predictive of the change in FM. However, aerobic fitness was found to be a significant predictor of the change in FM, with a negative relationship observed between fitness and FM.[6] These four studies have yielded somewhat similar results. The differences in findings as to the predictors of weight or fat gain from these studies could be due to differences in samples (boys, girls, age, normal or overweight at baseline) and methods of analysis of the data (adjusting or not adjusting for FFM).

ADOLESCENCE

In the MIT growth and development study,[9] EE was measured in the premenarcheal period, and body composition, dietary intake, and physical activity were measured annually until 4 years after menarche with a mean follow-up period of 7.1 ± 2.6 years. A linear mixed-effects model was used to evaluate the longitudinal relationship between BMI z-score and percent body fat, and measures of baseline RMR, activity EE, and TEE after adjusting for potential covariates including physical activity, age, age at menarche, and diet composition. RMR was not related to change in percent body fat or BMI z-score. A small positive relationship of activity EE and TEE with BMI z-score but not percent body fat was observed. When the results were stratified by parental overweight, the findings were unchanged for RMR. TEE and activity EE were positively related to BMI z-score in girls of overweight parents. These data do not support the hypothesis that low energy expenditure is a risk factor for weight gain in girls during adolescence.[9]

ENERGY EXPENDITURE IN CHILDREN WITH DEVELOPMENTAL DISABILITIES

Obesity is associated with several developmental disabilities including spastic quadraparesis, spina bifida, Down syndrome, and Prader–Willi syndrome. Research on body composition in children with developmental disabilities is limited. However, studies have shown that children, adolescents, and young adults with developmental disabilities have alterations in body composition.[42-44] Studies designed to examine the energy needs and relationship of energy expenditure and obesity in children and adolescents with developmental disabilities are discussed below. Most of these studies have very small sample sizes limiting the generalizability of the findings.

CEREBRAL PALSY

Cerebral palsy (CP) is a syndrome that is caused by damage to the brain during pregnancy, delivery, or shortly after birth.[45] Individuals with CP experience a number of motor problems including spasticity (tight muscles), nonfunctional movements, rigidity (severe spasticity), and poor balance. They may also have difficulties with speech, hearing, and/or vision and seizures, and may have learning disabilities or mental retardation. There are several types of cerebral palsy including spastic quadraparesis, spastic diplegia, hemiplegia, ataxia, and athetosis. Diagnosis is made based on neurological signs, abnormalities in muscle tone, and the presence of abnormal motor patterns and posture.[45] Spastic quadraparesis (SQCP) is one type of cerebral palsy that has been associated with obesity although some children with SQCP have significant limitations that cause feeding difficulties and thus result in undernutrition.

Table 8.3 summarizes the findings of studies reporting EE measures in children with CP and other syndromes. Stallings et al.[46] measured energy expenditure in 61 nonambulatory children and adolescents with SQCP, some of whom were undernourished, and 37 typically developing children. In children with SQCP who had reduced fat stores, RMR adjusted for body composition was found to be significantly lower than age-matched controls. In children with SQCP who had adequate fat stores, RMR did not differ from controls. Children with low fat stores had resting energy expenditure (REE) 88 ± 20% of that predicted from the WHO equation[47] while children with adequate fat stores had REE 101 ± 18% of that predicted from the WHO equation. Bandini et al.[48] found that RMR and FFM in a group of nine adolescents with CP (five SQCP, one athetoid, two diplegia, one

TABLE 8.3
Energy Expenditure in Children and Adolescents with Developmental Disabilities

N	Type of Disability	Characteristics of Study Participants (Age, Gender)	RMR Predicted from WHO Equation (%)	Physical Activity Level (Ambulatory)	Physical Activity Level (Nonambulatory)	Ref.
9	Cerebral palsy	18.6 ± 1.1 8 F 1 M	100.0 ± 1.0[a]	1.79 ± 0.29 (3)	1.23 ± 0.16 (6)	48
10	Cerebral palsy	8.2 ± 1.2 F 7.8 ± 1.6 M 5 F 5 M	N/A	1.59 ± 0.18 (9)	1.29 (1)	49
61	Cerebral palsy	9.0 ± 4.3 31 F 30 M	All: 91 ± 20 Low fat store group 88 ± 20 Adequate fat 101 ± 18	N/A	1.23 ± 0.36 Low fat store group 1.07 ± 0.27	46
13	Cerebral palsy	8.4 ± 4.4 5 F 8 M	79.0 ± 21	N/A	N/A	50
10	Spina bifida	16.6 ± 1.6 F 17.9 ± 0.5 M 7 F 3 M	85.0 ± 11.0	1.51 ± 0.06 (4)	1.20 ± 0.22 (5)	48
9	Down syndrome	8 ± 2 4 F 5 M	79.5 ± 10.4%	1.85 ± 0.23	N/A	60
10	Prader–Willi-syndrome	16 ± 4 5 F 5 M	N/A	N/A	N/A	61
10	Prader–Willi syndrome	11.7 ± 3.5 5F 5 M	N/A	1.33 ± 0.21	N/A	62
17	Prader–Willi syndrome	11.9 ± 3.4 10 F 7 M	N/A	1.33 ± 0.15	N/A	63

[a] Mean ± SD: () = N; N/A = not available.

hemiplegia) were significantly lower than in a group of typically developing adolescents. Yet, RMR in absolute terms was not significantly different from that predicted from the WHO equation (100.0 ± 1.0%). When comparing children with spastic diplegia to controls (each n = 10), van den Berg Emons et al.[49] reported that FFM and SMR expressed per kilogram FFM were similar among children with CP and controls. By contrast, Azcue et al.[50] reported a lower RMR and less FFM in children with SQCP (n = 13) than in controls (n = 21). RMR in these children were considerably lower than that predicted by WHO equations 79 ± 21%.

Overall, these studies suggest that RMR is lower in children and adolescents with CP and is a result of a decrease in FFM. There appears to be a wide variability in RMR, however, and the use of the WHO equations to calculate individual RMR may lead to a significant overestimation of energy needs. Azcue et al.[50] have speculated that there may be two different populations with SQCP: one whose REE is normal in relation to body cell mass and one whose REE is reduced in relation to body cell mass. These differences may be related to the site of the central nervous system lesion.[50]

In three studies described above,[46,48,49] TEE was also measured. In two studies,[46,48] TEE was found to be significantly lower in children with CP than in typically developing children and adolescents of the same age. In contrast, TEE expressed per kilogram FFM was not significantly different from controls in another study.[49] In the studies by Stallings et al.[46] and van den Berg Emons et al.,[49] PAL was significantly lower than controls. In the study by Bandini et al.,[48] PAL was significantly lower than controls but only for subjects who could not ambulate and not significantly different from those subjects who were ambulatory. This may be due to an increase in energy required for the subjects with CP who could ambulate because of poor efficiency and the increased work needed to perform the activity. Rose et al.[51] have demonstrated higher heart rates and slower walking speeds in ambulatory children with CP, suggesting a higher workload. The differences observed between studies might be due to the different age groups studied and the small sample sizes.

Overall, these findings suggest that individuals with CP have a lower energy requirement, not higher, as has often been suggested. Limited physical activity due to impairments in mobility, weak muscles, and hypotonia would be expected to decrease energy expenditure.

SEVERE CENTRAL NERVOUS SYSTEM IMPAIRMENT

Several studies[52,53] have been conducted to investigate the energy needs of children with severe central nervous system (CNS) impairment. Dickerson et al.[52] report RMR in adolescents with severe neurodevelopmental disabilities who were tube fed to be $80 \pm 11\%$ of that predicted from the WHO equations.[47] Bandini et al.[53] measured RMR in 12 persons (mean age 18.6 ± 6.2 years) with severe CNS impairment who were fed exclusively by gastrostomy feedings. These subjects were studied in the postprandial state, thus RMR included both RMR and the thermic effect of food. RMR was $63.7 \pm 18\%$ of that predicted from the WHO equations. Because these subjects were nonambulatory and totally dependent on caretakers for all their activities of daily living, RMR and the thermic effect of food were assumed to be equivalent to daily energy needs. Energy intake adjusted for changes in body weight was found to be a valid method to determine energy requirements in these individuals.

Many children with severe oral–motor problems are fed through a gastrostromy tube. When these children are fed orally, they may not receive adequate intake and may become malnourished. When fed via a gastrostromy tube, however, they may be at risk for obesity due to their lower energy requirements and lack of guidelines for energy intake. In the care of a child with severe physical disabilities, lower energy needs must be considered to prevent excessive weight gain and the development of obesity. It should also be noted that there is wide variability of energy requirements in these children. When possible, measurements of RMR would be helpful to establish energy needs. Additionally, it is necessary to emphasize the importance of monitoring protein and micronutrient intake to prevent nutritional deficiencies on these low calorie intakes.

SPINA BIFIDA

Spina bifida is a birth defect in which the neural tube fails to close and part of the spinal cord and surrounding nerves do not develop properly. Children with spina bifida can have difficulties with ambulation, and bladder and bowel control; they are often of short stature.[44,54,55] Obesity in this group of children is a common problem.[43,54,56]

Despite the high prevalence of obesity in children with spina bifida, only two studies have examined EE and physical activity in these children.[48,57] Fat-free mass, RMR, and TEE were significantly lower in adolescents with spina bifida than in a comparison group of typically developing adolescents.[48] The WHO equation overestimated RMR by 15%. The mean activity factor for nonambulatory children was 1.20 compared with 1.51 in ambulatory children. In another study by van den Berg Emons et al.,[57] low activity levels (as measured by accelerometry) were observed in ambulatory and nonambulatory adolescents and young adults with spina bifida in comparison with healthy age-matched subjects. These studies are limited by their small sample size but suggest that energy requirements are reduced in adolescents with spina bifida due to a reduction in FFM and/or a decrease in energy spent on physical activity.

Down Syndrome

Down syndrome (DS) is a developmental disorder caused by the presence of an extra chromosome 21 and is characterized by mental retardation, cardiac and thyroid disorders, and orthopedic problems.[58] Children with DS are of shorter stature than other children their age, and specific growth charts are available to monitor growth in children with DS. Obesity is common among children with DS;[59] however, little research has been done to determine the relationship of EE to obesity in this population.

In one study, Luke et al.[60] measured RMR (n = 9) and TEE (n = 12) in children with DS (mean age 8.0 years). RMR in children with DS was significantly lower than RMR of control children after adjusting for FFM, yet PAL (1.85 ± 0.23) was not significantly different from controls. Measured RMR was an average of 79.5% of RMR predicted from the WHO equations. Energy expenditure was not predictive of body fatness after a 1-year follow-up. However, the sample size was too small to determine conclusively whether low metabolic rate could be responsible for obesity in children with DS.

Prader–Willi Syndrome

Prader–Willi syndrome (PWS) is a complex genetic disorder caused by an abnormality of the chromosome 15 and is highly associated with obesity.[42] Major characteristics of PWS include hypotonia at birth, failure to thrive in infancy, poor suck and swallowing reflexes during early infancy, developmental delays, behavioral difficulties, hypogonadism, and delayed or diminished puberty.[42] Individuals with PWS have disordered satiety in that they do not experience the sensation of fullness after eating, which often results in hyperphagia, obsession with food, weight gain that is rapid or excessive between ages 1 to 6, and obesity.[42] Although only a few studies have examined the relationship of EE and obesity in this population, all have consistently shown that persons with PWS have reduced energy requirements.

Schoeller et al.[61] measured FFM and TEE in children and adolescents with PWS. TEE was significantly lower in the subjects with PWS than obese controls. After normalizing TEE for body size, TEE was lower in the subjects with PWS and reflected less energy spent on physical activity. Davies and Joughin[62] studied 10 children with PWS. Although there was no significant difference between TEE and RMR in children with PWS, the PAL value was 1.33 ± 0.21 in children with PWS and was significantly lower than in typically developing children 1.53 ± 0.23. Similarly, in a study by van Mill et al.,[63] FFM and BMR were lower in children with PWS than in a group of control children matched for sex and bone age, but there was no difference in BMR when adjusted for FFM. Their findings suggest that the lower RMR is a result of a decrease in FFM. Activity EE and PAL were also significantly lower in the subjects with PWS.[63] The lower FFM and the reduced energy spent on activity contribute to the reduced energy needs of this population. These findings of a reduced energy need in conjunction with the hyperphagia increase the risk for obesity in this population.

There are other less studied genetic disorders associated with obesity such as the Bardet–Biedl syndrome, Albright hereditary osteodystrophy, Cohen syndrome, and Borjeson–Forssman–Lehmann syndrome.[64] Studies of energy expenditure are limited or absent in these groups. Overall studies of children and adolescents with developmental disabilities are limited by small samples sizes. Nonetheless, most of the studies reported suggest that persons with cerebral palsy, spina bifida, Down syndrome, and Prader–Willi syndrome have reductions in FFM, RMR, and TEE. These studies suggest that the energy requirements of persons with these developmental disabilities are lower than those of their typically developing peers.

PHYSICAL ACTIVITY

Physical activity has been promoted as a lifelong positive health behavior in children and adolescents.[65] Current data on physical activity levels in children are few. One study of over 4000 children from ages 8 to 16 years showed that approximately 20% of U.S. children do not exercise vigorously more than twice per week, with these inactivity rates higher in girls (26%) than in boys (17%).[66] The Centers for Disease Control and Prevention (CDC)[67] recommends that students in kindergarten through grade 12 (ages 5 to 18 years) have comprehensive, daily physical education. However, only 60% of high school students are enrolled in physical education classes, with only 25% taking daily physical education.[68] This has increased slightly. The 2001 Youth Risk Behavior Surveillance System Survey (YRBSS) reported that 32.2% took physical education classes daily, with approximately 52% of students in grades 9 to 12 enrolled in physical education classes.[69] The current recommendation for children is to accumulate a minimum of 60 min of moderate and vigorous physical activity each day.[18] Recently, the National Association for Sport and Physical Education and the Council on Physical Education for Children also recommended at least 60 min and up to several hours per day on most days of the week.[70] The activity should be age appropriate, and long periods of inactivity are discouraged.[70]

Research has documented low physical activity levels of adolescents,[68] particularly in girls.[71] Furthermore, a precipitous decline in physical activity levels in adolescent girls was recently reported, with almost no physical activity reported by ages 18 and 19 years.[72] In the recent YRBSS survey, 31.2% of high school students reported no vigorous activity lasting 20 min or more during three of the seven preceding days.[69] Insufficient levels of physical activity in U.S. children may therefore lead to increases in adiposity.

The new DRIs recommend a PAL of 1.6 to prevent excess weight gain.[18] This means that to move from a very sedentary (PAL of 1.4) to an active lifestyle (PAL > 1.6), children and adolescents must participate in moderately intense activity a total of 60 min/d. Longitudinal studies are needed to monitor physical activity levels and normal growth patterns.

Several studies have been conducted in children using doubly labeled water to assess physical activity level.[73–78] A review by Torun et al.[73] indicated that the PAL ranges from 1.38 to 1.51 in studies including children 2.5 to 5.5 years. In a recent study of 3-year-old Caucasian children, Reilly et al.[78] reported a PAL of 1.60 in boys and 1.52 in girls.

In the review by Torun et al.,[73] the range of PALs from several studies for boys 6 to 13 years of age was 1.71 to 1.86, with a mean of 1.79 ± 0.06.[73] Correspondingly for girls 6 to 13 years of age, the range was 1.69 to 1.90, with a mean of 1.80 ± 0.12.[73] For adolescents over the age of 14 years, the mean for boys was 1.84 ± 0.05 (range 1.79 to 1.88) and for girls 1.69 ± 0.03 (range 1.67 to 1.69).[73]

Several studies have suggested that reduced physical activity plays a significant role in the etiology of childhood obesity.[41,79] In the Framingham Children's Study, preschool children with low levels of physical activity gained substantially more subcutaneous fat than did more active children.[80] In a 3-year longitudinal analysis of preschool children, increases in children's leisure activity and higher baseline aerobic activity were associated with decreases in body mass index.[81] This suggested that accelerated weight gain in preschool children could be modified by participation in physical activity.[81]

Studies of longitudinal changes in energy spent on physical activity are limited. In children followed from age 5 to 9.5 years, a decrease in TEE was observed in the girls, but TEE increased in the boys.[82] A decrease in activity EE in girls between 6.5 and 9.5 years of age occurred, where activity EE values dropped by 50%.[82] The lower TEE (and consequently activity EE) as the girls get older and increase their body weight is unusual and warrants further investigation. In contrast, Salbe et al.[41] studied obese Native American children at age 5 and again at age 10. Weight more than doubled over the 5 years, and activity EE increased over that period. In African-American and Caucasian adolescents with a mean age of 12.7 years, energy expenditure by doubly labeled water was measured over a 2-year period.[83] Despite an increase in body weight, average TEE did not change over the 2-year period; however, RMR increased slightly and activity EE decreased significantly.[83] This reduction in activity (measured by doubly labeled water) during adolescence would agree with self-report declines in activity in girls from 10 to 18 years of age.[72]

FUTURE DIRECTIONS

The relationship between EE and weight gain has been fairly well studied in infants, children, and adolescents, and the general consensus is that a lower energy expenditure is not predictive of weight gain. Little has been done with preschool age children and those with developmental disabilities. In addition, boys have not been studied over the pubertal period. Studies of ethnically diverse children and adolescents are warranted given the high rates of obesity in African-American, Hispanic, and Native American children. More studies are needed to determine the relationship between parental overweight, and fitness and body weight gain during childhood. Another potential area of research would be to conduct longitudinal studies into young adulthood. It would be also interesting to track children for a longer follow-up period; only one study[9] followed girls throughout the period of adolescent development. Given that energy expenditure studies are costly, this may be impractical. However, the length of the reviewed studies is typically less than 4 years.

Further improvements to the methodology used to assess activity levels in children and adolescents are needed to clarify age-related changes in activity. The discrepancies in findings of activity levels in children and adolescents may be due to the expression of the data or the inability of current methods to accurately assess physical activity. Further research is warranted to determine the best measure to assess physical activity in children.

SUMMARY

There is a consensus among the literature that maintenance of body weight and composition is highly important in terms of health consequences for children. Therefore, many different interventions have been implemented at clinical centers, schools, and the home to evaluate the influences of energy expenditure on obesity. Regulation of body weight is influenced by many factors. The energy needs of infants, children, and adolescents differ. Part of this is influenced by the energy requirement of physical activity. Because physical activity levels vary so much, not only across these age groups, but in individuals within an age group, many studies have focused on the role that energy expenditure, and in particular the physical activity component of energy expenditure, plays in energy balance and regulation of body weight. There has clearly been a focus on what component of energy expenditure may be important in the development of obesity.

The effects of growth and maturation on the outcomes make it difficult to concisely provide an overall conclusion from these studies. In addition, studies have used varied measures of energy expenditure and physical activity, making comparisons more difficult. However, it is certain that the increasing prevalence of obesity in the United States warrants attention. Energy expenditure and physical activity clearly plays a role in the regulation of body weight.

REFERENCES

1. Roberts SB, Savage J, Coward WA, Chew B, Lucas A. Energy expenditure and intake in infants born to lean and overweight mothers. *New Engl J Med.* 1988;318: 461–466.
2. Davies PSW, Day JME, Lucas A. Energy expenditure in early infancy and later body fatness. *Int J Obes.* 1991;15: 727–731.
3. Wells JC, Stanley M, Laidlaw AS, Day JM, Davies PS. The relationship between components of infant energy expenditure and childhood body fatness. *Int J Obes.* 1996;20: 848–853.
4. Stunkard AJ, Berkowitz RI, Stallings VA, Schoeller DA. Energy intake, not energy output, is a determinant of body size in infants. *Am J Clin Nutr.* 1999;69(3): 524–530.
5. Goran MI, Shewchuk R, Gower BA, Nagy TR, Carpenter WH, Johnson RK. Longitudinal changes in fatness in white children: no effect of childhood energy expenditure. *Am J Clin Nutr.* 1998;67(2): 309–316.
6. Johnson MS, Figueroa-Colon R, Herd SL, Fields DA, Sun M, Hunter GR, Goran MI. Aerobic fitness, not energy expenditure predicts increasing adiposity in African-American and Caucasian children. *Pediatrics.* 2000;106: e50–e56.
7. Figueroa-Colon R, Arani RB, Goran MI, Weinsier RL. Paternal body fat is a longitudinal predictor of changes in body fat in premenarcheal girls. *Am J Clin Nutr.* 2000;71: 829–834.
8. Treuth MS, Butte NF, Sorkin JD. Predictors of body fat gain in non-obese girls with a familial predisposition to obesity. *Am J Clin Nutr.* 2003;78: 1212–1218.
9. Bandini LG, Must A, Phillips SM, Naumova EN, Dietz WH. Relation of body mass index and body fatness to energy expenditure: longitudinal changes from pre-adolescence through adolescence *Am J Clin Nutr.* 2004;80: 1262–1269.
10. Griffiths M, Payne PR. Energy expenditure in small children of obese and non-obese parents. *Nature.* 1976;260: 698–700.
11. Goran MI, Treuth MS. Energy expenditure, obesity, and physical activity in children. *Pediatr Clin North Am.* 2001;48(4): 931–953.
12. Mayer J, Marshall JJ, Vitale JU, Christensen JH, Mashayki MB, Stare FJ. Exercise, food intake, and body weight in normal rats and genetically obese adult mice. *Am J Physiol.* 1954;177: 544–548.
13. Mayer J, Roy P, Mitra KP. Relation between calorie intake, body weight and physical work: studies in an industrial male population in West Bengal. *Am J Clin Nutr.* 1956;4: 169–175.
14. Westerterp KR. Alterations in energy balance with exercise. *Am J Clin Nutr.* 1998;68:970S–974S.
15. Schulz LO, Schoeller DA. A compilation of total daily energy expenditures and body weights in healthy adults. *Am J Clin Nutr.* 1994;60(5): 676–681.
16. Schoeller DA. Balancing energy expenditure and body weight. *Am J Clin Nutr.* 1998;68:956S–961S.
17. Spadano JL, Must A, Bandini LG, Dallal GE, Dietz WH. Energy cost of physical activites in 12-y-old girls: MET values and the influence of body weight. *Int J Obes.* 2003;27: 1528–1533.
18. Institute of Medicine, National Academy of Sciences. *Dietary Reference Intakes for Energy, Carbohydrate, Fiber, Fat, Fatty Acids, Cholesterol, Protein, and Amino Acids (Macronutrients).* National Academy Press, Washington, DC, 2002.
19. Baumgartner RN, Roche AF, Himes JH. Incremental growth tables: supplementary to previously published charts. *Am J Clin Nutr.* 1986;43: 711–722.
20. Hashke F. Body composition during adolescence. In: *Body Composition Measurements in Infants and Children: Report of the 98th Ross Conference on Pediatric Research.* Columbus, OH: Ross Laboratories, 1989: pp. 76–83.
21. Goran MI, Sun M. Total energy expenditure and physical activity in prepubertal children: recent advances based on the application of the doubly labeled water method. *Am J Clin Nutr.* 1998;68(Suppl): 944S–949S.
22. Goran MI. Energy expenditure, body composition, and disease risk in children and adolescents. *Proc Nutr Soc.* 1997;56: 195–209.
23. Ekelund U, Yngve A, Grage S, Westerterp K, Sjostrom M. Body movement and physical activity energy expenditure in children and adolescents: how to adjust for differences in body size and age. *Am J Clin Nutr.* 2004;79(5): 851–856.

24. Wells JCK, Cole TJ, Davies PSW. Total energy expenditure and body composition in early infancy. *Arch Dis Child*. 1996;75: 423–426.

25. Wells JCK, Hinds A, Davies PSW. Free-living energy expenditure and behavior in late infancy. *Arch Dis Child*. 1997;76: 490–494.

26. Maffeis C, Schutz Y, Micciolo R, Zoccante L, Pinelli L. Resting metabolic rate in six-to ten-year-old obese and nonobese children. *J Pediatr*. 1993;122: 556–562.

27. Bandini LG, Schoeller DA, Dietz WH. Energy expenditure in obese and nonobese adolescents. *Pediatr Res*. 1990;27: 198–203

28. DeLany JP, Harsh DW, Kime J, Kumler J, Melancon L, Bray GA. Energy expenditure in lean and obese pubertal children. *Obes Res*. 1995;3: 67–72.

29. Molnar D, Schutz Y. The effect of obesity, age, puberty and gender on resting metabolic rate in children and adolescents. *Eur J Pediatr*. 1997;156: 376–381.

30. Treuth MS, Figueroa-Colon R, Hunter GR, Weinsier RL, Butte NF, Goran MI. Energy expenditure and physical fitness in overweight vs non-overweight prepubertal girls. *Int J Obes*. 1998;22(5): 440–447.

31. Wurmser H, Laessle R, Jacob K, Langhard S, Uhl H, Angst A, et al. Resting metabolic rate in preadolescent girls at high risk of obesity. *Int J Obes*. 1998;22: 793–799.

32. Goran MI, Carpenter WH, McGloin A, Johnson R, Hardin JM, Weinsier RL. Energy expenditure in children of lean and obese parents. *Am J Physiol*. 1995;268: E917–E924.

33. Treuth MS, Butte NF, Wong WW. Effects of familial predisposition to obesity on energy expenditure in multiethnic prepubertal girls. *Am J Clin Nutr*. 2000;71: 893–900.

34. Bandini LG, Must A, Spadano JL, Dietz WH. Relationship of body composition, parental overweight, pubertal stage and ethnicity to energy expenditure among premenarcheal girls. *Am J Clin Nutr*. 2002;76(5): 1040–1047.

35. Morrison JA, Alfaro MP, Khoury P. Thorton BB, Daniels SR. Determinants of resting energy expenditure in young black girls and young white girls. J Ped 1996;129: 637–642.

36. Spadano JL, Must A, Bandini LG, Dallal GE, Dietz WH. Does menarche mark a period of elevated resting metabolic rate? *Am J Physiol*. 2004;286: E456–E452.

37. Kaplan AS, Zemel BS, Stallings VA. Differences in resting energy expenditure in prepubertal black children and white children. *J Pediatr*. 1996;129: 643–647.

38. Wong WW, Butte NF, Ellis KJ, Hergenroeder AC, Hill RB, Stuff JE, Smith E. Pubertal African-American girls expend less energy at rest and during physical activity than Caucasian girls. *J Clin Endocrinol Metab*. 1999;84: 906–911.

39. Yanovski SZ, Reynolds JC, Boyle AJ, Yanovski JA. Resting metabolic rate in African-American and Caucasian girls. *Obes Res*. 1997;5: 321–325.

40. Sun M, Gower BA, Nagy TR, Trowbridge CA, Dezenberg C, Goran MI. Total, resting, and activity-related energy expenditures are similar in Caucasian and African-American children. *Am J Physiol*. 1998;274(2 Pt 1): E232–E237.

41. Salbe AD, Weyer C, Harper I, Lindsay RS, Ravussin E, Tataranni PA. Assessing risk factors for obesity between childhood and adolescence: II. Energy metabolism and physical activity. *Pediatrics*. 2002;110(2 Pt 1): 307–314.

42. Holm VA, Cassidy SB, Butler MG, Hanchett JM, Greenswag LR, Whitman BY, Greenberg F. Prader–Willi Syndrome: consensus diagnostic criteria. *Pediatrics*. 1991;91(2): 398–402.

43. Fiore P, Picco P, Castagnola E, Palmieri A, Levato L, Gremmo M, et al. Nutritional survey of children and adolescents with myelomeningocele (MMC): Overweight associated with reduced energy intake. *Eur J Ped Surgery*.1998;8: 34–36(suppl 1).

44. Hayes-Allen MC, Tring FC. Obesity: another hazard for spina bifida children. *Br J Prev Soc Med*. 1973;27: 192–196.

45. UCP Research & Educational Foundation. *Cerebral Palsy — Facts & Figures*. Washington, DC: UCP Research & Educational Foundation, 2001.

46. Stallings VA, Zemel BS, Davies JC, Cronk CE, Charney EB. Energy expenditure of children and adolescents with severe disabilities: a cerebral palsy model. *Am J Clin Nutr*. 1996;64: 627–634.

47. World Health Organization, Energy and protein requirements: report of a joint FAO/WHO/UNU meeting. Geneva: World Health Organization,1985: 71–78.

48. Bandini LG, Schoeller DA, Fukagawa NK, Wykes LJ, Dietz WH. Body composition and energy expenditure in adolescents with cerebral palsy or myelodysplasia. *Pediatr Res.* 1991;29(1): 70–77.
49. van den Berg-Emons HJ, Saris WH, de Barbanson DC, Westerterp KR, Huson A, van Baak MA. Daily physical activity of schoolchildren with spastic diplegia and of healthy control subjects. *J Pediatr.* 1995;127(4): 578–584.
50. Azcue MP, Zello GA, Levy LD, Pencharz PB. Energy expenditure and body composition in children with spastic quadripelgic cerebral palsy. *J Pediatr.* 1996;129(6): 870–876.
51. Rose J, Medeiros JM, Parker R. Energy cost index as an estimate of energy expenditure of cerebral-palsied children during assisted ambulation. *Dev Med Child Neurol.* 1985;27: 485–490.
52. Dickerson RN, Brown RO, et al. Measured energy expenditure of tube-fed patients with severe neurodevelpmental disabilites. *J Am Coll Nutr.* 1999;18: 61–68.
53. Bandini LG, Puelzl-Quinn H, Morelli JA, Fukagawa NK. Estimation of energy requirements in persons with severe central nervous system impairment. *J Pediatr.* 1995;126(51): 28–32.
54. Hayes-Allen MC. Obesity and short stature in children with myelomeningocele. *Dev Med Child Neurol.* 1972;4(Suppl)27: 59–64.
55. Polito C, Delgaizo D, Del Gaizo D, Gi Manso G, Stabile D, Del Gado RD. Children with myelom-eninocele have shorter stature, greater body-weight, and lower bone-mineral content than healthy-children. *Nutrition Res.* 1995;15(11): 1605–1611.
56. Shepherd K, Roberts D, Golding S, Thomas BJ, Shepherd RW. Body composition in myelomenin-gocele. *Am J Clin Nutr.* 1991;53: 1–6.
57. van den Berg Emons, HJ, Hendrika J, Bussman B, Brobbel AS, Roebroeck ME, van Meeteren J, Stam IIJ. Everyday physical activity in adolescents and young adults with meningomyelocele as measured with a novel activity monitor. *J Pediatr.* 2001;139: 880–886.
58. The University of South Dakota School of Medicine and Health Sciences Center for Disabilities. 2003. *Developmental Disabilities Handbook*, extracted from www.usd.ed. Accessed July 2004.
59. Chumlea WC, Cronk CE. Overweight among children with Trisomy 21. *J Ment Defic Res.* 1981;25: 275–280.
60. Luke A, Roizen NJ, Sutton M, Schoeller DA. Energy expenditure in children with Down syndrome: Correcting metabolic rate for movement. *J Pediatr* 1994;125(51): 829–838.
61. Schoeller DA, Levitsky LL, Bandini LG, Dietz WW, Walczak A. Energy expenditure and body composition in Prader–Willi syndrome. *Metabolism.* 1988;37(2): 115–120.
62. Davies PSW, Joughin C. Using stable isotopes to assess reduced physical activity of individuals with Prader–Willi syndrome. *Am J Mental Retardation.* 1993;98: 349–353.
63. van Mill EA, Westerterp KR, Gerver WJ, Curfs LM, Schrander-Stumpel CT, Kester AD, Saris WH. Energy expenditure at rest and during sleep in children with Prader–Willi syndrome is explained by body composition. *Am J Clin Nutr.* 2000;71: 752–756.
64. Gunay-Aygun M, Cassidy SB, Nicholls RD. Prader Willi and other syndromes associated with obesity and mental retardation. *Behav Genet.* 1997;27: 307–324.
65. Kohl HW, Hobbs KE. Development of physical activity behaviors among children and adolescents. *Pediatrics.* 1998;101: 549–554.
66. Andersen RE, Crespo CJ, Bartlett SJ, Cheskin LJ, Pratt M. Relationship of physical activity and television watching with body weight and level of fatness among children. *JAMA.* 1998;279: 938–42.
67. Centers for Disease Control and Prevention. Guidelines for school and community programs to promote lifelong physical activity among young people. *Morbid Mortal Wkly Rept.* 1997;46(No RR-6): 1–36.
68. United States, Department of Health and Human Services (USDHHS), Public Health Service, Center for Disease Control and Prevention (CDC), Guidelines for school and community programs to promote lifelong physical activity among young people, *Morbid Mortal Wkly Rept.* 1997;46: 1.
69. CDC. Youth risk behavior surveillance — United States, 2001. *Morbid Mortal Wkly Rept.* 2002;51(SS04): 1–64.
70. NASPE (National Association for Sport and Physical Education), Council on Physical Education for Children. Reston, VA: Author. *Physical Activity for Children: A Statement of Guidelines for Children Ages 5–12.* 2nd ed. 2004.

71. Kimm SYS, Glynn NW, Kriska AA, Fitzgerald SL, Aaron DJ, Similo SL, et al. Longitudinal changes in physical activity in a biracial cohort during adolescence. *Med Sci Sports Exerc.* 2000;32(8): 1445–1454.

72. Kimm SY, Glynn NW, Kriska AM, Barton BA, Kronsberg SS, Daniels SR, et al. Decline in physical activity in black girls and white girls during adolescence. *N Engl J Med.* 2002;347(1)(0): 709–715.

73. Torun B, Davies PSW, Livingstone MBE, Paolisso M, Sackett R, Spurr GB. Energy requirements and dietary recommendations for children and adolescents 1 to 18 years old. *Eur J Clin Nutr.* 1998;50(1): S37–S80.

74. Fontvielle AM, Harper IT, Ferraro RT, Spraul M, Ravussin E. Daily energy expenditure by five-year-old children, measured by doubly labeled water. *J Pediatr.* 1993;123: 200–207.

75. Goran MI, Carpenter WH, McGloin A, Johnson R, Hardin MJ, Weinsier RL. Energy expenditure in children of lean and obese parents. *Am J Physiol.* 1995;268: E917–E925.

76. Davies PSW, Livingstone MBE, Prentice AM, Coward WA, Jagger SE, Stewart C, et al. Total energy expenditure during childhood and adolescence. *Proc Nutr Soc.* 1991;50: 14A.

77. Davies PS, Wells JC, Fieldhouse CA, Day JM, Lucas A. Parental body composition and infant energy expenditure. *Am J Clin Nutr.* 1995;61: 1026–1029.

78. Reilly JJ, Jackson DM, Montgomery C, Kelly LA, Slater C, Grant S, Payton JY. Total energy expenditure and physical activity in young Scottish children: mixed longitudinal study. *Lancet.* 2004;363: 211–212.

79. Eck LH, Klesges RC, Hanson CL, Slawson D. Children at familial risk for obesity: an examination of dietary intake, physical activity and weight status. *Intl J Obes.* 1992;16: 71–78.

80. Moore LL, Nguyen US, Rothman KJ, Cupples LA, Ellison RC. Preschool physical activity level and change in body fatness in young children. The Framingham Children's Study. *Am J Epidmiol.* 1995;142(9): 982–988.

81. Klesges RC, Klesges LM, Eck LH, Shelton ML. A longitudinal analysis of accelerated weight gain in preschool children. *Pediatrics.* 1995;95(1): 131–132.

82. Goran MI, Gower BA, Nagy TR, Johnson RK. Developmental changes in energy expenditure and physical activity in children: Evidence for a decline in physical activity in girls before puberty. *Pediatrics.* 1998;101: 887–891.

83. DeLany JP, Bray GA, Harsha DW, Volaufova J. Energy expenditure in African American and white boys and girls in a 2-y follow-up of the Baton Rouge Children's Study. *Am J Clin Nutr.* 2004:79(2): 268–273.

9 Endocrine Disorders Associated with Pediatric Obesity

Cong Ning and Jack A. Yanovski

CONTENTS

INTRODUCTION

Among the causes of childhood overweight are a number of endocrine disorders that present with weight gain or excessive adiposity as major clinical features (Table 9.1). While some early studies of overweight children referred for metabolic or endocrine evaluation found that over 20% of obesity in children and adolescents with age between 5 and 20 years had an underlying endocrine disorder, today children with identifiable endocrinopathies are believed to make up only a small minority of children referred for evaluation of overweight. For example, the prevalence of pediatric hypothyroidism,[1] the most common of the classical endocrine disorders traditionally associated with obesity, is approximately 0.14%; this prevalence can be contrasted with the prevalence of a body mass index (BMI) in the 95th percentile or more, which in the United States now exceeds 15% in 6 to 19 year olds.[2] Nevertheless, knowledge of the endocrine diseases associated with

TABLE 9.1
Endocrine Disorders That Present with Obesity in Pediatric Population

Hypothyroidism
Cushing's syndrome
Growth hormone deficiency and growth hormone resistance
Hyperinsulinemia
Leptin deficiency
Leptin receptor deficiency
Mutations in proopiomelanocortin
Mutations in prohormone convertase 1
Mutations in melanocortin-4 receptor
Mutation in neurotrophic tyrosine kinase receptor 2 (TrkB)
Hypothalamic obesity
Selected genetic syndromes with major endocrine phenotypes that are associated with obesity
Pseudohypoparathyroidism
Bardet–Biedl syndromes
Prader–Willi syndrome
Beckwith–Wiedemann syndrome

obesity is essential for the evaluation and treatment of overweight children and adolescents. In this chapter, we briefly discuss endocrine disorders that are part of the differential diagnosis of pediatric obesity.

ENDOCRINE DISORDERS ASSOCIATED WITH PEDIATRIC OBESITY

HYPOTHYROIDISM

Thyroid hormones play an important role in energy metabolism via several mechanisms: (1) increasing food intake, which in turn increases the thermic effect of food; (2) accelerating metabolic synthetic and catabolic rates as well as stimulating multiple energy-requiring processes such as ion cycling and metabolic substrate transport; and (3) increasing thermogenesis by amplifying the effect of adrenergic stimulation on uncoupling protein activation in brown adipose and other tissues.[3] Overall the effect of thyroid hormones on energy balance is to increase energy expenditure, and thyroid hormone deficiency in adults is associated with a 15 to 30% increase in body weight. In children with hypothyroidism, BMI may be increased by approximately one standard deviation unit.[4,5]

Although much of the weight gained with hypothyroidism is believed to be water retained,[6] due to increased capillary permeability,[7] decreased energy expenditure is also believed to contribute to the development of obesity in patients with hypothyroidism. In one study of hypothyroid mice, heat production from Ca^{2+} cycling during contraction in skeletal muscle accounted for 40 to 50% of the increased energy expenditure after correction of hypothyroidism.[8] The thermic effect of food, which accounts for approximately 10% of total daily energy expenditure, is also generally decreased in hypothyroidism. Although only 20 to 25% of resting energy expenditure is thyroid hormone–dependent, resting energy expenditure may be very sensitive to minimal changes of thyroid hormone levels. In a study of adult patients with hypothyroidism who were being treated with thyroid hormone, resting energy expenditure decreased about 15% when thyroid stimulating hormone (TSH) increased between 0.1 to 10 mU/L.[9] By contrast, obese adults with subclinical hypothyroidism (mildly elevated TSH but normal free thyroxine [T4] concentrations) have no metabolic or body composition differences from obese adults with normal TSH levels,[10] suggesting that as long as free T4 is maintained at the individual's set point, no defects in energy expenditure should be anticipated.

Numerous abnormalities in the hypothalamic–pituitary–thyroid axis have been described as causing hypothyroidism. Because of neonatal screening programs, congenital hypothyroidism is usually treated within the first 3 months of life and is not a cause of excessive weight gain unless adherence to prescribed thyroid hormone is problematic. The most common cause of acquired hypothyroidism during the childhood and adolescent period is Hashimoto (chronic autoimmune) thyroiditis. Excess weight gain with poor linear growth is the most common early clinical presentation in children with acquired primary hypothyroidism or central hypothyroidism. Because children with hypothyroidism usually have diminished linear growth, weight frequently does not exceed the 95th percentile,[11] but BMI may be high. Any overweight child with a diminution of linear growth should be evaluated for the possibility of hypothyroidism with measurement of both serum TSH and free T4 concentrations.

Most patients with hypothyroidism respond well to synthetic thyroxine replacement. Successful treatment reverses the symptoms and signs of hypothyroidism within a short period. Of note, in adults, excess adiposity does not invariably respond to appropriate thyroid hormone replacement,[12,13] even in those with severe hypothyroidism. Few data are available regarding the weight response in children treated for hypothyroidism, but the accelerated linear growth of children who are treated for hypothyroidism appears to lead to a diminished BMI.[4]

GROWTH HORMONE DEFICIENCY

Although BMI is negatively associated with growth hormone (GH) secretion,[14] and in obese children the 24-hour secretion of GH, the nocturnal GH peak,[15] and GH response to various pharmacological stimuli are diminished,[16–19] GH deficiency is rarely diagnosed in severely overweight children because these abnormalities usually are reversed following successful weight reduction. Nevertheless, GH deficiency is part of the differential diagnosis of pediatric overweight: children with GH deficiency have altered body composition, with greater fat mass and decreased lean mass, and generally have high weight for their low height. In GH-deficient children and adults, there is generally excess intra-abdominal adiposity and decreased lean body mass. Adult patients who had childhood growth hormone deficiency but who were no longer treated with GH have more features of the metabolic syndrome[20] and higher rates of cardiovascular morbidity and mortality than control groups. Therefore, GH deficiency in childhood is believed to be a significant risk factor for the metabolic syndrome in adulthood.

GH has profound metabolic effects on energy expenditure and metabolism. GH inhibits lipoprotein lipase, increases hormone sensitive lipase, and stimulates adipocyte lipolysis.[21] GH stimulates protein synthesis and increases fat-free mass (both muscle and bone mass). GH also appears to have a body composition–independent effect on energy expenditure: GH deficient adults treated with GH increase their resting metabolic rate to a greater extent than would be predicted based upon their changes in lean body mass.[22] Children and adults with growth hormone resistance caused by GH receptor defects (Laron syndrome) also have increased body adiposity that is not fully reversed by treatment with (insulin-like growth factor) IGF-1.[23]

Any defect in the hypothalamic–pituitary–somatotropic axis can cause growth hormone deficiency. Most children with isolated GH deficiency during childhood and adolescence have no identified cause. Poor linear growth with somewhat better weight gain is the usual clinical presentation of children with GH deficiency. Because of their short stature, such children rarely have weight above the 95th percentile, but may have an elevated BMI. Children with diminution of their linear growth should be evaluated for the possibility of GH deficiency.

GH replacement increases resting energy expenditure and restores normal body fat distribution in GH-deficient patients.[22,24] In GH-deficient children, the change of body composition can be detected as early as 6 weeks after initiation of GH therapy.[25] In one study of adult patients with

GH deficiency, GH treatment reduced body fat by 27% with normalized IGF-1 level and decreased levels of ghrelin and leptin after 9 months of GH therapy.[26] Reduction of resting metabolic rate accompanies discontinuation of GH: in GH-deficient adolescents, resting metabolic rate decreased by 11.3 kJ/kg fat-free mass 2 weeks after stopping GH.[27] Discontinuation of GH in adolescents with GH deficiency after they have reached adult height results in an increase in the percentage of body fat from 7.4 to 9.4% and body fat mass from 3.8 to 5.8 kg at 2 months after termination of GH replacement.[28] In one study of adolescents with partial growth hormone deficiency who were treated with GH and then restudied 1 year after stopping GH, alteration of body composition toward greater adiposity was also noted.[29]

In summary, GH deficiency is associated with increased body fat mass, decreased skeletal muscle and bone mass, and the metabolic syndrome. Many of these abnormalities are rapidly reversed by GH treatment. Any short child with low growth velocity should undergo an evaluation by a pediatric endocrinologist for GH deficiency that may include measurement of skeletal maturation (bone age) and provocative GH stimulation testing.

CUSHING'S SYNDROME

The clinical features of Cushing's syndrome are caused by tissue exposure to excess cortisol. Iatrogenic Cushing's syndrome is the most common etiology for Cushing's syndrome because of the widespread use of glucocorticoids for management of asthma and other chronic medical problems, although the exact prevalence of iatrogenic Cushing's syndrome is not well established in children. Endogenous Cushing's syndrome has an estimated prevalence of approximately 1 per million in children. Thus, while the diagnosis is frequently entertained in significantly overweight children, this disorder is rarely the cause of excessive weight gain in children or adolescents. In infants and children younger than 7 years, adrenal tumors are the most common cause of endogenous hypercortisolism. In older children, the most common cause is Cushing's disease due to an adrenocorticotropic hormone (ACTH)-producing pituitary adenoma.

Glucocorticoids affect metabolism through several mechanisms, including an increase in hepatic glucose production by stimulation of gluconeogenesis, an increase in postinsulin receptor muscle insulin resistance,[30] and stimulation of lipoprotein lipase in adipocytes, which in turn increases fat accumulation. Glucocorticoids are also required for the differentiation of adipose stromal cells to mature adipocytes. Glucocorticoids are powerful modulators of fat deposition. Adrenal insufficiency can ameliorate most genetic models of obesity — for example, adrenalectomy in the ob/ob mouse prevents the development of obesity.[31]

Cushing's syndrome is associated with central obesity, which indicates that glucocoticoids also play an important role in regulating adipose tissue distribution. Glucocorticoid receptor (GR) is expressed in adipose tissue with higher levels of mRNA for the GR in omental adipocytes. The activity of the enzyme 11β-hydroxysteroid dehydrogenase (11β-HSD) is believed to be a key factor that affects action of glucocorticoids on various tissues. There are two isoforms of 11β-HSD (11β-HSD1 and 11β-HSD2) that are involved in the interconversion of hormonally active cortisol to inactive cortisone. 11β-HSD1 is expressed in high abundance in adipose tissue, specifically in omental adipose tissue,[32] where it is believed to increase the local effects of cortisol on adipose tissue by converting inactive cortisone to active cortisol. In transgenic mice that have overexpression of 11β-HSD1 in adipocytes, there is a threefold increase in the accumulation of visceral adipose tissue, increased lipid accumulation, and an increase in adipocyte size.[33]

Of children with Cushing's syndrome, 80 to 90% present with excess weight gain and low linear growth velocity.[34,35] Therefore, evaluation of Cushing's syndrome should be carried out in all patients with abnormal weight gain and poor linear growth.[36,37] In children, the clinician must be prepared to consider the diagnosis without many of the features often seen in adults. Most children with Cushing's syndrome have been reported to have global rather than centripetal obesity, preserved skin thickness, no striae, and normal proximal muscular strength. Even though the most

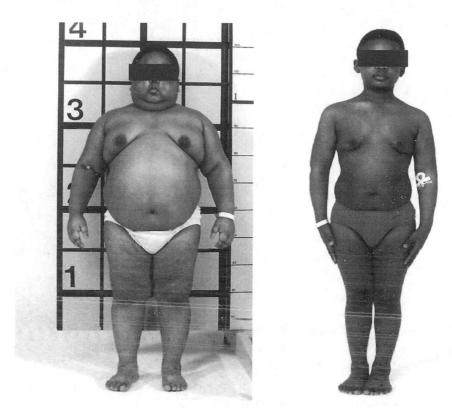

FIGURE 9.1 Pediatric Cushing disease before and after treatment for a pituitary adenoma.

common presentation of Cushing's syndrome in children is poor linear growth, often with a decrease in height percentile over time as the weight percentile increases, hypercortisolemic children with virilizing adrenal carcinoma may show growth acceleration or a normal growth velocity, so the absence of growth failure should not be used as evidence to exclude the diagnosis of Cushing's syndrome should there be other suggestive features.[38] The obesity of children with Cushing's syndrome is reversible when the underlying cause is removed (Figure 9.1).

Children suspected to have Cushing's syndrome should be evaluated by a pediatric endocrinologist. The diagnosis can be confirmed by measurement of urinary free cortisol concentrations as well as measurement of serum cortisol at 8 A.M. after administration of dexamethasone at 11 P.M. the previous night. Proper interpretation of urinary free cortisol measurement requires it to be normalized using the body surface area of the child.[39] Dexamethasone should be administered according to the child's body surface area ($0.3 \ \mu g/m^2$), with a maximum dose of 1 mg.[40]

INSULINOMA

Insulinoma is an extremely rare disease in children.[41] It has an estimated incidence in adults of 4 per 5,000,000 people per year,[42] with less than 10% of cases occurring before 20 years of age.[43] The characteristic clinical feature is frequent episodes of nonketotic hypoglycemia, accompanied by weight gain.

The clinical characteristics of insulinoma in childhood are similar to those described for adults: approximately 18 to 39% of adult patients present with excess weight gain.[44] An increase in energy intake in order to avoid hypoglycemic symptoms is presumed to be the main reason for the weight gain in patients with insulinoma, and food ingestion relieves symptoms in as many as 71% of adult patients.[45] Those with insulinoma may present with neurologic disorders, especially seizure disorders and neuroglycopenic symptoms, including confusion, personality change, or bizarre behavior.

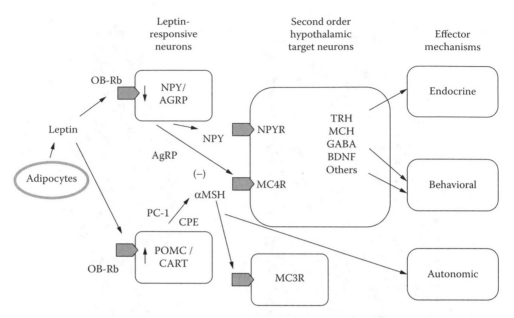

FIGURE 9.2 A simplified model of leptin signaling. The ligands leptin, POMC, and CART; the receptors for leptin, melanocortins, and BDNF; and the enzyme PC1 have been found to have function-altering mutations associated with obesity in children. Mutations in the ligands and receptors for NPY, AgRP, CPE, and MCH have been found to cause excessive weight gain when mutated in rodents but have not been convincingly shown to be associated with human obesity. OB-Rb, the signal-transducing form of the leptin receptor; NPY, neuropeptide Y; AGRP, agouti related protein; POMC, proopiomelanocortin; CART, cocaine–amphetamine related transcript; PC 1, prohormone convertase 1; CPE, carboxypeptidase E; αMSH, α-melanocyte stimulating hormone; NPYR, neuropeptide Y receptor; MC3R, melanocortin 3 receptor; MC4R, melanocortin 4 receptor; TRH, thyrotropin-releasing hormone; MCH, melanin concentrating hormone; GABA, gamma amino butyric acid; BDNF, brain-derived neurotrophic factor.

Autonomic symptoms such as diaphoresis or tremulousness may also be reported. Surgery is the primary treatment for insulinoma. Although few data are available in children, adult patients usually lose weight after successful treatment.

HYPOTHALAMIC OBESITY

The hypothalamus controls energy homeostasis by regulating food intake and energy expenditure through multiple mechanisms. Early animal studies showed that lesions of the ventromedial hypothalamic nucleus (VMH) led to hyperphagia and obesity whereas lesions in lateral hypothalamic area (LHA) caused anorexia and weight loss.[46,47] In humans, children who develop hypothalamic damage affecting these regions frequently have clinical symptoms of hyperphagia and morbid obesity that are difficult to control and clearly unrelated to the adequacy of their pituitary hormone replacement.[20,48]

Over the last 10 years, there has been an explosion of information regarding the orexigenic and anorectic peptides produced by neurons localized in hypothalamus that constitute the proximal leptin-responsive neuropeptidergic circuitry regulating food intake and body weight (Figure 9.2). In an effort to explain the neuroendocrine causes of the hypothalamic obesity syndrome, we briefly review several of these peptidergic systems.

The main regions in the hypothalamus involved in energy homeostasis are the arcuate nucleus (ARC), VMH, paraventricular nucleus (PVN), dorsomedial hypothalamic nucleus (DMH), and LHA. These regions can integrate the information about meal size, nutrient composition, and adipocyte stores from peripheral and central signals, and regulate food intake and energy expenditure through the anterior pituitary, descending autonomic pathways, and other brain regions.

Neuropeptide Y (NPY), which is synthesized by neurons located in the ARC, is among the most powerful orexigenic peptides. The melanocortins, peptides cleaved from pro-opimelanocortin (POMC) and which are also produced in the ARC, have opposite actions to NPY (greater details are given in the Disorders of the Leptin Signaling Pathway section). Other neuropeptides expressed in the hypothalamus, including the cocaine–amphetamine-related transcript (CART), agouti-related peptide (AGRP), orexins, melanin concentrating hormone (MCH), and brain-derived neurotrophic factor (BDNF), also have effects on food intake and body weight.[49–54]

Some peripheral signals produced from the gastrointestinal tract, such as cholescystokinin (CCK), glucagonlike peptide (GLP)-1, and peptide (YY3)-36, are found to decrease food intake when administered intracerebroventricularly,[55–57] via the activation of their individual receptors located in the VMH, PVN, and ARC.[58–60] Ghrelin, a growth hormone–releasing peptide produced mainly in the stomach, acts on hypothalamic pathways to stimulate food intake and fat accumulation.[61] Glucose-sensitive neurons, abundant in the LHA, and glucose-responsive neurons, abundant in the VMH, are considered to be involved in mediating the effects of changes in blood glucose concentrations on food intake. Insulin also appears to modulate energy balance via hypothalamic effects. Like leptin, intracerebroventricular insulin is an anti-obesity hormone that acts via insulin receptors, which are concentrated in the hypothalamus,[62,63] especially in the ARC region, to control food intake. Circulating insulin enters the central nervous system via a saturable transport system.[64] Intracerebroventricular infusion of insulin decreases food intake, while injection of insulin antibodies into the VMH stimulates food intake. Mice with a neuron-specific disruption of the insulin receptor (IR) gene develop hyperphagia in females and obesity with increased adiposity, mild insulin resistance, elevated insulin levels, dyslipidemia, and gonadal failure in both sexes.[65] Mice with deletion of the insulin receptor substrate-2 (IRS-2 KO) have a similar phenotype.[66] The anti-obesity effect of central insulin is mediated, at least in part, by inhibitory effects on NPY neurons and stimulation of the POMC signaling pathway, quite similar to those effects induced by leptin administration. Conversely, in IRS-2 KO mice, a decrease in arcuate nucleus mRNA expression of POMC in both sexes and an increase in expression of AgRP and NPY in female mice[67] are found. Those changes in hypothalamic NPY, AGPR, and POMC expression may contribute to the development of hyperphagia and obesity with disrupted insulin signaling in the brain. In addition to regulation of food intake, insulin may affect energy expenditure through the sympathetic nervous system. In the same study of IRS-2 KO mice, decreased uncoupling protein 1 (UCP1) mRNA expression in brown adipose tissue with defective thermoregulation in both sexes was found.[67]

Hypothalamic obesity may be caused by any process that causes damage to the hypothalamus, including congenital midline defects and acquired lesions (caused by tumor, trauma, or inflammatory disease) or as a consequence of treatment for such lesions (surgery or irradiation). Obesity occurs in approximately 50% of children treated surgically for craniopharyngioma.[20,48,68] The size of the hypothalamic area that is damaged is positively related to the risk for the abnormal BMI increase in children surviving brain tumors.[69] In one study of children with craniopharyngioma, the prevalence of obesity increased from 27% (6/21) preoperatively to 62% (13/21) 1 year after surgery.[70] Approximately 44% develop severe obesity (BMI-SD score > 3).[20,48]

Patients with hypothalamic obesity appear to be at risk for development of aspects of the insulin-resistance dysmetabolic syndrome,[71] including dyslipidemia, impaired glucose homeostasis, and nonalcoholic steatohepatitis. In one case series, liver cirrhosis or fibrosis was observed in 8 of 10 such patients who underwent liver biopsy for significant abnormalities in liver function tests.[72]

There are few data studying actual food intake of children with hypothalamic obesity. In one study, compared with 26 healthy, age- and BMI-matched German children, 19 German children with hypothalamic obesity did not consume more calories according to 7-day food diaries but had significantly reduced activity (measured by accelerometry), particularly during leisure time.[73]

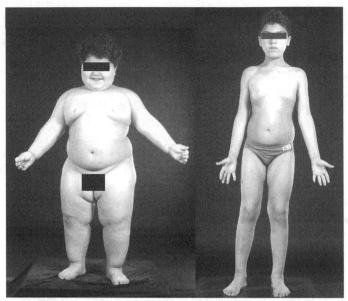

Age 3 yr, 42 kg   Age 7 yr, 32 kg

FIGURE 9.3 Leptin deficiency before (age 3 year, 42 kg) and after (age 7 year, 32 kg) treatment. (Photographs generously provided by IS Farooqi and S O'Rahilly, University of Cambridge, England.)

Free leptin concentrations in patients with hypothalamic obesity are higher and appear to increase with a greater slope as BMI increases than is observed in patients with nonsyndromic obesity, suggesting absence of feedback and central leptin insensitivity.[74] Patients with hypothalamic obesity may also be at risk for alterations in cortisol metabolism that may augment the effect of corticosteroids. The ratios of free and conjugated urinary cortisol to cortisone and their metabolites (tetrahydrocortisol +5 α-tetrahydrocortisol/tetrahydrocortisone, dihydrocortisols/dihydrocortisones, and cortols/cortolones) have been reported to be significantly higher in the urine of patients with hypothalamic obesity after a dose of hydrocortisone acetate. These data suggest augmented 11β-hydroxysteroid dehydrogenase type 1 activity, which would convert inactive 11β-ketosteroids to active 11β-OH glucocorticoids and possibly predispose hypothalamic obesity patients who take glucocorticoids to obesity.[75]

Disorders of the Leptin Signaling Pathway

Several monogenetic neuroendocrine disorders of the leptin signaling pathway that are associated with severe early-onset obesity in childhood have been uncovered over the past 10 years (Figure 9.3). These neuroendocrine disorders include leptin deficiency, leptin receptor mutations, POMC deficiency, prohormone convertase 1 (PC1) deficiency, and melanocortin-4 receptor (MC4R) mutations. Each of these disorders is briefly presented.

Leptin Deficiency and Leptin Receptor Mutations

Leptin, a hormone made primarily by adipocytes and which was isolated in 1994,[76] is involved in the regulation of food intake, energy expenditure, and energy balance in humans. The primary neuroendocrine role of leptin is to convey information about the status of adipocyte triglyceride content, along with the energy and macronutrient content of recent intake, to the hypothalamic centers that control energy intake[77] via leptin receptors. Leptin acts in the ARC to reduce food intake by inhibiting secretion of neuropeptide NPY, one of the most potent stimulators of food intake, and stimulating neurons that produce α-MSH, which inhibits food intake. Low leptin leads to reduced energy expenditure, suppression of anabolic processes, and increased appetite. Circulating leptin concentrations are highly correlated with indices of body fat content in human[78–80] and animals.[78,81] There is a gender difference in circulating leptin levels, with three- to fourfold higher concentrations in girls and women than in boys and men with a comparable body mass index.[82–84] Studies in animals and humans have demonstrated that insulin increases leptin gene expression and leptin secretion *in vitro* and *in vivo* and that glucose infusion increases plasma leptin levels.[85–87]

Leptin deficiency due to homozygous mutation in the leptin gene[88,89] or leptin resistance due to homozygous mutation in the leptin receptor gene[90] are associated with marked hyperphagia and severe early-onset obesity in humans because of increased energy intake that is due to decreased leptin effect on energy balance. Patients with either leptin deficiency or leptin resistance present with normal birth weight, but have rapid weight gain in the first few months of life, with severe hyperphagia and aggressive behavior when denied food. Basal temperature and resting metabolic rate appear normal. Cortisol concentrations in either condition are generally normal, and patients are normoglycemic with mildly raised plasma insulin, but pubertal development is impaired in both conditions. In those with leptin receptor mutation, but not in those with leptin deficiency, there appears to be hypothalamic hypothyroidism as well as mild growth retardation, with impaired basal and stimulated growth hormone secretion and decreased insulinlike growth factor 1 (IGF-1) and IGF binding protein-3 (IGF-BP-3) concentrations.[90] Heterozygous mutations of the leptin gene result in a partial deficiency syndrome characterized by increased body adiposity,[91] but heterozygous leptin receptor deficiency is without phenotype other than increased serum leptin.[90,92] In patients with congenital leptin deficiency, treatment with recombinant leptin therapy results in decreased weight and fat mass (Figure 9.3), reduced hyperphagia,[93,94] and correction of deficits of the neuroendocrine, reproductive, metabolic, and immune systems associated with leptin deficiency.[94,95]

Proopiomelanocortin (POMC) Deficiency

Human POMC is a 267 amino acid long precursor protein. The cleavage of POMC by the prohormone convertases PC1 and PC2 produces several bioactive peptides including α-melanocyte stimulating hormone (α-MSH), ACTH, β-lipotropin, and β-endorphin. Recent studies indicated that POMC expression in the ARC of the hypothalamus is important in regulation of appetite and energy homeostasis and that the interactions between POMC-derived peptide α-MSH and the melanocortin receptors, MC4R and MC3R, play a key role in this process. Overfeeding and peripheral leptin infusions induce the synthesis of POMC and its cleavage product α-MSH in the ARC, which then activates the MC4R located in the PVN and lateral hypothalamus.[96] Activation of MC4R primarily suppresses food intake. Animal studies show that mice lacking POMC-derived peptides are obese with defective adrenal development and altered pigmentation.[97]

Inactivation mutations of the POMC gene result in an exceedingly rare and complex disease due to lack of POMC-derived bioactive peptides. Few patients with either compound heterozygous or homozygous mutations in the POMC gene have been identified since the first children from Germany were described in 1998.[98–100] Clinical features of children with POMC deficiency include hyperphagia and severe obesity from early infancy (due to deficient MC3R and MC4R signaling), adrenal insufficiency (deficient MC2R signaling), and red hair pigmentation (deficient MC1R signaling). Heterozygous parents have normal adrenal function and do not have obesity or red hair pigmentation, which indicates that this disease has an autosomal recessive mode of inheritance.

Most studies find little evidence for abnormalities of POMC in otherwise normal overweight children.[101–103] A recently identified[104] heterozygous missense mutation in a POMC cleavage site results in an aberrant α-MSH/β-endorphin fusion peptide that was able to bind MC4R with an affinity similar to that of α- and β-MSH but had a markedly reduced ability to activate the receptor. This polymorphism appears to have a slightly increased prevalence among overweight than nonoverweight individuals (0.88% of a group of subjects with early-onset obesity and 0.22% of normal-weight controls).[104]

Prohormone Convertase 1 (PC1) Mutation

PC1 and PC2 are of particular importance for hypothalamic POMC processing[105,106] although other processing enzymes such as prohormone convertase PACE4 may play a role in POMC cleavage.[107] PC1 cleaves POMC into corticotropin and β-lipotropin at pairs of dibasic amino acid residues. ProSAAS, a neuroendocrine peptide precursor, inhibits PC1.[108] Transgenic mice expressing pro-SAAS are obese and hyperglycemic.[109]

Two patients (one child and one adult) with compound heterozygous mutations in PC1 have been identified.[110,111] The clinical features of those two patients were severe early onset obesity, marked small-intestinal absorptive dysfunction, postprandial hypoglycemia and hypoinsulinemia (due to decreased cleavage of proinsulin), hypocortisolemia secondary to ACTH deficiency (due to decreased cleavage of POMC), and elevated levels of prohormones including proinsulin, pro-glucagon, and POMC. In a 43-year-old adult patient with PC1 mutation, hypogonadotropic hypogonadism due to diminished processing has been also described.[110] The inability to cleave POMC is a likely mechanism for the obesity of these patients.

Melanocortin Receptor Gene Mutations

Both the MC3R and the MC4R appear to be important regulators of energy homeostasis via interactions with α-MSH. MC4R-knockout mice have severe obesity with hyperinsulinemia and hyperphagia;[94,112] heterozygous mice are also affected with an intermediate phenotype. MC4R-knockout mice do not respond to the anorectic effect of a melanocortin agonist.[113] These data indicate that the MC4R is important in mediating the effects of melanocortins on appetite.

MC3R knockout mice have increased fat mass and reduced lean mass. MC3R knockout mice are not hyperphagic.[114,115] These data suggest that MC3R regulates energy homeostasis by increasing feeding efficiency. Mice with defects in both MC3R and MC4R are heavier than mice lacking only the MC4R, suggesting these receptors affect body weight via different mechanisms.[113]

Human MC4R mutations appear to be the most common monogenic form of severe human obesity and are reported to occur in 4 to 5.1% of obese referral populations.[116–119] To date, approximately 30 different MC4R mutations have been associated with obesity. Patients with MC4R receptor mutations are characterized with severe early onset of obesity, increased linear growth (at least during childhood), severe hyperinsulinemia, and hyperphagia.[119] An obese phenotype is also present in some of those with heterozygous MC4R mutations.

Mutation of the TrkB (BDNF) Receptor

Yeo at al.[120] have described a nondysmorphic 8-year-old male who presented with global developmental delay including impaired short-term memory, abnormal pain sensation, and obesity. He had a heterozygous mutation of TrkB, the receptor for brain derived neurotrophic factor (BDNF). This boy had normal birth weight, but gained weight rapidly after age 6 months. Hypotonia was found at 6 weeks of age, and his subsequent course was notable for delayed motor and language milestones. Speech and language were particularly affected, and he did not speak until age 5 years. Absence seizures occurred in the second and third years of life. Yeo et al. subsequently screened 288 children with early-onset obesity and developmental delay, finding 5 with missense mutations of the TrkB receptor.

BDNF is believed to be downstream of MC4R in the leptin signaling pathway. *BDNF* is expressed at high levels in the ventromedial hypothalamus, where its expression is regulated by nutritional state and by MC4R signaling. Fasting suppresses VMH *BNDF* mRNA expression.[121] While homozygous *BNDF* deletion is embryologically lethal, *BDNF* heterozygous mice are obese,[122,123] as are mice in which the *BDNF* gene has been deleted, specifically in excitatory neurons.[124] Mice with conditional *BNDF* brain knockouts are hyperactive, hyperleptinemic, and hyperinsulinemic, and they have increased linear growth.[124,125] Both central and peripheral administration of *BDNF* decreases food intake, increases energy expenditure, and ameliorates the hyperinsulinemia and hyperglycemia of diabetic *db/db* mice, who lack functional leptin receptors,[124–128] and CSF *BDNF* infusion suppresses the hyperphagia and excessive weight gain observed on higher-fat diets in mice with deficient MC4R signaling.[121] In addition, mouse mutants that express the *BDNF* receptor TrkB at a quarter of the normal amount have hyperphagia and excessive weight gain on higher-fat diets.[121]

Because only one TrkB mutation has been studied for its functional effects on receptor signaling, it remains unclear to what extent such mutations may explain obesity in children with neurocognitive deficits. Thus far, no mutations in *BDNF* have been described in association with pediatric obesity.

GENETIC SYNDROMES PRESENTING AS ENDOCRINE DISORDERS THAT ARE ASSOCIATED WITH OBESITY

PSEUDOHYPOPARATHYROIDISM (PHP) TYPE IA

Among the four types of PHP (Ia, Ib, Ic, and II), obesity is a common feature in patients with PHP Ia. PHP Ia is an autosomal dominant disease, which is caused by heterozygous inactivating mutations in the gene encoding for Gsa, the α-subunit of G-protein signaling complex.[129,130] It is characterized by target organ unresponsiveness to multiple hormones, including thryotropin (TSH), parathyroid hormone (PTH), luteinizing hormone (LH), follicle stimulating hormone (FSH,) and growth hormone–releasing hormone (GHRH,)[131–133] and features of Albright's osteodystrophy (AHO). AHO is associated with developmental abnormalities that include a round face, short adult stature, obesity, brachydactyly, ectopic ossifications, and mental retardation.

Several mechanisms are considered to contribute to the development of obesity in patients with PHP Ia. The disorder is marked by decreased intracellular cyclic adenosine monophosphate (cAMP) levels and resistance to epinephrine,[134,135] phenomena that reduce adipocyte lipolysis. Reduced lipolytic response to epinephrine by 67% was found in Gsa-deficient children, as compared with controls.[135] A reduced Gsa function can also cause accelerated differentiation of fibroblasts to adipocytes.[136] GH deficiency, which is reported in 66 to 69% of patients with PHP type Ia,[132,133] may also contribute to the obesity. In one study, all GH deficient patients with PHP Ia demonstrated obesity and low serum concentrations of IGF-1 vs. none of the GH-sufficient subjects.[133] Although hypothyroidism is a very common finding among patients with PHP Ia, thyroid hormones seem to exert less effect on the development of obesity. Patients with PHP Ia presenting with congenital hypothyroidism continue excessive weight gain after adequate replacement of thyroxine.[137]

BARDET–BIEDL SYNDROMES (BBS)

BBS is the term used to refer to a series of heterogeneous autosomal recessive disorder characterized by pigmentary retinopathy, obesity, dental anomalies, brachydactyly and polydactyly, hypogenitalism, mental retardation, hypertension, and renal disorders. Mutations in at least six different genes (BBS1, BBS2, BBS4, BBS6, BBS7, BBS8) have been identified.[138–144] BBS is a rare disorder with a prevalence at 1:125,000 in the U.K. population[145] and 1:160,000 in Switzerland,[146] but it is relatively higher in specific isolated populations where consanguinity is more common.[147,148]

The prevalence of obesity (BMI ≥ 30 kg/m^2) in the BBS population is substantially higher (56%)[149] than in the general population (20%). The obesity usually begins in early childhood and is progressive with age.[150,151] Although obesity in BBS adults is usually associated with the trunk and proximal limbs and less frequently the face,[152] it has been described as having a diffuse and nonspecific distribution during the early life.[153] The mechanism of obesity in BBS is still not well understood. Patients with BBS show no differences of body fat or absolute resting metabolic rate compared with general obese populations.[154] It has been suggested that carriers of a BBS mutation are predisposed to obesity,[155,156] but a study that screened for BBS1 mutations in Newfoundland (an area with a high incidence of BBS1 mutations) showed no difference in prevalence of heterozygous BBS1 mutations in normal control and obese groups.[157]

PRADER–WILLI SYNDROME

Prader–Willi Syndrome (PWS), first described in 1956, is a complex human genetic disease that arises from lack of expression of paternally inherited imprinted genes on chromosome 15q11-q13, either secondary to a deletion of the paternal allele or because of uniparental maternal disomy of chromosome 15.[158] PWS is characterized by neonatal hypotonia and failure to thrive during infancy,[159–161] which is then followed by severe hyperphagia and early childhood obesity (arising generally after the age of 1 year). Among the abnormal eating behaviors observed in PWS are food stealing and foraging. Increased body fat with decreased fat-free mass is described in PWS patients, even in PWS infants with low body weight.[162] Onset of obesity usually begins between 1 to 6 years and progresses through adolescence into adulthood life if behavioral management is not undertaken. Children with PWS frequently have mental retardation, hypogonadism, short stature, and dysmorphic features. The prevalence of PWS is reported to be approximately 1:16,000 to 1:26,000.[163–165]

PWS is said to be the most common human genetic syndrome causing obesity. The obesity in PWS is likely caused by unbalanced energy metabolism, including higher energy intake and abnormal energy expenditure, possibly caused by multiple mechanisms. Hyperphagia with increased appetite in PWS patients has been proposed to be caused by abnormal hypersecretion of ghrelin, a circulating 28-amino acid neuropeptide that is synthesized mainly in the antrum of the stomach. Ghrelin receptors are located in the hypothalamus, particularly in NPY/AgRP neurons.[166] Although the orexigenic hypothalamic effect of ghrelin is primarily mediated through NPY/AgRP neurons, recent studies suggest that it also engages orexin neurons[167,168] and may act at other brain regions such as the caudal brainstem.[169] Ghrelin administration can stimulate food intake and increase adiposity in rodents.[61,170] In humans, ghrelin also stimulates appetite and increases food intake, at least in the short term.[171] Ghrelin levels are found to be inversely correlated with BMI, age, and insulin concentrations in normal children[172] and are lower in many patients after gastric bypass surgery[173] than those who lose weight through nonsurgical means. An extremely high ghrelin level is measured in patients with anorexia nervosa and decreases with weight gain.[174] In patients with PWS, markedly increased fasting plasma ghrelin levels are demonstrated (about 3- to 4.5-fold higher compared with obese subjects with similar BMI). Fasting ghrelin levels in patients with PWS are reported to be not significantly different[172] or 2.5-fold higher compared with normal lean controls.[175] The mechanism causing elevated ghrelin in PWS is not clear, but it is unlikely to be due to impaired GH–ghrelin feedback because systemic ghrelin levels in subjects with GH deficiency are not modified by 1 year of GH replacement therapy.[176]

GH insufficiency, which is a very common finding in PWS patients, is also considered to contribute, at least in part, to the development of obesity in PWS patients. In adults with PWS, GH replacement for 12 months decreased body fat by 2.5% and increased lean body mass by 2.5 kg.[177] In children with PWS, GH therapy improved body composition and growth velocity as well.[178,179] Several studies have found low 24-h energy expenditure, reduced physical activity, and reduced resting metabolic rate in patients with PWS, each of which has been considered a potential contributor to the development of obesity in PWS. However, resting metabolic rate appears to be normal after correction for both fat-free mass and fat mass, indicating that a low resting metabolism rate (RMR) may not be a primary abnormality of PWS contributing to obesity.[178,180,181]

Leptin levels in PWS follow the general patterns observed in individuals with nonsyndromic obesity, which indicates that leptin does not play a causative role in the obesity of PWS.[182] The circulating plasma leptin levels in male nonobese patients with PWS are about five times those of a nonobese control group.[183]

Beckwith–Wiedemann Syndrome (BWS)

BWS, first recognized in 1964, is a prototypic imprinting disorder resulting from mutations or epigenetic alterations in genes from an imprinted cluster at chromosome 11p15.5. Loss of imprinting of the insulinlike growth factor 2 (IGF-2) gene is frequently observed in BWS, as is reduced cyclin-dependent kinase inhibitor gene *CDKN1C* expression related to loss of maternal allele–specific methylation of the differentially methylated region KvDMR1. The majority of BWS cases occur sporadically. The familial form occurs in approximately 15% of patients in an autosomal dominant pattern, with variable expressivity and incomplete penetrance. The incidence of BWS is reported to be approximately 1:13,700 births.[184] The clinical features of BWS are macroglossia, abdominal wall defects, prenatal and postnatal overgrowth, visceromegaly, hemihyperplasia, ear anomalies, and neonatal hypoglycemia (secondary to pancreatic β-cell hyperplasia). Children with Beckwith–Wiedemann Syndrome have a 7 to 21% risk for the development of embryonic malignancies, most notably Wilms' tumor, although a wide variety of benign and malignant tumors including hepatoblastoma, adrenocortical carcinoma, rhabdomyosarcoma, and neuroblastoma have been reported.[185–187]

Although *CDKN1C* deficiency may caused placental overgrowth in BWS, which may contribute to overgrowth of the embryo,[188] transgenic mice with overexpression of IGF-2 exhibit most of the symptoms of BWS.[189] Variations in the phenotype of the disorder may be associated with different genotypes, but overexpression of IGF-2 is most frequently associated with overgrowth and obesity in BWS.[190]

SUMMARY

The prevalence of obesity in pediatric populations has increased dramatically over the last 30 years, and as a result, significant obesity caused by endocrine disorders makes up an ever decreasing fraction of overweight children. Because obesity caused by endocrinopathy is reversible with successful treatment, early diagnosis and initiation of treatment in endocrine obesity remains important. However, in the absence of suggestive signs or symptoms, extensive endocrine testing is not indicated for overweight children.

ACKNOWLEDGMENTS

Supported by HD00641 (NICHD) to JAY. JAY is a commissioned officer in the United States Public Health Service, NIH, DHHS

REFERENCES

1. Hunter I, Greene SA, MacDonald TM, Morris AD. Prevalence and aetiology of hypothyroidism in the young. *Arch Dis Child*. 2000;83: 207–210.
2. Ogden CL, Flegal KM, Carroll MD, Johnson CL. Prevalence and trends in overweight among US children and adolescents. 1999–2000. *JAMA*. 2002;288: 1728–1732.
3. Krotkiewski M. Thyroid hormones in the pathogenesis and treatment of obesity. *Eur J Pharmacol*. 2002;440: 85–98.
4. Teng L, Bui H, Bachrach L, Lee P, Gagne N, Deal C, Wilson DM. Catch-up growth in severe juvenile hypothyroidism: treatment with a GnRH analog. *J Pediatr Endocrinol Metab*. 2004;17: 345–354.

5. Darendeliler F, Yildirim M, Bundak R, Sukur M, Saka N, Gunoz H. Growth of children with primary hypothyroidism on treatment with respect to different ages at diagnosis. *J Pediatr Endocrinol Metab.* 2001;14: 207–210.

6. Villabona C, Sahun M, Roca M, Mora J, Gomez N, Gomez JM, et al. Blood volumes and renal function in overt and subclinical primary hypothyroidism. *Am J Med. Sci.* 1999;318: 277–280.

7. Wheatley T, Edwards OM. Mild hypothyroidism and oedema: evidence for increased capillary permeability to protein. *Clin Endocrinol* (Oxf). 1983;18: 627–635.

8. Leijendekker WJ, van Hardeveld C, Elzinga G. Heat production during contraction in skeletal muscle of hypothyroid mice. *Am J Physiol.* 1987;253: E214–E220.

9. al-Adsani H, Hoffer LJ, Silva JE. Resting energy expenditure is sensitive to small dose changes in patients on chronic thyroid hormone replacement. *J Clin Endocrinol Metab.*1997;82: 1118–1125.

10. Tagliaferri M, Berselli ME, Calo G, Minocci A, Savia G, Petroni ML, et al. Subclinical hypothyroidism in obese patients: relation to resting energy expenditure, serum leptin, body composition, and lipid profile. *Obes Res.* 2001;9: 196–201.

11. Abbassi V, Rigterink E, Cancellieri RP. Clinical recognition of juvenile hypothyroidism in the early stage. *Clin Pediatr* (Phila). 1980;19: 782–786.

12. Hoogwerf BJ, Nuttall FQ. Long-term weight regulation in treated hyperthyroid and hypothyroid subjects. *Am J Med.* 1984;76: 963–970.

13. Pears J, Jung RT, Gunn A. Long-term weight changes in treated hyperthyroid and hypothyroid patients. *Scott Med J.* 1990;35: 180–182.

14. Chemaitilly W, Trivin C, Souberbielle JC, Brauner R. Assessing short-statured children for growth hormone deficiency. *Horm Res.* 2003;60: 34–42.

15. Meistas MT, Foster GV, Margolis S, Kowarski AA. Integrated concentrations of growth hormone, insulin C-peptide and prolactin in human obesity. *Metabolism.* 1982;31: 1224–1228.

16. Bell JP, Donald RA, Espiner EA. Pituitary response to insulin-induced hypoglycemia in obese subjects before and after fasting. *J Clin Endocrinol Metab.* 1970;31: 546–551.

17. Copinschi G, Wegienka LC, Hane S, Forsham PH. Effect of arginine on serum levels of insulin and growth hormone in obese subjects. *Metabolism.* 1967;16: 485–491.

18. Mims RB, Stein RB, Bethune JE. The effect of a single dose of L-dopa on pituitary hormones in acromegaly, obesity, and in normal subjects. *J Clin Endocrinol Metab.* 1973;37: 34–39.

19. Topper E, Gil-Ad I, Bauman B, Josefsberg Z, Laron Z. Plasma growth hormone response to oral clonidine as compared to insulin hypoglycemia in obese children and adolescents. *Horm Metab Res.* 1984;16(Suppl 1): 127–130.

20. Srinivasan S, Ogle GD, Garnett SP, Briody JN, Lee JW, Cowell CT. Features of the metabolic syndrome after childhood craniopharyngioma. *J Clin Endocrinol Metab.* 2004;89: 81–86.

21. Dietz J, Schwartz J. Growth hormone alters lipolysis and hormone-sensitive lipase activity in 3T3-F442A adipocytes. *Metabolism.* 1991;40: 800–806.

22. Snel YE, Doerga ME, Brummer RJ, Zelissen PM, Zonderland ML, Koppeschaar HP. Resting metabolic rate, body composition and related hormonal parameters in growth hormone-deficient adults before and after growth hormone replacement therapy. *Eur J Endocrinol.* 1995;133: 445–450.

23. Laron Z. Consequences of not treating children with laron syndrome (primary growth hormone insensitivity). *J Pediatr Endocrinol Metab.* 2001;14(Suppl 5): 1243–1248;discussion 1261–1262.

24. Gregory JW, Greene SA, Jung RT, Scrimgeour CM, Rennie MJ. Changes in body composition and energy expenditure after six weeks' growth hormone treatment. *Arch Dis Child.* 1991;66: 598–602.

25. Hoos MB, Westerterp KR, Gerver WJ. Short-term effects of growth hormone on body composition as a predictor of growth. *J Clin Endocrinol Metab.* 2003;88: 2569–2572.

26. Eden Engstrom B, Burman P, Holdstock C, Karlsson FA. Effects of growth hormone (GH) on ghrelin, leptin, and adiponectin in GH-deficient patients. *J Clin Endocrinol Metab.* 2003;88: 5193–5198.

27. Cowan FJ, Evans WD, Gregory JW. Metabolic effects of discontinuing growth hormone treatment. *Arch Dis Child.* 1999;80: 517–523.

28. Kohno H, Ueyama N, Honda S. Unfavourable impact of growth hormone (GH) discontinuation on body composition and cholesterol profiles after the completion of height growth in GH-deficient young adults. *Diabetes. Obes Metab.* 1999;1: 293–296.

29. Tauber M, Jouret B, Cartault A, Lounis N, Gayrard M, Marcouyeux C, et al. Adolescents with partial growth hormone (GH) deficiency develop alterations of body composition after GH discontinuation and require follow-up. *J Clin Endocrinol Metab.* 2003;88: 5101–5106.

30. Block NE, Buse MG. Effects of hypercortisolemia and diabetes on skeletal muscle insulin receptor function in vitro and in vivo. *Am J Physiol.* 1989;256: E39–E48.

31. Naeser P. Effects of adrenalectomy on the obese-hyperglycemic syndrome in mice (gene symbol ob). *Diabetologia.* 1973;9: 376–379.

32. Bujalska IJ, Kumar S, Hewison M, Stewart PM. Differentiation of adipose stromal cells: the roles of glucocorticoids and 11beta-hydroxysteroid dehydrogenase. *Endocrinology.* 1999;140: 3188–3196.

33. Masuzaki H, Paterson J, Shinyama H, Morton NM, Mullins JJ, Seckl JR, Flier JS. A transgenic model of visceral obesity and the metabolic syndrome. *Science.* 2001;294: 2166–2170.

34. Magiakou MA, Mastorakos G, Oldfield EH, Gomez MT, Doppman JL, Cutler GB, Jr., et al. Cushing's syndrome in children and adolescents. Presentation, diagnosis, and therapy. *N Engl J Med.* 1994;331: 629–636.

35. Devoe DJ, Miller WL, Conte FA, Kaplan SL, Grumbach MM, Rosenthal SM, Wilson CB, Gitelman SE. Long-term outcome in children and adolescents after transsphenoidal surgery for Cushing's disease. *J Clin Endocrinol Metab.* 1997;82: 3196–3202.

36. Lee PA, Weldon VV, Migeon CJ. Short stature as the only clinical sign of Cushing's syndrome. *J Pediatr.* 1975;86. 89–91.

37. Streeten DH, Faas FH, Elders MJ, Dalakos TG, Voorhess M. Hypercortisolism in childhood: short-comings of conventional diagnostic criteria. *Pediatrics.* 1975;56: 797–803.

38. Lee PD, Winter RJ, Green OC. Virilizing adrenocortical tumors in childhood: eight cases and a review of the literature. *Pediatrics.* 1985;76: 437–444.

39. Gomez MT, Malozowski S, Winterer J, Vamvakopoulos NC, Chrousos GP. Urinary free cortisol values in normal children and adolescents. *J Pediatr.* 1991;118: 256–258.

40. Hindmarsh PC, Brook CG. Single dose dexamethasone suppression test in children: dose relationship to body size. *Clin Endocrinol (Oxf).* 1985;23: 67–70.

41. Jaksic T, Yaman M, Thorner P, Wesson DK, Filler RM, Shandling B. A 20-year review of pediatric pancreatic tumors. *J Pediatr. Surg.* 1992;27: 1315–1317.

42. Dolan JP, Norton JA. Occult insulinoma. *Br J Surg.* 2000;87: 385–387.

43. Stefanini P, Carboni M, Patrassi N, Basoli A. Beta-islet cell tumors of the pancreas: results of a study on 1,067 cases. *Surgery.* 1974;75. 597–609

44. Harrington MG, McGeorge AP, Ballantyne JP, Beastall G. A prospective survey for insulinomas in a neurology department. *Lancet.* 1983;1: 1094–1095.

45. Dizon AM, Kowalyk S, Hoogwerf DJ. Neuroglycopenic and other symptoms in patients with insulinomas. *Am J Med.* 1999;106: 307–310.

46. Hetherington AW. Hypothalamic lesions and adiposity in the rat. *Anat Rec.* 1940;78: 149–172

47. Anand BK. Localization of feeding center in the hypothalamus of the rat. *Proc Soc Exp Biol Med.* 1951;11: 323–324.

48. Muller HL, Bueb K, Bartels U, Roth C, Harz K, Graf N, et al. Obesity after childhood craniopharyngioma — German multicenter study on pre-operative risk factors and quality of life. *Klin Padiatr.* 2001;213: 244–249.

49. Kernie SG, Liebl DJ, Parada LF. BDNF regulates eating behavior and locomotor activity in mice. *Embo J.* 2000;19: 1290–1300.

50. Nakagawa T, Ono-Kishino M, Sugaru E, Yamanaka M, Taiji M, Noguchi H. Brain-derived neurotrophic factor (BDNF) regulates glucose and energy metabolism in diabetic mice. *Diabetes Metab Res Rev.* 2002;18: 185–191.

51. Lawrence CB, Celsi F, Brennand J, Luckman SM. Alternative role for prolactin-releasing peptide in the regulation of food intake. *Nat Neurosci.* 2000;3: 645–646.

52. Lawrence CB, Ellacott KL, Luckman SM. PRL-releasing peptide reduces food intake and may mediate satiety signaling. *Endocrinology.* 2002;143: 360–367.

53. Roland BL, Sutton SW, Wilson SJ, Luo L, Pyati J, Huvar R, et al. Anatomical distribution of prolactin-releasing peptide and its receptor suggests additional functions in the central nervous system and periphery. *Endocrinology.* 1999;140: 5736–5745.

54. Lawrence CB, Williams T, Luckman SM. Intracerebroventricular galanin-like peptide induces different brain activation compared with galanin. *Endocrinology.* 2003;144: 3977–3984.

55. Degen L, Matzinger D, Drewe J, Beglinger C. The effect of cholecystokinin in controlling appetite and food intake in humans. *Peptides.* 2001;22: 1265–1269.

56. Donahey JC, van Dijk G, Woods SC, Seeley RJ. Intraventricular GLP-1 reduces short- but not long-term food intake or body weight in lean and obese rats. *Brain Res.* 1998;779: 75–83.

57. Batterham RL, Cowley MA, Small CJ, Herzog H, Cohen MA, Dakin CL, et al. Gut hormone PYY(3–36) physiologically inhibits food intake. *Nature.* 2002;418: 650–654.

58. Dourish CT, Rycroft W, Iversen SD. Postponement of satiety by blockade of brain cholecystokinin (CCK-B) receptors. *Science.* 1989;245: 1509–1511.

59. Kanse SM, Kreymann B, Ghatei MA, Bloom SR. Identification and characterization of glucagon-like peptide-1 7–36 amide-binding sites in the rat brain and lung. *FEBS Lett.* 1988;241: 209–212.

60. Schwartz MW, Morton GJ. Obesity: keeping hunger at bay. *Nature.* 2002;418: 595–597.

61. Tschop M, Smiley DL, Heiman ML. Ghrelin induces adiposity in rodents. *Nature.* 2000;407: 908–913.

62. Wilcox BJ, Matsumoto AM, Dorsa DM, Baskin DG. Reduction of insulin binding in the arcuate nucleus of the rat hypothalamus after 6-hydroxydopamine treatment. *Brain Res.* 1989;500: 149–155.

63. Baskin DG, Wilcox BJ, Figlewicz DP, Dorsa DM. Insulin and insulin-like growth factors in the CNS. *Trends Neurosci.* 1988;11: 107–111.

64. Baura GD, Foster DM, Porte D, Jr Kahn SE, Bergman RN, Cobelli C, Schwartz MW. Saturable transport of insulin from plasma into the central nervous system of dogs *in vivo*. A mechanism for regulated insulin delivery to the brain. *J Clin Invest.* 1993;92: 1824–1830.

65. Bruning JC, Gautam D, Burks DJ, Gillette J, Schubert M, Orban PC, et al. Role of brain insulin receptor in control of body weight and reproduction. *Science.* 2000;289: 2122–2125.

66. Tobe K, Suzuki R, Aoyama M, Yamauchi T, Kamon J, Kubota N, et al. Increased expression of the sterol regulatory element-binding protein-1 gene in insulin receptor substrate-2(-/-) mouse liver. *J Biol Chem.* 2001;276: 38337–38340.

67. Masaki T, Chiba S, Noguchi H, Yasuda T, Tobe K, Suzuki R, et al. Obesity in insulin receptor substrate-2-deficient mice: disrupted control of arcuate nucleus neuropeptides. *Obes Res.* 2004;12: 878–885.

68. Hoffman HJ, De Silva M, Humphreys RP, Drake JM, Smith ML, Blaser SI. Aggressive surgical management of craniopharyngiomas in children. *J Neurosurg.* 1992;76: 47–52.

69. Lustig RH, Post SR, Srivannaboon K, Rose SR, Danish RK, Burghen GA, et al. Risk factors for the development of obesity in children surviving brain tumors. *J Clin Endocrinol Metab.* 2003;88: 611–616.

70. Sorva R. Children with craniopharyngioma. Early growth failure and rapid postoperative weight gain. *Acta Paediatr Scand.* 1988;77: 587–592.

71. Srinivasan S, Ogle GD, Garnett SP, Briody JN, Lee JW, Cowell CT. Features of the metabolic syndrome after childhood craniopharyngioma. *J Clin Endocrinol Metab.* 2004;89: 81–86.

72. Adams LA, Feldstein A, Lindor KD, Angulo P. Nonalcoholic fatty liver disease among patients with hypothalamic and pituitary dysfunction. *Hepatology* 2004;39: 909–914.

73. Harz KJ, Muller HL, Waldeck E, Pudel V, Roth C. Obesity in patients with craniopharyngioma: assessment of food intake and movement counts indicating physical activity. *J Clin Endocrinol Metab.* 2003;88: 5227–5231.

74. Patel L, Cooper CD, Quinton ND, Butler GE, Gill MS, Jefferson IG, et al. Serum leptin and leptin binding activity in children and adolescents with hypothalamic dysfunction. *J Pediatr. Endocrinol Metab.* 2002;15: 963–971.

75. Tiosano D, Eisentein I, Militianu D, Chrousos GP, Hochberg Z. 11 Beta-hydroxysteroid dehydrogenase activity in hypothalamic obesity. *J Clin Endocrinol Metab.* 2003;88: 379–384.

76. Zhang Y, Proenca R, Maffei M, Barone M, Leopold L, Friedman JM. Positional cloning of the mouse obese gene and its human homologue. *Nature.* 1994;372: 425–432.

77. Havel PJ. Control of energy homeostasis and insulin action by adipocyte hormones: leptin, acylation stimulating protein, and adiponectin. *Curr Opin Lipidol.* 2002;13: 51–59.

78. Maffei M, Halaas J, Ravussin E, Pratley RE, Lee GH, Zhang Y, et al. Leptin levels in human and rodent: measurement of plasma leptin and ob RNA in obese and weight-reduced subjects. *Nat Med.* 1995;1: 1155–1161.

79. Considine RV, Sinha MK, Heiman ML, Kriauciunas A, Stephens TW, Nyce MR, et al. Serum immunoreactive-leptin concentrations in normal-weight and obese humans. *N Engl J Med.* 1996;334: 292–295.

80. Havel PJ, Kasim-Karakas S, Mueller W, Johnson PR, Gingerich RL, Stern JS. Relationship of plasma leptin to plasma insulin and adiposity in normal weight and overweight women: effects of dietary fat content and sustained weight loss. *J Clin Endocrinol Metab.* 1996;81: 4406–4413.

81. Ahren B, Mansson S, Gingerich RL, Havel PJ. Regulation of plasma leptin in mice: influence of age, high-fat diet, and fasting. *Am J Physiol.* 1997;273: R113–120.

82. Hassink SG, Sheslow DV, de Lancey E, Opentanova I, Considine RV, Caro JF. Serum leptin in children with obesity: relationship to gender and development. *Pediatrics.* 1996;98: 201–203.

83. Hickey MS, Israel RG, Gardiner SN, Considine RV, McCammon MR, Tyndall GL, et al. Gender differences in serum leptin levels in humans. *Biochem Mol Med.* 1996;59: 1–6.

84. Havel PJ, Kasim-Karakas S, Dubuc GR, Mueller W, Phinney SD. Gender differences in plasma leptin concentrations. *Nat Med.* 1996;2: 949–950.

85. Havel PJ. Role of adipose tissue in body-weight regulation: mechanisms regulating leptin production and energy balance. *Proc Nutr Soc.* 2000;59: 359–371.

86. Utriainen T, Malmstrom R, Makimattila S, Yki-Jarvinen H. Supraphysiological hyperinsulinemia increases plasma leptin concentrations after 4 h in normal subjects. *Diabetes.* 1996;45: 1364–1366.

87. Saad MF, Khan A, Sharma A, Michael R, Riad-Gabriel MG, Boyadjian R, et al. Physiological insulinemia acutely modulates plasma leptin. *Diabetes.* 1998;47: 544–549.

88. Montague CT, Farooqi IS, Whitehead JP, Soos MA, Rau H, Wareham NJ, et al. Congenital leptin deficiency is associated with severe early-onset obesity in humans. *Nature.* 1997;387: 903–908.

89. Strobel A, Issad T, Camoin L, Ozata M, Strosberg AD. A leptin missense mutation associated with hypogonadism and morbid obesity. *Nat Genet.* 1998;18: 213–215.

90. Clement K, Vaisse C, Lahlou N, Cabrol S, Pelloux V, Cassuto D, et al. A mutation in the human leptin receptor gene causes obesity and pituitary dysfunction. *Nature.* 1998;392: 398–401.

91. Farooqi IS, Keogh JM, Kamath S, Jones S, Gibson WT, Trussell R, et al. Partial leptin deficiency and human adiposity. *Nature.* 2001;414: 34–35.

92. Lahlou N, Issad T, Lebouc Y, Carel JC, Camoin L, Roger M, Girard J. Mutations in the human leptin and leptin receptor genes as models of serum leptin receptor regulation. *Diabetes* 2002;51: 1980–1985.

93. Farooqi IS, Jebb SA, Langmack G, Lawrence E, Cheetham CH, Prentice AM, et al. Effects of recombinant leptin therapy in a child with congenital leptin deficiency. *N Engl J Med.* 1999;341: 879–884.

94. Licinio J, Caglayan S, Ozata M, Yildiz BO, de Miranda PB, O'Kirwan F, et al. Phenotypic effects of leptin replacement on morbid obesity diabetes mellitus, hypogonadism, and behavior in leptin-deficient adults. *Proc Natl Acad Sci USA.* 2004;101: 4531–4536.

95. Farooqi IS, Matarese G, Lord GM, Keogh JM, Lawrence E, Agwu C, et al. Beneficial effects of leptin on obesity T cell hyporesponsiveness, and neuroendocrine/metabolic dysfunction of human congenital leptin deficiency. *J Clin Invest.* 2002;110: 1093–1103.

96. Hagan MM, Rushing PA, Schwartz MW, Yagaloff KA, Burn P, Woods SC, et al. Role of the CNS melanocortin system in the response to overfeeding. *J Neurosci.* 1999;19: 2362–2367.

97. Yaswen L, Diehl N, Brennan MB, Hochgeschwender U. Obesity in the mouse model of pro-opiomelanocortin deficiency responds to peripheral melanocortin. *Nat Med.* 1999;5: 1066–1070.

98. Krude H, Biebermann H, Luck W, Horn R, Brabant G, Gruters A. Severe early-onset obesity, adrenal insufficiency and red hair pigmentation caused by POMC mutations in humans. *Nat Genet.* 1998;19: 155–157.

99. Krude H, Gruters A. Implications of proopiomelanocortin (POMC) mutations in humans: the POMC deficiency syndrome. *Trends Endocrinol Metab.* 2000;11:15–22.

100. Krude H, Biebermann H, Schnabel D, Tansek MZ, Theunissen P, Mullis PE, et al. Obesity due to proopiomelanocortin deficiency: three new cases and treatment trials with thyroid hormone and ACTH4-10. *J Clin Endocrinol Metab.*2003;88: 4633–4640.

101. Feng N, Adler-Wailes D, Elberg J, Chin JY, Fallon E, Carr A, et al. Sequence variants of the pomc gene and their associations with body composition in children. *Obes Res.* 2003;11: 619–24.

102. Echwald SM, Sorensen TI, Andersen T, Tybjaerg-Hansen A, Clausen JO, Pedersen O. Mutational analysis of the proopiomelanocortin gene in Caucasians with early onset obesity. *Int J Obes Relat Metab Disord.* 1999;23: 293–298.

103. Miraglia del Giudice E, Cirillo G, Santoro N, D'Urso L, Carbone MT, Di Toro R, Perrone L. Molecular screening of the proopiomelanocortin (POMC) gene in Italian obese children: report of three new mutations. *Int J Obes Relat Metab Disord.* 2001;25: 61–67.

104. Challis BG, Pritchard LE, Creemers JW, Delplanque J, Keogh JM, Luan J, et al. A missense mutation disrupting a dibasic prohormone processing site in pro-opiomelanocortin (POMC) increases susceptibility to early-onset obesity through a novel molecular mechanism. *Hum Mol Genet.* 2002;11: 1997–2004.

105. Thomas L, Leduc R, Thorne BA, Smeekens SP, Steiner DF, Thomas G. Kex2-like endoproteases PC2 and PC3 accurately cleave a model prohormone in mammalian cells: evidence for a common core of neuroendocrine processing enzymes. *Proc Natl Acad Sci USA.* 1991;88: 5297–5301.

106. Benjannet S, Rondeau N, Day R, Chretien M, Seidah NG. PC1 and PC2 are proprotein convertases capable of cleaving proopiomelanocortin at distinct pairs of basic residues. *Proc Natl Acad Sci USA.* 1991;88: 3564–3568.

107. Dong W, Marcinkiewicz M, Vieau D, Chretien M, Seidah NG, Day R. Distinct mRNA expression of the highly homologous convertases PC5 and PACE4 in the rat brain and pituitary. *J Neurosci.* 1995;15: 1778–1796.

108. Fricker LD, McKinzie AA, Sun J, Curran E, Qian Y, Yan L, et al. Identification and characterization of proSAAS, a granin-like neuroendocrine peptide precursor that inhibits prohormone processing. *J Neurosci.* 2000;20: 639–648.

109. Wei S, Feng Y, Che FY, Pan H, Mzhavia N, Devi LA, et al. Obesity and diabetes in transgenic mice expressing proSAAS. *J Endocrinol.* 2004;180: 357–368.

110. Jackson RS, Creemers JW, Ohagi S, Raffin-Sanson ML, Sanders L, Montague CT, et al. Obesity and impaired prohormone processing associated with mutations in the human prohormone convertase 1 gene. *Nat Genet.* 1997;16: 303–306.

111. Jackson RS, Creemers JW, Farooqi IS, Raffin-Sanson ML, Varro A, Dockray GJ, et al. Small-intestinal dysfunction accompanies the complex endocrinopathy of human proprotein convertase 1 deficiency. *J Clin Invest.* 2003;112: 1550–1560.

112. Chen D, Garg A. Monogenic disorders of obesity and body fat distribution. *J Lipid Res.* 1999;40: 1735–1746.

113. Marsh DJ, Hollopeter G, Huszar D, Laufer R, Yagaloff KA, Fisher SL, et al. Response of melanocortin-4 receptor-deficient mice to anorectic and orexigenic peptides. *Nat Genet.* 1999;21: 119–122.

114. Fehm HL, Smolnik R, Kern W, McGregor GP, Bickel U, Born J. The melanocortin melanocyte-stimulating hormone/adrenocorticotropin(4-10) decreases body fat in humans. *J Clin Endocrinol Metab.* 2001;86: 1144–1148.

115. Butler AA, Kesterson RA, Khong K, Cullen M.J, Pelleymounter MA, Dekoning J, et al. A unique metabolic syndrome causes obesity in the melanocortin-3 receptor-deficient mouse. *Endocrinology.* 2000;141: 3518–3521.

116. Hinney A, Schmidt A, Nottebom K, Heibult O, Becker I, Ziegler A, et al. Several mutations in the melanocortin-4 receptor gene including a nonsense and a frameshift mutation associated with dominantly inherited obesity in humans. *J Clin Endocrinol Metab.* 1999;84: 1483–1486.

117. Ho G, MacKenzie RG. Functional characterization of mutations in melanocortin-4 receptor associated with human obesity. *J Biol Chem.* 1999;274: 35816–35822.

118. Vaisse C, Clement K, Durand E, Hercberg S, Guy-Grand B, Froguel P. Melanocortin-4 receptor mutations are a frequent and heterogeneous cause of morbid obesity. *J Clin Invest.* 2000;106: 253–262.

119. Farooqi IS, Keogh JM, Yeo GS, Lank EJ, Cheetham T, O'Rahilly S. Clinical spectrum of obesity and mutations in the melanocortin 4 receptor gene. *N Engl J Med.* 2003;348: 1085–1095.

120. Yeo GS, Connie Hung CC, Rochford J, Keogh J, Gray J, Sivaramakrishnan S, et al. A de novo mutation affecting human TrkB associated with severe obesity and developmental delay. *Nat Neurosci.* 2004;7: 1187–1189.

121. Xu B, Goulding EH, Zang K, Cepoi D, Cone RD, Jones KR, et al. Brain-derived neurotrophic factor regulates energy balance downstream of melanocortin-4 receptor. *Nat Neurosci.* 2003;6: 736–742.

122. Lyons WE, Mamounas LA, Ricaurte GA, Coppola V, Reid SW, Bora SH, et al. Brain-derived neurotrophic factor-deficient mice develop aggressiveness and hyperphagia in conjunction with brain serotonergic abnormalities. *Proc Natl Acad Sci USA*. 1999;96: 15239–15244.

123. Kernie SG, Liebl DJ, Parada LF. BDNF regulates eating behavior and locomotor activity in mice. *Embo J*. 2000;19: 1290–1300.

124. Rios M, Fan G, Fekete C, Kelly J, Bates B, Kuehn R, et al. Conditional deletion of brain-derived neurotrophic factor in the postnatal brain leads to obesity and hyperactivity. *Mol Endocrinol*. 2001;15: 1748–17457.

125. Ono M, Ichihara J, Nonomura T, Itakura Y, Taiji M, Nakayama C, Noguchi H. Brain-derived neurotrophic factor reduces blood glucose level in obese diabetic mice but not in normal mice. *Biochem Biophys Res Commun*. 1997;238: 633–637.

126. Nakagawa T, Tsuchida A, Itakura Y, Nonomura T, Ono M, Hirota F, et al. Brain-derived neurotrophic factor regulates glucose metabolism by modulating energy balance in diabetic mice. *Diabetes*. 2000;49: 436–444.

127. Nonomura T, Tsuchida A, Ono-Kishino M, Nakagawa T, Taiji M, Noguchi H. Brain-derived neurotrophic factor regulates energy expenditure through the central nervous system in obese diabetic mice. *Int J Exp Diabetes Res*. 2001;2: 201–209.

128. Nakagawa T, Ono-Kishino M, Sugaru E, Yamanaka M, Taiji M, Noguchi H. Brain-derived neurotrophic factor (BDNF) regulates glucose and energy metabolism in diabetic mice. *Diabetes Metab Res Rev*. 2002;18: 185–191.

129. Patten JL, Johns DR, Valle D, Eil C, Gruppuso PA, Steele G, et al. Mutation in the gene encoding the stimulatory G protein of adenylate cyclase in Albright's hereditary osteodystrophy. *N Engl J Med*. 1990;322: 1412–1419.

130. Miric A, Vechio JD, Levine MA. Heterogeneous mutations in the gene encoding the alpha-subunit of the stimulatory G protein of adenylyl cyclase in Albright hereditary osteodystrophy. *J Clin Endocrinol Metab*. 1993;76: 1560–1568.

131. Fitch N. Albright's hereditary osteodystrophy: a review. *Am J Med. Genet*. 1982;11: 11–29.

132. Mantovani G, Maghnie M, Weber G, De Menis E, Brunelli V, Cappa M, et al. Growth hormone-releasing hormone resistance in pseudohypoparathyroidism type ia: new evidence for imprinting of the Gs alpha gene. *J Clin Endocrinol Metab*. 2003;88: 4070–4074.

133. Germain-Lee EL, Groman J, Crane JL, Jan de Beur SM, Levine MA. Growth hormone deficiency in pseudohypoparathyroidism type 1a: another manifestation of multihormone resistance. *J Clin Endocrinol Metab*. 2003;88: 4059–4069.

134. Kaartinen JM, Kaar ML, Ohisalo JJ. Defective stimulation of adipocyte adenylate cyclase, blunted lipolysis, and obesity in pseudohypoparathyroidism 1a. *Pediatr Res*. 1994;35: 594–597.

135. Carel JC, Le Stunff C, Condamine L, Mallet E, Chaussain JL, Adnot P, et al. Resistance to the lipolytic action of epinephrine: a new feature of protein Gs deficiency. *J Clin Endocrinol Metab*. 1999;84: 4127–4131.

136. Wang HY, Watkins DC, Malbon CC. Antisense oligodeoxynucleotides to GS protein alpha-subunit sequence accelerate differentiation of fibroblasts to adipocytes. *Nature*. 1992;358: 334–337.

137. Ong KK, Amin R, Dunger DB. Pseudohypoparathyroidism — another monogenic obesity syndrome. *Clin Endocrinol* (Oxf). 2000;52: 389–391.

138. Badano JL, Ansley SJ, Leitch CC, Lewis RA, Lupski JR, Katsanis N. Identification of a novel Bardet–Biedl syndrome protein BBS7, that shares structural features with BBS1 and BBS2. *Am J Hum Genet*. 2003;72: 650–658.

139. Mykytyn K, Braun T, Carmi R, Haider NB, Searby CC, Shastri M, et al. Identification of the gene that, when mutated, causes the human obesity syndrome BBS4. *Nat Genet*. 2001;28: 188–191.

140. Katsanis N, Beales PL, Woods MO, Lewis RA, Green JS, Parfrey PS, et al. Mutations in MKKS cause obesity, retinal dystrophy and renal malformations associated with Bardet–Biedl syndrome. *Nat Genet*. 2000;26: 67–70.

141. Slavotinek AM, Stone EM, Mykytyn K, Heckenlively JR, Green JS, Heon E, et al. Mutations in MKKS cause Bardet–Biedl syndrome. *Nat Genet*. 2000;26: 15–16.

142. Nishimura DY, Searby CC, Carmi R, Elbedour K, Van Maldergem L, Fulton AB, et al. Positional cloning of a novel gene on chromosome 16q causing Bardet–Biedl syndrome (BBS2). *Hum Mol Genet*. 2001;10: 865–874.

143. Mykytyn K, Nishimura DY, Searby CC, Shastri M, Yen HJ, Beck JS, et al. Identification of the gene (BBS1) most commonly involved in Bardet–Biedl syndrome, a complex human obesity syndrome. *Nat Genet.* 2002;31: 435–438.

144. Ansley SJ, Badano JL, Blacque OE, Hill J, Hoskins BE, Leitch CC, et al. Basal body dysfunction is a likely cause of pleiotropic Bardet–Biedl syndrome. *Nature.* 2003;425: 628–633.

145. Beales PL, Warner AM, Hitman GA, Thakker R, Flinter FA. Bardet–Biedl syndrome: a molecular and phenotypic study of 18 families. *J Med Genet.* 1997;34: 92–98.

146. Klein D, Ammann F. The syndrome of Laurence-Moon-Bardet–Biedl and allied diseases in Switzerland. Clinical, genetic and epidemiological studies. *J Neurol Sci.* 1969;9: 479–513.

147. Green JS, Parfrey PS, Harnett JD, Farid NR, Cramer BC, Johnson G, et al. The cardinal manifestations of Bardet–Biedl syndrome, a form of Laurence-Moon-Biedl syndrome. *N Engl J Med.* 1989;321: 1002–1009.

148. Farag TI, Teebi AS. High incidence of Bardet–Biedl syndrome among the Bedouin. *Clin Genet.* 1989;36: 463–464.

149. Beales PL, Elcioglu N, Woolf AS, Parker D, Flinter FA. New criteria for improved diagnosis of Bardet–Biedl syndrome: results of a population survey. *J Med Genet.* 1999;36: 437–446.

150. Dekaban AS, Parks JS, Ross GT. Laurence-Moon syndrome: evaluation of endocrinological function and phenotypic concordance and report of cases. *Med Ann Dist Columbia.* 1972;41: 687–694.

151. Bauman ML, Hogan GR. Laurence-Moon-Biedl syndrome. Report of two unrelated children less than 3 years of age. *Am J Dis Child.* 1973;126: 119–126.

152. Hrynchak PK. Bardet–Biedl syndrome. *Optom Vis Sci.* 2000;77: 236–243.

153. O'Dea D, Parfrey PS, Harnett JD, Hefferton D, Cramer BC, Green J. The importance of renal impairment in the natural history of Bardet–Biedl syndrome. *Am J Kidney Dis.* 1996;27: 776–783.

154. Grace C, Beales P, Summerbell C, Jebb SA, Wright A, Parker D, Kopelman P. Energy metabolism in Bardet–Biedl syndrome. *Int J Obes Relat Metab Disord.* 2003;27: 1319–1324.

155. Croft JB, Swift M. Obesity, hypertension, and renal disease in relatives of Bardet–Biedl syndrome sibs. *Am J Med. Genet.* 1990;36: 37–42.

156. Croft JB, Morrell D, Chase CL, Swift M. Obesity in heterozygous carriers of the gene for the Bardet–Biedl syndrome. *Am J Med. Genet.* 1995;55: 12–15.

157. Fan Y, Rahman P, Peddle L, Hefferton D, Gladney N, Moore SJ, et al. Bardet–Biedl syndrome 1 genotype and obesity in the Newfoundland population. *Int J Obes Relat Metab Disord.* 2004;28: 680–684.

158. Nicholls RD, Knepper JL. Genome organization, function, and imprinting in Prader–Willi and Angelman syndromes. *Annu Rev Genomics Hum Genet.* 2001;2: 153–175.

159. Butler MG. Prader–Willi syndrome: current understanding of cause and diagnosis. *Am J Med Genet.* 1990;35: 319–332.

160. Holm VA, Cassidy SB, Butler MG, Hanchett JM, Greenswag LR, Whitman BY, Greenberg F. Prader–Willi syndrome: consensus diagnostic criteria. *Pediatrics.* 1993;91: 398–402.

161. Morgan JB, Rolles CJ. The nutrition and growth over a 10 month period of an infant with the Prader–Willi syndrome. *Hum Nutr Appl Nutr.* 1984;38: 304–307.

162. Bekx MT, Carrel AL, Shriver TC, Li Z, Allen DB. Decreased energy expenditure is caused by abnormal body composition in infants with Prader–Willi Syndrome. *J Pediatr.* 2003;143: 372–376.

163. Burd L, Vesely B, Martsolf J, Kerbeshian J. Prevalence study of Prader–Willi syndrome in North Dakota. *Am J Med. Genet.* 1990;37: 97–99.

164. Smith A, Egan J, Ridley G, Haan E, Montgomery P, Williams K, Elliott E. Birth prevalence of Prader–Willi syndrome in Australia. *Arch Dis Child.* 2003;88: 263–264.

165. Vogels A, Van Den Ende J, Keymolen K, Mortier G, Devriendt K, Legius E, Fryns JP. Minimum prevalence, birth incidence and cause of death for Prader–Willi syndrome in Flanders. *Eur J Hum Genet.* 2004;12: 238–240.

166. Zigman JM, Elmquist JK. Minireview: From anorexia to obesity — the yin and yang of body weight control. *Endocrinology.* 2003;144: 3749–3756.

167. Olszewski PK, Li D, Grace MK, Billington CJ, Kotz CM, Levine AS. Neural basis of orexigenic effects of ghrelin acting within lateral hypothalamus. *Peptides.* 2003;24: 597–602.

168. Toshinai K, Date Y, Murakami N, Shimada M, Mondal MS, Shimbara T, et al. Ghrelin-induced food intake is mediated via the orexin pathway. *Endocrinology.* 2003;144: 1506–1512.

169. Faulconbridge LF, Cummings DE, Kaplan JM, Grill HJ. Hyperphagic effects of brainstem ghrelin administration. *Diabetes*. 2003;52: 2260–2265.

170. Wren AM, Small CJ, Ward HL, Murphy KG, Dakin CL, Taheri S, et al. The novel hypothalamic peptide ghrelin stimulates food intake and growth hormone secretion. *Endocrinology*. 2000;141: 4325–4328.

171. Wren AM, Seal LJ, Cohen MA, Brynes AE, Frost GS, Murphy KG, et al. Ghrelin enhances appetite and increases food intake in humans. *J Clin Endocrinol Metab*. 2001;86: 5992.

172. Haqq AM, Farooqi IS, O'Rahilly S, Stadler DD, Rosenfeld RG, Pratt KL, et al. Serum ghrelin levels are inversely correlated with body mass index, age, and insulin concentrations in normal children and are markedly increased in Prader–Willi syndrome. *J Clin Endocrinol Metab*. 2003;88: 174–178.

173. Cummings DE, Weigle DS, Frayo RS, Breen PA, Ma MK, Dellinger EP, Purnell JQ. Plasma ghrelin levels after diet-induced weight loss or gastric bypass surgery. *N Engl J Med*. 2002;346: 1623–1630.

174. Otto B, Cuntz U, Fruehauf E, Wawarta R, Folwaczny C, Riepl RL, et al. Weight gain decreases elevated plasma ghrelin concentrations of patients with anorexia nervosa. *Eur J Endocrinol*. 2001;145: 669–673.

175. Cummings DE, Clement K, Purnell JQ, Vaisse C, Foster KE, Frayo RS, et al. Elevated plasma ghrelin levels in Prader Willi syndrome. *Nat Med*. 2002;8: 643–644.

176. Janssen JA, van der Toorn FM, Hofland LJ, van Koetsveld P, Broglio F, Ghigo E, et al. Systemic ghrelin levels in subjects with growth hormone deficiency are not modified by one year of growth hormone replacement therapy. *Eur J Endocrinol*. 2001;145: 711–716.

177. Hoybye C, Hilding A, Jacobsson H, Thoren M. Growth hormone treatment improves body composition in adults with Prader–Willi syndrome. *Clin Endocrinol* (Oxf). 2003;58: 653–661.

178. Carrel AL, Myers SE, Whitman BY, Allen DB. Benefits of long-term GH therapy in Prader–Willi syndrome: a 4-year study. *J Clin Endocrinol Metab*. 2002;87: 1581–1585.

179. Myers SE, Davis A, Whitman BY, Santiago JV, Landt M. Leptin concentrations in Prader–Willi syndrome before and after growth hormone replacement. *Clin Endocrinol* (Oxf). 2000;52: 101–105.

180. Goldstone AP, Brynes AE, Thomas EL, Bell JD, Frost G, Holland A, et al. Resting metabolic rate, plasma leptin concentrations, leptin receptor expression, and adipose tissue measured by whole-body magnetic resonance imaging in women with Prader Willi syndrome. *Am J Clin Nutr*. 2002;75: 468–475.

181. Schoeller DA, Levitsky LL, Bandini LG, Dietz WW, Walczak A. Energy expenditure and body composition in Prader–Willi syndrome. *Metabolism*. 1988;37: 115–120.

182. Bueno G, Moreno LA, Pineda I, Campos J, Ruibal JL, Juste MG, et al. Serum leptin concentrations in children with Prader–Willi syndrome and non syndromal obesity. *J Pediatr Endocrinol Metab*. 2000;13: 425–430.

183. Butler MG, Moore J, Morawiecki A, Nicolson M. Comparison of leptin protein levels in Prader–Willi syndrome and control individuals. *Am J Med Genet*. 1998;75: 7–12.

184. Mannens M, Alders M, Redeker B, Bliek J, Steenman M, Wiesmeyer C, et al. Positional cloning of genes involved in the Beckwith–Wiedemann syndrome, hemihypertrophy, and associated childhood tumors. *Med Pediatr Oncol*. 1996;27: 490–494.

185. Sotelo-Avila C, Gonzalez-Crussi F, Fowler JW. Complete and incomplete forms of Beckwith–Wiedemann syndrome: their oncogenic potential. *J Pediatr*. 1980;96: 47–50.

186. Schneid H, Vazquez MP, Vacher C, Gourmelen M, Cabrol S, Le Bouc Y. The Beckwith–Wiedemann syndrome phenotype and the risk of cancer. *Med Pediatr Oncol*. 1997;28: 411–415.

187. Weksberg R, Nishikawa J, Caluseriu O, Fei YL, Shuman C, Wei C, et al. Tumor development in the Beckwith–Wiedemann syndrome is associated with a variety of constitutional molecular 11p15 alterations including imprinting defects of KCNQ1OT1. *Hum Mol Genet*. 2001;10: 2989–3000.

188. Takahashi K, Kobayashi T, Kanayama N. p57(Kip2) regulates the proper development of labyrinthine and spongiotrophoblasts. *Mol Hum Reprod*. 2000;6: 1019–1025.

189. Sun FL, Dean WL, Kelsey G, Allen ND, Reik W. Transactivation of Igf2 in a mouse model of Beckwith–Wiedemann syndrome. *Nature*. 1997;389: 809–815.

190. Engel JR, Smallwood A, Harper A, Higgins MJ, Oshimura M, Reik W, et al. Epigenotype-phenotype correlations in Beckwith–Wiedemann syndrome. *J Med Genet*. 2000;37: 921–926.

10 Physical Activity and Adiposity in Children and Adolescents

Paule Barbeau, Bernard Gutin, and Melinda S. Sothern

CONTENTS

INTRODUCTION

We begin this chapter by reviewing what is known about the determinants of physical activity in youth and the role of physical activity in the etiology of pediatric obesity. We then summarize what is known from nonexperimental studies about the relations of physical activity with body composition and preclinical markers for future cardiovascular disease and type 2 diabetes in youths. Next, we review experimental studies of physical activity and its effects on body composition and energy expenditure. Experimental studies provide the clearest evidence of causal relations. Although a distinction can be drawn between the terms *physical activity* (i.e., all movement that elevates energy expenditure) and *exercise* (more structured and intense activity), for purposes of this chapter they are used interchangeably to refer to movement associated with various degrees of energy expenditure.

DETERMINANTS OF PHYSICAL ACTIVITY IN YOUTHS

The determinants influencing physical activity are numerous and reviewed in detail in other chapters of this volume. They include personal, social, and environmental factors. Some of these factors are addressed briefly here.

GENDER, RACE, AND MATURATION

Gender and race have been found to be determinants of physical activity in children. Reviews by Sallis et al.[1,2] reported that (1) boys are more active than girls;[3,4] this is supported by data showing that even as young as 5 to 6 years of age, cardiovascular fitness was approximately 5% higher in boys compared with girls,[5] and (2) whites seem to be more active in aerobic activities than blacks or Mexican Americans,[4] which is consistent with recent data[4,6,7] showing that even after controlling for body fatness, cardiovascular fitness was 15 to 17% lower in black youths compared with white youths. Furthermore, it is well established that physical activity tends to decline during adolescence,[8,9] particularly among girls.[10]

INTRAPERSONAL AND INTERPERSONAL FACTORS

A detailed review of the behavioral determinants of physical activity is presented in Chapter 14. Briefly, a review of 11 prospective studies of predictors in youths[11-21] indicated that high levels of physical activity were predicted by (1) enjoyment of physical activity, (2) positive parental and peer social support and influence, (3) specific self-efficacy to exercise regularly, (4) parental modeling (e.g., parent physical activity levels), (5) preference for physically active behaviors, and (6) history of participation in competitive sport and better grades in physical education classes. Furthermore, a 1-year increase in overweight prevalence in the National Longitudinal Study of Adolescent Health was associated with increased television or video viewing among white boys and girls, and a decrease in moderate to vigorous physical activity in boys and girls of all racial groups.[22]

COMMUNITY LEVEL FACTORS

A detailed review of the community determinants of physical activity is presented in Chapter 16. Factors at the community level that are related to physical activity may include access to, and availability of, supervised facilities and equipment, and age-appropriate programs.[12,15,23,24] Another important factor may be community design[25] and area of residence.[26,27]

SUMMARY

Several factors may influence physical activity levels. Whereas behavioral determinants may be to some extent modifiable, other determinants such as gender and race are not. It is important when assessing physical activity behavior and when developing interventions to consider all associated factors, including modifiable and nonmodifiable determinants.

PHYSICAL ACTIVITY, PHYSICAL FITNESS, ADIPOSITY, AND HEALTH

NONEXPERIMENTAL STUDIES

Many of the health problems associated with obesity, such as cardiovascular disease and type 2 diabetes, manifest themselves in the form of morbidity and mortality during the adult years. However, the origins of these problems can be traced to childhood. Because lifestyle habits are to some degree formed early in life and track into adulthood,[28] effective early intervention may have lifelong impact. In the United Kingdom, it was shown that active adults tended to have been active as children, and sedentary adults who had been active as children were more likely to be persuaded to become active.[29] In addition, body weight lost in weight control intervention programs is more likely to be sustained in children than in adults.[30]

Because pediatric obesity and poorer fitness have increased in prevalence over the last 10 to 15 years,[31-33] the implications for future public health are worrisome. One illustration of the seriousness of the secular trend to increased obesity is the parallel increase in the incidence of type 2 diabetes and obesity among youngsters in Cincinnati over a 10-year period.[34] Support for the positive influence of physical activity in this scenario is provided by the results of prospective studies that found favorable changes in risk factors in those children who improved the most in physical fitness.[35–37]

Because physical activity, cardiovascular fitness, and adiposity are interrelated,[38,39] studies that measure only adiposity and find relations to risk factors[40] may be partly obscuring the role of physical activity and physical fitness. It seems that physical activity and fitness exert independent influences on risk factors, even when adiposity is controlled statistically.[36,38,39,41,42] However, for other risk factors it seems that physical activity and physical fitness tend to exert much of their favorable effect on risk factors through their influence on adiposity. For example, in a sample of 1092 third-grade children, obesity was associated with higher systolic blood pressure and total cholesterol, whereas self-reported physical activity levels were not related to the risk factors.[43] We found that both low cardiovascular fitness and high body fatness were correlated with unfavorable risk factor levels in 7 to 11 year olds;[44] however, when multiple regression was applied, only percent fat explained a significant independent proportion of the variance in the risk factors. We followed this study with one in which weight was controlled experimentally rather than statistically; that is, cardiovascular fitness was expressed as submaximal heart rate during the weight-supported task of supine cycling,[45] thus dissociating fitness from weight (and fatness). We found that percent fat was significantly related to unfavorable levels of systolic blood pressure, triacylglycerol, high density lipoprotein cholesterol, the ratio of total to high density lipoprotein cholesterol, and insulin, whereas cardiovascular fitness was not significantly correlated with any of the risk factors. These findings are consistent with preliminary results from a recent project in which both fatness and fitness explained variability in risk factors when considered by themselves, but fatness tended to eliminate fitness from the equation when they were entered together.[46]

The evidence reviewed is consistent with the notions that several major "adult" health problems actually have their origins in childhood, and that excess adipose tissue is associated with preclinical markers for some of these diseases. Furthermore, the associations of physical activity and cardiovascular fitness with health seem to be mediated by adiposity. However, causal inferences drawn from the results of nonexperimental designs must be considered very tentative until supported by experimental studies that determine the extent to which changes in fatness are followed by changes in the fatness-related preclinical markers.

EXPERIMENTAL STUDIES: PREVENTION

Although cross-sectional and longitudinal cohort studies can provide a foundation for hypotheses concerning the relations among physical activity, adiposity, and health, only controlled experiments can apply rigorous tests of the hypotheses. For example, knowing that in free-living youths there is a cyclic relationship between inactivity, weight gain, more inactivity, more weight gain, and so on may be less illuminating than seeing what happens when youths increase or decrease their physical activity level.

Indirect support for the value of physical activity early in life comes from experimental studies on animals that have shown physical training to prevent obesity[47] and to greatly attenuate development of the metabolic syndrome.[48] Although it is reasonable to formulate hypotheses from animal studies, the complexity of the growing human requires that the hypotheses be tested directly in children at different stages of maturity. Few studies have used physical activity interventions to prevent obesity or attenuate the deposition of undesirable levels of adipose tissue in youths, although this is an area of research that is growing. A few reviews have been published on this topic.[49–52]

There are few published randomized controlled studies that have used physical activity interventions to try to prevent obesity or attenuate the deposition of undesirable adipose tissue in youths. Published studies based in elementary schools have provided mixed results. One of the largest trials, the Child and Adolescent Trial for Cardiovascular Health (CATCH) study, was a 3-year intervention that focused mainly on modifying the school environment to increase moderate to vigorous physical activity during physical education classes and decrease the fat content of the school lunch offerings. Despite showing increases in moderate to vigorous physical activity during physical education classes, there was no significant effect on body mass index or skinfolds.[53] The 8-week Cardiovascular Health in Children (CHIC) Study compared a "usual health instruction" with a classroom-based health education curriculum intervention with an enhanced physical education intervention. Despite a greater increase in total self-reported physical activity in the physical education schools compared with the health education schools, there were no significant differences in the changes in body mass index or skinfolds at the school level.[54] The Girls Health Enrichment Multi-site Studies (GEMS) included 12-week pilot studies that assessed the effect of a summer camp that included physical activity,[55] an after-school physical activity intervention,[56] or after-school dance classes[57] on body mass index in young black girls. These interventions did not result in any significant differences in change in body mass index, although for the most part the changes were in the expected direction. A multicomponent 3-year study in elementary schools in Greece that included an enhanced physical education component found a greater increase in physical activity and a smaller increase in body mass index (BMI) in the intervention schools compared with the control schools.[58]

Large-scale, multisite studies in middle schools also have yielded mixed results. Planet Health, a 2-year study, included components aimed at increasing physical activity, decreasing television viewing, and improving dietary behaviors. Results showed that the prevalence of obesity was reduced in the intervention schools compared with the control schools, but only in girls.[59] CHIC II, which included an 8-week intervention where schools were randomized to exercise only, education only, exercise and education, or a control group, found that although there was no significant difference between the groups for change in body mass index, the two groups that received exercise had a significantly smaller increase in skinfolds compared with the education only and control groups.[60] Active Winners, an 18-month after-school and summer physical activity program that aimed at increasing physical activity, found no differences in physical activity levels between the intervention and control groups;[61] measures of adiposity were not available. The Middle-School Physical Activity and Nutrition (M-SPAN) study, a 2-year intervention that included components aimed at increasing physical activity during physical education and throughout the school day also failed to show a significant difference in physical activity levels between intervention and control schools; however, body mass index decreased significantly in boys, but not in girls.[62]

Preliminary results of two after-school interventions in elementary schools conducted at the Medical College of Georgia for children who vary over the spectrum of adiposity (July 2004) suggest that favorable effects on adiposity are seen when children engage in moderate to vigorous physical activity for more than 80 min/d; children in the intervention group who attended the sessions more often showed greater reductions in adiposity (see abstracts in Refs. 63 and 64).

In summary, published physical activity intervention studies have shown mixed results on changes in physical activity behavior, adiposity, and cardiovascular risk factors. However, most of these studies did not specifically target vigorous physical activity and several included physical activity sessions that were shorter than recommended for children. In addition, few studies targeted weight status or adiposity as the primary outcome variable. Thus, the impact of physical activity intervention studies on obesity prevention in youth remains understudied. Please see Table 10.1 for a summary of the studies in this section.

EXPERIMENTAL STUDIES: TREATMENT

This section includes pediatric weight loss studies utilizing individual and family based counseling interventions, including physical activity and/or exercise and nutrition, in clinical or after school settings. The findings reported in a recent review article by Sothern[65] are also summarized. This

TABLE 10.1
Summary of Prevention/Intervention Studies

| No. Studies | Duration | Intervention Components | | | | Favorable Changes | | | Ref. |
		PE	Other PA	Summer Camp	Non-PA	PA	Adiposity	CVD Risk Factors[a]	
4	8 weeks–3 yr					2	2	TC (2) HDLC (1) BP (1)	54, 58, 105, 109
1	12 weeks			×		—	NS	—	55
1	18 months		×	×		NS	—	—	61
3	8 weeks–3 yr		×			—	2	—	56, 107, 111
1	2 yr	×	×			NS	Boys (1)	—	62
6	2–3 yr	×			×	4	Girls (1)	HDLC (1)	59, 101–104, 113
1	12 weeks		×		×	—	NS	—	57
1	7 months	×	×		×	—	NS	Glucose	114

Note: PE = physical education, PA = physical activity, CVD = cardiovascular disease, TC = total cholesterol, HDLC = high-density lipoprotein cholesterol, BP = blood pressure, NS = nonsignificant.

[a] Number in parentheses indicates how many studies showed favorable changes in the CVD risk factors listed.

review included studies that adhered to the following criteria: (1) study duration ≥ 8 weeks, (2) number of subjects 30 or more total (or 15 per group), and (3) published between 1980 and 2003.

We identified randomized and controlled trials and studies of other design that included increased physical activity and/or exercise in interventions to reduce weight status and/or adiposity in children and adolescents.[30, 66–94] Nine of the randomized controlled studies[71,73,76-79,81,82,93] and one controlled clinical observation[89] examined the independent contribution of differing types of exercise and/or physical activity interventions in group counseling interventions. Only one study[81] reported no additional advantage of adding increased physical activity and/or exercise to the weight loss intervention. Epstein and colleagues[81] examined the effect of diet plus lifestyle exercise versus diet only and waiting list control over 6 months. Both treatment groups had significant reductions in weight status and/or adiposity compared with controls. However, there were no significant differences in the reduction of weight status and/or adiposity between diet only and diet plus exercise groups at 6- or 12-month follow-up. In contrast, in a later study, Epstein and colleagues[78] reported that exercise enhanced the outcome of the short-term treatment of childhood overweight and encouraged improvements in fitness when compared with diet-only approaches. Epstein et al.[77] also examined the efficacy of three different types of exercise treatment programs for overweight children. They found no differences in the weight maintenance of overweight children participating in aerobic exercise, calisthenics, and lifestyle during the first year of treatment. However, during the second year follow-up, the lifestyle exercise group maintained the weight loss while the other subjects participating in calisthenics and aerobic exercise gained significant amounts of weight.

In a study of overweight adolescents, Becque and colleagues[70] reported a significant reduction in multiple cardiovascular risk factors using an exercise intensity of 60 to 80% of maximal heart rate and progressively increasing durations of walking, jogging, swimming, and aerobic dancing over 8 weeks in conjunction with dietary counseling versus an intervention of dietary plus behavior counseling. Sothern and colleagues[89] published results that the inclusion of regular resistance training in a program to prevent and treat pediatric overweight in preadolescent children is not only feasible, but also safe, and may contribute to increased retention at 1 year. However the study used nonconcurrent controls and, thus, was not randomized. Rocchini et al.[73] examined the effect of exercise alone vs. exercise plus diet and behavior modification and control. Both exercise alone and exercise plus diet and behavior groups illustrated significant reductions in weight status and/or adiposity versus controls.

Gutin et al. designed a study that used a modified cross-over design to see the effects of training and detraining in obese children.[95] The children were randomly assigned to participate in the physical training during the first or second 4-month periods of the 8-month experimental period. Measurements were made at baseline, after 4 months and after 8 months; therefore, it was possible to view the pattern of changes over an 8-month period during which the growing children participated in more or less regular exercise. The three-point data were analyzed using time by group analyses of variance to determine the effects of the training and detraining. Figure 10.1 shows that for percent fat (the primary outcome variable), the time by group interaction was significant and the pattern was as predicted; i.e., Group 1 declined in percent fat during the period of training and increased somewhat during the next 4 months, while Group 2 remained stable during the first 4 months and declined during the 4 months when they engaged in the training. It is noteworthy that the declines in percent fat were due to significant declines in fat mass, along with (nonsignificant) increases in fat-free mass during the periods of training. This is in contrast to the reductions in fat-free mass that occur when dieting alone was used for weight control.[96] Furthermore, as shown in Figure 10.2 Panel A, during the first 4-month period, the control group had a significant decrease in visceral adipose tissue compared with an increase in the PT group 2.[72]

Almost no information is available concerning the optimal dose of physical activity for treatment of childhood obesity.[97] With respect to exercise intensity, if total energy used during the exercise sessions is the critical factor in producing an energy deficit, then simply lengthening low intensity sessions would allow a youth to use the same amount of energy as would be used in a shorter

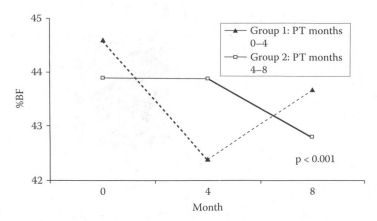

FIGURE 10.1 Least squares means for percent body fat (%BF) over the three time points of the study. Group 1 engaged in physical training (PT) for the first 4 months of the intervention period and Group 2 engaged in PT for the second 4 months of the intervention period; the thickened lines denote the periods of training for each group. The *p* value is for the group by time interaction in the analysis of variance. (From Gutin B, Owens T, Okuyama T, Riggs S, Ferguson M, Litaker M. *Obes Res.* 1999;7: 208–214.)

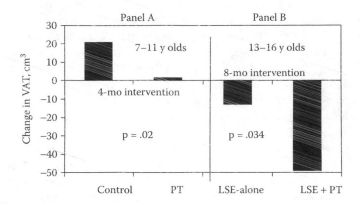

FIGURE 10.2 Panel A: Changes in visceral adipose tissue (VAT) over a 4-month period in physical training (PT) and control groups. The control group increased significantly more than PT group in both fat depots. Panel B: Changes in VAT over an 8-month period in groups that engaged in life-style education (LSE) alone or LSE + PT (low-intensity and high-intensity PT) grouped together. (From Gutin B, Barbeau P, Yin Z. *Quest.* 2004;56: 120–141.)

session of higher intensity. Savage et al.[98] used this approach with prepubertal boys and found skinfold fat to decline similarly in the low and high intensity groups, even though the high intensity training resulted in a clearer improvement in cardiovascular fitness.

However, even when the energy expenditure during the exercise sessions is controlled, there are reasons to suspect that higher intensity exercise may be more efficacious in reducing fatness if the intervention continues for a longer period than the typical 2 to 4 months. First, postexercise metabolism may be greater following higher intensity exercise; the small amount of extra energy used following each session may gradually accumulate to meaningful levels over long periods. Second, if high intensity training increases cardiovascular fitness more effectively.[98] then the youth would be able progressively to use up more energy in a given amount of training time, eventually leading to greater fat loss.

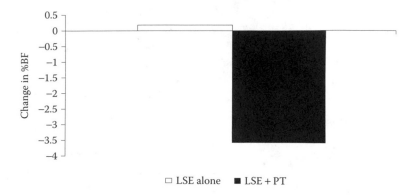

□ LSE alone　■ LSE + PT

FIGURE 10.3 Changes in percent body fat (%BF) over an 8-month period in groups that engaged in life-style education (LSE) alone, LSE + PT (low-intensity and high-intensity PT) grouped together. (From Gutin B, Barbeau P, Owens S, Lemmon CR, Bauman M, Allison J, Kang HS, Litaker MS. *Am J Clin Nutr.* 2002;75: 818–826.)

To explore these issues, Gutin et al. conducted an 8-month intervention study in which obese adolescents engaged in lifestyle education alone, lifestyle education plus low intensity physical training, or lifestyle education plus high intensity training; the energy expended in the training sessions was designed to be held constant by having the low intensity group continue for approximately 42 min while the high intensity group exercised for approximately 30 min per session. The changes in adiposity were not significantly different between the moderate and high intensity groups. However, as shown in Figure 10.3 and Figure 10.2 Panel B, compared with lifestyle education alone, those in the two physical training groups combined reduced their percent body fat as well as their visceral adipose tissue levels, respectively.[71] Moreover, within the exercise groups, those individuals who attended more often and who used up more energy in the physical training sessions showed greater reductions in adiposity, providing partial support for the idea that higher doses lead to greater reductions in fatness.

In summary, five studies have demonstrated an independent positive effect of different types of physical activity and/or exercise on weight status and/or adiposity in children and adolescents,[71,77,79,93,95] including visceral adiposity.[71,72] Short-term studies were mixed concerning the effect of structured versus lifestyle exercise. And only two long-term studies in young children[77,80] and one long-term study in adolescents[71] compared different physical activity and/or exercise interventions.

EXPERIMENTAL STUDIES: CARDIOVASCULAR DISEASE RISK FACTORS

Some studies of the effects of physical activity on cardiovascular risk factors have failed to provide clear evidence that the PT was effective,[99] leading some to say that exercise does not improve these aspects of cardiovascular health in children.[99] Although it may be true that exercise is ineffective in altering the very early etiology of cardiovascular disease, a conclusive judgment is not warranted because some of the null results may have been due to study limitations.[100]

Several physical activity intervention studies of varying lengths (8 weeks to 2 years) that targeted physical education resulted in increased amounts of moderate to vigorous physical activity during physical education classes[101–105] or increases in daily physical activity outside of school hours.[54,68–70,73,75,76,85,88,91,98,106-111] However, some of these interventions did not result in significant changes in body composition.[104,112–114] Despite this, some studies showed a significant improvement in cholesterol levels,[76,85,88,104,107–110] capillary glucose,[114] insulin,[106] lipids,[76,88,91,106,110] and blood pressure.[69,70,73,85,105,110] Although physical education interventions have been shown to increase physical activity, it has been harder to demonstrate improvement in body fatness, fitness, or cardiovascular risk factors. It is possible that the increases in physical activity, although significant, were not large enough to elicit significant changes in fatness. Alternately, it may be that the intensity of the physical activity was not high enough or the duration long enough, or of the proper type (i.e., aerobic) to elicit increases in fitness. In contrast, most of the studies that demonstrated favorable effects on cardiovascular disease risk factors were not conducted during school time, thus allowing for greater blocks of time and the involvement of parents in some cases. Thus, interventions that lasted longer than the typical 2 to 3 months, and/or that led to substantial reductions in body fatness, seemed more likely to elicit improvements in obesity-associated cardiovascular disease risk factors. Please see Table 9.2 for a summary of the studies in this section.

DECREASING SEDENTARY BEHAVIORS

A few studies examined an intervention that included reducing sedentary behaviors (e.g., TV watching). Two studies conducted by Robinson and others reported interventions that successfully decreased television viewing time and adiposity in children. One of these interventions combined a family-based television viewing reduction program with a school-based physical activity intervention;[57] the other consisted of classroom education on television viewing.[115] In a 4-month plus 1-year follow-up study by Epstein and others,[82] reducing sedentary behaviors was shown to be superior over increasing physical activity and/or exercise in promoting maintenance of weight loss in overweight children. In a more recent small clinical trial (n = 18), Roemmich et al.[116] compared the effect of feedback and reinforcement for physical activity with a control group that did not receive feedback or reinforcement. The intervention group wore accelerometers and accumulated counts that were converted to television access time. The control group also wore accelerometers, but had free access to television. The intervention group had a 24% increase in physical activity, which was significantly greater than in the control group. Interestingly, although television time decreased in the intervention group but increased in the control group, the difference between the groups was not statistically significant.

SUMMARY

Obesity prevention studies that used physical activity interventions have yielded conflicting results. Differing exercise intensities and program durations may be partly responsible for these results. On the other hand, treatment interventions that included programs to increase physical activity and/or exercise resulted in significant reductions in weight status and/or adiposity in children and adolescents. It is unclear whether lifestyle or structured approaches are more effective. Using a treatment intervention that includes a program to decrease sedentary behaviors may result in significant reductions in weight status and/or adiposity in children and adolescents; however, further research is needed.

DIRECTIONS FOR FUTURE RESEARCH

We need more information concerning the optimal exercise dose for body composition and other aspects of health. Relatively little is known about how much, what modality, or what intensity of physical activity is most efficacious in altering cardiovascular health in people of any age, and especially little is known about this matter in children. The same can be said about visceral adipose tissue. The data are already suggesting that the recommendations for adults, i.e., 30 min/d of moderate activity, are inadequate for children. Recent recommendations from various groups recommend that children obtain at least 1 h of moderate to vigorous physical activity each day.[117,118]

In deciding how to alter lifestyle to improve body composition, it is necessary to consider both physical activity and diet together. Therefore, efficacy studies of interactions between different

TABLE 10.2
Summary of Treatment Intervention Studies

No. Studies	Duration	Intervention Components					Favorable Changes		Ref.
		Supervised PA	Behavior Modification	Home PA	Family	Other/Non-PA	Adiposity	CVD Risk Factors[a]	
1	1 yr						1		87
1	10–20 weeks		×		×	×	1	TC, LDLC, TG (1)	88
5	8 weeks–18 months		×	×	×	×	5	TC, HDLC, TG (1)	68, 76, 81, 89, 137
1	10–20 weeks	×		×		×	1	—	90
11	8 weeks–15 months		×	×	×	×	8	NS	66, 67, 69, 74, 75, 77, 79, 84, 92–94
2	20 weeks–2 yr	×	×			×	NS	BP (1)	70, 85
2	20 weeks–4 months		×	×		×	2	BP (1)	73, 82
2	2 months–1 yr	×	×		×	×	2	TG (1)	78, 91
1	3–6 months	×		×		×	1	—	86
5	11 weeks–1 yr	×					2	HDLC (2) TC (1) INS, TG (1)	72, 95, 98, 106, 108
1	8 months	×	×				1	TG, BP (1)	71, 110

Note: PA = physical activity, CVD = cardiovascular disease, TC = total cholesterol, LDLC = low-density lipoprotein cholesterol, HDLC = high-density lipoprotein cholesterol, TG = triglycerides, BP = blood pressure, INS = insulin, NS = nonsignificant.

[a] Number in parentheses indicates how many studies showed favorable changes in the CVD risk factors listed.

exercise doses and different types of diets are needed to provide a stronger scientific foundation for school or community interventions.

An issue related to the concept of exercise intensity, about which very little is known, is the role of resistance training in weight control programs. It does seem clear that resistance training can help youths to improve their muscular strength[119] and endurance,[120] thereby helping their performance and future participation in sports and dance activities. In a recent meta-analysis of 30 pediatric obesity treatment studies that included an exercise intervention, LeMura and Maziekas[121] found that significant improvements in body composition were associated with programs that included both moderate aerobic exercise and high-repetition resistance training. Because strength training usually involves taking the muscle group close to, or all the way to, momentary failure, it is high in intensity even though the overall energy expended may not be as high as in aerobic training sessions. The high intensity of the exercise, and the resulting increases in muscle (i.e., lean) tissue, may lead to favorable changes in body composition. Moreover, the intense muscular activity may enhance insulin action and improve cardiovascular disease and type 2 diabetes risk status, independent of body fatness or cardiovascular fitness.[122]

Several studies show that vigorous exercise training elicits positive alterations in the metabolic profiles of children and adolescents and are associated with reduced adiposity.[5,52,63,64,71,95,106,110,123–126] When resistance training is combined with moderate aerobic training and diet, several studies show positive improvements in lipid profiles, body composition, and aerobic fitness.[89,91,121] Recent studies in adults report that differences in the characteristics of muscle composition are related to insulin resistance, muscle oxidative enzymatic capacity, systemic adiposity, and, more importantly, VO_2 max.[127] The adult research literature suggests that regular exercise training (over 6 months) improves fat oxidation (increased oxidative enzymes), glucose metabolism (increased number of glucose transporters and glucose into triglycerides), mitochondrial function, sympathetic nervous system activity (improved catecholamine stimulation response), and lipoprotein lipase activity, which may, indirectly, positively affect metabolic profiles.[128–131] The benefits of aerobic exercise training in adult type 2 diabetic patients are well established.[132] Vigorous training and the resulting enhancement of aerobic fitness may, therefore, provide a protective mechanism in children and adolescents at risk for obesity and type 2 diabetes.[65,133] However, the role of vigorous exercise training in the prevention of obesity and metabolic disease has not been thoroughly examined in children and adolescents.

SUMMARY

It is becoming clear that already in young children, excess total body and visceral adiposity are linked to unfavorable levels of preclinical markers for "adult" diseases such as cardiovascular disease and type 2 diabetes. Data from cross-sectional and nonexperimental longitudinal studies suggest that physical activity and fitness during childhood have favorable effects on these preclinical markers, with much of the effect mediated by the influence of physical activity on body composition. However, randomized trials of controlled physical training over periods of several months have produced mixed results, with some failing to provide evidence of favorable changes in these preclinical markers.

One way to reconcile these somewhat discrepant results is to postulate that the nonexperimental studies allow the uncovering of causal relations that emerge after several years of exposure to the detrimental effects of inactivity or excess fatness, while short-term experimental studies do not produce an increase in activity over a long enough period for favorable changes in the preclinical markers to take place. The other possibility is that physical activity has a limited or negligible causal effect on preclinical markers during childhood[99] and the relations found in the nonexperimental studies are due to the common influence of some other factor, such as a genetic predisposition to be active, fit, or lean on the one hand and to have favorable levels of the risk markers on the other. Longer-term experimental studies that include higher doses of physical activity are needed to clarify the true impact of physical activity.

In considering the relation of physical activity to health in youths, it is necessary to note that physical activity poses some risks in the form of sports injuries. In fact, Aaron and Laporte[134] suggest that many of the purported benefits of regular physical activity in youth are myths ("an active child is a healthy child"; "an active child will be an active adult"), and that on balance the risk of injury and related medical costs outweigh the potential benefits of physical activity for most youth. However, as we have seen in this chapter, the evidence of a beneficial effect of physical activity on the body composition and health of children is rapidly accumulating. In addition, longitudinal projects such as the Amsterdam Study[28] have shown tracking from adolescence into adulthood of variables such as physical activity, body composition, and cardiovascular risk factors.

The secular trend toward greater child and adolescent obesity over the last three decades[31,33,135] suggests that past public health efforts to improve activity and diet behaviors have been overcome by societal trends toward less activity and/or greater intake of high-fat foods. To date, programs that have taken a public health approach in school and community settings have had only modest success in altering diet, physical activity, and preclinical markers of adult diseases (e.g., Luepker et al.[53]). However, the recent Surgeon-General's report[136] shows that the scientific evidence linking physical activity to health is convincing. Perhaps this increasing recognition of the importance of physical activity will energize governmental, community, and privately owned agencies to sponsor more research on these topics, providing an improved foundation for the development of more effective interventions. Meanwhile, there is enough known to encourage parents, health professionals, teachers, and legislators to implement measures to increase physical activity of our children, thereby contributing to their present and future health.

REFERENCES

1. Sallis JF, Prochaska JJ, Taylor WC. A review of correlates of physical activity of children and adolescents. *Med Sci Sports Exerc.* 2000;32: 963–975.
2. Sallis JF. Age-related decline in physical activity: a synthesis of human and animal studies. *Med Sci Sports Exerc.* 2000;32: 1598–1600.
3. Trost SG, Pate RR, Dowda M, Saunders R, Ward DS, Felton G. Gender differences in physical activity and determinants of physical activity in rural fifth grade children. *J Sch Health.* 1996;66: 145–150.
4. Kann L, Kinchen SA, Williams BI, Ross JG, Lowry R, Hill CV, et al. Youth risk behavior surveillance — United States, 1997. *Morb Mortal Wkly Rep.* 1998;47: 1–89.
5. Gutin B, Basch C, Shea S, Contento I, DeLozier M, Rips J, et al. Blood pressure, fitness, and fatness in 5- and 6-year-old children. *JAMA.* 1990;264: 1123–1127.
6. Pivarnik JM, Bray MS, Hergenroeder AC, Hill RB, Wong WW. Ethnicity affects aerobic fitness in U.S. adolescent girls. *Med Sci Sports Exerc.* 1995;27: 1635–1638.
7. Trowbridge CA, Gower BA, Nagy TR, Hunter GR, Treuth MS, Goran MI. Maximal aerobic capacity in African-American and Caucasian children. *Am J Physiol Endocrinol Metab.* 1997;273: 145–150.
8. Janz KF, Mahoney LT. Three-year follow-up of changes in aerobic fitness during puberty: the Muscatine study. *Res Quart Exerc Sport.* 1997;68: 1–9.
9. Pate RR, Long BJ, Heath G. Descriptive epidemiology of physical activity in adolescents. *Pediatr Exerc Sci.* 1994;6: 434–447.
10. Grunbaum J, Kann L, Kinchen S, Ross J, Hawkins J, Lowry R, et al. Youth risk behavior surveillance — United States, 2003. *Morbity Mortality Wkly Rep.* 2004;53: 1–96.
11. Trost SG, Pate RR, Ward DS, Saunders R, Riner W. Correlates of objectively measured physical activity in preadolescent youth. *Am J Prev Med.* 1999;17: 120–126.
12. Barnett TA, O'Loughlin J, Paradis G. One- and two-year predictors of decline in physical activity among inner-city schoolchildren. *Am J Prev Med.* 2002;23: 121–128.
13. Prochaska JJ, Sallis JF, Sarkin JA, Calfas KJ. Examination of the factor structure of physical activity behaviors. *J Clin Epidemiol.* 2000;53: 866–874.

14. Reynolds KD, Killen JD, Bryson SW, Maron DJ, Taylor CB, Maccoby N, Farquhar JW. Psychosocial predictors of physical activity in adolescents. *Prev Med.* 1990;19: 541–551.

15. Trost SG, Pate RR, Saunders R, Ward DS, Dowda M, Felton G. A prospective study of the determinants of physical activity in rural fifth-grade children. *Prev Med.* 1997;26: 257–263.

16. Trost SG, Owen N, Bauman AE, Sallis JF, Brown W. Correlates of adults' participation in physical activity: review and update. *Med Sci Sports Exerc.* 2002;34: 1996–2001.

17. Sallis JF, Calfas KJ, Alcaraz JE, Gehrman C, Johnson MF. Potential mediators of change in a physical activity promotion course for university students: Project GRAD. *Ann Behav Med.* 1999;21: 149–158.

18. DiLorenzo TM, Stucky-Ropp RC, Vander Wal JS, Gotham HJ. Determinants of exercise among children. II. A longitudinal analysis. *Prev Med.* 1998;27: 470–477.

19. Baker CW, Little TD, Brownell KD. Predicting adolescent eating and activity behaviors: the role of social norms and personal agency. *Health Psychol.* 2003;22: 189–198.

20. Pender NJ. Motivation for physical activity among children and adolescents. *Ann Rev Nurs Res.* 1998;16: 139–172.

21. Epstein LH, Roemmich JN, Raynor HA. Behavioral therapy in the treatment of pediatric obesity. *Pediatr Clin N Am.* 2001;48: 981–993.

22. Gordon-Larsen P, Adair LS, Popkin BM. Ethnic differences in physical activity and inactivity patterns and overweight status. *Obes Res.* 2002;10: 141–706.

23. Sallis JF, Conway TL, Prochaska JJ, McKenzie TL, Marshall SJ, Brown M. The association of school environments with youth physical activity. *Am J Publ Health.* 2001;91: 618–620.

24. Thompson M, Flournoy R, Rubin V. Is your address affecting your health? In: American Public Health Association 131th Annual Meeting; San Francisco; APHA. Abstract 69827. Retrieved from http://apha.confex.com/apha/131am/techprogram/paper_69827.htm.

25. Frank LD, Engelke PO, Schmid TL. Health and community design: the impact of built environment on physical activity. Washington, DC: Island Press; 2003.

26. Brownson RC, Baker EA, Housemann RA, Brennan LK, Bacak SJ. Environmental and policy determinants of physical activity in the United States. *Am J Publ Health.* 2001;91: 1995–2003.

27. Brownson RC, Eyler AA, King AC, Brown DR, Shyu YL, Sallis JF. Patterns and correlates of physical activity among US women 40 years and older. *Am J Publ Health.* 2000;90: 264–270.

28. Kemper H, van Mechelen W. Physical fitness and the relationship to physical activity. In: Kemper H, Ed. *The Amsterdam Growth Study.* Champaign: Human Kinetics; 1995: 174–188.

29. James WPT. Chapter discussion. In: Chadwick DJ, Cardew G, Eds. The Origins and Consequences of Obesity. Chichester: Wiley; 1996: 252–253.

30. Epstein LH, Valoski AM, Kalarchian MA, McCurley J. Do children lose and maintain weight easier than adults: a comparison of child and parent weight changes from six months to ten years. *Obes Res.* 1995;3: 411–417.

31. Troiano RP, Flegal KM, Kuczmarski RJ, Campbell SM, Johnson CL. Overweight prevalence and trends for children and adolescents — The National Health and Nutrition Examination Surveys, 1963–1991. *Arch Pediatr Adolesc Med* 1995;149: 1085–1091.

32. Kuntzleman CT. Childhood fitness: what is happening? What needs to be done. *Prev Med.* 1993;22: 520–532.

33. Hedley AA, Ogden CL, Johnson CL, Carroll MD, Curtin LR, Flegal KM. Prevalence of overweight and obesity among US children, adolescents, and adults, 1999–2002. *JAMA.* 2004;291: 2847–2850.

34. Pinhas-Hamiel O, Dolan LM, Daniels SR, Standiford D, Khoury PR, Zeitler P. Increased incidence of non-insulin-dependent diabetes mellitus among adolescents. *J Pediatr.* 1996;128: 608–615.

35. Hofman A, Walter HJ. The association between physical fitness and cardiovascular risk factors in children in a five-year follow-up study. *Int J Epidemiol.* 1989;18: 830–835.

36. Shea S, Basch CE, Gutin B, Stein AD, Contento IR, Irigoyen M, Zybert P. The rate of increase in blood pressure in children 5 years of age is related to changes in aerobic fitness and body mass index. *Pediatrics.* 1994;94: 465–470.

37. McMurray RG, Harrell JS, Bangdiwala SI, Hu J. Tracking of physical activity and aerobic power from childhood through adolescence. *Med Sci Sports Exerc.* 2003;35: 1914–1922.

38. Schmitz KH, Jacobs DR, Jr., Hong CP, Steinberger J, Moran A, Sinaiko AR. Association of physical activity with insulin sensitivity in children. *Int J Obes Relat Metab Disord.* 2002;26: 1310–1316.

39. Gutin B, Yin Z, Humphries M, Hoffman W, Kang H, Gower B, Barbeau P. Both body fatness and cardiovascular fitness are related to fasting insulin in black and white teen-agers. *J Pediatr.* 2004;145: 737–743.

40. Weiss R, Caprio S. A tale of twins and insulin resistance. *J Pediatr.* 2004;144: 567–568.

41. Craig SB, Bandini LG, Lichtenstein AH, Schaefer EJ, Dietz WH. The impact of physical activity on lipids, lipoproteins, and blood pressure in preadolescent girls. *Pediatrics.* 1996;98: 389–395.

42. Suter E, Hawes MR. Relationship of physical activity, body fat, diet, and blood lipid profile in youths 10–15 yr. *Med Sci Sports Exerc.* 1993;25: 748–754.

43. McMurray RG, Harrell JS, Levine AA, Gansky SA. Childhood obesity elevates blood pressure and total cholesterol independent of physical activity. *Int J Obes Relat Metab Disord.* 1995;19: 881–886.

44. Gutin B, Islam S, Manos T, Cucuzzo N, Smith C, Stachura ME. Relation of percentage of body fat and maximal aerobic capacity to risk factors for atherosclerosis and diabetes in black and white seven-to eleven-old children. *J Pediatr.* 1994;125: 847–852.

45. Gutin B, Owens S, Treiber F, Islam S, Karp W, Slavens G. Weight-independent cardiovascular fitness and coronary risk factors. *Arch Pediatr Adolesc Med.* 1997;151: 462–265.

46. Gutin B, Yin Z, Humphries M, Bassali R, Le N, Daniels S, Barbeau P. Relations of body fatness and cardiovascular fitness to lipid profile in black and white adolescents. *Pediatr Res.* 2005; 58: 78–82.

47. Oscai L. Exercise and obesity: emphasis on animal models. In: Gisolfi C, Lamb D, Eds. *Perspectives in Exercise Science and Sports Medicine: Youth, Exercise and Sport.* Indianapolis, IN: Benchmark Press; 1989: 273–292.

48. Reaven G. Role of insulin resistance in human disease. *Diabetes.* 1988;37: 1595–1607.

49. Campbell K, Waters E, O'Meara S, Summerbell C. Interventions for preventing obesity in childhood. A systematic review. *Obes Rev.* 2001;2: 149–157.

50. Reilly JJ. Assessment of childhood obesity: national reference data or international approach? *Obes Res.* 2002;10: 838–840.

51. Campbell K, Waters E, O'Meara S, Kelly S, Summerbell C. Interventions for preventing obesity in children. *Cochrane Database Syst Rev.* 2002: CD001871.

52. Gutin B, Barbeau P, Yin Z. Exercise interventions for prevention of obesity and related disorders in youths. *Quest.* 2004;56: 120–141.

53. Luepker RV, Perry CL, McKinlay SM, Nader PR, Parcel GS, Stone EJ, et al. Outcomes of a field trial to improve children's dietary patterns and physical activity. The Child and Adolescent Trial for Cardiovascular Health. CATCH collaborative group. *JAMA.* 1996;275: 768–776.

54. Harrell JS, McMurray RG, Bangdiwala SI, Frauman AC, Gansky SA, Bradley CB. Effects of a school-based intervention to reduce cardiovascular disease risk factors in elementary-school children: the Cardiovascular Health in Children (CHIC) study. *J Pediatr.* 1996;128: 797–805.

55. Baranowski T, Baranowski JC, Cullen KW, Thompson DI, Nicklas T, Zakeri IE, Rochon J. The fun, food, and fitness project (FFFP): the Baylor GEMS pilot study. *Ethn Dis.* 2003;13: S30–S39.

56. Story M, Sherwood NE, Himes JH, Davis M, Jacobs DR, Jr., Cartwright Y, et al. An after-school obesity prevention program for African-American girls: the Minnesota GEMS pilot study. *Ethn Dis.* 2003;13: S54–64.

57. Robinson TN, Killen JD, Kraemer HC, Wilson DM, Matheson DM, Haskell WL, et al. Dance and reducing television viewing to prevent weight gain in African-American girls: the Stanford GEMS pilot study. *Ethn Dis.* 2003;13: S65–S77.

58. Manios Y, Moschandreas J, Hatzis C, Kafatos A. Evaluation of a health and nutrition education program in primary school children of Crete over a three-year period. *Prev Med.* 1999;28: 149–159.

59. Gortmaker SL, Peterson K, Wiecha J, Sobol AM, Dixit S, Fox MK, Laird N. Reducing obesity via a school-based interdisciplinary intervention among youth: Planet Health. *Arch Pediatr Adolesc Med.* 1999;153: 409–418.

60. McMurray RG, Harrell JS, Bangdiwala SI, Bradley CB, Deng S, Levine A. A school-based intervention can reduce body fat and blood pressure in young adolescents. *J Adolesc Health.* 2002;31:125–132.

61. Pate RR, Saunders RP, Ward DS, Felton G, Trost SG, Dowda M. Evaluation of a community-based intervention to promote physical activity in youth: lessons from Active Winners. *Am J Health Promot.* 2003;17: 171–182.

62. Sallis JF, McKenzie TL, Conway TL, Elder JP, Prochaska JJ, Brown M, et al. Environmental interventions for eating and physical activity. A randomized controlled trial in middle schools. *Am J Prev Med*. 2003;24: 209–217.

63. Barbeau P, Litaker MS, Howe CA, Gutin B. Changes in body composition after a 10-mo physical activity intervention in 8–12 y old black girls in the MCG APEX study (abstract). *Can J Appl Physiol*. 2002;27(Suppl): S3.

64. Gutin B, Yin Z, Hanes JC, Moore JB, Johnson M, Barbeau P, et al. The Medical College of Georgia (MCG) FitKid Project: result of a physical activity intervention during the 3rd grade on cardiovascular risk factors. *Obes Res*. 2004;12(Suppl).

65. Sothern MS. Obesity prevention in children: physical activity and nutrition. *Nutrition*. 2004;20: 704–708.

66. Golan M, Fainaru M, Weizman A. Role of behaviour modification in the treatment of childhood obesity with the parents as the exclusive agents of change. *Int J Obes Relat Metab Disord*. 1998;22: 1217–1224.

67. Graves T, Meyers A, Clark L. An evaluation of parental problem-solving training in the behavioral treatment of childhood obesity. *J Consult Clin Psychol*. 1988;56: 246–250.

68. Flodmark C, Ohlsson T, Ryden O, Sveger T. Prevention of progression to severe obesity in a group of obese schoolchildren treated with family therapy. *Pediatrics*. 1993;91: 880–884.

69. Brownell KD, Kelman JH, Stunkard AJ. Treatment of obese children with and without their mothers: changes in weight and blood pressure. *Pediatrics*. 1983;71: 515–523.

70. Becque M, Katch V, Rocchini A, Marks C, Moorehead C. Coronary risk incidence of obese adolescents: reduction by exercise plus diet interventions. *Pediatrics*. 1988;81: 605–612.

71. Gutin B, Barbeau P, Owens S, Lemmon CR, Bauman M, Allison J, et al. Effects of exercise intensity on cardiovascular fitness, total body composition, and visceral adiposity of obese adolescents. *Am J Clin Nutr*. 2002;75: 818–826.

72. Owens S, Gutin B, Allison J, Riggs S, Ferguson M, Litaker M, Thompson W. Effect of physical training on total and visceral fat in obese children. *Med Sci Sports Exerc*. 1999;31: 143–148.

73. Rocchini AP, Katch V, Anderson J, Hinderliter J, Becque D, Martin M, Marks C. Blood pressure in obese adolescents: effect of weight loss. *Pediatrics*. 1988;82: 16–23.

74. Saelens BE, Sallis JF, Wilfley DE, Patrick K, Cella JA, Buchta R. Behavioral weight control for overweight adolescents initiated in primary care. *Obes Res*. 2002;10: 22–32.

75. Wadden T, Stunkard A, Rich L, Rubin K, Sweidel G, McKinney S. Obesity in black adolescent girls: a controlled clinical trial of treatment by diet, behavior modification, and parental support. *Pediatrics*. 1990;85: 345–352.

76. Epstein LH, Kuller LH, Wing RR, Valoski A, McCurley J. The effect of weight control on lipid changes in obese children. *Am J Dis Child*. 1989;143: 454–457.

77. Epstein LH, Wing RR, Koeske R, Valoski A. A comparison of lifestyle exercise, aerobic exercise, and calisthenics on weight loss in obese children. *Behav Ther*. 1985;16: 345–356.

78. Epstein LH, Wing RR, Penner BC, Kress MJ. Effect of diet and controlled exercise on weight loss in obese children. *J Pediatr*. 1985;107: 358–361.

79. Epstein LH, Paluch RA, Raynor HA. Sex differences in obese children and siblings in family-based obesity treatment. *Obes Res*. 2001;9: 746–753.

80. Epstein LH, Valoski A, Wing RR, McCurley J. Ten-year outcomes of behavioral family-based treatment for childhood obesity. *Health Psychol*. 1994;13: 373–383.

81. Epstein LH, Wing RR, Koeske R, Valoski A. Effects of diet plus exercise on weight change in parents and children. *J Consult Clin Psychol*. 1984;52: 429–437.

82. Epstein LH, Valoski AM, Vara LS, McCurley J, Wisniewski L, Kalarchian MA, et al. Effects of decreasing sedentary behavior and increasing activity on weight change in obese children. *Health Psychol*. 1995;2: 109–115.

83. Epstein LH, Valoski A, Wing RR, McCurley J. Ten-year follow-up of behavioral, family-based treatment for obese children. *JAMA*. 1990;264: 2519–2523.

84. Chen W, Chen S, Hsu H. Counseling clinic for pediatric weight reduction: Program formulation and follow-up. *J Formos Med Assoc*. 1997;96: 59–62.

85. Resnicow K, Yaroch AL, Davis A, Wang DT, Carter S, Slaughter L, et al. GO GIRLS! Results from a nutrition and physical activity program for low-income, overweight African American adolescent females. *Health Educ Behav.* 2000;27: 616–631.

86. Eliakim A, Kaven G, Berger I, Friedland O, Wolach B, Nemet D. The effect of a combined intervention on body mass index and fitness in obese children and adolescents — a clinical experience. *Eur J Pediatr.* 2002;161: 449–454.

87. Sothern MS, Hunter S, Suskind RM, Brown R, Udall JN, Jr., Blecker U. Motivating the obese child to move: the role of structured exercise in pediatric weight management. *South Med J.* 1999;92: 577–584.

88. Sothern M, Despeney B, Brown R, Suskind R, Udall J, Blecker U. Lipid profiles of obese children and adolescents before and after significant weight loss: differences according to sex. *South Med J.* 2000;93: 278–282.

89. Sothern M, Loftin M, Udall J, Suskind R, Ewing T, Tang S, Blecker U. Safety, feasibility and efficacy of a resistance training program in preadolescent obese children. *Am J Med Sci.* 2000;319: 370–375.

90. Sothern M, Udall J, Suskind R, Vargas A, Blecker U. Weight loss and growth velocity in obese children after very low calorie diet, exercise and behavior modification. *Acta Paediatrica.* 2000;89: 1036–1043.

91. Brown R, Sothern M, Suskind R, Udall J, Blecker U. Racial differences in the lipid profiles of obese children and adolescents before and after significant weight loss. *Clin Pediatr* (Phila). 2000;39: 427–431.

92. Mellin LM, Slinkard LA, Irwin CE, Jr. Adolescent obesity intervention: validation of the SHAPE-DOWN program. *J Am Diet Assoc.* 1987;87: 333–338.

93. Epstein L, Paluch R, Gordy C, Dorn J. Decreasing sedentary behaviors in treating pediatric obesity. *Arch Pediatr Adolesc Med.* 2000;154: 220–226.

94. Epstein LH, Paluch RA, Gordy CC, Saelens BE, Ernst MM. Problem solving in the treatment of childhood obesity. *J Consult Clin Psychol.* 2000;68: 717–721.

95. Gutin B, Owens T, Okuyama T, Riggs S, Ferguson M, Litaker M. Effect of physical training and its cessation on percent fat and bone density of obese children. *Obes Res.* 1999;7: 208–214.

96. Schwingshandl J, Borkenstein M. Changes in lean body mass in obese children during a weight reduction program: effect on short term and long term outcome. *Int J Obes Relat Metab Disord.* 1995;19: 752–755.

97. Bar-Or O, Foreyt J, Bouchard C, Brownell KD, Dietz WH, Ravussin E, et al. Physical activity, genetic, and nutritional considerations in childhood weight management. *Med Sci Sports Exerc.* 1998;30: 2–10.

98. Savage MP, Petratis MM, Thomson WH, Berg K, Smith JL, Sady SP. Exercise training effects on serum lipids of prepubescent boys and adult men. *Med Sci Sports Exerc.* 1986;18: 197–204.

99. Rowland T. Is there a scientific rationale supporting the value of exercise for the present and future cardiovascular health of children? The con argument. *Pediatr Exerc Sci.* 1996;8: 303–309.

100. Gutin B, Owens S. Is there a scientific rationale supporting the value of exercise for the present and future cardiovascular health of children. *Pediatr Exerc Sci.* 1996;8: 294–302.

101. Sallis JF, McKenzie TL, Alcaraz JE, Kolody B, Faucette N, Hovell MF. The effects of a 2-year physical education program (SPARK) on physical activity and fitness in elementary school students. Sports, Play and Active Recreation for Kids. *Am J Public Health.* 1997;87: 1328–1334.

102. Luepker RV, Perry CL, McKinlay SM, Nader PR, Parcel GS, Stone EJ, et al. Outcomes of a field trial to improve children's dietary patterns and physical activity. The Child and Adolescent Trial for Cardiovascular Health. CATCH collaborative group. *JAMA.* 1996;275: 768–776.

103. Simons-Morton BG, Parcel GS, Baranowski T, Forthofer R, O'Hara NM. Promoting physical activity and a healthful diet among children: results of a school-based intervention study. *Am J Public Health.* 1991;81: 986–991.

104. Donnelly JE, Jacobsen DJ, Whatley JE, Hill JO, Swift LL, Cherrington A, et al. Nutrition and physical activity program to attenuate obesity and promote physical and metabolic fitness in elementary school children. *Obes Res.* 1996;4: 229–243.

105. Hansen H, Froberg K, Hyldebrandt N, Nielson J. A controlled study of eight months of physical training and reduction of blood pressure in children: the Odense schoolchild study. *BMJ.* 1991;303: 682–685.

106. Ferguson MA, Gutin B, Le N-A, Karp W, Litaker M, Humphries M, et al. Effect of exercise training and its cessation on components of the insulin resistance syndrome in obese children. *Int J Obes Relat Metab Disord.* 1999;22: 889–895.

107. Harrell JS, Gansky SA, McMurray RG, Bangdiwala SI, Frauman AC, Bradley CB. School-based interventions improve heart health in children with multiple cardiovascular disease risk factors. *Pediatrics.* 1998;102: 371–380.

108. Sasaki J, Shindo M, Tanaka H, Ando M, Arakawa K. A long-term aerobic exercise program decreases the obesity index and increases the high density lipoprotein cholesterol concentration in obese children. *Int J Obes Relat Metab Disord.* 1987;11: 339–345.

109. Blessing D, Keith R, Williford H, Blessing M, Barskdale J. Blood lipid and physiological responses to endurance training in adolescents. *Pediatr Exerc Sci.* 1995;7: 199–202.

110. Kang HS, Gutin B, Barbeau P, Owens S, Lemmon CR, Allison J, et al. Physical training improves insulin resistance syndrome markers in obese adolescents. *Med Sci Sports Exerc.* 2002;34: 1920–1927.

111. Yin Z, Gutin B, Hanes JC, Moore JB, Johnson M, Barbeau P, et al. The Medical College of Georgia (MCG) FitKid Project: result of a physical activity intervention during the 3rd grade on cardiovascular risk factors (abstract). *Obes Res.* 2004;12(Suppl): A7.

112. Luepker RV. How physically active are American children and what can we do about it. *Int J Obes Relat Metab Disord.* 1999;23 Suppl 2: S12–17.

113. Caballero B, Clay T, Davis SM, Ethelbah B, Rock BH, Lohman T, et al. Pathways: a school-based, randomized controlled trial for the prevention of obesity in American Indian schoolchildren. *Am J Clin Nutr.* 2003;78: 1030–1038.

114. Trevino RP, Yin Z, Hernandez A, Hale DE, Garcia OA, Mobley C. Impact of the Bienestar school-based diabetes mellitus prevention program on fasting capillary glucose levels: a randomized controlled trial. *Arch Pediatr Adolesc Med.* 2004;158: 911–917.

115. Robinson TN. Reducing children's television viewing to prevent obesity: a randomized controlled trial. *JAMA.* 1999;282: 1561–1567.

116. Roemmich JN, Gurgol CM, Epstein LH. Open-loop feedback increases physical activity of youth. *Med Sci Sports Exerc.* 2004;36: 668–673.

117. Corbin CB. *Physical Activity Guide for Children: A Statement of Guidelines for Children Ages 5–12,* 2nd Edition. Reston, VA: American Alliance for Health, Physical Education, Recreation & Dance, 2004.

118. Public Health Agency of Canada and the Canadian Society for Exercise Physiology Physiology HCaCSfE. *Canada's Physical Activity Guide.* Ottawa: Health Canada, 2002.

119. Treuth MS, Hunter GR, Pichon C, Figueroa-Colon R, Goran MI. Fitness and energy expenditure after strength training in obese prepubertal girls. *Med Sci Sports Exerc.* 1998;30: 1130–1136.

120. Payne VG, Morrow JR, Johnson L, Dalton SN. Resistance training in children and youth: a meta-analysis. *Res Quart Exerc Sport.* 1997;68: 80–88.

121. LeMura LM, Maziekas MT. Factors that alter body fat, body mass, and fat-free mass in pediatric obesity. *Med Sci Sports Exerc.* 2002;34: 487–496.

122. Hurley BF, Hagberg JM, Goldberg AP, Seals DR, Ehsani AA, Brennan RE, Holloszy JO. Resistive training can reduce coronary risk factors without altering VO_2 max or percent body fat. *Med Sci Sports Exerc.* 1988;20: 150–154.

123. Gutin B, Cucuzzo N, Islam S, Smith C, Stachura ME. Physical training, lifestyle education, and coronary risk factors in obese girls. *Med Sci Sports Exerc.* 1996;28: 19–23.

124. Gutin B, Ramsey L, Barbeau P, Cannady W, Ferguson M, Litaker M, Owens S. Plasma leptin concentrations in obese children: changes during 4-mo periods with and without physical training. *Am J Clin Nutr.* 1999;69: 388–394.

125. Barbeau P, Gutin B, Litaker MS, Ramsey LT, Cannady WE, Allison J, et al. Influence of physical training on plasma leptin in obese youths. *Can J Appl Physiol.* 2003;28: 382–396.

126. Dionne. I. The association between vigorous physical activities and fat deposition in male adolescents. *Med Sci Sports Exerc.* 2000;32: 392–395.

127. Kelley DE, Goodpaster B, Wing RR, Simoneau JA. Skeletal muscle fatty acid metabolism in association with insulin resistance, obesity, and weight loss. *Am J Physiol.* 1999;277: E1130–1141.

128. Kelley DE, Goodpaster BH. Effects of physical activity on insulin action and glucose tolerance in obesity. *Med Sci Sports Exerc.* 1999;31: S619–623.

129. Tonkonogi M, Krook A, Walsh B, Sahlin K. Endurance training increases stimulation of uncoupling of skeletal muscle mitochondria in humans by non-esterified fatty acids: an uncoupling-protein-mediated effect? *Biochem J.* 2000;351(Pt 3): 805–810.

130. Poehlman ET, Denino WF, Beckett T, Kinaman KA, Dionne IJ, Dvorak R, Ades PA. Effects of endurance and resistance training on total daily energy expenditure in young women: a controlled randomized trial. *J Clin Endocrinol Metab.* 2002;87: 1004–1009.

131. Horowitz JF, Leone TC, Feng W, Kelly DP, Klein S. Effect of endurance training on lipid metabolism in women: a potential role for PPARalpha in the metabolic response to training. *Am J Physiol Endocrinol Metab.*2000;279: E348–355.

132. Sothern MS, Loftin M, Suskind RM, Udall JN, Blecker U. The health benefits of physical activity in children and adolescents: implications for chronic disease prevention. *Eur J Pediatr.* 1999;158: 271–274.

133. Sothern MS, Gordon ST. Prevention of obesity in young children: a critical challenge for medical professionals. *Clin Pediatr* (Phila). 2003;42: 101–111.

134. Aaron DJ, Laporte RE. Physical activity, adolescence, and health: an epidemiological perspective. In: Holloszy J, Ed. *Exercise and Sports Sciences Reviews.* Baltimore, MD: Williams & Wilkins; 1997: 391–405.

135. Freedman DS, Srinivasan SR, Valdez RA, Williamson DF, Berenson GS. Secular increases in relative weight and adiposity among children over two decades: the Bogalusa Study. *Pediatrics.* 1997;99: 420–426.

136. U.S. Department of Health and Human Services, Centers for Disease Control and Prevention. Physical activity and health: a report from the Surgeon General. Atlanta, GA: U.S. Department of Health and Human Services, Centers for Disease Control and Prevention, National Center for Chronic Disease Prevention and Health Promotion; 1996.

11 Puberty, Insulin Resistance, and Type 2 Diabetes

Barbara A. Gower and Sonia Caprio

CONTENTS

OVERVIEW

Type 2 diabetes is occurring with increasing frequency among adolescents. Physiological changes that occur during the pubertal transition may precipitate the disease among individuals who are at risk for type 2 diabetes for other reasons (e.g., obesity, ethnicity). This chapter reviews the physiological changes that occur with puberty in the context of how they contribute to insulin resistance and/or risk for type 2 diabetes. In addition, the additive effects of obesity and ethnicity on risk for adolescent type 2 diabetes are discussed.

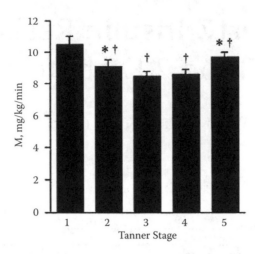

FIGURE 11.1 Insulin resistance (*M*) by Tanner stage, adjusted for sex and BMI. A lower *M* value represents greater insulin resistance. Data are expressed as mean + SE. *P < 0.05 compared with preceding Tanner stage; †P < .05 compared with Tanner stage 1. (Reproduced with permission from Moran A, Jacobs DR, Jr, Steinberger J, Hong C-P, Prineas R, Luepker R et al. *Diabetes*. 1999;48: 2039–2044.).

PUBERTAL INSULIN RESISTANCE

PHYSIOLOGY

The pubertal transition is associated with a transient decline in insulin sensitivity of up to 30%, which resolves upon completion of the pubertal transition[1–5] (Figure 11.1). Because pediatric type 2 diabetes often appears during midpuberty, it has been hypothesized that this transient depression in insulin sensitivity contributes to the risk for impaired glucose tolerance and type 2 diabetes. This may be particularly true among youth who have a preexisting risk for type 2 diabetes from other factors (e.g., obesity, family history). Although the extent to which pubertal insulin resistance contributes to adolescent type 2 diabetes has not been quantified, it is noteworthy that relative to adults, children progress more rapidly to frank type 2 diabetes; whereas adults commonly remain in a state of impaired glucose tolerance for 10 years, children can be diagnosed with type 2 diabetes at age 13 years or younger. This difference in rate of disease progression between the two age groups suggests that the etiology may differ and perhaps that pubertal insulin resistance makes a significant contribution to adolescent type 2 diabetes.

MECHANISM OF PUBERTAL INSULIN RESISTANCE

Although the proximate cause of pubertal insulin resistance has not been determined with certainty, it seems to be related to changes in growth hormone (GH). The pubertal elevation in GH, in conjunction with other hormones, stimulates anabolic growth. However, GH also promotes lipolysis, and GH administration is associated with both an elevation in circulating free fatty acids (FFA) and a decrease in insulin sensitivity.[6] Furthermore, elevation in FFA is associated with skeletal muscle resistance to insulin-stimulated glucose uptake.[7] These observations have led to the development of the hypothesis that GH, through stimulation of FFA or other mechanisms, is responsible for pubertal insulin resistance.

The temporal profile of GH over the course of puberty also parallels that of pubertal insulin resistance. Among girls, GH increases significantly by Tanner stage II and peaks at Tanner stage IV; among boys, GH does not increase until Tanner stage IV.[8] In both sexes, the GH secretion rate decreases to prepubertal levels by Tanner stage V. The profile of GH contrasts with that of testosterone, estradiol, and adrenal androgens, which also increase throughout puberty, but do not decline at the conclusion of the pubertal transition. In addition, experimental administration of neither testosterone[9] nor dihydrotestosteorne[10] affects insulin sensitivity in adolescents with delayed puberty. Thus, when considering the endocrine changes that occur throughout puberty, it appears that GH is more likely than other hormones to be responsible for pubertal insulin resistance.

CHARACTERISTICS OF PUBERTAL INSULIN RESISTANCE

Few studies using appropriate methodology have been conducted to characterize the extent to which pubertal insulin resistance at the whole-body level affects individual physiological processes such as hepatic glucose production, and protein and lipid metabolism. Use of stable isotope techniques has clarified that whereas insulin stimulation of skeletal muscle glucose uptake is impaired during puberty, insulin inhibition of hepatic glucose production is not.[11] Additional research, using the euglycemic clamp, documented insulin resistance at the level of insulin-stimulated glucose uptake, but not at the level of amino acid or protein metabolism, as assessed with stable isotopically labeled leucine administration.[12] Adolescents did not differ from adults with respect to basal or insulin-suppressed plasma concentrations of total amino acids, leucine flux, or leucine oxidation. Under clamp conditions, insulin acted primarily to inhibit protein breakdown in both adolescents and adults.

In a second study involving protein metabolism, observation of leucine flux using stable isotopes indicated that whole-body proteolysis was lower in pubertal relative to prepubertal children; likewise, protein oxidation as assessed with indirect calorimetry was lower among the pubertal individuals.[13] In contrast, protein synthesis did not differ with pubertal status, suggesting that skeletal muscle accrual during puberty is primarily due to a decrease in protein utilization. However, in this study, insulin-stimulated inhibition of proteolysis was lower among pubertal children, indicating that pubertal insulin resistance may extend to aspects of protein metabolism. Differences between studies may have been due to the presence or absence of a prepubertal comparison group.

Further research involving clamp methodology and stable isotopic techniques also indicated that total body lipolysis and fat oxidation among pubertal children were higher than among prepubertal children or adults. In addition, insulin suppression of fat oxidation was lower among pubertal children when compared with prepubertal children and adults.[5] Both lipolysis and fat oxidation were correlated with circulating insulin-like growth factor (IGF-1) concentrations. The increase in lipid availability may contribute to the increased energy needed to fuel rapid growth and lean tissue deposition.

The magnitude of pubertal insulin resistance appears to be unaffected by the degree of adiposity. In longitudinal observation, the tertile of body fat percentage did not affect the magnitude of the reduction in insulin sensitivity that was observed as the children progressed from Tanner stage I to Tanner stage III (30, 33, and 36% reduction in insulin sensitivity in the first, second, and third tertile, respectively).[2] However, insulin sensitivity was lower in the fatter children regardless of pubertal stage.

Taken together, it appears that pubertal insulin resistance may affect multiple aspects of fuel metabolism. Nonetheless, pubertal metabolism appears optimized to permit or promote anabolic growth.

TIMING

The timing of the onset of puberty differs with ethnicity, being earlier among African Americans when compared with Caucasians. Thus, the occurrence of pubertal insulin resistance is likely to occur earlier among African Americans compared with Caucasians. Whether, and the extent to which, this difference contributes to ethnic differences in diabetes risk has not been established.

Data from 17,077 U.S. girls aged 3 to 12 years evaluated at physicians' offices have shown that the average age of the transition to Tanner stage II using breast development is 9.96 ± 1.82 years among Caucasian girls, and 8.87 ± 1.93 years among African American girls.[14] Likewise, National Health and Nutrition Examination Survey (NHANES III) data indicated that African American girls had an earlier median age at entry into Tanner breast stage II than their Caucasian counterparts.[15] Hispanic girls were intermediate, and did not differ from Caucasians with respect to age at entry to Tanner stage II. Hispanic boys entered Tanner stage II later than African American boys, based on genitalia development, but did not differ from Caucasian boys. On average, girls entered puberty earlier than boys by approximately 1.5 years. Regardless of ethnicity or gender, children traversed puberty in ~5 to 6 years. Among girls, obesity was associated with earlier puberty; this association was stronger among Caucasians than African Americans and did not explain earlier puberty among African Americans as compared with Caucasians.[16]

The earlier initiation of puberty among African Americans suggests an earlier depression of insulin sensitivity (S_i). Our data among African American and Caucasian children have shown that despite a similar mean age of ~11 years, African-American children were more developmentally advanced than Caucasian children (mean Tanner stage of III for African Americans and II for Caucasians).[17] In this study, insulin sensitivity was significantly lower among African Americans compared with Caucasians, but the individual contributions of ethnicity and Tanner stage were not evaluated. Longitudinal data have shown that when matched for Tanner stage rather than age, African American and Caucasian children show a similar 32% depression in insulin sensitivity as they progress from Tanner stage I to Tanner stage III or IV.[2] African admixture is negatively associated with S_i throughout the pubertal transition.[18]

There is some evidence that African Americans and Caucasians differ regarding the ability to compensate for pubertal insulin resistance with an increase in insulin secretion. Despite a 30% depression in S_i among African American adolescents compared with prepubertal children, first and second phase insulin secretion did not differ.[19] In contrast, among Caucasian adolescents, both first and second phase insulin secretions are higher during puberty than prior to puberty.[3] However, another study reported no interaction with race (African American and Caucasian) on the change in acute insulin response to glucose (AIRg), a proxy index of first-phase insulin secretion, during the pubertal transition.[2] Both African American and Caucasian adolescents similarly failed to fully compensate for pubertal insulin resistance with an increase in AIRg, resulting in a lower disposition index (S_i × AIRg (acute insulin response to glucose); an index of insulin action) among children at Tanner stage III or IV than among the same individuals at Tanner stage I. Thus, although beta cell function may decline disproportionately among African American compared with Caucasian adolescents, further research is needed to verify this possibility.

In summary, because of the combined effects of ethnicity and gender, African American girls enter puberty earlier than other gender–ethnic subgroups, and therefore are exposed to the associated depression in insulin sensitivity earlier. Superimposed on this scenario is a preexisting depression in insulin sensitivity due to African American ethnicity. African American girls may therefore be at greater risk than other gender–ethnic subgroups for type 2 diabetes. With the additional insult of obesity, the prevalence of which is 26.2% among African American adolescent girls,[111] the risk for type 2 diabetes would increase further yet. This scenario may explain existing epidemiological data indicating that African American girls are, in fact, the gender–ethnic subgroup with the highest prevalence of type 2 diabetes.[20]

EPIDEMIOLOGY OF TYPE 2 DIABETES IN CHILDREN AND ADOLESCENTS

THE CHANGING FACE OF TYPE 2 DIABETES

Type 2 diabetes is a serious and common metabolic disorder affecting 6.6% of the population in United States.[21] The prevalence of this disorder has increased dramatically over the past two decades and continues to rise. Until recently, type 2 diabetes occurred mainly after the fourth decade of life. Thus, aging was considered as one of the major risk factors for its onset.[22] More recently, however, an unprecedented emergence of type 2 diabetes in youth has been recognized, primarily (but not exclusively) affecting minority populations.[23–25] Undoubtedly, this phenomenon parallels the alarming increase in the prevalence of obesity in children and adolescents. Indeed, most children and adolescents presenting with type 2 diabetes are severely obese.[23] The majority of these children have a family history of type 2 diabetes. Obesity and family history of diabetes seem to have a synergistic effect because the impact of obesity on risk for type 2 diabetes is much greater in children with a positive family history.

EPIDEMIOLOGY: IS THE INCREASED PREVALENCE REAL OR ARE WE JUST DETECTING MORE TYPE 2 DIABETES NOW?

Information on the prevalence of type 2 diabetes in childhood and adolescence is sparse in contrast to the wealth of data in adults. Moreover, little is known about the natural history and pathophysiology of type 2 diabetes in youth. Over the past 20 years, in Japan, type 2 diabetes incidence increased 10-fold in children aged 6 to 12 years: 0.2 per 100,000 per year from 1976 to 1980 vs. 2.0 per 100,000 per year from 1991 to 1995. Similarly, over the same period, type 2 diabetes incidence doubled among 12 to 13 year olds: 7.3 vs. 13.9 per 100,000 per year.[25] In Pima Indians aged 15 to 19 years, the prevalence of type 2 diabetes markedly increased from 2.4% in males and 2.7% in females in 1967 to 1976 to 3.8% in males and 5.3% in females in 1987 to 1996.[26,27] In other ethnic groups, the prevalence rates have more than doubled over the past two decades. Particularly disconcerting is the increasing prevalence in African American and Hispanic children and adolescents. These reported prevalence rates are likely an underestimate of the true magnitude of the problem because the disease is often underdiagnosed or misclassified. Indeed, Fagot-Campagna estimated that the proportion of cases misclassified as type 1 diabetes among African Americans was 17% among boys and 27% among girls.[28] However, at the population level, the prevalence of type 2 diabetes among children is only ~1% or less.[28]

PREVALENCE OF IMPAIRED GLUCOSE TOLERANCE (PREDIABETES) AMONG OBESE YOUTH

In adults, type 2 diabetes develops over long periods and most, if not all, patients initially have impaired glucose tolerance (IGT), which is an intermediate stage in the natural history of type 2 diabetes.[29] With appropriate changes in life style and/or pharmacologic intervention, progression from IGT to frank diabetes in adults can be delayed or prevented.[30,31] Thus, great emphasis has recently been placed on the early detection of IGT in adults.

The emergence of type 2 diabetes in childhood or adolescence may suggest, however, a different progression of events in the dynamics of the deterioration of glucose metabolism. Until recently it was unclear whether the onset of diabetes in youth was preceded by a prediabetes stage, as occurs in adults. Sinha et al.[32] undertook a study to determine the prevalence of IGT in a multiethnic cohort of obese children and adolescents. Using a clinic-based population of 55 obese children and 112 obese adolescents, IGT was detected in 25% of the obese children and 21% of obese adolescents. Subsequent studies by Weiss at al.[33] in a larger cohort of moderately and severely obese children and adolescents demonstrated that the prevalence of IGT increases with worsening obesity.

However, among overweight Latino children living in the United States, the prevalence of IGT was 27% regardless of the degree of obesity.[34,35] Similar high prevalence rates have been reported in obese children from Thailand and Philippines,[36,37] whereas lower prevalence rates were found in obese children in France.[38]

RISK FACTORS ASSOCIATED WITH IGT AND TYPE 2 DIABETES IN YOUTH

The unabated rise in the prevalence of obesity is one, if not the major, cause for the marked increase in the frequency of type 2 diabetes in both children and adults. Severe obesity is also a risk factor for IGT in youth. Obesity may be a stronger indicator of diabetes risk among children than adults because obesity causes earlier expression of the genetic susceptibility to diabetes. Most, if not all, youngsters with diabetes are obese and have acanthosis nigricans and elevated triglycerides. The link between diabetes and obesity may be the presence of insulin resistance that is commonly found in these two disorders.[39] Insulin resistance, in this context, is defined as a defect in insulin-stimulated glucose uptake, primarily by skeletal muscle. Despite much work, it is still unclear what causes insulin resistance. It is clear, however, that insulin resistance is very important in the etiology of diabetes for the following reasons: (1) it is found in the majority of patients with overt diabetes,[40] (2) it is only partially reversible by any form of treatment,[39] (3) it can be traced back through earlier stages of IGT,[41] and (4) it predicts subsequent development of the disease with remarkable consistency in both the prediabetic and normoglycemic states.[42] Insulin resistance, as indicated by the surrogate marker of the homeostasis model assessment, was found to be the best predictor of 2-h plasma glucose in our cohort of obese children and adolescents.[32] Other predictor factors were the fasting proinsulin level, the 2-h insulin level, and the fasting insulin level.[32]

However, insulin resistance alone is rarely the cause of type 2 diabetes. In some individuals, sustained elevation in insulin secretion can compensate indefinitely for insulin resistance. In order for frank type 2 diabetes to develop, the beta cell must fail to secrete adequate insulin to compensate for the insulin resistance.[43] Thus, it is generally believed that a combination of insulin resistance and impaired beta cell function ultimately leads to the development of type 2 diabetes among adults. This hypothesis is supported by data from Mexican Americans,[44] Pima Indians,[45] and Latino women with gestational diabetes.[46] In all cases, a low level of insulin secretion, relative to ambient insulin sensitivity, independently predicted subsequent development of type 2 diabetes.

Insulin resistance and impaired beta cell function may have different etiologies, as suggested by a recent study of 72 predominantly Latino children.[47] Among this group of eighth-grade students, insulin resistance was best predicted by obesity; in contrast, impaired beta cell function was best predicted by family history of type 2 diabetes. Thus, a combination of obesity and genetic factors may be required for type 2 diabetes to develop among children (as well as adults).

As has been discussed, pubertal status can affect insulin resistance, independent of obesity status. In addition, as is discussed later in this chapter, racial ancestry has independent effects on insulin resistance. It is thus likely that the adverse effects of obesity, ethnicity, and puberty may combine to produce a severe degree of insulin resistance that requires maximal beta cell function to maintain euglycemia. Once at this stage, further weight gain and a low level of physical activity may exacerbate insulin resistance and precipitate progression to IGT, beta cell failure, and type 2 diabetes.

CONTRIBUTION OF OBESITY TO INSULIN RESISTANCE

BODY COMPOSITION AND ABDOMINAL FAT DISTRIBUTION

Obesity is the most common cause of insulin resistance in childhood. As in adults, however, among children, total fat explains only about 50% of the variance in insulin resistance. Abnormal fat distribution, particularly intraabdominal fat accumulation, has been found to be a strong determinant of insulin action, independent of overall adiposity.[48,49] Particularly in adults, visceral adiposity is an independent risk factor for the development of type 2 diabetes and cardiovascular disease, and therefore represents a major public health problem. Similar studies in obese children and adults that have examined *in vivo* insulin action and secretion, and their relationship to fat distribution suggest that increased visceral fat, hyperinsulinemia, and insulin resistance are closely linked abnormalities that are expressed early in the natural history of obesity.[50]

It should be noted, however, that at least in adults, increased accumulation of subcutaneous abdominal fat also has been found to be associated with insulin resistance.[51] Visceral and subcutaneous fat differ in their biological responses; visceral fat is more resistant to insulin and has increased sensitivity to cathecholamines.[52] In favor of the important role of visceral fat is the recent report by Klein et al.,[53] which demonstrated that removal of large volume of subcutaneous abdominal fat by liposuction resulted in a considerable decrease in body weight but did not have a significant effect on insulin sensitivity in skeletal muscle. In addition, liposuction had no significant effects on blood pressure, fasting concentrations of glucose, insulin, or lipids, or plasma markers of inflammation. Goodpaster et al.,[54] in a weight loss intervention trial, found that the decrease in visceral adiposity was the body composition change that best predicted the improvement in insulin sensitivity after weight loss.

Visceral fat is generally considered to account for only 10% of overall adipose tissue mass. Therefore, it is puzzling as to why and how this relatively small depot of adipose tissue correlates so strongly with insulin resistance. It has been proposed that the metabolic abnormalities associated with visceral adipose tissue relate to its release of fatty acids directly into the portal circulation. Fatty acid flux to the liver affects hepatic extraction of insulin, increases hepatic glucose production, and stimulates the synthesis and secretion of triglycerides.[55,56] Moreover, it is possible that visceral fat is especially active in the release of adipocytokines, such as TNF-α and interleukin-6, which are known to alter insulin action in muscle tissue.[57–59]

It is conceivable, however, that the ratio of visceral to subcutaneous adipose tissue also may be an important variable in explaining insulin resistance. Indeed, individuals with type 2 diabetes tend to have a higher proportion of visceral to subcutaneous fat than healthy individuals. Although the subcutaneous abdominal fat mass is larger than the visceral fat mass, lipolysis is more readily suppressed in the former, and it may secrete less adipokines, which are known to alter insulin action.

It is possible that subcutaneous fat, including abdominal subcutaneous fat, plays a necessary role in lipid storage and thereby contributes to a healthy metabolic profile. A shift in fat distribution from subcutaneous to visceral may therefore result in metabolic disturbance. Consistent with this hypothesis, obese adolescents with IGT had significantly less abdominal subcutaneous fat (460 ± 47 cm^2) compared with obese adolescents with normal glucose tolerance (626 ± 39 cm^2, $p = 0.016$; $p = 0.04$ adjusted for total body fat) (Table 11.1). Visceral fat tended to be higher in the IGT group (70 ± 11 cm^2) than in the normal glucose tolerant (NGT) group (47 ± 6 cm^2, $p = 0.065$, adjusted for total body fat). The ratio of visceral to subcutaneous fat was 100% higher in the IGT subjects (0.15 ± 0.02) vs. the NGT subjects (0.07 ± 0.008, $p = 0.002$). Representative MRIs from one boy with NGT, and a boy with IGT, are shown in Figure 11.2. Both the enlarged visceral depot ($r = 0.63$, $p < 0.01$) and the visceral-to-subcutaneous ratio ($r = 0.66$, $p < 0.01$) were inversely related to insulin-stimulated glucose metabolism.

These results support the hypothesis that insulin resistance is associated with an altered distribution of abdominal fat. Furthermore, these data are consistent with results obtained in both human and animal models of lipodystrophy,[60–62] in which there is an absence of subcutaneous adipose tissue. These conditions are associated with elevated circulating concentrations of lipids and their accumulation in both myocytes and the visceral adipose depot. Thus, the ability to store excess triglyceride in peripheral subcutaneous fat may play a role in regulating insulin sensitivity, and ultimately may protect against the development of type 2 diabetes. Consistent with this hypothesis is the evidence derived from the use of thiazolidinediones, which improve insulin sensitivity while increasing subcutaneous abdominal fat but decreasing the visceral and liver fat depots.[63,64]

TABLE 11.1

Visceral and Subcutaneous Abdominal Fat in Children with Normal (NGT) and Impaired (IGT) Glucose Tolerance (mean ± SD)

	Caucasian, African American, Hispanic[a,b]		Hispanic[c]	
	NGT; n = 14	IGT; n = 14	NGT; n = 87	IGT; n = 35
Age (yr)	14 ± 2	13 ± 3	11 ± 2	11 ± 2
BMI (kg/m²)	39.3 ± 5.5	37.0 ± 5.8	27.9 ± 5.5	28.3 ± 7.6
% body fat	43.0 ± 1.2	42.0 ± 2.0	37.9 ± 0.07	36.3 ± 0.01
Visceral (cm²)	47 ± 6	70 ± 11	47 ± 18	46 ± 22
Subcut. abd. (cm²)	626 ± 39	460 ± 47	316 ± 136	296 ± 132
Visc.:subcut.	0.07 ± 0.01	0.15 ± 0.02[d]	0.18 ± 0.18	0.17 ± 0.06

[a] NGT: n = 4 Caucasian, 5 African-American, 5 Hispanic; IGT: n = 5 Caucasian, 3 African-American, 6 Hispanic.
[b] Weiss R, Fufour S, Taksali S, Tamborlane WV, Petersen KF, Bonadonna R et al. *Lancet.* 2003;362: 951–957.
[c] Goran MI, Bergman RN, Avila Q, Watkins M, Ball GDC, Shaibi GQ et al. *J Clin Endocrinol Metab.* 2004;89: 207–212.
[d] *P* < 0.01 vs. NGT.

Subject A
NGT boy, age 13
Percent body fat: 39.0

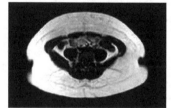

Visceral fat area: 30 cm²
Subcutaneous fat area: 520 cm²
Visceral/subcutaneous: 0.057

Subject B
IGT boy, age 9
Percent body fat: 42.3

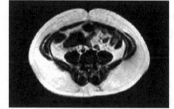

Visceral fat area: 85 cm²
Subcutaneous fat area: 394 cm²
Visceral/subcutaneous: 0.215

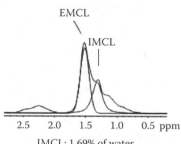

IMCL: 1.69% of water
EMCL: 2.93% of water

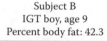
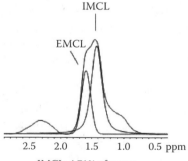

IMCL: 4.71% of water
EMCL: 3.46% of water

FIGURE 11.2 Transverse abdominal MRI scans (L4 vertebral level 1; fat appears white with T1 weighting) and ¹H-NMR soleus muscle spectra from an obese boy with NGT (Subject A) and an obese boy with IGT (Subject B). The subjects have similar amounts of total body fat, but there is more visceral fat and less subcutaneous fat in the subject with IGT (B) compared with the matched control (A). Muscle lipid partitioning also was substantially different, with greater IMCL and similar EMCL in the IGT subject (B) compared with the respective control (A).

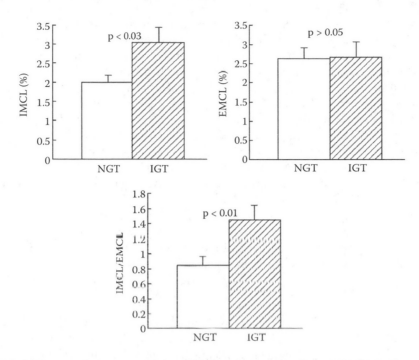

FIGURE 11.3 Differences in intramyocellular (IMCL) and extramyocellular (EMCL) lipid content and the IMCL-to-EMCL ratio in obese children and adolescents with normal (NGT) and impaired (IGT) glucose tolerance.

However, it should be pointed out that not all studies involving children have indicated an association between body fat distribution and risk factors for type 2 diabetes. Among healthy Caucasian and African American children, total fat and subcutaneous abdominal fat were both inversely related to insulin sensitivity and explained similar amounts of variance.[65] In contrast, visceral fat was not independently related to insulin sensitivity. In addition, among overweight Hispanic youth, visceral and subcutaneous abdominal fat did not differ between those with normal glucose tolerance and those with impaired glucose tolerance (Table 11.1).[35] Differences among studies may be due to the degree or duration of obesity of the subjects, or to ethnic or racial differences in the determinants of glucose tolerance.

SKELETAL MUSCLE TRIGLYCERIDE AND INSULIN RESISTANCE

Although adipose tissue is the major depot of body fat and the main source of FFA delivered to the circulation for utilization at distant sites (e.g., skeletal muscle, heart), increased intramyocellular lipid content has been recognized recently as an important factor modulating insulin action.[66,67] Intramuscular triglyceride stores are elevated among adult patients with type 2 diabetes and correlate with insulin resistance.[68] More importantly, increased intramyocellular lipid content has been found in the offspring of individuals with type 2 diabetes.[69] Using proton nuclear magnetic resonance (^{1}H-NMR) spectroscopy, Sinha et al.[70] were the first to report that obese adolescents have increased intramyocellular lipid content, which strongly correlated with insulin resistance, independent of overall adiposity. Employing the same techniques, Weiss et al.[33] found that the intramyocellular (IMCL) lipid content of the soleus muscle was 30% higher in obese adolescents with IGT (3.04 ± 0.43) vs. NGT (1.99 ± 0.19, $p < 0.03$), whereas no between-group difference was found in the extramyocellular (EMCL) lipid depots (Figure 11.3). Consequently, the ratio of IMCL to EMCL was significantly greater in the IGT (1.45 ± 0.20) vs. NGT group (0.85 ± 0.11, $p < 0.01$). Representative spectra from one boy with NGT and one boy with IGT are shown in Figure 11.2.

The study by Weiss et al.[33] is the first spectroscopic demonstration that intramyocellular lipid accumulation is associated with insulin resistance in children with prediabetes, thus further supporting the view that increased lipid content in myocytes is a marker of impaired insulin action.[71] Indeed, abnormalities in insulin signaling have been found to arise as a result of an overaccumulation of various lipid moieties in myocytes, such as long-chain fatty acyl-CoA (LC-CoA), which has been shown to interfere directly with insulin signaling and glucose transport.[72–75] Further evidence of cause and effect between IMCL and insulin resistance is provided by a study by Greco et al.,[76] showing that selective depletion of IMCL stores restored normal insulin sensitivity in obese adults, despite a persistent excess of total body fat mass. More recently, Houmard et al.[77] reported that a reduction in intramuscular LC-CoA content may be responsible for the enhanced insulin sensitivity observed with weight loss in obese individuals. What causes the accumulation of triglycerides in the myocytes is unclear. Defects in muscle fatty acid oxidation, increased FA flux to muscle, or both have been considered as potential factors leading to accumulation of fat in the myocytes.[67] Studies by Simoneau and Kelley[78,79] indicate that the metabolic capacity of skeletal muscle in obese adults appears to be organized toward fat esterification rather than oxidation.[79] Moreover, muscle fatty acid binding and transport proteins may be altered in obesity and type 2 diabetes.[79]

Adiponectin

The discovery of leptin in 1994 has dramatically changed the view of adipose tissue in the regulation of energy balance.[80] Adipose tissue secretes several proteins that act as potential regulators of glucose and lipid homeostasis.[80] These proteins have been collectively referred to as adipocytokines because of their structural similarity with cytokines.[81]

Among these adipocytokines, Acrp30, known as adiponectin, is unique in that it is reduced in obesity, in contrast to the markedly increased levels of many other adipocytokines (e.g., leptin[80] and TNF-α[82,83]). Of note, the decline in circulating adiponectin levels coincided with the onset of insulin resistance and the development of diabetes in monkeys.[84] Adiponectin gene expression and plasma levels correlated with the insulin-sensitive state in both rodents and obese adults.[84–87] Administration of adiponectin to mice consuming a high-fat diet led to an improvement of insulin sensitivity, which was associated with decreased muscle and liver triglyceride content and increased fat oxidation in muscle.[87–89] Thus, dysregulation in the synthesis and/or secretion of adiponectin from the adipose tissue may play a role in the pathogenesis of insulin resistance in both obesity and type 2 diabetes.

Most studies regarding the link between adiponectin and insulin resistance have been performed in rodents, nonhuman primates, and adult subjects with obesity and type 2 diabetes. There is little information on circulating levels of adiponectin in pediatrics, despite the profound influence of obesity on insulin and glucose metabolism in this age group. Adiponectin was assessed within a group of nonobese and obese adolescents, and its relationship with total body fat, central adiposity, whole-body insulin sensitivity (assessed by the insulin clamp technique), and muscle lipid content (determined by ^{1}H-NMR spectroscopy) was explored.[90] All measures of obesity, including BMI, percentage total fat, intraabdominal and subcutaneous fat (measured by MRI) as well as IMCL and EMCL lipid content were greater in the obese group than in the nonobese group. Circulating plasma adiponectin levels were significantly lower in obese (9.2 ± 1.1 µg/mL) than nonobese (14.3 ± 1.6 µg/mL, $P < 0.001$) adolescents. These differences remained significant after adjusting for gender ($P < 0.002$ for both IMCL and adiponectin). Plasma adiponectin concentrations were inversely related to percentage total body fat ($r = -0.48$, $P < 0.05$), but not to subcutaneous abdominal or visceral fat volume. Of particular interest, a strong inverse relationship was observed between plasma adiponectin levels and IMCL content ($r = -0.73$, $P < 0.001$); this relationship persisted after controlling for percentage total fat and central adiposity ($r = -0.63$, $P < 0.001$). This association was stronger when tested only within the obese subjects ($r = -0.78$, $P < 0.001$) and was nonsignificant when tested within the nonobese subjects. Plasma adiponectin levels were positively related to insulin sensitivity ($r = 0.52$, $P < 0.02$). This relationship was preserved when controlling for free fatty acids ($r = 0.42$, $P = 0.05$), yet was lost when controlling for triglycerides. Of particular note, the relationship between adiponectin and insulin sensitivity was completely lost after adjusting for IMCL ($r = 0.13$, $P < 0.56$). Likewise, the relationship between insulin sensitivity and IMCL became insignificant after adjusting for adiponectin levels ($r = -0.40$, $P < 0.07$). Thus, among adolescents, the putative modulatory effect of adiponectin on insulin sensitivity appears to be mediated via the accumulation of IMCL and plasma triglyceride levels.

In a larger cohort of children and adolescents, Weiss et al.[33] recently reported that adiponectin levels decreased with increasing degree of obesity, and that these levels were lowest in subjects with highest level of insulin resistance. Of note, lower levels of adiponetin were found in obese adolescents with prediabetes compared with weight-matched adolescents with normal glucose tolerance.[33]

Regulation of adiponectin production, including the mechanisms for the reduction in adiponectin levels in obesity and type 2 diabetes, has yet to be fully elucidated.

CONTRIBUTION OF ETHNICITY TO RISK FOR TYPE 2 DIABETES

From an epidemiological perspective, within the United States, children and adolescents of ethnic minority groups are more likely to acquire type 2 diabetes than children and adolescents of European descent.[23–25] This difference pertains to individuals of African ancestry (African American), Native American ancestry, and Hispanic ancestry (primarily Mexican American). The basis for ethnic differences in disease risk has not been entirely determined, but existing information indicates that both genetic factors and lifestyle may contribute. Ethnicity is such a profound risk factor for type 2 diabetes among youth that the American Diabetes Association recommends screening children at or above the 85th percentile for BMI if they also are an ethnic minority (American Indian, Black, Hispanic, or Asian/Pacific Islander) and have one additional risk factor (e.g., family history, acanthosis nigricans).[91]

AFRICAN AMERICANS

Based on existing data, it appears that relative to Caucasian children and adolescents, African American children and adolescents (1) are less sensitive to insulin-stimulated glucose uptake, (2) have a greater first-phase beta-cell insulin secretory response to a glucose challenge, and (3) have a lower degree of hepatic insulin clearance, both on a percentage basis and in absolute terms. These processes are to some extent related and to some extent independent of each other. All may contribute to risk for type 2 diabetes. Importantly, these differences are independent of adiposity. Thus, although greater adiposity among African American youth is likely to explain a portion of the greater disease incidence, the physiological differences in aspects of insulin action are likely to be genetic.

Insulin Sensitivity

Studies using several techniques to directly assess insulin-stimulated glucose uptake have indicated that African American children and adolescents are less insulin sensitive than Caucasian children and adolescents. Using the tolbutamide-modified intravenous glucose tolerance test (IVGTT), Gower et al. reported 42% lower S_i among African American compared with Caucasian prepubertal children,[65] and 45% lower S_i among adolescents (mean Tanner stage 3).[17] In both cases, neither body composition (adiposity) nor body fat distribution (visceral or subcutaneous abdominal fat) accounted for the ethnic difference (Figure 11.4). Using similar methodology, Goran et al. reported 35% lower S_i among young African American compared with Caucasian children (Tanner stages 1 to 3) who did not differ with respect to adiposity.[92] Similarly, S_i as assessed with the euglycemic

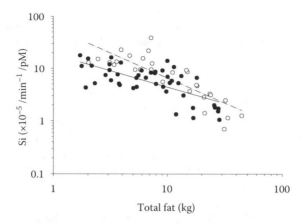

FIGURE 11.4 Insulin sensitivity vs. total fat in African American (●) and Caucasian (○) prepubertal children. (Reproduced with permission from Gower BA, Nagy TR, Goran MI. *Diabetes*. 1999;48: 1515–1521.).

clamp has been observed to be approximately 22% lower among prepubertal African American children compared with Caucasian children[81] (14.8 ± 1.0 vs. 18.9 ± 1.4 μmol·min^{-1}·kg^{-1}FFM, $P < 0.05$). Among adolescents, the insulin sensitivity index, as determined with the hyperglycemic clamp, was lower in African Americans compared with Caucasians with similar mean body mass index.[93]

To begin to determine if this ethnic difference in S_i is due to genetic or environmental factors, a study was undertaken in which the term "ethnicity" was replaced in statistical models with two new terms: African genetic admixture (ADM) and socioeconomic status (SES).[18] African ADM is a continuous variable ranging from 0 to 100 that reflects the proportion of an individual's genes that is of African ancestry. Using data from 125 children and adolescents, it was determined that S_i was inversely related to African ADM; it was not related to SES, determined by questionnaire. In agreement with a nonenvironmental basis for the ethnic difference in S_i, previous research showed that it was not explained by diet[94] or physical activity, although S_i was higher among more active children.[95] However, other research has indicated that the dietary fat-to-carbohydrate intake ratio, which is higher among African Americans compared with Caucasians, is associated with both insulin sensitivity and clearance, as determined with euglycemic clamp.[81]

Insulin Secretion

Insulin secretion can be estimated using several techniques, with those involving measurement of C-peptide providing the most robust estimates. Because insulin, but not C-peptide, is subject to hepatic extraction, peripheral C-peptide concentration more directly reflects pancreatic secretion than does peripheral insulin. Using C-peptide modeling, Gower et al. reported twofold greater first-phase insulin secretion among African American as opposed to Caucasian adolescents.[17] This difference could not be accounted for by individual differences in insulin sensitivity and was, therefore, not simply compensatory for relative insulin resistance in the African American group. Similarly, among both prepubertal children[96] and adolescents,[93] insulin secretion as estimated with the hyperglycemic clamp (mean of five insulin measures during the first 15 min) was determined to be greater among African Americans compared with BMI-matched Caucasians.

During the IVGTT, AIRg, which is the incremental (above basal) area under the insulin curve for the first 10 min of the test, serves as a proxy measure of first-phase insulin secretion. Using this outcome, it was determined that at any given degree of S_i, AIRg among African American prepubertal children was twofold (girls; 1646 ± 590 vs. 792 ± 514 μIU /mL × 10 min, mean ± SD) to threefold (boys; 2214 ± 2215 vs. 773 ± 431 μIU/mL × 10 min) higher than among Caucasian

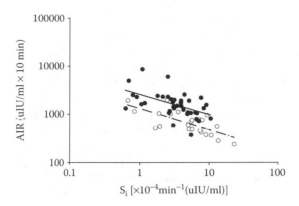

FIGURE 11.5 Acute insulin response to glucose (AIRg) vs. insulin sensitivity in African American (●) and Caucasian (○) prepubertal children.

prepubertal children (Figure 11.5). Looking longitudinally across the pubertal transition, African genetic admixture was independently related to AIRg.[18] The higher AIRg among African Americans is physiologically relevant. During an IVGTT, glucose declines faster and reaches a lower nadir[17] among African Americans compared with Caucasians. Thus intravenous glucose tolerance is greater among African Americans (3.81 + 1.64 %/min) compared with Caucasians (2.44 ± 1.01 %/min; $P < 0.01$), leading to the paradoxical situation that African Americans, relative to Caucasians, have lower S_i but higher i.v. glucose tolerance.

To extend these observations, mathematical modeling of C-peptide data from an IVGTT was used to better estimate insulin secretion and clearance. With this methodology, it was determined that African genetic admixture was associated with a unique insulin secretory profile characterized by a greater proportion of insulin secreted during the first phase and a lesser proportion secreted during the second phase.[97] In this study, higher SES, independent of ADM, was associated with lower insulin secretion throughout the IVGTT.

In contrast, Goran et al. reported that greater AIRg among African American compared with Caucasian children was not associated with greater insulin secretion.[92] This study also involved C-peptide modeling in conjunction with an IVGTT. Neither first- nor second-phase secretion differed between the two groups.

Although the proximate mechanism for greater beta cell sensitivity to glucose among African Americans is not known, it may occur secondary to greater secretion of glucagon-like peptide-1 (GLP-1). This gut-derived hormone is released in response to glucose, and augments glucose-stimulated insulin secretion from the pancreas, both on an acute and chronic[98,99] basis. Studies in obese adults have indicated that both fasting and postchallenge GLP-1 concentrations are higher among African Americans compared with Caucasians.[100] It remains to be determined whether GLP-1 is higher among African American compared with Caucasian children, and whether higher GLP-1 among African Americans explains greater first-phase insulin secretion.

Insulin Clearance

Insulin clearance is difficult to assess directly. One relatively robust method involves mathematical modeling of C-peptide and insulin data. Using the extended-combined model of Watanabe et al., insulin clearance was assessed in a group of 94 African American and Caucasian children and adolescents.[97] Data were collected over 4 years, during which subjects received an IVGTT annually. A mixed model approach was used to account for the effect of pubertal stage, age, and multiple testing of subjects. Results indicated that insulin clearance was inversely related to African ADM when expressed as percent of hormone secreted ($P < .05$), as well as when expressed as absolute mass of hormone extracted by the liver ($P < .05$). Using the same approach, Goran et al. reported that African American children had ~25 percent lower hepatic insulin extraction than both Caucasian and Hispanic children, who did not differ from each other.[92] Similar conclusions were reached by Arslanian et al.[101] and Uwaifo et al.[102] in prepubertal children, using the euglycemic and hyperglycemic clamps, respectively. The euglycemic clamp provides an estimate of clearance by dividing the insulin infusion rate during the clamp by the measured increase in peripheral insulin concentration above baseline. Uwaifo et al.[102] used the C-peptide to insulin molar ratio during the clamp to estimate clearance. The C-peptide to insulin molar ratio can give an approximation of clearance but has several pitfalls.[103] Lower clearance among African American compared with Caucasian adolescents was reported previously in a study that used the ratio of the C-peptide and insulin areas-under-the-curve over the course of a 180-min IVGTT.[17]

Free Fatty Acids

Free fatty acids may influence both insulin sensitivity and beta cell function.[104] A relative increase in FFA may reflect a decrease in sensitivity of adipose tissue to the antilipolytic effect of insulin.

Several published reports exist regarding ethnic differences in FFA among children. Goran et al. reported that fasting (basal) FFAs were positively correlated with second phase insulin secretion, and inversely correlated with insulin sensitivity among African American children, but not among Caucasian or Hispanic children; basal FFA did not differ with ethnicity in this study.[92] Gower et al. found that higher peak insulin following an intravenous glucose challenge was associated with lower FFA during an IVGTT among Caucasian and African American children matched for S_i.[105] In addition, African American children had lower postchallenge FFA than Caucasians, a difference that disappeared after adjusting for peak insulin. Danadian et al. reported that basal lipolysis was 40% lower among African American vs. Caucasian children, and that this difference persisted after adjusting for basal insulin, which was higher among African Americans.[106] Thus, although African Americans have higher basal and postchallenge insulin and, in some studies, lower FFA, when compared with Caucasians, it is not clear whether these various outcomes are mechanistically linked.

Summary

In summary, relative to Caucasians, African Americans have lower S_i, higher first-phase insulin secretion, and lower insulin clearance. These differences are independent of body composition and fat distribution. As children, African Americans have relatively robust beta-cell function, which actually exceeds that seen among Caucasian children matched for S_i, leading to an increased rate of glucose disposal as reflected in greater intravenous glucose tolerance. The physiological cause of the greater first-phase insulin secretion among African Americans is not known, but may be due to greater GLP-1. Whether this relatively robust beta-cell responsiveness ultimately could lead to pancreatic exhaustion remains to be determined. The mechanistic basis for lower S_i among African Americans likewise is not known but may occur secondary to higher ambient insulin concentrations. On an acute basis, relatively high concentrations of insulin, whether due to greater insulin secretion or lesser clearance, may lead to the development of insulin resistance over time within an individual. It is also possible that from an evolutionary perspective, relative hyperinsulinemia resulted in a reduction in S_i across generations as an adaptation to avoid hypoglycemia. Thus, it is possible that ethnic differences in aspects of insulin secretion, clearance, and sensitivity represent inherent differences in insulin–glucose homeostasis. It will be important to determine whether any of these differences confer risk for type 2 diabetes, and if so, whether they are modifiable.

NATIVE AMERICANS

The incidence of type 2 diabetes among American Indian and First Nation youth is a serious concern. As documented in a recent review article,[107] the prevalence per 1000 children and adolescents was 14.1 among Navajo aged 12 to 19; 22.3 among Pima aged 10 to 14; 50.9 among Pima aged 15 to 19; 11.1 among Cree and Ojibway aged 4 to 19; and 36 among Cree and Ojibway girls aged 10 to 19 (no boys in this age range were reported to have type 2 diabetes).

Pima Indians residing in the United States have the highest prevalence of type 2 diabetes in the world,[108] a statistic that extends to children and adolescents. As of 1981, incident type 2 diabetes among Pima children aged 5 to 14 years was 1 in 1000 person years; among those aged 15 to 25 years, it was 9 in 1000 person-years.[109] All Pima children aged 5 years and older are routinely screened for type 2 diabetes. More recent figures[110] indicate that the prevalence of the disease among girls aged 15 to 19 is over 5%, and among boys aged 15 to 19 years is 4%. This was the highest reported prevalence of pediatric type 2 diabetes at this time. Prevalence rates increased two- to threefold over the 30 years preceding the study.

However, the relative contributions of obesity, lifestyle, genetics, and the intrauterine environment to this ethnic disparity in disease risk are not clear. It has been estimated that 40% of type 2 diabetes across Pima individuals aged 5 to 34 could be attributed to effects of the intrauterine environment.[110] Among those aged 5 to 14, close to 100% of the cases were associated with a mother with type 2 diabetes. This association could not be explained by maternal obesity. Perhaps maternal hyperglycemia or hyperinsulinemia act to "program" one or more aspect of offspring physiology (e.g., pancreatic function). The 30-year increase in prevalence of pediatric type 2 diabetes in this population was statistically attributable to the increases in gestational diabetes and offspring obesity. Thus, it is possible that to some extent, obesity and diabetes beget obesity and diabetes.

The Pima Indians are not the only Native American group afflicted with pediatric type 2 diabetes. In Manitoba, the prevalence of the disease[111] among Native American children aged 7 to 14 years is 0.53 per 1000.

Because the Pimas have been studied more extensively than other groups, most of what is known regarding pediatric type 2 diabetes among Native Americans is derived from this population. Pima Indian children show elevated fasting insulin relative to Caucasian children matched for age and weight.[112] It is not clear whether this relative hyperinsulinemia occurs independent of, or secondary to, insulin resistance. Nor is it clear whether this relative hyperinsulinemia is a risk factor for the development of type 2 diabetes. Among Pima children and adolescents aged 5 to 19 years, fasting insulin concentration was significantly associated with development of subsequent diabetes; however, fasting insulin did not independently predict disease development after accounting for relative body weight (body weight divided by age- and sex-specific standard weight for height). In this population, relative body weight and 2-hour plasma glucose concentration following a glucose challenge were the best predictors of subsequent development of type 2 diabetes.

MEXICAN AMERICANS OR HISPANICS

Relatively little information is available with respect to robust measures of insulin dynamics and action in children of Mexican or Hispanic ancestry. Goran et al. reported that Hispanic children aged 10.0 ± 1.9 years had lower insulin sensitivity when compared with Caucasian children matched for BMI; S_i did not differ between Hispanic and African American children.[92] Although BMI did not differ with ethnicity, percent body fat was significantly higher among the Hispanic children relative to the other two groups (Hispanic: 32.7%; Caucasian: 25.7%; African American: 25.2%). Nevertheless, lower insulin sensitivity among Hispanics compared with Caucasians was statistically independent of adiposity.

Using C-peptide modeling from IVGTT data, it was further determined that first-phase insulin secretion was slightly, but not significantly, higher among Hispanic children relative to the other two groups. Second-phase insulin secretion was lower among African American compared with Hispanic children, who did not differ from Caucasians. Hepatic insulin extraction (percent of that secreted) was significantly lower among African Americans relative to the other two groups. Taken together, these data suggest that Hispanic ethnicity, relative to Caucasian, is associated with impaired insulin sensitivity, but not with alteration in insulin secretion or clearance. However, when compared with African Americans, Hispanics appear to compensate differently for a similar degree of insulin resistance; whereas African Americans show increased first-phase insulin secretion and decreased insulin clearance, Hispanics show greater second-phase insulin secretion.

Several studies have used less robust measures to assess diabetes risk among Hispanic children. Among 403 third-grade children in the Houston, TX, area, Mexican American individuals were more likely than Caucasians to have three or more risk factors for the insulin resistance syndrome (elevations in insulin, triglycerides, systolic blood pressure, or BMI, or depression in HDL-C, relative to the population median); this was particularly true among boys.[113]

Among Hispanic children, measures of obesity were positively associated with fasting insulin even at the young age of 2 to 3 years, and fasting insulin was independently associated with C-reactive protein, a marker of inflammation that is associated with risk for cardiovascular disease.[114]

Data from NHANES III showed that glycosylated hemoglobin was 6 to 9 times higher among Hispanic and African American youth aged 6 to 24 years when compared with Caucasian youth; however, these differences were not independent of BMI, which was likewise higher among the ethnic minority groups.[115]

Family history appears to play a large role in determining type 2 diabetes among Hispanic youth; in one study, 87% of Hispanic children with type 2 diabetes had a positive family history of the disease, and 80% had at least one first-degree relative with the disease.[116] In this study, the frequency of children with type 2 diabetes who were Hispanic (67%) exceeded the expected frequency based on demographic data (20%), suggesting a higher frequency among the Hispanic population. It has been suggested that a combination of Mexican and Native American genes is partially responsible for the high incidence of type 2 diabetes among Hispanics.[117]

CONCLUDING REMARKS

Although obesity and insulin resistance are risk factors for type 2 diabetes, for frank type 2 diabetes to occur, the beta cell must cease to produce insulin in a quantity sufficient to compensate for insulin resistance. Beta cell failure occurs in only a subset of insulin resistant individuals, perhaps those with a genetic predisposition. However, to date, it has not been possible, through genetic analysis or other means, to identify those individuals predisposed to beta cell failure. The identification of a marker for future beta cell failure that could be used to identify youth at risk for type 2 diabetes would be extremely useful. Whether any of the observed ethnic differences discussed in this section will prove to be such a marker remains to be determined, and likely will require both epidemiological and longitudinal study.

REFERENCES

1. Amiel SA, Sherwin RS, Simonson DC, Lauritano AA, Tamborlane WV. Impaired insulin action in puberty. A contributing factor to poor glycemic control in adolescents with diabetes. *N Engl J Med.* 1986;315: 215–219.
2. Goran MI, Gower BA. Longitudinal study on pubertal insulin resistance. *Diabetes.* 2002;50: 2444–2450.

3. Caprio S, Plewe G, Diamond MP, Simonson DC, Boulware SD, Sherwin RS, et al. Increased insulin secretion in puberty: a compensatory response to reductions in insulin sensitivity. *J Pediatr.* 1989;114: 963–967.

4. Moran A, Jaccobs DR Jr, Steinberger J, Hong C-P, Prineas R, Luepker R, et al. Insulin resistance during puberty. Results from clamp studies in 357 children. *Diabetes.* 1999;48: 2039–2044.

5. Arslanian S, Kalhan SC. Correlations between fatty acid and glucose metabolism. Potential explanation of insulin resistance of puberty. *Diabetes.* 1994;43: 908–914.

6. Piatti PM, Monti LD, Conti CM, Magni F, Galli-Klienle M, Fochesato E, et al. Mediation of the hepatic effects of growth hormone by its lipolytic activity. *J Clin Endocrinol Metab.* 1999;84: 1658–1663.

7. Boden G, Lebed B, Schatz M, Homko C, Lemieux S. Effects of acute changes of plasma free fatty acids on intramyocellular fat content and insulin resistance in healthy subjects. *Diabetes.* 2001;50: 1612–1617.

8. Albertsson-Wikland K, Rosberg S, Karlberg J, Groth T. Analysis of 24-hour growth hormone profiles in healthy boys and girls of normal stature: relation to puberty. *J Clin Endocrinol Metab.* 1994;78: 1195–1201.

9. Arslanian S, Suprasongsin C. Testosterone treatment in adolescents with delayed puberty: changes in body composition, protein, fat and glucose metabolism. *J Clin Endocrinol Metab.* 1997;82: 3213–3220.

10. Saad RJ, Keenan BS, Danadian K, Lewy V, Arslanian S. Dihydrotestosterone treatment in adolescents with delayed puberty: does it explain insulin resistance of puberty? *J Clin Endocrinol Metab.* 2001;86: 4881–4886.

11. Amiel SA, Caprio S, Sherwin RS, Plewe G, Haymond MW, Tamborlane WV. Insulin resistance of puberty: a defect restricted to peripheral glucose metabolism. *J Clin Endocrinol Metab.* 1991;72: 277–282.

12. Caprio S, Cline G, Boulware S, Permnente C, Shulman GI, Sherwin RS, et al. Effects of puberty and diabetes on metabolism of insulin-sensitive fuels. *Am J Physiol (Endocrinol Metab).* 1994;266: E885–E891.

13. Arslanian S, Kalhan SC. Protein turnover during puberty in normal children. *Am J Physiol (Endocrinol Metab).* 1996;270: E79–E84.

14. Herman-Giddens ME, Slora EJ, Wasserman RC, Bourdony CJ, Bhapkar MV, Koch GG, et al. Secondary sexual characteristics and menses in young girls seen in office practice: a study from the pediatric research in office settings network. *Pediatrics.* 1997;99: 505–512.

15. Sun SS, Schubert CM, Chumlea WC, Roche AF, Kulin HE, Lee PA, et al. National estimates of the timing of sexual maturation and racial differences among US children. *Pediatrics.* 2002;110. 911–919.

16. Kaplowitz PB, Slora EJ, Wasserman RC, Pedlow SE, Herman-Giddens ME. Earlier onset of puberty in girls: relation to increased body mass index and race. *Pediatrics.* 2001;108: 347–353.

17. Gower BA, Granger WM, Franklin F, Shewchuk RM, Goran MI. Contribution of insulin secretion and clearance to glucose-induced insulin concentration in African-American and Caucasian children. *J Clin Endocrinol Metab.* 2002;87: 2218–2224.

18. Gower BA, Fernandez JR, Beasley TM, Shriver MD, Goran MI. Using genetic admixture to explain racial differences in insulin-related phenotypes. *Diabetes.* 2003;52: 1047–1051.

19. Saad RJ, Danadian K, Arslanian S. Insulin resistance of puberty in African-American children: lack of a compensatory increase in insulin secretion. *Pediatr Diabetes.* 2002;3: 4–9.

20. Pinhas-Hamiel O, Dolan LM, Daniels SR, Standiford D, Khoury PR, Zeitler P. Increased incidence of non-insulin-dependent diabetes mellitus among adolescents. *J Pediatr.* 1996;128: 608–615.

21. King H, Aubert RE, Herman WH. Global burden of diabetes, 1995–2025: prevalence, numerical estimates, and projections. *Diabetes Care.* 1998;21: 1414–1431.

22. Zimmet PZ. The pathogenesis and prevention of diabetes in adults. *Diabetes Care.* 1995;18: 1050–1064.

23. Rosenbloom A, Joe J, Young RS, Winter NE. Emerging epidemic of type 2 diabetes in youth. *Diabetes Care.* 1999;22: 345–354.

24. Dabelea D, Pettitt DJ, Jones KL, Arslanian S. Type 2 diabetes mellitus in minority children and adolescents. An emerging problem. *Endocrine Metab Clinics N Am.* 1999;28: 709–729.

25. Kitagawa T, Owada M, Urakami T, Yamauchi K. Increased incidence of non-insulin-dependent diabetes mellitus among Japanese schoolchildren correlates with an increased intake of animal protein and fat. *Clin Pediatr.* 1998;33: 111–115.

26. Dabelea D, Hanson RL, Bennett PH, Roumain J, Knowler WC, Pettitt DJ. Increasing prevalence of type 2 diabetes in American Indian children. *Diabetologia.* 1998;41: 904–910.

27. Alberti G, Zimmet PZ, Shaw J, Bloomgarden Z, Kaufman F, Silink M. Type 2 diabetes in the young: the evolving epidemic. *Diabetes Care.* 2004;27: 1798–1811.

28. Fagot-Campagna A, Saaddine JB, Flegal KM, Beckles GL. Diabetes, impaired fasting glucose, and elevated HbA1c in US adolescents: the third National Health and Nutrition examination survey. *Diabetes Care.* 2001;24: 834–837.

29. Edelstein SL, Knowler WC, Bain RP, Barrett-Connor E, Dowse GK, Haffner SM, et al. Predictors of progression from impaired glucose tolerance to NIDDM: an analysis of six prospective studies. *Diabetes.* 1997;46: 701–710.

30. Knowler WC, Barrett-Connor E, Fowler SE, Hamman RF, Lachin JM, Walker EA, et al. Reduction in the incidence of type 2 diabetes with lifestyle intervention or metformin. *N Engl J Med.* 2002;346: 393–403.

31. Tuomilehto J, Lindstrom J, Eriksson JG, Valle TT, Hamalainen H, Ilanne-Parikka P, et al. Prevention of type 2 diabetes mellitus by changes in lifestyle among subjects with impaired glucose tolerance. *N Engl J Med.* 2001;344: 1343–1350.

32. Sinha R, Fisch G, Teague B, Tamborlane WV, Banyas B, Allen K, et al. Prevalence of impaired glucose tolerance among children and adolescents with marked obesity. *N Engl J Med.* 2002;346: 802–810.

33. Weiss R, Fufour S, Taksali S, Tamborlane WV, Petersen KF, Bonadonna R, et al. Pre-type 2 diabetes in obese youth: a syndrome of impaired glucose tolerance, severe insulin resistance and altered myocellular and abdominal fat partitioning. *Lancet.* 2003;362: 951–957.

34. Cruz ML, Weigensberg M, Huang TTK, Ball G, Shaibi GQ, Goran MI. The metabolic syndrome in overweight Hispanic youth and the role of insulin sensitivity. *J Clin Endocrinol Metab.* 2004;89: 108–113.

35. Goran MI, Bergman RN, Avila Q, Watkins M, Ball GDC, Shaibi GQ, et al. Impaired glucose tolerance and reduced beta-cell function in overweight Latino children with a positive family history for type 2 diabetes. *J Clin Endocrinol Metab.* 2004;89: 207–212.

36. Keamseng C, Likitmaksul S, Kiattisakthavee P, et al. Risk of metabolic disturbance and diabetes development in Thai obese children. 29th Annual Meeting of the International Society for Pediatric and Adolescent Diabetes. 2003; Saint-Malo, France. *J Pediatr Endocrinol Metab.* 20003;16(Suppl 4): 919–955.

37. Lee W, Tang J, Karim H, et al. Abnormalities of glucose tolerance in severely obese Singapore children. 29th Annual Meeting of the International Society for Pediatric and Adolescent Diabetes. 2003; Saint-Malo, France. *J Pediatr Endocrinol Metab.* 20003;16(Suppl 4): 919–955.

38. Tounian P, Aggoun Y, Dubern B, et al. Presence of increased stiffness of the common carotid artery and endothelial dysfunction in severely obese children: a prospective study. *Lancet.* 2001;358: 1400–1404.

39. DeFronzo R. Pathogenesis of type 2 diabetes: metabolic and molecular implications for identifying diabetes genes. *Diabetes Rev.* 1997;5: 177–269.

40. Ferrannini E. Insulin resistance versus insulin deficiency in NIDDM: problems and prospects. *Endocr Rev.* 1998;19: 447–490.

41. Perseghin G, Ghosh S, Gerow K, Shulman GI. Metabolic defects in lean nondiabetic offspring of NIDDM patients. *Diabetes.* 1997;46: 1001–1009.

42. Martin BC, Warram JH, Krowleski AS, Bergman RN, Soeldner JS, Kahn RC. Role of glucose and insulin resistance in the development of type 2 diabetes mellitus: results of a 25 year follow-up study. *Lancet.* 1992;340: 925–929.

43. Buchanan TA. Pancreatic beta-cell loss and preservation in type 2 diabetes. *Clin. Therap.* 2003;25 (Suppl B): B32–B46.

44. Haffner SM, Miettinen H, Gaskill SP, Stern MP. Decreased insulin secretion and increased insulin resistance are independently related to the 7-year risk of NIDDM in Mexican Americans. *Diabetes.* 1995;44: 1386–1391.

45. Lillioja S, Mott DM, Spraul M, Ferraro R, Foley JE, Ravussin E, et al. Insulin resistance and insulin secretory dysfunction as precursors of non-insulin-dependent diabetes mellitus. Prospective studies of Pima Indians. *N Engl J Med*. 1993;329: 1988–1992.

46. Buchanan TA, Xiang AH, Kjos SL, Trigo E, Lee WP, Peters RK. Antepartum predictors of the development of type 2 diabetes in Latino women 11–26 months after pregnancies complicated by gestational diabetes. *Diabetes*. 1999;48: 2430–2436.

47. Rosenbaum M, Nonas C, Horlick M, Fennoy I, Vargas I, Schachner H, et al. Beta-cell function and insulin sensitivity in early adolescence: association with body fatness and family history of type 2 diabetes mellitus. *J Clin Endocrinol Metab*. 2004;89: 5469–5476.

48. Carey DG, Jenkins AB, Campbell LV, Freund J, Chisholm DJ. Abdominal fat and insulin resistance in normal and overweight women: Direct measurements reveal a strong relationship in subjects at both low and high risk of NIDDM. *Diabetes*. 1996;45: 633–638.

49. Despres JP. The insulin resistance-dyslipidemic syndrome of visceral obesity. Effect on patient risk. *Obes Res*. 1998;6 (Suppl 1): 8S-17S.

50. Caprio S, Hyman LD, Limb C, McCarthy S, Lange R, Sherwin RS, et al. Central adiposity and its metabolic correlates in obese adolescent girls. *Am J Physiol*. 1995;269: E118–E126.

51. Abate N, Garg A, Peshock RM, Stray-Gundersen J, Grundy SM. Relationships of generalized and regional adiposity to insulin sensitivity in men. *J Clin Invest*. 1995;96: 88–98.

52. Wajchenberg BL. Subcutaneous and visceral adipose tissue: their relation to the metabolic syndrome. *Endocr Rev*. 2000;21: 697–738.

53. Klein S, Fontana L, Young L, Coggan A, Kilo C, Patterson B, et al. Absence of an effect of liposuction on insulin action and risk factors for coronary heart disease. *N Engl J Med*. 2004;350: 2549–2557.

54. Goodpaster BH, Kelley DE, Wing RR, Meier A, Thaete FL. Effects of weight loss on insulin sensitivity in obesity: influence of regional adiposity. *Diabetes*. 1999;48: 839–847.

55. Jensen MD, Haymond MW, Rizza RA, Cryer PE, Miles JM. Influence of body fat distribution on free fatty acid metabolism in obesity. *J Clin Invest*. 1989;83: 1168–1173.

56. Montague CT, O'Rahilly S. The perils of portliness: causes and consequences of visceral adiposity. *Diabetes*. 2000;49: 883–888.

57. Sethi JK, Hotamisligil GS. The role of TNF alpha in adipocyte metabolism. *Sem Cell Dev Biol*. 1999;10: 10–29.

58. Lang CH, Dobrescu C, Bagby CJ. Tumor necrosis factor alpha impairs insulin action on peripheral glucose disposal and hepatic glucose output. *Endocrinology*. 1992;130: 43–52.

59. Bastard JP, Maachi M, Van Nhieu JT, Jardel C, Bruckert E, Grimaldi A, et al. Adipose tissue IL-6 content correlates with resistance to insulin activation of glucose uptake *in vivo* and *in vitro*. *J Clin Endocrinol Metab*. 2002;87: 2084–2089.

60. Lewis GF, Carpentier A, Adeli K, Giacca A. Disordered fat storage and mobilization in the pathogenesis of insulin resistance and type 2 diabetes. *Endocr Rev*. 2002;23: 201–229.

61. Gan SK, Samaras K, Thompson CH, Kraegen EW, Carr A, Cooper DA, et al. Altered myocellular and abdominal fat partitioning predict disturbance in insulin action in HIV protease inhibitor-related lipodystrophy. *Diabetes*. 2002;51: 3163–3169.

62. Kim JK, Gavrilova O, Chen Y, Reitman ML, Shulman GI. Mechanism of inulin resistance in A-ZIP/F-1 fatless mice. *J Biol Chem*. 2000;275: 8456–8460.

63. Akazawa S, Sun F, Ito M, Kawasaki E, Eguchi K. Efficacy of troglitizone on body fat distribution in type 2 diabetes. *Diabetes Care*. 2000;23: 1067–1071.

64. Petersen KF, Oral EA, Dufour S, Befroy D, Ariyan C, Yu C, et al. Leptin reverses insulin resistance and hepatic steatosis in patients with severe lipodystrophy. *J Clin Invest*. 2002;109: 1345–1350.

65. Gower BA, Nagy TR, Goran MI. Visceral fat, insulin sensitivity, and lipids in prepubertal children. *Diabetes*. 1999;48: 1515–1521.

66. McGarry JD. Dysregulation of fatty acid metabolism in the etiology of type 2 diabetes. *Diabetes*. 2002;51: 7–18.

67. Kelley DE, Mandarino LJ. Fuel selection in human skeletal muscle in insulin resistance: a re-examination. *Diabetes*. 2000;49: 677–683.

68. Stein DT, Szczepaniak LS, Dobbins RL, McGarry JD. Increasing intramyocellular triglyceride stores are associated with impaired glucose tolerance and NIDDM. *Diabetes*. 1999;48(Suppl 1): 287A.

69. Perseghin G, Ghosh S, Gerow K, Shulman GI. Metabolic defects in lean nondiabetic offspring of NIDDM patients: a cross-sectional study. *Diabetes*. 1997;46: 1001–1009.

70. Sinha R, Dufour S, Peterson KF, LeBon V, Enoksson S, Ma Y-Z, et al. Assessment of skeletal muscle triglyceride content by 1H nuclear magnetic resonance spectroscopy in lean and obese adolescents. *Diabetes*. 2002;51: 1022–1027.

71. Shulman GI. Cellular mechanisms of insulin resistance. *J Clin Invest*. 2000;106: 171–176.

72. Itani SI, Ruderman NB, Schmieder F, Boden G. Lipid-induced insulin resistance in human muscle is associated with changes in diacylglycerol, protein kinase C, and IKB-alpha. *Diabetes*. 2002;51: 2005–2011.

73. Dresner A, Laurent D, Marcucci N, Griffin M, Dufour S, Cline GW, et al. Effects of free fatty acids on glucose transport and IRS-1 associated phosphatidylinositol 3-kinase activity. *J Clin Invest*. 1999;103: 253–259.

74. Griffin M, Marcucci MJ, Cline GW, Bell K, Barucci N, Lee D, et al. Free fatty acid-induced insulin resistance is associated with activation of protein kinase C theta and alterations in the insulin signaling cascade. *Diabetes*. 1999;48: 1270–1274.

75. Yu C, Chen Y, Cline G, Zhang D, Zong H, Wang Y, et al. Mechanism by which fatty acids inhibit insulin activation of insulin receptor substrate-1 (IRS-1)-associated phosphatidylinositol 3-kinase activity in muscle. *J Biol Chem*. 2002;52: 50230–50236.

76. Greco AV, Mingrone G, Giancaterini A, Manco M, Morroni M, Cinti S, et al. Insulin resistance in morbid obesity. Reversal with intramyocellular fat depletion. *Diabetes*. 2002;51: 144–151.

77. Houmard JA, Tannez CJ, Yu C, Cunningham PG, Pories WJ, MacDonald KG, et al. Effects of weight loss on insulin sensitivity and intramuscular long-chain fatty acyl-CoAs in morbidly obese subjects. *Diabetes*. 2002;51: 2959–2963.

78. Simoneau JA, Veerkamp JH, Turcotte LP, Kelley DE. Markers of capacity to utilize fatty acids in human skeletal muscle: relation to insulin resistance and obesity and effects of weight loss. *FASEB J*. 1999;13: 2051–2060.

79. Kelley DE, Simoneau JA, Goodpaster BH, Troost F. Defects of skeletal muscle fatty acid metabolism in obesity. *Obes Res*. 1997;4: 215.

80. Zhang Y, Proenca R, Maffei M, Barone M, Leopold L, Friedman JM. Positional cloning of the mouse obese gene and its human homologue. *Nature*. 1994;372: 425–432.

81. Saltiel AR. You are what you secrete. *Nature Med*. 2001;7: 887–888.

82. Hotamisligil GS. The role of TNF receptors in obesity and insulin resistance. *J Int Med*. 1999;245: 621–625.

83. Arita Y, Kihara S, Ouchi N, Takahashi Y, Maeda K, Miyagawa JI, et al. Paradoxical decrease of an adipose-specific protein, adiponectin, in obesity. *Biochem Biophys Res Comm*. 1999;257: 79–83.

84. Hotta K, Funahashi T, Bodkin NL, Ortmeyer HK, Arita Y, Hansen BC, et al. Circulating concentrations of the adipocyte protein adiponectin: a decrease in parallel with reduced insulin senstitivity during the progression of type 2 diabetes in Rhesus monkeys. *Diabetes*. 2001;50: 1126–1133.

85. Hu E, Liang P, Spiegelman BM. Adipo Q is a novel adipose-specific gene dysregulated in obesity. *J Biol Chem*. 1996;271: 10697–10703.

86. Weyer C, Funahashi T, Tanaka S, Hotta K, Matsuzawa Y, Pratley RE, et al. Hypoadiponectinemia in obesity and type 2 diabetes: close association with insulin resistance and hyperinsulinemia. *J Clin Endocrinol Metab*. 2001;86: 1930–1935.

87. Comuzzie AG, Funahashi T, Sonnenberg G, Martin LJ, Jacob HJ, Black AE, et al. The genetic basis of plasma variation in adiponectin, a global endophenotype for obesity and the metabolic syndrome. *J Clin Endocrinol Metab*. 2001;86: 4321–4325.

88. Yamauchi T, Kamon J, Waki H, Terauchi Y, Kubota N, Hara K, et al. The fat-derived hormone adiponectin reverses insulin resistance associated with both lipoatrophy and obesity. *Nature Med*. 2001;7: 887–888.

89. Fruebis J, Tsao TS, Javorschi S, Ebbets-Reed D, Erickson MR, Yen FT, et al. Proteolytic cleavage product of 30-kDa adipocyte complement-related protein increases fatty acid oxidation in muscle and causes weight loss in mice. *Proc Natl Acad Sci*. 2001;98: 2005–2010.

90. Weiss R, Dufour S, Groszmann A, Petersen KF, Dziura J, Taksali S, et al. Low adiponectin levels in adolescent obesity: a marker of increased intramyocellular lipid accumulation. *J Clin Endocrinol Metab*. 2003;88: 2014–2018.

91. American Diabetes Association. Type 2 diabetes in children and adolescents. *Pediatrics*. 2000;105: 671–680.

92. Goran MI, Bergman RN, Cruz ML, Watanabe R. Insulin resistance and associated compensatory responses in African-American and Hispanic children. *Diabetes Care*. 2002;25: 2184–2190.

93. Arslanian S, Suprasongsin C. Differences in the *in vivo* insulin secretion and sensitivity of healthy black versus white adolescents. *J Pediatr*. 1996;129: 440–443.

94. Lindquist CH, Gower BA, Goran MI. Role of dietary factors in ethnic differences in early risk of cardiovascular disease and type 2 diabetes. *Am J Clin Nutr*. 2000;71: 725–732.

95. Ku C-Y, Gower BA, Hunter GR, Goran MI. Racial differences in insulin secretion and sensitivity in prepubertal children: role of physical fitness and physical activity. *Obes Res*. 2000;8: 506–515.

96. Arslanian S, Suprasongsin C, Janosky JE. Insulin secretion and sensitivity in black versus white prepubertal healthy children. *J Clin Endocrinol Metab*. 1997;82: 1923–1927.

97. Phadke R, Watanabe M, Fernandez JR, Goran MI, Gower BA. African genetic admixture is associated with a unique secretory profile in children and adolescents. *Obes Res*. 2004;12(5): A72.

98. Fehmann HC, Goke R, Bachle R, Wagner B, Arnold R. Priming effect of glucagon like peptide 1 amide, GIP, and cholecystokinin at the isolated perfused rat pancreas. *Biochim Biophys Acta*. 1991;1091: 356–363.

99. Drucker DJ. Minireview: the glucagon-like peptides. *Endocrinology*. 2001;142: 521–527.

100. Velasquez-Mieyer PA, Cowan PA, Umpierrez GE, Lustig RH, Cashion AK, Burghen GA. Racial differences in glucagon-like peptide-1 (GLP-1) concentration and insulin dynamics during oral glucose tolerance test in obese subjects. *Int J Obes*. 2003;27: 1359–1364.

101. Arslanian S, Saad R, Lewy V, Danadian K, Janosky JE. Hyperinsulinemia in African-American children. Decreased insulin clearance and increased insulin secretion and its relationship to insulin sensitivity. *Diabetes*. 2002;51: 3014–3019.

102. Uwaifo GI, Nguyen TT, Keil MF, Russell DL, Nicholson JC, Bonat SH, et al. Differences in insulin secretion and sensitivity of Caucasian and African American prepubertal children. *J Pediatr*. 2002;140: 673–680.

103. Polonsky KS, Rubenstein AH. C-peptide as a measure of the secretion and hepatic extraction of insulin. Pitfalls and limitations. *Diabetes*. 1984;33: 486–494.

104. Boden G. Effects of free fatty acids (FFA) on glucose metabolism: significance for insulin resistance and type 2 diabetes. *Exp Clin Endocrinol Diabetes*. 2003;111: 121–124.

105. Gower BA, Herd SL, Goran MI. Anti-lipolytic effects of insulin in African American and white prepubertal children. *Obes Res*. 2001;9: 224–228.

106. Danadian K, Lewy V, Janosky JE, Arslanian S. Lipolysis in African-American children: is it a metabolic risk factor predisposing to obesity? *J Clin Endocrinol Metab*. 2001;86: 3022–3026.

107. Fagot-Campagna A, Pettitt DJ, Engelgau MM, Burrows NR, Geiss LS, Valdez R, et al. Type 2 diabetes among North American children and adolescents: an epidemiological review and a public health perspective. *J Pediatr*. 2000;136: 664–672.

108. Knowler WC, Bennett PH, Hamman RF, Miller M. Diabetes incidence and prevalence in Pima Indians: a 19-fold greater incidence than in Rochester, Minnesota. *Am J Epidemiol*. 1978;108: 497–505.

109. Knowler WC, Pettitt DJ, Savage PJ, Bennett PH. Diabetes incidence in Pima Indians: Contributions of obesity and parental diabetes. *Am J Epidemiol*. 1981;113: 144–156.

110. Dabelea D, Knowler WC, Pettitt DJ. Effect of diabetes in pregnancy on offspring: follow-up research in the Pima Indians. *J Maternal-Fetal Med*. 2000;9: 83–88.

111. Dean HJ, Mundy RL, Moffatt M. Non-insulin dependent diabetes mellitus in Indian children in Manitoba. *Can Med Assoc J*. 1992;147: 52–57.

112. Pettitt DJ, Moll PP, Knowler WC, Mott DM, Nelson RG, Saad MF, et al. Insulinemia in children at low and high risk of NIDDM. *Diabetes Care*. 1993;16: 608–615.

113. Batey LS, Goff DC, Jr., Tortolero SR, Nichaman MZ, Chan W, Chan FA, et al. Summary measures of the insulin resistance syndrome are adverse among Mexican-American versus non-Hispanic white children. *Circulation*. 1997;96: 4319–4325.

114. Shea S, Aymong E, Zybert P, Shamoon H, Tracy RP, Deckelbaum RJ, et al. Obesity, fasting plasma insulin, and C-reactive protein levels in healthy children. *Obes Res*. 2003;11: 95–103.

115. Winkleby MA, Robinson TN, Sundquist J, Kraemer HC. Ethnic variation in cardiovascular diesease risk factors among children and young adults. Findings from the Third National Health and Nutrition Examination Survey, 1988–1994. *JAMA*. 1999;281: 1006–1013.

116. Glaser NS, Jones KL. Non-insulin dependent diabetes mellitus in Mexican-American children. *West J Med*. 1998;168: 11.

117. Gardner LI Jr, Stern MP, Haffner SM, Gaskill SP, Hazuda HP, Relethford JH, et al. Prevalence of diabetes in Mexican Americans. Relationship to percent of gene pool derived from native American sources. *Diabetes*. 1984;33: 86–92.

12 Metabolic Syndrome in Children and Adolescents

Martha L. Cruz

CONTENTS

INTRODUCTION

Obesity in childhood has significant short- and long-term impact on the health and well-being of children and adolescents. Several reports have linked childhood obesity to type 2 diabetes in youth,[1] impaired glucose tolerance,[2,3] hypertension, dyslipidemia,[4,5] polycystic ovary syndrome,[6] and more recently, nonalcoholic fatty liver disease.[7,8] The clustering of abnormalities associated with obesity are collectively known as the metabolic syndrome. Although the components of the metabolic syndrome were first described over 40 years ago, it was only recently that both the World Health Organization and the U.S. Cholesterol Education Program Adult Treatment Panel III (ATP III)[9] provided a clinical definition of the syndrome. These criteria, although similar in that they focus on obesity, dyslipidemia, hyperglycemia. and hypertension, differ in the individual constituents and threshold levels. The uniform case definition of the syndrome has promoted epidemiological investigations to establish the prevalence and characteristics of the syndrome across different adult populations.[10–16]

In adults, the metabolic syndrome is an entity that places individuals at risk of type 2 diabetes[15,16] and cardiovascular disease[13,14] that is associated with increased cardiovascular disease mortality.[13,14] The findings from studies in adults coupled with the obesity epidemic in childhood have resulted in a new interest in the study of the metabolic syndrome in youth and on its potential impact on the health and well-being of children and adolescents.

Recent studies[17,18] have shown the prevalence rate of the metabolic syndrome among overweight children is as high as 30%. Although, no studies to date have directly explored the impact of the metabolic syndrome on disease outcomes in childhood, autopsy studies in youth have shown that several metabolic risk factors are related to the early stages of coronary atherosclerosis.[5,19] Therefore, the high prevalence of the metabolic syndrome among overweight youth coupled with the epidemic increase in childhood obesity could lead to premature heart disease, type 2 diabetes, and nonalcoholic fatty liver disease. This chapter (1) provides evidence to show that the metabolic syndrome is highly prevalent among overweight children and may be more pronounced in certain ethnic minorities, (2) examines the underlying pathophysiology of the syndrome during childhood and argues that the underlying defect is likely to be obesity coupled with insulin resistance, (3) examines available evidence linking the metabolic syndrome (and its individual components) with disease outcomes, and (4) suggests strategies for screening, prevention, and treatment of the syndrome in youth.

PREVALENCE OF THE METABOLIC SYNDROME IN OVERWEIGHT CHILDREN AND ADOLESCENTS

The impact of obesity on metabolic risk factors in childhood has been subject of study for several decades. During the 1990s multiple large population-based studies demonstrated that obese youth had elevated levels of triglycerides and LDL cholesterol, and low levels of HDL cholesterol.[20,21] The Bogalusa Heart Study, a community-based study of risk factors for cardiovascular disease in black and white youth, pooled data from 9167 subjects aged 5 to 17 years.[20] These investigators found that overweight (defined as a body mass index (BMI) > 85th percentile) children and adolescents were 2.4, 3.0, 3.4, 7.1, and 4.5 times more likely to have adverse levels of cholesterol, LDL cholesterol, HDL cholesterol, triglycerides, and blood pressure, respectively.[20] More recently, investigators have examined the clustering of metabolic abnormalities in both normal weight and obese children. Although, studies have reported relatively low prevalence rates of the metabolic syndrome among children of different ages,[22–25] a very different picture emerges when prevalence rates are expressed by degree of adiposity.[17,18,22] For instance, recent data from the Third National Health and Nutrition Examination Survey (NHANES III), showed that the prevalence of the metabolic syndrome was 28.7% in overweight adolescents (BMI ≥ 95th percentile) compared with 6.1% in adolescents at risk for overweight (BMI ≥ 85th but lower than 95th percentile) and 0.1% in those with a BMI below the 85th percentile.[22] In overweight adolescents, 89% had at least one abnormality of the metabolic syndrome and more than half (56%) had two abnormalities.[22] The individual prevalence of abdominal obesity, high triglycerides, low HDL cholesterol, and high blood pressure in overweight adolescents was 74.5, 51.8, 50, and 11.2%, respectively. High fasting glucose (defined as glucose > 110 mg/dL) was present in 2.6% of overweight adolescents. In this NHANES III adolescent population, the vast majority (80%) of youth who were classified as having the metabolic syndrome were also classified as being overweight based on a BMI > 95th percentile. In view of the increasing rise in childhood overweight, the overall prevalence of the metabolic syndrome in childhood is likely to be higher than that estimated from NHANES III data. For instance, in a clinical-based population, Weiss et al.[18] reported a prevalence of 39 and 49.7% in obese adolescents above the 97th and 99th percentile for BMI. Thus, the prevalence of the metabolic syndrome is clearly related to increasing severity of obesity.

The prevalence of the metabolic syndrome appears to be influenced by ethnicity. In U.S. adults, the prevalence rates are higher among Hispanics (31.9%) and lower among blacks (21.6%) compared with whites (23.8%).[11] Likewise, the prevalence of the metabolic syndrome in U.S. adolescents was highest among Hispanics (5.6%) and lowest among blacks (2.0%) compared with white adolescents (4.8%).

Among Hispanic adolescents, the high prevalence of the metabolic syndrome may be a consequence of obesity. The prevalence of overweight in Hispanic youth has approximately doubled in the last 10 years, such that 23.4% of Hispanic adolescents are now overweight compared with 12.7% of whites.[26]

We recently explored the prevalence of the metabolic syndrome in a group of overweight Hispanic children (aged 8 to 13 years) with a family history for type 2 diabetes.[17] The metabolic syndrome was defined as the presence of three or more of the following abnormalities: abdominal obesity (waist circumference ≥ 90th percentile for age, gender, and ethnicity from NHANES III), hypertriglyceridemia (triglycerides ≥ 90th percentile for age and gender),[27] low HDL cholesterol (HDL cholesterol ≤ 10th percentile for age and gender),[27] hypertension (systolic or diastolic blood pressure > 90th percentile adjusted for height, age, and gender[28]) and finally, impaired glucose tolerance.[29] Using this definition, we found that 30% of overweight Hispanic children with a family history for type 2 diabetes have the metabolic syndrome.[17] Furthermore, 9 out of 10 Hispanic overweight children with a family history for type 2 diabetes have at least one feature of the metabolic syndrome.[17]

Although the prevalence of obesity among African American adolescents in the United States is also high (23.6%), paradoxically African American children and adolescents have a lower prevalence of the metabolic syndrome[22-24] at least when a similar definition of ATP III is used. This is not entirely surprising because African American youth (like adults) have lower triglycerides and higher HDL cholesterol levels compared with their white counterparts.[23] These findings suggest that the impact of obesity on the components of the metabolic syndrome may vary by ethnic group as has been shown to be the case in South Asians.[30]

ETIOLOGY OF THE METABOLIC SYNDROME IN CHILDHOOD

The role of obesity on the metabolism of lipids and glucose, regulation of blood pressure, thrombotic and fibrinolytic processes, and inflammatory reactions is evident in both adults[31] and children.[32] However, obesity probably is necessary but not sufficient by itself to produce the metabolic syndrome. Other factors must come into play, such as aging and genetic susceptibility.

ROLE OF INSULIN RESISTANCE

Perhaps, the most accepted hypothesis, and one that is supported by prospective studies, is that obesity coupled with increased susceptibility to insulin resistance[33-36] may be the key underlying abnormality of the metabolic syndrome. The role of obesity and insulin resistance in the etiology of the metabolic syndrome has been recently explored in children through cross-sectional and prospective studies.[17,18,25,37] The Cardiovascular Risk in Young Finns Study was one of the first groups to explore the childhood predictors of the metabolic syndrome. To do this, the investigators established the relationship between fasting insulin at baseline and the development of the metabolic syndrome 6 years later in a cohort of 1865 children and adolescents ages 6 to 18. In this study the metabolic syndrome was defined as having high triglyceride and high blood pressure (> 75th percentile) and low HDL-cholesterol (< 25th percentile).[25] The results from this study showed that baseline insulin concentration was higher in children who subsequently developed metabolic syndrome, lending support to the view that insulin resistance precedes the development of the metabolic syndrome in childhood.[25] Because obesity in childhood is closely associated with insulin resistance, it would have been important to establish that the development of the metabolic syndrome in children and adolescents was related to an increase in adiposity over the 6-year period.

More recently, researchers from the Bogalusa Heart Study attempted to disentangle the relative contribution of childhood obesity (measured via BMI) versus insulin resistance (measured via fasting insulin) to the adulthood risk of developing the metabolic syndrome.[37] For an average of 11.6 years, 718 children aged 8 to 17 years at baseline, were followed. The metabolic syndrome was defined as having the four factors — BMI, fasting insulin, systolic (or mean arterial) blood pressure, and triglyceride/HDL ratio — in the highest quartile for age, gender, ethnicity, and study year.[37] Significant positive trends were seen between childhood BMI as well as insulin quartiles and the incidence of clustering in adulthood. Children in the top quartile of BMI and insulin versus those in the bottom quartile were 11.7 and 3.6 times more likely to develop clustering, respectively, as adults. A high childhood BMI was significantly associated with the incidence of clustering in adulthood even after adjustment for childhood insulin levels. However, in this study, adjustment for childhood BMI eliminated the influence of insulin on the incidence of clustering in adulthood. Thus, in this bi-ethnic, community-based study, childhood obesity (measured via BMI) was more closely associated with the presence of the metabolic syndrome in adulthood than was fasting insulin. These findings suggest that obesity in childhood precedes the development of the metabolic syndrome in adulthood.

Although obesity in childhood may be more closely associated with the development of the metabolic syndrome than insulin resistance is, the question remains as to why some obese children develop the metabolic syndrome and others do not. The recent NHANES III data on the prevalence of the metabolic syndrome among U.S. adolescents found that approximately 30% of overweight children (BMI > 95th percentile) have the metabolic syndrome while the remaining 70% do not.[22] We recently addressed this issue in a cohort (n =126) of overweight Hispanic adolescents (mean BMI percentile 97 ± 2.9; age 8 to 13 years) with a family history for type 2 diabetes.[17] We hypothesized that in overweight Hispanic children, insulin resistance would be more closely associated with the metabolic syndrome than overall adiposity. In this study, insulin sensitivity was measured via the frequently sampled intravenous glucose tolerance test and minimal modeling, and overall adiposity was measured by dual energy x-ray absorptiometry (DEXA).[17] We found that insulin sensitivity (after adjustment for differences in adiposity) was 62% lower in overweight youth with the metabolic syndrome compared with overweight youth without the metabolic syndrome. Furthermore, in multivariate regression analysis, insulin sensitivity, but not fat mass, was independently and negatively related to triglycerides and blood pressure and positively related to HDL cholesterol.[17] These results suggest that the effect of adiposity on lipids and blood pressure control is mediated via insulin resistance.

Our findings in overweight Hispanic youth are in agreement with previous results in which directly measured insulin sensitivity has been shown to be independently associated with the separate components of the metabolic syndrome.[38,39] For instance, we previously reported that after adjustment for differences in body composition (fat and lean tissue mass), insulin sensitivity (measured by the frequently sampled intravenous tolerance test) was negatively associated with systolic blood pressure in a mixed cohort of African American and white prepubertal children with a wide varying degrees of adiposity.[38] Insulin sensitivity measured via the euglycemic insulin clamp has also been shown to be correlated with fasting triglycerides and HDL cholesterol in white children and adolescents (n = 357; mean age ~13 years) and this relationship remained after adjustment for BMI.[39]

Despite significant differences in the definition of the metabolic syndrome and in the pediatric populations studied, collectively, the above findings suggest that both obesity and insulin resistance contribute to the development of the metabolic syndrome during childhood.

ROLE OF INFLAMMATION AND ADIPOCYTOKINES

Inflammation and hypercoagulability predispose individuals to atherothrombosis and are important features of the metabolic syndrome.[40] Obesity is associated with subclinical chronic inflammation as evidenced by increased levels of IL-6, TNF, CRP, and leptin and decreased levels of adiponectin.[41,42] The dysregulation in adipocytokine production is thought by some to be the missing link between obesity and insulin resistance.[41-43] IL-6, which is considered the central mediator of inflammatory response, is released from visceral and subcutaneous fat subsequent to sympathetic nervous system activation. It is considered that approximately 25 to 30% of systemic IL-6 is derived from adipose tissue. Visceral fat releases approximately 2 to 3 times more IL-6 than subcutaneous adipose tissue. IL-6 delivery to the liver via the portal vein increases CRP production in the liver such that IL-6 coupled with free fatty acids are considered key players in the relationship between obesity and disease risk. Adiponectin, which belongs to the soluble defense collagen family, has been shown to be positively correlated with insulin sensitivity and HDL cholesterol levels in adults. Adiponectin levels are low in subjects with diabetes, in normal first-degree relatives of diabetic patients, and in nondiabetic obese individuals.[40]

Few studies have examined the relationship between adiposity, insulin resistance, and inflammatory markers in children. Recently, the impact of adolescent obesity on circulating adiponectin levels and the relationship between adiponectin and insulin sensitivity were examined in a small group of obese and nonobese adolescents.[44] Plasma adiponectin levels were shown to be lower in obese adolescents and were related to insulin resistance, independent of total body fat and central adiposity.[44] In two different studies, childhood adiposity was associated with higher levels of the proinflammatory markers, CRP and IL-6.[18,45] Although adiponectin has been shown to be inversely related to plasma triglyceride levels and CRP to HDL cholesterol levels, it is unclear if these relationships are independent of insulin sensitivity. Of greater importance is establishing whether dysregulation of inflammatory cytokines is causative or a consequence of insulin resistance. A recent study in adult first-degree relatives of type 2 diabetics aimed to partially answer this question. Although relatives of type 2 diabetic subjects had 20% lower insulin sensitivity (measured via the insulin clamp) than controls with no family history for diabetes, they were not different in terms of CRP or adiponectin. These findings suggest that adiposity probably interacts with insulin resistance to raise CRP levels and do not support role of inflammation in the development of insulin resistance.[46] Studies designed to address longitudinally the relationship between obesity, inflammation, and insulin resistance are clearly needed to answer such questions.

IMPACT OF THE METABOLIC SYNDROME ON DISEASE OUTCOMES IN CHILDHOOD

PREMATURE CARDIOVASCULAR DISEASE AND TYPE 2 DIABETES

In adults, the metabolic syndrome is a risk factor for type 2 diabetes and cardiovascular disease,[9] which is associated with increased cardiovascular disease mortality.[13] Although, no studies to date have directly explored the impact of the metabolic syndrome on disease outcomes in childhood, autopsy studies in youth have shown that cardiovascular risk factors (including obesity, high blood pressure, high triglycerides, and low HDL cholesterol) are related to the early stages of coronary atherosclerosis.[5,19] Furthermore, the extent of lesions increases markedly with the presence of multiple risk factors.[5] Therefore, the high prevalence of the metabolic syndrome among overweight youth coupled with the epidemic increase in childhood obesity could lead to a disproportionate increase in cardiovascular disease in adulthood.

Type 2 diabetes has already emerged as critical health problem in overweight adolescents,[1,2] as discussed in Chapter 11. It remains to be determined if having the metabolic syndrome in addition to impaired fasting glucose or impaired glucose tolerance increases the subsequent risk of developing type 2 diabetes in the future.

NONALCOHOLIC FATTY LIVER DISEASE

Nonalcoholic fatty liver disease (NAFLD) encompasses the entire spectrum of liver disease, which includes simple hepatic steatosis without inflammation (which may not lead to progressive liver injury), nonalcoholic steatohepatitis (NASH), and the resulting cirrhosis (which may be devoid of steatosis). NAFLD is the most common liver disease in the United States.[47] In adults, insulin resistance is regarded as an essential factor for the development of NAFLD, and in turn, NAFLD is considered a feature of the metabolic syndrome.[48] In children, NAFLD has been shown to occur most commonly in conditions associated with insulin resistance, including obesity and type 2 diabetes.[7,49,50] A recent retrospective study found that children with biopsy-proven NAFLD were almost exclusively obese and had fasting hyperinsulinemia.[51] In another retrospective study, 83% of patients diagnosed with NASH were obese, 30% had elevated serum triglycerides, and 19% had elevated serum cholesterol.[7] These data suggest that NAFLD in childhood is also associated with an insulin resistant state and may be a further metabolic abnormality associated with the metabolic syndrome.

Finally, the question of whether cutoff values should be ethnic and gender specific needs to be addressed. We would like to propose that in developing a pediatric definition of the metabolic syndrome, three issues be considered: (1) individual components should be similar to those of adults for sake of comparison and to evaluate tracking; (2) current recommendations and cutoff values need to be developed or reevaluated, particularly for waist circumference, dyslipidemia, and perhaps hyperglycemia; and (3) the use of single cutoff values (as opposed to multiple cutoff values depending on gender, age, ethnicity) might be easier to apply but less sensitive in identifying children at risk. A working definition of the metabolic syndrome in childhood should certainly be put forth but will require consensus among both clinicians and scientists and hopefully will be developed in the near future.

STRATEGIES FOR SCREENING AND TREATMENT OF THE METABOLIC SYNDROME IN CHILDREN AND ADOLESCENTS

Despite the lack of a uniform definition of the metabolic syndrome in childhood, and the use of different cutoff values, the prevalence of the metabolic syndrome in childhood and adolescence is relatively low irrespective of the definition used. The exception is overweight youth. Recent studies have shown that the metabolic syndrome is strikingly high among overweight children and adolescents,[17,22] and suggest that Hispanic youth (predominantly of Mexican American ancestry) may be at increased risk compared with whites.[22] These findings suggest that although screening for the metabolic syndrome is probably not warranted in the pediatric population as a whole, screening of overweight children and adolescents, and particularly those belonging to specific minority groups, may be necessary. Although current pediatric guidelines recommend screening for obesity,[52] type 2 diabetes,[1] hypertension,[28] and dyslipidemias[53–56] in at-risk children and adolescents, they do so under the domain of individual pediatric specialties. Therefore, screening for the metabolic syndrome in overweight children and adolescents (as opposed to screening for individual disease outcomes related to the syndrome) may help simplify screening strategies and raise awareness, both at the physician level and in the individual member or family level, of the combined risk for both type 2 diabetes and cardiovascular disease among overweight youth. In addition, it may simplify the need for multiple recommendations and guidelines for the identification and treatment of overweight youth for separate diseases processes (e.g., obesity, hypertension, type 2 diabetes), which in reality overlap due to a shared pathophysiology. Although this may be viewed by some as cumbersome and difficult to implement, the current recommendations for screening already include screening for several features of the syndrome and all agree that overweight youth are at particular risk. The exception is waist circumference (for which there are no recommendations) and to a certain extent fasting lipids. Based on our current understanding of obesity, insulin resistance, and the metabolic syndrome, screening for adverse lipids should be instituted in all overweight children and adolescents. Support for this view is provided by the finding that adverse lipids (high triglycerides and low HDL cholesterol) are by far the most common risk factor associated with the metabolic syndrome in childhood[17,22] and appear to be due to underlying insulin resistance.[2] In summary, pediatric recommendations may need to be updated so that the existing multiple guidelines are more consistent and address the purpose of screening — identifying and treating children at risk. The development of a comprehensive guideline to screen and identify children with the metabolic syndrome might prove more useful in the prevention of the major disease outcomes related to the metabolic syndrome — type 2 diabetes and cardiovascular disease in childhood.

STRATEGIES FOR TREATMENT OF THE METABOLIC SYNDROME

The identification of children with the metabolic syndrome might help to direct treatment strategies by focusing on the underlying pathophysiology (e.g., insulin resistance) rather than on individual risk factors. We propose that targeting insulin resistance (as opposed to weight loss) may be more effective in preventing or delaying the onset of cardiovascular disease and type 2 diabetes in high-risk youth because strategies aimed at reducing body weight have been for the most part unsuccessful. For instance, insulin resistance and its associated risk factors may be improved directly or indirectly through specific exercise modalities, dietary interventions, and/or pharmacological agents without the need to make large changes in body fatness. For instance, a recent study showed that high intensity physical training for 8 months in overweight adolescents resulted in improvements in fasting plasma triglycerides, LDL particle size, and diastolic blood pressure even though there was little change in body fatness.[57] Alternatively, nonweight-bearing activities such as strength training may be more acceptable in overweight children and may serve to enhance long-term health.[58] Specific nutrients such as dietary fiber, for example, may improve insulin sensitivity and glucose homeostasis through various mechanisms related to decreased gastric emptying, increased fat oxidation, decreased hepatic output of glucose, and stimulation of GLP-1 secretion (reviewed in Pereira and Ludwig[59]). Support for this view comes from a recent report in which whole grain consumption was found to be associated with greater insulin sensitivity and lower body mass index in adolescents, and this association was stronger among the heaviest adolescents.[39] Other nutrients that may have beneficial effects on insulin sensitivity are the phytoestrogens. Nutritional intervention studies performed in animals and humans suggest that the ingestion of soy protein associated with isoflavones and flaxseed rich in lignans improves glucose control and insulin resistance (reviewed in Bhathena and Velasquez[60]). Finally, in very high risk, insulin-resistant children, pharmacotherapy may be indicated. A recent double-blind randomized trial in obese, insulin resistant youth, aged 12 to 19 years, treated with metformin for 6 months, showed significant improvements in glucose tolerance and fasting insulin.[61] Other agents that may prove beneficial in the treatment of insulin resistance in high risk youth are the thiazolidinediones, which are much more potent insulin sensitizers than metformin. Thiazolidinediones have been shown to improve insulin sensitivity, glucose tolerance, and cardiovascular risk factors in type 2 diabetes, impaired glucose tolerance, and nondiabetic insulin-resistant obese subjects.[62–65] In summary, more research needs to be conducted to establish the effectiveness of different types of interventions on insulin sensitivity in children. It is likely that beneficial and long-lasting health effects will be achieved only through the combined approaches that are gender, age and culturally sensitive.

CONCLUSIONS

In conclusion, the prevalence of the metabolic syndrome, although very low in normal weight children (BMI < 85th percentile), is high in those that are overweight (BMI > 95th percentile). Approximately 30% of overweight children have the metabolic syndrome and 9 out of 10 have at least one feature of the syndrome. The underlying insulin resistance of obesity seems to be an important pathophysiological event contributing to the syndrome, and this is already evident in childhood. Because the number of overweight children is increasing and it is evident that the pathology begins early in life, we advocate the creation of a definition of the metabolic syndrome in childhood with comprehensive screening of overweight children based partly on current pediatric guidelines. Future research is needed to investigate the effects of lifestyle and pharmacological interventions aimed at improving insulin resistance in overweight children.

ACKNOWLEDGMENTS

This work was supported by a National Institutes of Health grant R01 DK 59211.

REFERENCES

1. American Diabetes Association. Type 2 diabetes in children and adolescents. *Pediatrics*. 2000;105(3 Pt 1): 671–680.
2. Goran MI, Bergman RN, Avila Q, Watkins M, Ball GD, Shaibi GQ, et al. Impaired glucose tolerance and reduced beta-cell function in overweight Latino children with a positive family history for type 2 diabetes. *J Clin Endocrinol Metab*. 2004;89(1): 207–212.
3. Sinha R, Fisch G, Teague B, Tamborlane WV, Banyas B, Allen K, et al. Prevalence of impaired glucose tolerance among children and adolescents with marked obesity. *N Engl J Med*. 2002;346(11): 802–810.
4. Daniels SR, Morrison JA, Sprecher DL, Khoury P, Kimball TR. Association of body fat distribution and cardiovascular risk factors in children and adolescents. *Circulation*. 1999;99(4): 541–545.
5. Berenson GS, Srinivasan SR, Bao W, Newman WP, III, Tracy RE, Wattigney WA. Association between multiple cardiovascular risk factors and atherosclerosis in children and young adults. The Bogalusa Heart Study. *N Engl J Med*. 1998;338(23): 1650–1656.
6. Gulekli B, Turhan NO, Senoz S, Kukner S, Oral H, Gokmen O. Endocrinological, ultrasonographic and clinical findings in adolescent and adult polycystic ovary patients: a comparative study. *Gynecol Endocrinol*. 1993;7(4): 273–277.
7. Rashid M, Roberts EA. Nonalcoholic steatohepatitis in children. *J Pediatr Gastroenterol Nutr*. 2000;30(1): 48–53.
8. Fishbein MH, Miner M, Mogren C, Chalekson J. The spectrum of fatty liver in obese children and the relationship of serum aminotransferases to severity of steatosis. *J Pediatr Gastroenterol Nutr*. 2003;36(1): 54–61.
9. National Institutes of Health. The Third Report of the National Cholesterol Education Program Expert Panel on Detection, Evaluation, and Treatment of High Blood Cholesterol in Adults (Adult Treatment Panel III). 01–3670. 2001. Bethesda, MD, National Insitutes of Health. NIH Publication 01–3670.
10. Alexander CM, Landsman PB, Teutsch SM, Haffner SM. NCEP-defined metabolic syndrome, diabetes, and prevalence of coronary heart disease among NHANES III participants age 50 years and older. *Diabetes* 2003;52(5): 1210–1214.
11. Ford ES, Giles WH, Dietz WH. Prevalence of the metabolic syndrome among US adults: findings from the third National Health and Nutrition Examination Survey. *JAMA*. 2002;287(3): 356–359.
12. Meigs JB, Wilson PW, Nathan DM, D'Agostino RB, Sr., Williams K, Haffner SM. Prevalence and characteristics of the metabolic syndrome in the San Antonio Heart and Framingham Offspring Studies. *Diabetes*. 2003;52(8): 2160–2167.
13. Isomaa B, Almgren P, Tuomi T, Forsen B, Lahti K, Nissen M, et al. Cardiovascular morbidity and mortality associated with the metabolic syndrome. *Diabetes Care*. 2001;24(4): 683–689.
14. Lakka HM, Laaksonen DE, Lakka TA, Niskanen LK, Kumpusalo E, Tuomilehto J, et al. The metabolic syndrome and total and cardiovascular disease mortality in middle-aged men. *JAMA*. 2002;288(21): 2709–2716.
15. Laaksonen DE, Lakka HM, Niskanen LK, Kaplan GA, Salonen JT, Lakka TA. Metabolic syndrome and development of diabetes mellitus: application and validation of recently suggested definitions of the metabolic syndrome in a prospective cohort study. *Am J Epidemiol*. 2002;156(11): 1070–1077.
16. Hanson RL, Imperatore G, Bennett PH, Knowler WC. Components of the "metabolic syndrome" and incidence of type 2 diabetes. *Diabetes*. 2002;51(10): 3120–3127.

17. Cruz ML, Weigensberg MJ, Huang TT, Ball G, Shaibi GQ, Goran MI. The metabolic syndrome in overweight Hispanic youth and the role of insulin sensitivity. *J Clin Endocrinol Metab*. 2004;89(1): 108–113.

18. Weiss R, Dziura J, Burgert TS, Tamborlane WV, Taksali SE, Yeckel CW, et al. Obesity and the metabolic syndrome in children and adolescents. *N Engl J Med*. 2004;350(23): 2362–2374.

19. McGill HC, Jr., McMahan CA, Herderick EE, Zieske AW, Malcom GT, Tracy RE, et al. Obesity accelerates the progression of coronary atherosclerosis in young men. *Circulation*. 2002;105(23): 2712–2718.

20. Freedman DS, Dietz WH, Srinivasan SR, Berenson GS. The relation of overweight to cardiovascular risk factors among children and adolescents: the Bogalusa Heart Study. *Pediatrics*. 1999;103(6 Pt 1): 1175–1182.

21. Resnicow K, Futterman R, Vaughan RD. Body mass index as a predictor of systolic blood pressure in a multiracial sample of US schoolchildren. *Ethn Dis*. 1993;3(4): 351–361.

22. Cook S, Weitzman M, Auinger P, Nguyen M, Dietz WH. Prevalence of a metabolic syndrome phenotype in adolescents: findings from the third National Health and Nutrition Examination Survey, 1988–1994. *Arch Pediatr Adolesc Med*. 2003;157(8): 821–827.

23. Chen W, Srinivasan SR, Elkasabany A, Berenson GS. Cardiovascular risk factors clustering features of insulin resistance syndrome (syndrome X) in a biracial (black-white) population of children, adolescents, and young adults: the Bogalusa Heart Study. *Am J Epidemiol*. 1999;150(7): 667–674.

24. Chen W, Bao W, Begum S, Elkasabany A, Srinivasan SR, Berenson GS. Age-related patterns of the clustering of cardiovascular risk variables of syndrome X from childhood to young adulthood in a population made up of black and white subjects: the Bogalusa Heart Study. *Diabetes*. 2000;49(6): 1042–1048.

25. Raitakari OT, Porkka KV, Ronnemaa T, Knip M, Uhari M, Akerblom HK, et al. The role of insulin in clustering of serum lipids and blood pressure in children and adolescents. The Cardiovascular Risk in Young Finns Study. *Diabetologia*. 1995;38(9): 1042–1050.

26. Strauss RS, Pollack HA. Epidemic increase in childhood overweight, 1986–1998. *JAMA*. 2001;286(22): 2845–2848.

27. Hickman TB, Briefel RR, Carroll MD, Rifkind BM, Cleeman JI, Maurer KR, et al. Distributions and trends of serum lipid levels among United States children and adolescents ages 4–19 years: data from the Third National Health and Nutrition Examination Survey. *Prev Med*. 1998;27(6): 879–890.

28. Update on the 1987 Task Force Report on High Blood Pressure in Children and Adolescents: a working group report from the National High Blood Pressure Education Program. National High Blood Pressure Education Program Working Group on Hypertension Control in Children and Adolescents. *Pediatrics*. 1996;98(4 Pt 1): 649–658.

29. American Diabetes Association. Clinical practice recommendations 2002. *Diabetes Care* 2002;25 Suppl 1: S1–147.

30. McKeigue PM, Ferrie JE, Pierpoint T, Marmot MG. Association of early-onset coronary heart disease in South Asian men with glucose intolerance and hyperinsulinemia. *Circulation*. 1993;87(1): 152–161.

31. Grundy SM. What is the contribution of obesity to the metabolic syndrome? *Endocrinol Metab Clin North Am*. 2004;33(2): 267–282.

32. Goran MI, Ball GD, Cruz ML. Obesity and risk of type 2 diabetes and cardiovascular disease in children and adolescents. *J Clin Endocrinol Metab*. 2003;88(4): 1417–1427.

33. Reaven GM. Insulin resistance and compensatory hyperinsulinemia: role in hypertension, dyslipidemia, and coronary heart disease. *Am Heart J*. 1991;121(4 Pt 2): 1283–1288.

34. Reaven GM. Banting lecture 1988. Role of insulin resistance in human disease. *Diabetes*. 1988;37(12): 1595–1607.

35. Liese AD, Mayer-Davis EJ, Tyroler HA, Davis CE, Keil U, Duncan BB, et al. Development of the multiple metabolic syndrome in the ARIC cohort: joint contribution of insulin, BMI, and WHR. Atherosclerosis risk in communities. *Ann Epidemiol*. 1997;7(6): 407–416.

36. Ferrannini E, Muscelli E, Stern MP, Haffner SM. Differential impact of insulin and obesity on cardiovascular risk factors in non-diabetic subjects. *Int J Obes Relat Metab Disord*. 1996;20(1): 7–14.

37. Srinivasan SR, Myers L, Berenson GS. Predictability of childhood adiposity and insulin for developing insulin resistance syndrome (syndrome X) in young adulthood: the Bogalusa Heart Study. *Diabetes*. 2002;51(1): 204–209.

38. Cruz ML, Huang TTK, Johnson MS, Gower BA, Goran MI. Insulin sensitivity and blood pressure in black and white children. *Hypertension.* 2002;40(1): 18–22.

39. Sinaiko AR, Jacobs DR, Jr., Steinberger J, Moran A, Luepker R, Rocchini AP, et al. Insulin resistance syndrome in childhood: associations of the euglycemic insulin clamp and fasting insulin with fatness and other risk factors. *J Pediatr.* 2001;139(5): 700–707.

40. Devaraj S, Rosenson RS, Jialal I. Metabolic syndrome: an appraisal of the pro-inflammatory and procoagulant status. *Endocrinol Metab Clin North Am.* 2004;33(2): 431–53.

41. Yudkin JS, Kumari M, Humphries SE, Mohamed-Ali V. Inflammation, obesity, stress and coronary heart disease: is interleukin-6 the link? *Atherosclerosis.* 2000;148(2): 209–214.

42. Yudkin JS. Adipose tissue, insulin action and vascular disease: inflammatory signals. *Int J Obes Relat Metab Disord.* 2003;27(Suppl 3): S25–S28.

43. Despres JP. Inflammation and cardiovascular disease: is abdominal obesity the missing link? *Int J Obes Relat Metab Disord.* 2003;27(Suppl 3): S22–S24.

44. Weiss R, Dufour S, Groszmann A, Petersen K, Dziura J, Taksali SE, et al. Low adiponectin levels in adolescent obesity: a marker of increased intramyocellular lipid accumulation. *J Clin Endocrinol Metab.* 2003;88(5): 2014–2018.

45. Gillum RF. Association of serum C-reactive protein and indices of body fat distribution and overweight in Mexican American children. *J Natl Med Assoc.* 2003;95(7): 545–552.

46. Kriketos AD, Greenfield JR, Peake PW, Furler SM, Denyer GS, Charlesworth JA, et al. Inflammation, insulin resistance, and adiposity: a study of first-degree relatives of type 2 diabetic subjects. *Diabetes Care.* 2004;27(8): 2033–2040.

47. Falck-Ytter Y, Younossi ZM, Marchesini G, McCullough AJ. Clinical features and natural history of nonalcoholic steatosis syndromes. *Semin Liver Dis.* 2001;21(1): 17–26.

48. Marchesini G, Brizi M, Bianchi G, Tomassetti S, Bugianesi E, Lenzi M, et al. Nonalcoholic fatty liver disease: a feature of the metabolic syndrome. *Diabetes.* 2001;50(8): 1844–1850.

49. Baldridge AD, Perez-Atayde AR, Graeme-Cook F, Higgins L, Lavine JE. Idiopathic steatohepatitis in childhood: a multicenter retrospective study. *J Pediatr.* 1995;127(5): 700–704.

50. Tominaga K, Kurata JH, Chen YK, Fujimoto E, Miyagawa S, Abe I, et al. Prevalence of fatty liver in Japanese children and relationship to obesity. An epidemiological ultrasonographic survey. *Dig Dis Sci.* 1995;40(9): 2002–2009.

51. Schwimmer JB, Deutsch R, Rauch JB, Behling C, Newbury R, Lavine JE. Obesity, insulin resistance, and other clinicopathological correlates of pediatric nonalcoholic fatty liver disease. *J Pediatr.* 2003;143(4): 500–505.

52. Barlow SE, Dietz WH. Obesity evaluation and treatment: Expert Committee recommendations. The Maternal and Child Health Bureau, Health Resources and Services Administration and the Department of Health and Human Services. *Pediatrics.* 1998;102(3): E29.

53. National Cholesterol Education Program. Report of the Expert Panel on Blood Cholesterol Levels in Children and Adolescents. US Department of Health and Human Services. National Heart, Blood and Lung Institute. NIH Publication No. 91–2732, 1991.

54. Williams CL, Hayman LL, Daniels SR, Robinson TN, Steinberger J, Paridon S, et al. Cardiovascular health in childhood: a statement for health professionals from the Committee on Atherosclerosis, Hypertension, and Obesity in the Young (AHOY) of the Council on Cardiovascular Disease in the Young, American Heart Association. *Circulation.* 2002;106(1): 143–160.

55. Kavey RE, Daniels SR, Lauer RM, Atkins DL, Hayman LL, Taubert K. American Heart Association guidelines for primary prevention of atherosclerotic cardiovascular disease beginning in childhood. *Circulation.* 2003;107(11): 1562–1566.

56. Steinberger J, Daniels SR. Obesity, insulin resistance, diabetes, and cardiovascular risk in children: an American Heart Association scientific statement from the Atherosclerosis, Hypertension, and Obesity in the Young Committee (Council on Cardiovascular Disease in the Young) and the Diabetes Committee (Council on Nutrition, Physical Activity, and Metabolism). *Circulation.* 2003;107(10): 1448–1453.

57. Kang HS, Gutin B, Barbeau P, Owens S, Lemmon CR, Allison J, et al. Physical training improves insulin resistance syndrome markers in obese adolescents. *Med Sci Sports Exerc.* 2002;34(12): 1920–1927.

58. Bernhardt DT, Gomez J, Johnson MD, Martin TJ, Rowland TW, Small E, et al. Strength training by children and adolescents. *Pediatrics*. 2001;107(6): 1470–1472.

59. Pereira MA, Ludwig DS. Dietary fiber and body-weight regulation. Observations and mechanisms. *Pediatr Clin North Am*. 2001;48(4): 969–980.

60. Bhathena SJ, Velasquez MT. Beneficial role of dietary phytoestrogens in obesity and diabetes. *Am J Clin Nutr*. 2002;76(6): 1191–1201.

61. Freemark M, Bursey D. The effects of metformin on body mass index and glucose tolerance in obese adolescents with fasting hyperinsulinemia and a family history of type 2 diabetes. *Pediatrics*. 2001;107(4): art-e55.

62. Antonucci T, Whitcomb R, McLain R, Lockwood D, Norris RM. Impaired glucose tolerance is normalized by treatment with the thiazolidinedione troglitazone. *Diabetes Care*. 1997;20(2): 188–193.

63. Ghazzi MN, Perez JE, Antonucci TK, Driscoll JH, Huang SM, Faja BW, et al. Cardiac and glycemic benefits of troglitazone treatment in NIDDM. The Troglitazone Study Group. *Diabetes*. 1997;46(3): 433–439.

64. Miyazaki Y, Mahankali A, Matsuda M, Mahankali S, Hardies J, Cusi K, et al. Effect of pioglitazone on abdominal fat distribution and insulin sensitivity in type 2 diabetic patients. *J Clin Endocrinol Metab*. 2002;87(6): 2784–2791.

65. Yamasaki Y, Kawamori R, Wasada T, Sato A, Omori Y, Eguchi H, et al. Pioglitazone (AD-4833) ameliorates insulin resistance in patients with NIDDM. AD-4833 Glucose Clamp Study Group, Japan. *Tohoku J Exp Med*. 1997;183(3): 173–183.

13 Behavioral Aspects of Food Intake: Implications and Potential Targets for Overweight Prevention

Tanja V.E. Kral, Meredith S. Dolan, Julia Kerns, and Myles S. Faith

CONTENTS

INTRODUCTION

"Food is fun, fundamental, frightening, and far-reaching."[1] That is to say, food has a fundamental and pervasive role in the lives of children, fueling essential biological functions for growth and development while serving an integral role in children's peer relations. This is especially true as children undergo dramatic biological and psychosocial transitions during puberty, when the influences of parents on children's food choices gradually diminish and those of peers gradually augment. Eating behavior is critical for attaining successful energy balance (see Chapters 7 and 8), and so efforts to modify unhealthy eating behaviors in children (i.e., those that promote excessive energy intake) will likely be critical for successful prevention initiatives. To this end, it is important to understand the controls of a child's eating behavior — especially those that can be more readily transformed to achieve healthier intake patterns. This, however, as any parent or child caregiver knows, is no simple task. Children are often picky in their food choices, usually prefer foods they find palatable, and can resist efforts of parents and caregivers to promote healthy eating behaviors. Hence, identifying the controls of a child's eating behavior — ones that can be modified and accepted by children — is of the utmost importance.

This chapter addresses the behavioral aspects of food intake in children, focusing on the controls of a child's eating behavior. We emphasize modifiable factors that in theory if not practiced, could be changed to support initiatives to prevent overweight in children. The chapter emphasizes *breadth* rather than *depth* of topic coverage, underscoring the range of modifiable influences that can improve a child's eating behavior. Following this introduction, the second section presents the rationale for targeting small but sustainable changes in a child's eating behavior to help support overweight prevention initiatives. Noting that childhood overweight results from very subtle but sustained energy imbalances, this section suggests that modest, sustainable changes in children's eating practices may help to curb excess weight gain in children. The third section reviews the effects of specific food presentation strategies, including the influence of portion sizes, frequency of food exposure, and role modeling. The fourth section reviews the effects of specific food properties, including the influence of glycemic index, sugar-sweetened beverage intake, and energy density (kilocalories per gram). The fifth section reviews the effects of familial feeding styles and meal patterns, including parental feeding styles, family meals and TV viewing, and snacking practices. Finally, we review a list of refined child eating traits that may offer targets for prevention initiatives in growing children (i.e., energy compensation ability, eating in the absence of hunger). We conclude by summarizing the literature and providing thoughts for future research.

MODIFYING EATING BEHAVIOR FOR OVERWEIGHT PREVENTION: CAN SMALL CHANGES HELP ACHIEVE ENERGY BALANCE?

The development of overweight in growing children occurs from a daily energy imbalance (between intake and expenditure) as subtle as 2%, if sustained over time. This is the equivalent of ~125 kJ/day, or ~30 kcal/day.[2] As Goran[2] notes, this energy imbalance can be rectified by substituting physical activity for 15 min/day of television viewing. Expressed in terms of food intake, this subtle energy imbalance is even more striking. Table 13.1 presents the corresponding energy equivalent

---

TABLE 13.1
Energy Equivalents of 30 kcal from Popular Children's Snack Foods

2 Barnum's Animal Crackers
1/3 Chips Ahoy! Chocolate Chip Cookie
8 Plain M&Ms
1/3 cup Pepsi or Coca-Cola
3 Ruffles Potato Chips
0.15 cups Orville Redenbacher's Light Microwave Popcorn
6 Rold Gold Tiny Pretzel Twists

Source: Adapted from Borushek A. *The Doctor's Pocket Calorie Fat & Carbohydrate Counter.* Costa Mesa, CA: Family Health Publications; 2004.

---

of 30 kcal from popular child snack foods.[3] The table illustrates that all else being equal, and assuming no compensatory changes in energy expenditure, modest but sustained changes in child daily energy intake may have a potent effect on curbing excess weight gain in growing children. For these very reasons, expert guidelines for obesity prevention often recommend that young children who are at risk for overweight maintain their current body weight, capitalizing on their increasing height velocity to prevent the onset of overweight.[4] Such efforts do not necessarily require aggressive restrictions in children's daily energy intake and, in principle, can be achieved by substituting foods of lower energy density for foods of higher energy density.

EFFECTS OF FOOD PRESENTATION STRATEGIES

PORTION SIZES

Young children appear to have an innate ability to regulate energy intake[5–7] such that they generally maintain a consistent level of energy intake across meals. However, children's ability to self-regulate energy intake may be undermined by "supersizing" the portion sizes of foods that are served to them. Portion sizes of foods that are sold at restaurants, fast-food outlets, take-out establishments, and supermarkets have increased considerably over the past few decades.[8] There has also been a trend for individuals and families to consume more and more meals away from home.[9] These trends are concerning given evidence that portion size changes can affect energy intake. In studies that systematically varied the amount of food served to young adult participants, food and energy intake significantly increased with increasing portion sizes.[10] This finding held true for a variety of foods including both amorphous foods (i.e., foods with no distinct shape)[11,12] as well as unit-type foods such as sandwiches.[13]

Whether children overeat in response to increasing portion sizes appears to depend on their age. A study conducted in 3- and 5-year-old preschool children was designed to investigate the effects of portion size on children's food intake.[14] Children of both age groups were served macaroni and cheese for lunch on three different occasions. The portion size of the lunch entrée was varied (small = 150 g, medium = 263 g, and large = 376 g for 3-year-old children; small = 225 g, medium = 338 g, and large = 450 g for 5-year-old children) across three test days, and children were given *ad libitum* access to the respective lunch entrées. Results showed that 5-year-old children consumed a significantly greater amount of macaroni and cheese when served the large portion compared with when they were served the small portion. In 3 year olds, however, there was no effect of portion size on energy intake (see Figure 13.1). These younger children ate similar amounts of the lunch entrée on all three occasions, regardless of the portion size served. Findings from this experiment demonstrate that as children get older they may become more responsive to environmental cues, such as the portion size of foods, rather than internal hunger and satiety cues, when determining the amount of food they consume.

In a follow-up study, Fisher et al.[15] repeatedly exposed 3- to 5-year-old children to large portions of a macaroni and cheese lunch entrée. Children were served two series of four lunches, which were separated by 2 weeks. During one series an age-appropriate portion (i.e., reference portion) was served to children; during the other series a large portion (i.e., double the reference portion) was served. On separate test meal occasions that followed each of the two lunch series, children were asked to self-serve their own food from a serving bowl that contained the large portion of the lunch entrée. Results indicated that doubling the age-appropriate portion of an entrée increased children's entrée intake by 25% and increased their total lunch intake (i.e., energy from entrée plus other items) by 15%. On the other hand, when children were allowed to serve themselves, they consumed 25% *less* energy compared with when they were being served a large entrée portion.

Findings from a recently published cross-sectional study are in concordance with these laboratory-based findings. McConahy et al.[16] evaluated the relationship between food intake behaviors and total energy intake among children aged 2 to 5 years old participating in the Continuing Survey

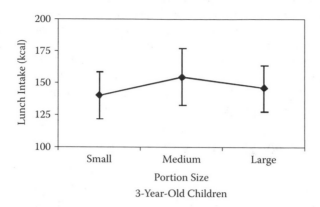

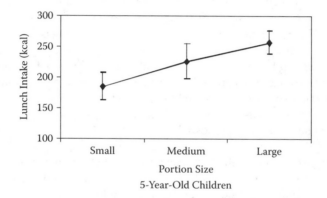

FIGURE 13.1 Effects of portion size servings on *ad libitum* lunch intake in 3-year-old children (upper panel) and 5-year-old children (lower panel). (Data from Rolls BJ, Engell D, Birch LL. *J Am Dietetic Assoc.* 2000;100(2): 232–234.)

of Food Intakes by Individuals, 1994–1996, 1998 (CSFII 94–96, 98). Children's dietary intake was measured by two 24-h dietary recalls. The results showed that the portion size of 10 commonly eaten foods was a significant predictor of energy intake, explaining nearly 20% of the variance in energy intake.

In conclusion, evidence is emerging that young children's energy intake can be influenced by the portion sizes of foods served to them, as is the case for adults. These findings suggest the potential merits of providing children with age-appropriate portion sizes and allowing children to self-serve their own food as overweight prevention strategies.

FREQUENCY OF FOOD EXPOSURE

As weaning infants are being introduced to solid foods, all foods are novel to them at first. The initial reaction of children to novel foods typically is one of rejection. The unwillingness of children to eat novel foods has been referred to as "neophobia."[17] It is by repeated exposure to novel foods and the experience of positive or negative postingestive consequences that children begin to establish food preferences and aversions.[1]

From a developmental perspective, it is desirable to give children access to a variety of foods to ensure adequate nutrient intake. Children who exhibit high levels of neophobia tend to be less willing to try new foods.[18] A study conducted by Falciglia et al.[19] found that 8- to 10-year-old

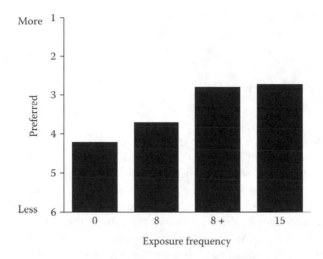

FIGURE 13.2 Effects of frequency of novel food exposure on young children's preference ratings for those foods. (Adapted from Sullivan SA, Birch LL. *Dev. Psychol.* 1990;26(4): 546–551.)

children who showed high levels of neophobia consumed a significantly less varied diet than did children who exhibited an average or high willingness to try new foods.

One potential strategy to reduce food neophobia in children is through repeated exposure to novel foods, as the frequency of exposure to novel foods can alter children's food acceptance and food preferences. To investigate this phenomenon, Sullivan and Birch[20] repeatedly exposed 4- to 5-year-old children to one of three initially novel food items (i.e., salty tofu, sweet tofu, or plain tofu). Results indicated that increased exposure to flavored tofu significantly increased children's preferences for that tofu version, with 8 to 15 exposures being optimal for this shift in preference to occur (see Figure 13.2).

In a recent study by Wardle et al.,[21] 5- to 7-year-old children were randomly assigned to one of three groups: an exposure-based intervention, a reward-based intervention, or a no-treatment control group. Children in the exposure-based intervention group were encouraged to taste bite size sweet red pepper and then to rate their acceptance of the pepper, while children in the reward-based group were given a sticker if they tried at least one piece of red pepper. Results indicated that acceptance of red pepper was significantly greater in the exposure group compared with the control group. The reward-based group showed an intermediate level of change, which did not significantly differ from either the exposure-based intervention group or the control group. Because food preferences play a large role in determining intake,[22] interventions that aim to increase acceptance of low-energy nutrient-dense foods through repeated exposure may represent useful strategies to achieve improved long-term dietary changes.

Role Modeling

Another strategy to increase children's acceptance of a variety of foods is through role modeling or observational learning. Hendy and Raudenbush[23] found that modeling by a teacher was effective in influencing a child's food selections if the teacher was enthusiastic, rather than silent, about the experimental foods. However, the effectiveness of an enthusiastic teacher role model was nullified in the presence of a peer model who encouraged consumption of a different food. Another study[24] demonstrated that trained female peer models were more successful than trained peer males in increasing food acceptance among preschool children. Likewise, peer modeling was shown to have a greater influence on younger children than on older children.[22] Thus, modeling healthy eating behaviors can be an effective way to enhance food acceptance and increase the consumption of a variety of healthful foods (e.g., fruits, vegetables, whole grain products). However, the potency of this phenomenon may depend on a range of role model attributes (e.g., age, sex, personality, teacher vs. peer).

EFFECTS OF FOOD PROPERTIES

GLYCEMIC INDEX

A property of food known as the glycemic index (GI) has been the focus of several laboratory-based experiments (reviewed in more detail in Chapter 18). The ingestion of a low GI meal compared with a high GI meal has been shown to decrease feelings of hunger,[25,26] increase feelings of satiety,[27,28] and reduce energy intake.[29,30] The proposed mechanism of action by which the GI of foods is believed to exert its effects on hunger and satiety is by promoting pancreatic hormone secretion and subsequently altering the availability of metabolic fuels after the ingestion of a meal.

Studying the effects of GI on food intake and separating them from other potential influences (e.g., energy density or the volume of food) is a challenging task. The formulation of experimental meals demands skill and knowledge about specific properties of foods because the GI of a meal is easily affected by a multitude of factors that co-occur within a single meal (e.g., macronutrient composition and fiber content of accompanying foods in a meal). One of the challenges for nutritional science will be to disaggregate these influences on child appetite and food intake. Practically, low GI foods may have a role in overweight prevention by promoting nonrestrictive eating practices and increased consumption of lower energy-dense foods.

SUGAR-SWEETENED BEVERAGE INTAKE

Excess intake of sugar-sweetened beverages may promote excess weight gain in growing children and adolescents. Ludwig et al.[31] conducted a longitudinal study of 548 ethnically diverse 11- and 12-year-old children attending Boston schools; they were followed for 19 months. The researchers found a positive association between soda intake and excess weight gain, such that each additional serving of a sugar-sweetened beverage was associated with an additional increase in body mass index (BMI; kg/m^2) of 0.024 kg/m^2 over 19 months. Potential mechanisms for this association were not tested, but they may involve the high GI of sugar-sweetened beverages or the ingestion of excess energy from soda. To the extent that children do not compensate for the energy consumed from sugar-sweetened beverages, this will result in a positive energy balance.

More recently, Newby et al.[32] tested whether daily intake of sugar-sweetened beverages, fruit juices, diet sodas, and milk promoted excess weight gain over 1 and 2 years in 9- to 14-year-old children. Beverage intake was measured by a semiquantitative food frequency questionnaire, and BMI was calculated from self-reported weight and height, ascertained in 1996, 1997, and 1998. Results indicated that among boys each additional serving of a sugar-sweetened beverage consumed was significantly associated with an additional 0.004 kg/m^2 gain in BMI over 1 year. Boys who increased their sugar-sweetened beverage intake from the prior year by 2 or more servings per day showed a significantly greater 1-year BMI gain than boys whose sugar-sweetened beverage intake remained unchanged. Among girls, comparable patterns of results were observed, although the effects were smaller and did not reach statistical significance. Among both sexes, the association between sugar-sweetened beverage intake and weight (gain) was eliminated after controlling for total energy intake. This suggests that the mechanism by which sugar-sweetened beverage intake promotes overweight is by introducing extra calories into the diet.

That sugar-sweetened beverage consumption can influence weight gain in children was demonstrated in a randomized trial by James et al.[33] The investigators examined whether a school-based educational program aimed to reduce carbonated beverage consumption could prevent excess weight gain in 7- to 11-year-old children. Classrooms were randomly assigned to a control group or an

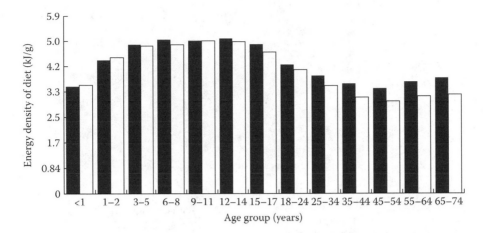

FIGURE 13.3 Age-related changes in the energy density levels of self-selected diets in a national sample of children and adults (■ Males; □ Females). (From Drewnowski A. *Proc Nutrition Soc.* 2000;59(2): 239–244. Reprinted with permission.)

intervention group, in which the benefits of a healthy diet and decreased consumption of "fizzy" drinks were taught. After 12 months, the percentage of overweight children increased by 0.75% in the control group compared with a 0.02% decrease in the intervention group. These results provide experimental evidence that interventions targeting decreased soft drink consumption can effectively decrease the risk of excess weight gain in children.

ENERGY DENSITY

The energy density (kilocalorie per gram) of foods influences energy intake, as demonstrated by studies that systematically varied the energy density of single meals served in the laboratory while holding macronutrient composition and palatability similar. These studies showed that increasing the energy density of the diet consistently promoted increased energy intake during the meal in young adults.[34,35] Comparable laboratory experiments with children are needed, although existing data implicate the importance of energy density in controlling children's energy intake. Data from the National Health and Nutrition Examination Surveys (NHANES) suggest developmental differences in the energy density of self-selected diets across the lifespan. Drewnowski[36] summarizes that young children exhibit a high preference for energy-dense foods, which may foster their growth and development. As shown in Figure 13.3, the energy density of self-selected diets reaches its peak during later childhood and adolescence, and then gradually declines during adulthood.

Children have a predisposition for learning to prefer foods that are high in energy density over those which are more energy dilute. In a series of elegant studies, Birch and colleagues[37–39] repeatedly exposed 2- to 5-year-old children to fixed amounts of foods and drinks that differed in flavors and were either high or low in fat content and energy density. Results indicated that children more readily developed preferences for flavors associated with high energy–dense foods and drinks.

In a cross-sectional study, Martí-Henneberg and colleagues[40] observed that energy intake, food volume, and energy density in the diet, measured by 24-h dietary recalls, progressively increased between 1 to 2 years and 13 to 15 years of age. The age-related increases in energy density were 47% and 33% for boys and girls, respectively. Toward the end of puberty and early adulthood (21 to 30 years of age), the investigators observed a significant decrease in dietary energy density in both sexes. These findings agree with the observation that food preferences undergo a shift during adolescence and early adulthood away from sweet foods toward a more varied diet that includes more energy-diluted foods such as fruits and vegetables.[41,42]

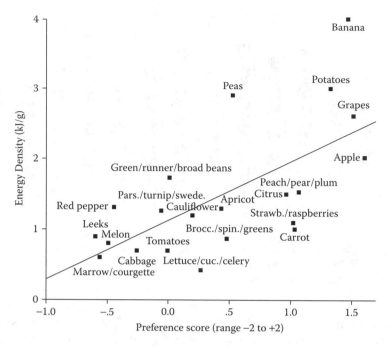

FIGURE 13.4 Association between children's reported preferences for fruits and vegetables and the energy densities of those foods. (From Gibson EL, Wardle J. *Appetite*. 2003;41(1): 97–98. Reprinted with permission from Elsevier.)

Children's learned preference for foods of a higher energy density has also been found in a study which examined preferences for fruits and vegetables. Gibson and Wardle[43] showed that children between the ages of 4 and 5 years showed a greater preference for fruits and vegetables that are relatively higher in energy density compared with those of relatively lower energy density. As shown in Figure 13.4, children's preference scores for fruits and vegetables were significantly positively correlated with the energy density of the foods. Inspection of the graph reveals that the foods most highly preferred by children were not only higher in energy density but also contained more sugar and therefore were sweeter in taste.

A question that remains to be clarified is whether one can dissociate a preference for more energy-dense foods from a preference for sweeter foods (i.e., those with a high sugar content) such as fruits. When Gibson and Wardle controlled for total sugar content in vegetables, the positive relationship between food preferences and the energy density of food remained significant. Foods of high energy density are often higher in fat and sugar, which enhances the taste and texture of the food. Thus, a rigorous discussion about children's preferences for energy-dense foods needs to be tied to a broader discussion concerning the development of food preferences during childhood.

EFFECTS OF FAMILIAL FEEDING STYLES AND MEAL PATTERNS

PARENTAL FEEDING STYLES

Parental feeding strategies may influence the development of children's eating patterns, their ability to regulate food intake, and ultimately their weight status. Specifically, a series of laboratory and observational studies reveal that excessive parental restriction of children's eating is associated with increased energy intake and body weight in children.[22] Johnson and Birch[6] conjecture that parental efforts to focus children's attention on external cues (e.g., food portion size and rewards) may undermine children's ability to respond to internal hunger and satiety signals. Restricting access to highly palatable snack foods has also been shown to increase children's preferences and requests for such forbidden foods,[44] and has been shown to promote increased eating in the absence of hunger in children.[45]

A recent review of the literature examined 19 studies testing the association between parental feeding strategies and child energy intake and weight status.[46] This review surveyed a variety of caregiver feeding styles, including restriction of child eating, using food incentives to calm the child, providing structure during feeding interactions, emotional feeding, and instrumental feeding. Results of the review indicated that restriction of child eating — but no other feeding domain — was consistently associated with increased child energy intake and weight status. That is, parents who were more restrictive of children's eating at meals tended to have children who consumed excess energy at meals and were heavier.

The association between restriction of child eating and child weight status appears to be a bidirectional one, such that parental control is elicited by the child's excess body weight and this control, in turn, may exacerbate overeating by girls.[47] Indeed, the "detrimental" effects of feeding restriction appear to be most pronounced among the heaviest children[44] or children with a familial predisposition to obesity.[48] Thus, the underlying causal pathways are complicated and partially originate from the child's characteristics.

Practically, these findings suggest that caution may be warranted in the use of *excessive* or *aggressive* restriction of children's eating, especially when targeting young children who are not yet overweight. An alternative to restricting preferred foods is the use of reinforcement strategies to promote increased intake of healthier foods that are lower in energy density as a substitute. The clinical utility of this strategy was demonstrated in an obesity prevention study of 8- to 12-year-old children conducted by Epstein and colleagues.[49] The use of positive reinforcement strategies has been critical to the treatment of childhood obesity and may be equally important for prevention.

FAMILY MEALS AND TV VIEWING

An interesting study by Coon et al.[50] documented an impressive association between TV-viewing practices during family meals and children's food consumption patterns. Participating families were recruited from Maryland suburbs and included at least one child in the fourth to sixth grade. Parents reported whether the TV was usually on or usually off during breakfast, after-school snacks, and dinner meals at home. Child food intake was measured using 24-h dietary recalls. Compared with children whose families had the TV on during 0 or 1 meal/day, children whose families had the TV on during 1 or 2 meal/day consumed fewer daily servings of vegetables (means = 0.095 vs. 0.066), but increased daily servings of red meat (means = 0.040 vs. 0.080) and soda intake (means = 0.050 vs. 0.091). The two groups of children also differed in their intake of other food categories. Specifically, compared with children exposed to TV during 0 or 1 meal/day, children exposed to TV during 2 or 3 meals/day were less likely to consume fruits, vegetables, juice, and juice drinks during meals (mean daily servings = 0.340 vs. 0.259) and more likely to consume meat dishes (mean daily servings = 0.156 vs. 0.198) and pizza, snacks, and soda (mean daily servings = 0.104 vs. 0.163).

SNACKING PATTERNS

Snacking patterns appear to develop early in life, as suggested by a recent cross-sectional phone survey of 3022 parents of infants and toddlers aged 4 to 24 months. Results indicated that an infant dietary pattern that included breakfast, lunch, dinner, plus snacks emerged during the months 7 and 8 of life and was well established by months 9 to 11.[51] Infants and toddlers were fed seven times per day, on average, and the percentage of children consuming snacks increased with age. Afternoon snacks were consumed by over 80% of toddlers (12 to 24 months of age) and made up ~25% of their daily energy intake.

TABLE 13.2
Snacking among U.S. Children in 1977, 1989, and 1996

	Ages 2–5 y			Ages 6–11 y			Ages 12-18 y		
	1977	1989	1996	1977	1989	1996	1977	1989	1996
Snacks/day	1.73	1.87	2.29[a,b]	1.56	1.59	1.99[a,b]	1.60	1.62	1.97[a,b]
Grams/snack	158	167	153	200	205	195	275	298[a]	307
Kilocalories/ snack	171	187	175	231	250	243	296	320	318
Kilocalories from snacks	283	331[a]	378[a,b]	347	387	462[a,b]	460	496	612[a,b]

[a] Data point is significantly different from 1977 data point at the 0.01 level.

[b] Data point is significantly different from 1989 data point at the 0.01 level.

Source: Jahns L, Siega-Riz AM, Popkin BM. *J Pediatrics.* 2001;138(4): 493-498.

Jahns et al.[52] have shown that snacking behavior in U.S. children has steadily increased since 1977. Using dietary recall data from the Nationwide Food Consumption Survey (for 1977 to 1978) and the Continuing Survey of Food Intake by Individuals (for 1989 to 1991 and 1994 to 1996), they found that the number of snacks per day and kilocalories from snacks significantly increased over time. This was observed among children 2 to 5 years of age, 6 to 11 years of age, and 12 to 18 years of age. However, the total energy content per snack (kilocalories per snack) did not increase over time in any of the age groups (Table 13.2). Thus, although the total energy content of snacks per se has not increased over time, the number of daily snacking occurrences or events has increased and currently constitutes a large percentage of youth's total daily energy intake.

Despite these findings, excess intake of high-calorie snack foods does not appear to discriminate overweight from nonoverweight adolescents.[53] Especially striking are recent findings from a 10-year prospective study of 196 nonobese girls who were 8 to 12 years old at baseline.[54] Participants returned for annual anthropometry evaluations until 4 years after menarche. Results indicated that reported intake of high-calorie snack foods failed to predict change in BMI z-score or percent body fat across a variety of statistical models. Soda intake was the only variable that predicted excess weight gain over time. These findings underscore the importance of soda intake, perhaps more so than intake of energy-dense snack foods, in the onset and maintenance of childhood overweight. Reducing the consumption of sugar-sweetened beverages during daily snacks could represent an opportune target for prevention initiatives in children.

REFINED EATING TRAITS AND THEIR POTENTIAL ROLE IN THE PREVENTION OF OVERWEIGHT

As noted at the outset of this chapter, overweight can result from subtle but sustained imbalances between energy intake and output in growing children. Consequently, investigators have developed laboratory methodologies for measuring refined eating traits and patterns that may be informative for understanding the etiology of childhood overweight. These traits might also suggest novel avenues for developing overweight prevention initiatives. This section summarizes work on two particular eating traits: eating in the absence of hunger and energy compensation ability.

EATING IN THE ABSENCE OF HUNGER

Eating in the absence of hunger (EAH) refers to a propensity to consume energy from available snack foods despite (a) having recently completed a meal and (b) feeling full. Developed by Fisher and Birch,[55] the experimental paradigm for measuring EAH begins by providing the child participant *ad libitum* access to an experimental multi-item meal (typically lunch), after which the child indicates the extent to which he or she is full using a validated silhouette scale. Only children who report being full continue with the protocol, which involves tasting ~10 snack food (e.g., pretzels, crackers, chocolate candies) and then being allowed *ad libitum* access to consume as much of the snack foods as desired. EAH refers to the total amount of energy consumed from these snack foods — that is, the amount of food the child continues to eat despite indicating that he or she is full.

EAH appears to be a stable trait over time, at least among girls. Birch et al.[44] provided evidence that EAH scores were stable from 5 to 7 years of age, such that 64% of the girls who showed low EAH levels at age 5 continued to show low EAH levels at age 7, while 68% of the girls who showed high EAH levels at age 5 continued to show high EAH levels at age 7. EAH has also been linked cross-sectionally and prospectively to increased weight status among girls,[45] suggesting that this trait may be a behavioral mechanism by which positive energy balance is achieved and maintained in growing children. Studies suggest that increased parental restriction of a child's eating may promote EAH,[44,47] perhaps by drawing children's attention away from internal hunger and satiety cues and more toward external eating cues.

To the extent that EAH promotes weight gain in children, this suggests a potential avenue for prevention initiatives in children. These could include efforts to reduce the consumption of high energy–dense snacks between meals and, instead, to promote the consumption of water-rich, low energy-dense foods such as fruits and vegetables. This theory has not yet been tested, however, in the context of a controlled prevention trial.

Energy Compensation Ability ("Caloric Compensation")

If one were to measure a child's eating behavior at a series of discrete meals, energy intake may appear erratic and unrelated from one meal to the next. That is, food intake at any given meal may appear to be governed by momentary states of hunger and seem unsystematic. Despite this considerable meal-to-meal and even day-to-day variability, compelling evidence suggests that young children tend to regulate energy intake over prolonged periods. For example, Birch and colleagues[56] assessed the cumulative daily energy intake of 15 preschool children whose food intake was precisely measured over a 1-week period in the free-living environment. Results indicated that although meal-to-meal intake was relatively inconsistent (coefficient of variation = 30 to 44%), day-to-day total energy intake was much more consistent and stable (coefficient of variation = ~10%). Children's ability to adjust energy intake in response to changes in the energy content of previously consumed meals has been called "caloric compensation."

Controlled laboratory studies conducted over several decades demonstrate that the average preschool child, typically 2 to 5 years old, possesses adequate compensation abilities. In the typical research protocol, children visit a laboratory on two occasions to consume a multi-item lunch. These test meals are identical across visits. Prior to consuming the test meal (20 to 120 min, depending on the protocol), child participants consume a fixed amount or volume of a "preload" snack that is formulated to vary in energy density (i.e., a "low-energy" vs. "high-energy" preload). To the extent that children consume more energy at the subsequent meal following the low-energy preload compared with the high-energy preload, or reduce intake following the high-energy preload, this would support the theory that children possess an ability to compensate for energy.

In a review of 11 studies testing compensation ability in children, Birch and Fisher[57] found that the majority of the studies provided evidence for energy compensation ability in children. All studies of 2- to 5-year-old children showed that the average total energy intake was greater following the low-energy compared with the high-energy preload. The one study[58] that failed to show compensation studied 9- and 10-year-old children suggests that children may lose the ability to compensate as they grow older. That is, as children age, environmental and other social-cognitive factors (e.g., dieting, emotional factors, peer influences) may override an innate sensitivity to physiologically based hunger and satiety cues. The theory is appealing and needs to be investigated in prospective studies.

Although the *average* preschool child compensates well to maintain consistent energy intake levels, there is considerable between-child variability in this trait.[6,59] That is, some children appear to be more adept at compensating and regulating energy intake than are other children. Reasons for this interindividual variability are poorly understood, although excessive parental feeding control during meals may disrupt children's ability to compensate for energy intake.[47] Additional research is needed to identify determinants of the inability to compensate in some children because diminished compensation ability has been linked to increased child adiposity.[6]

Literature on compensation ability implicates another potentially novel avenue for prevention strategies in children, that is, "satiety training." Research suggests that training children to attend to internal feelings of hunger and fullness when eating, as opposed to external cues, can improve children's energy compensation abilities.[60] Moreover, we have shown that children can be trained to attend to internal feelings of hunger and fullness, and scale these sensations quantitatively.[61] Whether these skills could be used clinically to help children achieve better long-term energy balance is currently unknown.

MEASUREMENT CONSIDERATIONS AND RECOMMENDATIONS

The accurate measurement of dietary intake in children and adolescents is a challenging task and demands sophisticated skills and knowledge on the part of the researcher. Table 13.3 outlines examples of measurement strategies that are available to assess the effects of various environmental factors, properties of foods, and eating patterns on energy intake in children and adolescents. The references noted in the table provide detailed descriptions of the respective methods.[62–73]

TABLE 13.3
Types of Measurements to Assess Dietary Intake in Children and Adolescents

	Type of Measurement
	Environmental Factors
Portion size	Laboratory-based experiments;[14,15] experiments in naturalistic settings;[12] 24-h dietary recalls;[16] food records
	Properties of Foods
Energy density	Laboratory-based experiments;[34,35] experiments in naturalistic settings; 24-h dietary recalls; food records[62]
Glycemic index	Laboratory-based experiments[29,63]
Sugar-sweetened beverage intake	Experiments in naturalistic settings; 24-h dietary recalls;[50,64] food records; food frequency questionnaire[65]
	Eating Behaviors
Eating in the absence of hunger	Laboratory-based experiments[55]
Caloric compensation ability	Laboratory-based experiments[59,66]
Snacking	24-h dietary recall;[67] food records; food frequency questionnaire
	Home-Environmental Influences
Parental feeding styles	Self-report measures (questionnaires);[68,69] videotaped meal in laboratory setting[70]
Frequency of exposure	Laboratory-based experiments;[39] self-report measures (questionnaires)
Family meals and TV viewing	Self-report measures (questionnaires, interviews);[71] TV monitors
Role modeling	Laboratory-based experiments;[72] experiments in naturalistic settings;[24,73] self-report measures (questionnaires)

Studies that are conducted in a laboratory-based setting operate under a high level of control over experimental procedures and meals, and thus have the advantage of excluding many environmental influences that are known to affect eating behavior. The setup of a laboratory, though desirable, is costly and may not be accessible to many researchers.

An alternative option to assess dietary intake in children and adolescents is to administer one or more self-report measures such as food records, 24-h dietary recalls, and food frequency questionnaires (FFQs). The self-report of dietary intake is problematic in adults,[74,75] but has been shown to be even more so in children and adolescents[76] Not only are individuals prone to underreporting the type of food and the amount of food they eat, but they also have difficulty judging portion sizes of foods. There is evidence[76] that children's cognitive abilities to estimate portion sizes of foods or to remember the type of food they consumed are limited. Therefore, for children who are under the age of 8, it is typically the parent or primary caretaker who reports the child's intake. Beyond 8 to 10 years of age, there is evidence that children can reliably report prior day food intake with some assistance from their parents.[77,78] Even though children increasingly gain knowledge about the types of foods they eat as they age, their self-reported intakes are often flawed by inaccurate portion size estimations, omissions of foods or drinks (i.e., underreporting), or incorrect identification of foods.[76]

The following are practical recommendations to help improve the accuracy of three dietary intake methods (i.e., food records, 24-h dietary recalls, and FFQs) in children and adolescents.

FOOD RECORDS

- Design age-appropriate food record forms (e.g., provide clear structure and instructions).
- Conduct extensive training on how to complete food records (e.g., show examples, have child practice).
- Conduct extensive training on how to estimate the portion size of foods.[79]
- Provide digital scales to accurately weigh food portions.
- Use portion size aids and provide illustrations of commonly used household measures and dishes (e.g., cups, spoons, bowls, glasses), geometric shapes, and food-specific gram weight descriptions.[80]
- Have child or adolescent complete food records over an extended period (e.g., 3 to 7 days).
- Provide portable pocket-sized notebooks to encourage children to write down foods as they are eaten and then transfer the information to their food record as soon as possible.
- Consider innovative technologies (e.g., Palm Pilot) as recording tools.

24-HOUR DIETARY RECALLS

- Use multiple-pass method to limit extent of underreporting:[80]
  - Pass 1: "Quick List" (ask child or adolescent to recall everything he or she ate the previous day).
  - Pass 2: "Detailed description" (ask child or adolescent to clarify any foods mentioned in quick list; ask subject to provide information about type and amount of foods eaten).
  - Pass 3: "Review" (review list of foods provided by child or adolescent and probe for additional eating occasions; clarify portion sizes).

- Provide child or adolescent with three-dimensional food models that include common household measures (e.g., spoons, cups, bowls, glasses), common household items that can be compared with serving sizes of specific foods (e.g., 1 medium fruit = tennis ball, 1 serving of bread = CD case), and food-specific weight descriptions.

- Administer initial recall in person (to provide additional guidance); conduct subsequent recalls on the telephone.
- Have children or adolescents complete recalls on multiple randomly chosen days.

FOOD FREQUENCY QUESTIONNAIRES

Consider an age-appropriate questionnaire such as the Youth/Adolescent Questionnaire (YAQ), a self-administered food frequency questionnaire that is based on the validated adult Nurses' Health Study semiquantitative food frequency questionnaire. The questionnaire has been modified to include more youth-specific food choices (e.g., snack foods) and to make the format easier to complete by older children and adolescents[81,82] Copies of the YAQ can be obtained by contacting Helaine R. Rockett, Nutrition Research Manager at helaine.rockett@channing.harvard.edu.

CONCLUSION

Children's eating behavior is influenced by many factors in the free-living environment. A wide spectrum of influences can work in concert to shape children's short-term and long-term eating behavior and, ultimately, their weight status. In this chapter, we reviewed several of the more extensively researched controls of children's eating behavior. In principle and practice, these are modifiable influences that could potentially play a role in childhood overweight prevention. The daily energy deficit needed to induce a negative energy balance and to curb excess child weight gain is relatively small. Thus, the modifications necessary to support healthier eating practices in children may be achievable by targeting small but sustainable changes to foods and child feeding strategies rather than imposing dramatic dietary restrictions on children that they resist.

There is a need for further research on the behavioral aspects of eating behavior in children with combined findings from basic research into the biology of long-term energy balance. Many of the outstanding studies reviewed in this chapter address influences on children's *short-term* eating behavior. At the same time, understanding the controls of *longer-term* food intake will be necessary for understanding how to better reestablish energy balance and prevent excess weight gain in growing children. In order to identify significant predictors of excess weight gain and its prevention, it will be critical to study children's habitual eating behavior and food choices on a more long-term basis, in natural settings, and with respect for biological compensatory mechanisms.

REFERENCES

1. Rozin P. Food is fundamental, fun, frightening, and far-reaching. *Social Res.* 1999;66: 9–30.
2. Goran MI. Metabolic precursors and effects of obesity in children: a decade of progress, 1990–1999 *Am J Clin Nutr.* 2001;73(2): 158–171.
3. Borushek A. *The Doctor's Pocket Calorie Fat & Carbohydrate Counter.* Costa Mesa, CA: Family Health Publications; 2004.
4. Barlow SE, Dietz WH. Obesity evaluation and treatment: expert committee recommendations. The Maternal and Child Health Bureau, Health Resources and Services Administration and the Department of Health and Human Services. *Pediatrics.* 1998;102(3): E29.
5. Birch LL, Deysher M. Conditioned and unconditioned caloric compensation: evidence for self regulation of food intake by young children. *Learning and Motivation* 1985;16: 341–355.
6. Johnson SL, Birch LL. Parents' and children's adiposity and eating style. *Pediatrics.* 1994;94(5): 653–661.
7. Birch LL, Johnson SL, Jones MB, Peters JC. Effects of a nonenergy fat substitute on children's energy and macronutrient intake. *Am J Clin Nutr.* 1993;58(3): 326–333.
8. Young LR, Nestle M. The contribution of expanding portion sizes to the US obesity epidemic. *Am J Public Health.* 2002;92(2): 246–249.

9. French SA, Story M, Neumark-Sztainer D, Fulkerson JA, Hannan P. Fast food restaurant use among adolescents: associations with nutrient intake, food choices and behavioral and psychosocial variables. *Int J Obes Related Metabol Dis.* 2001;25(12): 1823–1833.

10. Rolls BJ. The supersizing of America: portion size and the obesity epidemic. *Nutr Today.* 2003;38(2): 42–53.

11. Rolls BJ, Morris EL, Roe LS. Portion size of food affects energy intake in normal-weight and overweight men and women. *Am J Clin Nutr.* 2002;76(6): 1207–1213.

12. Diliberti N, Bordi PL, Conklin MT, Roe LS, Rolls BJ. Increased portion size leads to increased energy intake in a restaurant meal. *Obes Res.* 2004;12(3): 562–568.

13. Rolls BJ, Roe LS, Meengs JS, Wall DE. Increasing the portion size of a sandwich increases energy intake. *J Am Diet Assoc.* 2004;104(3): 367–372.

14. Rolls BJ, Engell D, Birch LL. Serving portion size influences 5-year-old but not 3-year-old children's food intakes. *J Am Diet Assoc.* 2000;100(2): 232–234.

15. Fisher JO, Rolls BJ, Birch LL. Children's bite size and intake of an entree are greater with large portions than with age-appropriate or self-selected portions. *Am J Clin Nutr.* 2003;77(5): 1164 1170.

16. McConahy KL, Smiciklas-Wright H, Mitchell DC, Picciano MF. Portion size of common foods predicts energy intake among preschool-aged children. *J Am Diet Assoc.* 2004;104(6): 975–979.

17. Galloway AT, Lee Y, Birch LL. Predictors and consequences of food neophobia and pickiness in young girls. *J Am Diet Assoc.* 2003;103: 692–698.

18. Pliner P, Hobden K. Development of a scale to measure the trait of food neophobia in humans. *Appetite.* 1992;19(2): 105–120.

19. Falciglia GA, Couch SC, Gribble LS, Pabst SM, Frank R. Food neophobia in childhood affects dietary variety *J Am Diet Assoc.* 2000;100(12): 1474–1481.

20. Sullivan SA, Birch LL. Pass the sugar, pass the salt: experience dictates preference. *Dev Psychol.* 1990;26(4): 546–551.

21. Wardle J, Herrera ML, Cooke L, Gibson EL. Modifying children's food preferences: the effects of exposure and reward on acceptance of an unfamiliar vegetable. *Europ J Clin Nutrition.* 2003;57(2): 341–348.

22. Birch LL, Fisher JO. Development of eating behaviors among children and adolescents. *Pediatrics.* 1998;101(3 Pt 2): 539–549.

23. Hendy HM, Raudenbush B. Effectiveness of teacher modeling to encourage food acceptance in preschool children. *Appetite.* 2000;34(1): 61–76.

24. Hendy HM. Effectiveness of trained peer models to encourage food acceptance in preschool children. *Appetite.* 2002;39(3): 217–225.

25. Krotkiewski M. Effect of guar gum on body-weight, hunger ratings and metabolism in obese subjects. *Br J Nutrition.* 1984;52(1): 97 105.

26. Lavin JH, Read NW. The effect on hunger and satiety of slowing the absorption of glucose: relationship with gastric emptying and postprandial blood glucose and insulin responses. *Appetite.* 1995;25(1): 89–96.

27. Haber GB, Heaton KW, Murphy D, Burroughs LF. Depletion and disruption of dietary fibre. Effects on satiety, plasma-glucose, and serum-insulin. *Lancet.* 1977;2(8040): 679–682.

28. Gustafsson K, Asp NG, Hagander B, Nyman M, Schweizer T. Influence of processing and cooking of carrots in mixed meals on satiety, glucose and hormonal response. *Int J Food Sci Nutrition.* 1995;46(1): 3–12.

29. Ludwig DS, Majzoub JA, Al-Zahrani A, Dallal GE, Blanco I, Roberts SB. High glycemic index foods, overeating, and obesity. *Pediatrics.* 1999;103(3): E26.

30. Spitzer L, Rodin J. Effects of fructose and glucose preloads on subsequent food intake. *Appetite.* 1987;8(2): 135–145.

31. Ludwig DS, Peterson KE, Gortmaker SL. Relation between consumption of sugar-sweetened drinks and childhood obesity: a prospective, observational analysis. *Lancet.* 2001;357(9255): 505–508.

32. Newby PK, Peterson KE, Berkey CS, Leppert J, Willett WC, Colditz GA. Beverage consumption is not associated with changes in weight and body mass index among low-income preschool children in North Dakota. *J Am Diet Assoc.* 2004;104(7): 1086–1094.

33. James J, Thomas P, Cavan D, Kerr D. Preventing childhood obesity by reducing consumption of carbonated drinks: cluster randomised controlled trial. *BMJ.* 2004;328(7450): 1237.

34. Bell EA, Castellanos VH, Pelkman CL, Thorwart ML, Rolls BJ. Energy density of foods affects energy intake in normal-weight women. *Am J Clin Nutr.* 1998;67(3): 412–420.

35. Kral TV, Roe LS, Rolls BJ. Does nutrition information about the energy density of meals affect food intake in normal-weight women? *Appetite.* 2002;39(2): 137–145.

36. Drewnowski A. Sensory control of energy density at different life stages. *Proc Nutr Soc.* 2000;59(2): 239–244.

37. Birch LL, McPhee L, Steinberg L, Sullivan S. Conditioned flavor preferences in young children. *Physiol Behav.* 1990;47(3): 501–505.

38. Johnson SL, McPhee L, Birch LL. Conditioned preferences: young children prefer flavors associated with high dietary fat. *Physiol Behav.* 1991;50(6): 1245–1251.

39. Kern DL, McPhee L, Fisher J, Johnson S, Birch LL. The postingestive consequences of fat condition preferences for flavors associated with high dietary fat. *Physiol Behavior.* 1993;54(1): 71–76.

40. Martí-Henneberg C, Capdevila F, Arija V, Arija V, Perez S, Cuco G, et al. Energy density of the diet, food volume and energy intake by age and sex in a healthy population. *Europ J Clin Nutrition.* 1999;53(6): 421–428.

41. Drewnowski A. Sensory preferences for fat and sugar in adolescence and adult life. *Ann NY Acad Sci.* 1989;561: 243–250.

42. Birch LL, Sullivan SA. Measuring children's food preferences. *J School Health.* 1991;61(5): 212–214.

43. Gibson EL, Wardle J. Energy density predicts preferences for fruit and vegetables in 4-year-old children. *Appetite.* 2003;41(1): 97–98.

44. Birch LL, Fisher JO, Davison KK. Learning to overeat: maternal use of restrictive feeding practices promotes girls' eating in the absence of hunger. *Am J Clin Nutr.* 2003;78(2): 215–220.

45. Fisher JO, Birch LL. Eating in the absence of hunger and overweight in girls from 5 to 7 y of age. *Am J Clin Nutr.* 2002;76(1): 226–231.

46. Faith MS, Scanlon KS, Birch LL, Francis LA, Sherry B. Parent-child feeding strategies and their relationships to child eating and weight status. *Obes Res.* 2004;12(11): 1711–1722.

47. Birch LL, Fisher, JO. Mothers' child-feeding practices influence daughters' eating and weight. *Am J Clin Nutr.* 2000;71(5): 1054–1061.

48. Faith MS, Berkowitz RI, Stallings VA, Kerns J, Storey M, Stunkard AJ. Parental feeding attitudes and styles and child body mass index: prospective analysis of a gene-environment interaction. *Pediatrics.* 2004;114(4): E429–E436.

49. Epstein LH, Gordy CC, Raynor HA, Beddome M, Kilanowski CK, Paluch R. Increasing fruit and vegetable intake and decreasing fat and sugar intake in families at risk for childhood obesity. *Obesity Res.* 2001;9(3): 171–178.

50. Coon KA, Goldberg J, Rogers BL, Tucker KL. Relationship between use of television during meals and children's food consumption patterns. *Pediatrics.* 2001;107(1): E7.

51. Skinner JD, Ziegler P, Pac S, Devaney B. Meal and snack patterns of infants and toddlers. *J Am Diet Assoc.* 2004;104(1): 65–70.

52. Jahns L, Siega-Riz AM, Popkin BM. The increasing prevalence of snacking among US children from 1977 to 1996. *J Pediatr.* 2001;138(4): 493–498.

53. Bandini LG, Vu D, Must A, Cyr H, Goldberg A, Dietz WH. Comparison of high-calorie, low-nutrient-dense food consumption among obese and non-obese adolescents. *Obes Res.* 1999;7(5): 438–443.

54. Phillips SM, Bandini LG, Naumova EN, Cyr H, Colclough S, Dietz WH, Must A. Energy-dense snack food intake in adolescence: longitudinal relationship to weight and fatness. *Obes Res.* 2004;12(3): 461–472.

55. Fisher JO, Birch LL. Restricting access to foods and children's eating. *Appetite.* 1999;32(3): 405–419.

56. Birch LL, Johnson SL, Andresen G, Peters JC, Schulte MC. The variability of young children's energy intake. *New Engl J Med.* 1991;324(4): 232–235.

57. Birch LL, Fisher JO. Food intake regulation in children. Fat and sugar substitutes and intake. *Ann NY Acad Sci.* 1997;819: 194–220.

58. Anderson GH, Saravis S, Schacher R, Zlotkin S, Leiter LA. Aspartame: effect on lunch-time food intake, appetite, and hedonic response in children. *Appetite.* 1989;13: 93–103.

59. Faith MS, Keller KL, Johnson SL, Pietrobelli A, Matz PE, Must S, et al. Familial aggregation of energy intake in children. *Am J Clin Nutr.* 2004;79(5): 844–850.

60. Johnson SL. Improving preschoolers' self-regulation of energy intake. *Pediatrics*. 2000;106(6): 1429–1435.

61. Faith MS, Kermanshah M, Kissileff HR. Development and preliminary validation of a silhouette satiety scale for children. *Physiol Behav*. 2002;76(2): 173–178.

62. Cox DN, Mela DJ. Determination of energy density of freely selected diets: methodological issues and implications. *Int J Obes Related Metabol Dis*. 2000;24(1): 49–54.

63. Warren JM, Henry CJ, Simonite V. Low glycemic index breakfasts and reduced food intake in preadolescent children. *Pediatrics*. 2003;112(5): E414.

64. Harnack L, Stang J, Story M. Soft drink consumption among US children and adolescents: nutritional consequences. *J Am Diet Assoc*. 1999;99(4): 436–441.

65. Berkey CS, Rockett HR, Field AE, Gillman MW, Colditz GA. Sugar-added beverages and adolescent weight change. *Obes Res*. 2004;12(5): 778–788.

66. Birch LL, McPhee LS, Bryant JL, Johnson SL. Children's lunch intake: effects of midmorning snacks varying in energy density and fat content. *Appetite*. 1993;20(2): 83–94.

67. Jahns L, Siega-Riz AM, Popkin BM. The increasing prevalence of snacking among US children from 1977 to 1996. *J Pediatr*. 2001;138(4): 493–498.

68. Birch LL, Fisher JO, Grimm-Thomas K, Markey CN, Sawyer R, Johnson SL. Confirmatory factor analysis of the Child Feeding Questionnaire: a measure of parental attitudes, beliefs and practices about child feeding and obesity proneness. *Appetite*. 2001;36(3): 201 210.

69. Wardle J, Sanderson S, Guthrie CA, Rapoport L, Plomin R. Parental feeding style and the inter-generational transmission of obesity risk. *Obes Res*. 2002;10(6): 453–462.

70. Drucker RR, Hammer LD, Agras WS, Bryson S. Can mothers influence their child's eating behavior? *J Dev Behav Pediatr*. 1999;20(2): 88–92.

71. Melgar-Quinonez HR, Kaiser LL. Relationship of child-feeding practices to overweight in low income Mexican-American preschool-aged children. *J Am Diet Assoc*. 2004;104(7): 1110–1119

72. Tibbs T, Haire-Joshu D, Schechtman KB, Brownson RC, Nanney MS, Houston C, Auslander W. The relationship between parental modeling, eating patterns, and dietary intake among African-American parents. *J Am Diet Assoc*. 2001;101(5): 535–541.

73. Rotenberg KJ, Carte L, Speirs A. The effects of modeling dietary restraint on food consumption: do restrained models promote restrained eating? *Eating Behaviors*. 2005;6(1): 75–84.

74. Scagliusi FB, Polacow VO, Artioli GG, Benatti FB, Lancha AH, Jr. Selective underreporting of energy intake in women: magnitude, determinants, and effect of training. *J Am Diet Assoc*. 2003;103(10): 1306 1313.

75. Bedard D, Shatenstein B, Nadon S. Underreporting of energy intake from a self-administered food-frequency questionnaire completed by adults in Montreal. *Public Health Nutrition*. 2004;7(5): 675–681.

76. Livingstone MB, Robson PJ, Wallace JM. Issues in dietary intake assessment of children and adolescents. *Br J Nutrition*. 2004;92(2): S213–S222.

77. Lytle LA, Nichaman MZ, Obarzanek E, Glovsky E, Montgomery D, Nicklas T, et al. Validation of 24–hour recalls assisted by food records in third-grade children. The CATCH Collaborative Group. *J Am Diet Assoc*. 1993;93(12): 1431–1436.

78. Sobo EJ, Rock CL, Neuhouser ML, Maciel TL, Neumark-Sztainer D. Caretaker-child interaction during children's 24–hour dietary recalls: who contributes what to the recall record? *J Am Diet Assoc*. 2000;100(4): 428–433.

79. Weber JL, Cunningham-Sabo L, Skipper B, Lytle L, Stevens J, Gittelsohn J, et al. Portion-size estimation training in second- and third-grade American Indian children. *Am J Clin Nutr*. 1999;69(4): S782–S787.

80. Johnson RK, Driscoll P, Goran MI. Comparison of multiple-pass 24-hour recall estimates of energy intake with total energy expenditure determined by the doubly labeled water method in young children. *J Am Diet Assoc*. 1996;96(11): 1140–1144.

81. Rockett HR, Breitenbach M, Frazier AL, Witschi J, Wolf AM, Field AE, Colditz GA. Validation of a youth/adolescent food frequency questionnaire. *Prev Med*. 1997;26(6): 808–816.

82. Rockett HR, Wolf AM, Colditz GA. Development and reproducibility of a food frequency questionnaire to assess diets of older children and adolescents. *J Am Diet Assoc*. 1995;95(3): 336–340.

14 Behavioral Aspects of Physical Activity in Childhood and Adolescence

Donna Spruijt-Metz and Brian E. Saelens

CONTENTS

OVERVIEW AND INTRODUCTION

As our environment becomes more obesogenic, the central role of physical activity, sports, and exercise in the prevention and treatment of pediatric obesity has become increasingly evident.[1,2] However, not only do physical activity levels in youth decline steadily throughout puberty, there is increasing evidence that physical activity levels of youth have generally declined over the past several decades.[3,4]

There is thus a need to identify ways to help young people increase their physical activity levels. However, promotion of physical activity in youth is not straightforward and has not yielded success. The Ontario Public Health Association's *Review of Reviews*[5] synthesized the findings of

12 authoritative reviews of school- and community-based interventions to prevent pediatric obesity. In general, interventions tended to positively affect health-related knowledge and attitudes. However, impacts on physical activity were modest, and changes in physical activity were usually not substantial enough to decrease BMI, skinfolds, or other indicators of pediatric obesity. In addition, Resnicow and Robinson reviewed 16 school-based interventions to prevent cardiovascular disease. They found that 65% of the studies had positive effects on cognitive variables such as knowledge, while only 30% had any impact on physical activity, and only 16% affected adiposity outcomes.[6]

This chapter addresses important considerations for the development of effective physical activity interventions for children and adolescents. Current levels of physical activity are first contrasted with the recommended levels of physical activity for these populations. A brief overview of progress toward a comprehensive science of pediatric exercise behavior then prefaces an introduction to elements of theory. We argue the importance of basing interventions on good theories of health behavior and present six criteria for a "good" theory in this context. In proposing specific constructs to examine so that we can explain individual differences in children's physical activity, theory-based observational research more readily leads to theory-based intervention and more readily to accumulating a knowledge base regarding ways to intervene to increase children's physical activity. Featuring research using three of the most commonly employed theories of health behavior and one of the more recent ones, we review the progress and problems of promoting physical activity in demographically diverse youth.

RECOMMENDATIONS FOR CHILDREN'S PHYSICAL ACTIVITY

The short- and long-term health benefits of physical activity for children and adolescents are outlined in Chapters 9 and 11 of this book. The specific amount, intensity, and type of physical activity recommended for children's optimal health remains elusive. Given the lack of long-term studies needed to more clearly specify this recommendation for physical activity in childhood, such recommendations for children have often been derived from recommendations for adults' physical activity.[7] For example, objectives from *Healthy People 2010* for adolescents' physical activity[8] suggest recommended amounts, frequencies, and duration of physical activity levels similar to those for adults. Table 14.1 provides examples of recommendations for children's physical activity. Many have called for the development of more specific physical activity recommendations based on specific desired outcomes (e.g., weight control, bone health) for both adults and children.

TABLE 14.1
Recommendations for Physical Activity Specific to Children and Adolescents

Population	Type	Amount	Ref.
Adolescents	Moderate to vigorous intensity	Active daily and 3 or more sessions per week at least 20 minutes long	127
Young people	At least moderate intensity	60 min/day	128
Young people	Strength and flexibility	At least twice a week	128
Children	Not specified	60 min/day	129
Adolescents	Moderate intensity	30 min on at least 5 days/week	8
Adolescents	Vigorous intensity	20 min on at least 3 days/week	8
Children 5–12 years old	Not specified	At least 60 min and up to several hours; several bouts per day >15 min	130

OVERALL PREVALENCE AND GENERAL EPIDEMIOLOGY

Estimates of children's physical activity vary somewhat according to the population, the measure (e.g., self-report), and metric (e.g., average minutes or percentage above a recommended threshold) examined to document prevalence. Some general estimates regarding prevalence can be gleaned from existing data. Recent studies documenting physical activity prevalence in childhood are detailed in Table 14.2. Findings across most studies in Table 14.2 suggest that more than 60% of children engage in physical activity of at least moderate intensity three or more days a week, usually lasting more than 30 min each day. The percentage of children engaging in 60 min or more of physical activity each day (consistent with more recent recommendations for children's physical activity) is lower, with marked variability (30 to 100%) in prevalence estimates, in part based on the child's age. For example, Riddoch and colleagues estimate that more than 97% of 9 year olds average 60+ minutes of moderate to vigorous intensity exercise (MVPA) each day, with this percentage dropping to 62 to 82% for 15 year olds.[9] Based on accelerometer and heart rate data, the average child engages in about 50 to 200 min of physical activity of at least moderate intensity each day. The average MVPA minutes also vary with age, with younger children having higher values.

In addition to total physical activity time, intensity is another important consideration in physical activity prevalence estimates. Over 60% of children report engaging in vigorous physical activity three or more days per week.[10–12] Objective measures of physical activity call into question the absolute amount of time children spend in vigorous physical activity, with average vigorous time per day generally being less than 15 min.[13–15] Further, bouts of vigorous physical activity lasting more than 20 consecutive minutes are rare when assessing physical activity more objectively among children.[14] Given this, most studies report the combination of moderate and vigorous physical activity, but moderate intensity physical activity clearly predominates at least when self-report measures are not used.[14,15]

Approximately 20 to 25% of children report engaging in minimal physical activity[16,17] and 11.5% report no physical activity[12] during the previous week. These percentages of little or no physical activity, as well as the percentage of children meeting certain levels of physical activity throughout the week, are higher in older children and girls.

PROMOTING PHYSICAL ACTIVITY IN PEDIATRIC POPULATIONS

Until the 1990s, physical activity promotion research primarily sought to understand and intervene on person-level determinants of behavior.[18] Person-level determinants include sociodemographic (e.g., age, gender), cognitive (e.g., attitudes about physical activity), social-environmental (e.g., adult support received for physical activity), and behavioral (e.g., prior levels of physical activity) factors. Progress in the field was slow, and results of interventions were frequently negligible.[6,19] In 1992, Stokols published his seminal article delineating the need for social ecological approaches to health promotion and disease prevention.[20] Since that time, advances have been made toward a more transdisciplinary understanding of how the social, economic, political, and physical environments interact to affect child and adolescent physical activity.[21–24] The environment is one of the only things that has changed along with obesity — but what we don't understand are the mechanisms by which it affects behavior. Compelling evidence from the emergent literature on environmental correlates of physical activity show that comprehensive strategies including strategies to affect policy and physical and social environments must continue to incorporate individual correlates of physical activity in order to change behavior[25,26] (also see Chapters 16 and 17 of this volume). To work toward a comprehensive science of pediatric exercise promotion, we therefore need to include strategies to expand our understanding of how to motivate children and adolescents to be active on an individual level. This process ideally starts with and continues to develop theories of behavior and behavior change and their applicability to pediatric physical activity.

TABLE 14.2
Recent Prevalence Estimates of Children's Physical Activity

Sample	Measure	Metric	Overall results	Modifiers	Ref.
High school students (1997 YRBS)	Self-report of VPA in past 7 days	% 3+ days of 20+ min VPA	63.8%	Decline with age; males > females; higher in white than black or Hispanic	10
American 7–12 graders (n = 13157)	Self-report times per week in various physical activities of at least moderate intensity	1. Five times per week 2. Two times per week	1. 33.2% 2. 25.4% for males; 39.9% for females	1. Higher for males than females; ethnicity-related differences among females, with higher rates among non-Hispanic whites than other ethnicities	17
3–17-year-old children across 26 studies (n = 1883)	Heart rate reserve (HRR)	1. Min 20–40% HRR 2. Min 40–50% HRR 3. Min 50–60% HRR 4. Min 60–70% HRR	1. 128.0 min/day 2. 47.1 min/day 3. 29.3 min/day 4. 14.7 min/day	1. Decline with age, most marked in the 20–40% HRR minutes	13
American 1–12 graders (n = 375)	Accelerometer for 7 days	1. % 30 min MVPA on 5+ days/week 2. % 60 min MVPA on 5+ days/week 3. % 3+ days with 1 or more 20-min bout of VPA 4. Minutes of MVPA or VPA	1. 76.1–100.0% 2. 29.4–100.0% 3. 1.0–3.3% 4. 50–200+ min/day of MVPA; ~5–~32 min/day VPA	1 and 2. Decline with age, particularly from 7–9 to 10–12 grades; males > females only in 10–12 grades 4. Decline with age, particularly in MVPA from 1–3 to 4–6 grades; males > females in most grade categories, with most marked gender differences in VPA	14,131
Canadian 7–13 graders (n = 1477–2188)	1 and 2. Self-report of days of 20+ min vigorous during past 7 days	1. No vigorous 2. 3+ days/week vigorous	1. 13.7–15.3% 2. 63.1–66.4%	2. Decline with increasing age in % females getting 3+ days	11

Population	Measure	Result	Findings	Ref.

Chinese 6–18-year-old school children (n = 2675)	Self-report of MVPA in and out of school and through commuting to school in past 7 d
	1. Nonschool MVPA
	  a. % > 0
	  b. median (min/week)
	2. School MVPA
	  a. % > 0
	  b. median (min/week)
	3. Active commuting
	  a. % > 0
	  b. median (min/week)
		1a. 5–12%
		1b. 120–180 min
		
		2a. 68–75%
		2b. 90–110 min
		
		3a. 77–89%
		3b. 100–150 min
			1a. Increase with age; males > females
			
			2a. Decrease with age
			2b. Increase with age; males > females
			3a. Decrease with age
			3b. Increase with age
				132

American 9–13 year olds (n = 3120)	1. Self-report participation in organized physical activity in past 7 days 2. Self-report participation in free-time physical activity in past 7 days	1. 38.5% 2. 77.4%	1. Higher in white, non-Hispanic than black, non-Hispanic and Hispanic; higher with increasing parental education and income 2. Higher in males than females	16
European 9 and 15 year olds (n = 2185)	Accelerometer for 4 days 1. Average min MVPA/day 2. Percentage 60+ min MVPA/day	1. 142–200 min/day for 9 year olds, 60–110 min/day for 15 year olds 2. 97.4–97.6% of 9 year olds and 52.0–81.9% of 15 year olds	1. and 2. Males more active than females at both ages	9
American 11–15 year olds (n = 770)	Accelerometer for 7 days 1. Average min MPA/day 2. Average min VPA/day 3. Percentage 60+ min MVPA/day	1. 44.4–62.5 min/day 2. 4.2–12.4 min/day 3. 59% (boys), 34% (girls)		15
High school students (2003 YRBS) (n = 15214)	1. Self-report VPA in past 7 days 2. Self-report MPA in past 7 days 3. No MPA or VPA in past 7 days	1. 62.6% 2. 24.7% 3. 11.5%	1. and 2. Higher in males, non-Hispanic whites, and younger students 3. Higher among females, blacks, older students	12

Note: Includes studies published during or after 1999, with sufficiently large sample sizes (n > 300), that provide an estimate of overall (or through combination overall) physical activity engaged in by children and used a metric convertible to minutes or a minute threshold (e.g., step counts of a pedometer); MVPA = moderate to vigorous intensity physical activity; VPA = vigorous intensity physical activity; MPA = moderate intensity physical activity; min = minutes; YRBS = Youth Risk Behavior Surveillance

ELEMENTS OF BEHAVIORAL THEORY: CORRELATES, MEDIATORS, AND MODERATORS

Behavioral theories of pediatric physical activity are composed of a set of interrelated propositions about sociodemographic, social and environmental, personal, and/or behavioral factors that might explain and predict why young people do (or do not) engage in physical activity.[27,28] Research has shown that levels of physical activity in pediatric populations are related to a series of psychosocial variables (i.e., *correlates*)[29] and intervening causal variables (i.e., *mediators*).[30] Correlates may show strong statistical associations with physical activity in cross-sectional analyses but do not necessarily *cause* physical activity.[31] For instance, gender (male) is consistently and significantly associated with higher levels of physical activity across childhood and adolescence, but it is doubtful that gender (per se) *causes* physical activity.

On the other hand, the nature of a mediator is causal, and it has been persuasively argued that interventions to change physical activity levels work by affecting proposed intervening mediators.[19] For example, let's assume that self-efficacy was found to be positively related to physical activity levels in African American teenage girls,[32] thus making it a correlate of physical activity in this population. An intervention to change physical activity in this group might then be designed specifically to improve self-efficacy, and so to consequently increase levels of physical activity. To consider self-efficacy not only a correlate, but also a mediator of intervention effects, four criteria would have to be met.[33,34] First, the intervention would have to produce a change in the outcome variable — in this case, produce an increase in physical activity. Second, the intervention would have to have an effect on the proposed theoretical construct (the intervention would need to increase self-efficacy). Third, the proposed mediator (self-efficacy) would have to show a statistically significant relationship to physical activity when controlling for effects of the intervention. Fourth, we would need to demonstrate that the intervention-initiated changes in the proposed theoretical construct (self-efficacy) directly lead to (or cause) changes in physical activity. In this case, children whose self-efficacy increased more would need to show greater increases in physical activity than children whose self-efficacy did not increase as much. Only when these four criteria are fulfilled could self-efficacy be considered a mediator of physical activity change.

Another important consideration in theories, and therefore intervention, is the issue of *moderation*. Increasingly, we are finding that interventions do not work as well or in the same way across populations. That is, program effects may be moderated by certain features of a specific group. *Moderator* effects refer to characteristics of individuals or groups that significantly affect the strength or even direction of the relationship between a variable and outcome behavior.[35] For instance, a program targeting family participation in physical activity might work to increase physical activity in children but actually backfire in some adolescent populations,[36] thus making age a moderator of this intervention. Some correlates, such as developmental stage, gender, and ethnicity, may moderate program effects, but not all correlates are moderators. Furthermore, some "hard" correlates that are frequently treated as moderators — correlates that are not readily changeable (e.g., gender, ethnicity, socioeconomic status) — may actually be proxy variables for potential mediators. For instance, the gender effect on physical activity is in part likely a socialization effect that could conceivably be changed through targeted interventions, rather than an exclusively biologically sex-based and nonmodifiable phenomenon.

THE IMPERATIVE OF THEORY

Several authors have argued persuasively that interventions to change physical activity can only work through intervention on the appropriate mediating variables.[19,37] In other words, if programs to increase physical activity in youth are to be successful, they must be consistently designed based on viable theory that has been operationalized and measured according to rigorous scientific standards.[38] Theory helps to transform knowledge about behavior into effective strategies for interventions and, in turn, to understand how effective strategies work. Only through theory-based intervention research can research and practice be unified. A well-chosen theory will guide the development of an intervention at each phase, from conceptualization through planning, operationalization, implementation, measurement, and evaluation.[39] Conversely, without a knowledge of which variables affect physical activity behavior, we may be unable to explain why some interventions work while others do not, as well as be unable to generalize or replicate findings. Furthermore, the most thorough search for correlates in the natural environment may overlook important mediators and moderators of behavior because they might not occur in the natural environment. For instance, setting exercise goals may not be behavior that children typically undertake and will therefore not occur as a natural correlate of physical activity. However, theory may suggest that interventions to increase goal setting will increase physical activity, thus proposing the goal setting and the change in goal setting will mediate the intervention. Progress in our understanding of and ability to promote physical activity change depends upon rigorous application, testing, and refinement of theoretical principles of human behavior.[40]

"BORROWING" THEORIES

Physical activity research has generally "borrowed" theories from other realms of health-related behavior research, such as prevention of smoking and promotion of cancer screening. However, unlike smoking or getting a mammogram, physical activity is never an all-or-nothing proposal. You can't quit or refrain entirely. Even though many children are not active enough to derive health benefits from their physical activity, daily life typically requires some level of physical activity, if only to get from one place to another. It may not be appropriate to approach physical activity in the same way as on–off, yes–no dichotomous health-risk behaviors such as smoking or drug use (you do or you don't), or even in the same manner as other dichotomous positive health behaviors, such as obtaining health screenings.[41]

Another problem in current theory in pediatric physical activity is that we frequently "borrow" models of behavior from the adult literature. The social cognitive theory, theory of planned behavior, and health behavior model are the three theoretical models of human behavior that have guided most research on determinants of physical activity in youth to date. These models were developed to understand adult behavior and subsequently applied to children and adolescent populations. While these theories and models have contributed significantly to understanding physical activity behaviors in adolescents, much is missing of what we know about youths' perceptions of the world.[42] Current theories thus may fail to accommodate central issues such as cognitive and emotional development, which we know affect motivation for exercise, ability to understand messages, physical activity preferences, and correlates of physical activity.[29,43,44] Furthermore, their cognitive emphasis and central focus on competence or efficacy may limit the discussion of other important factors that motivate children and adolescents to be physically active.[45] Although certain concepts from these models may apply to youth, we cannot assume that the same factors that determine physical activity in adults will explain physical activity levels in youth.[46]

IDENTIFYING "GOOD" THEORIES

A good theory can guide development of interventions by delineating factors and determinants to be studied, by identifying facilitating situations and relevant processes, by guiding timing and sequencing, and by indicating possible methods of intervention and evaluation.[38,39,47] Theories provide information on what is needed to change specific behaviors, as well as what needs to be done to meet that need. For instance, social cognitive theory says that increased self-efficacy will increase physical activity, and suggests several mechanisms through which self-efficacy might be increased. The question is: Which theories are "good" theories for promoting physical activity in pediatric populations? Proposed here are six criteria for elements of a "good" theory of pediatric

TABLE 14.3
Six Criteria for a "Good" Theory of Physical Activity

1. Correlation	Constructs describe/predict physical activity
2. Moderation	Allows for consideration of relevant moderators (age, culture, gender)
3. Mediation	Constructs (1) impact physical activity and (2) are modifiable through intervention
4. Prescription	Prescribes or suggests viable avenues for behavior change
5. Elegance	The model is (1) parsimonious and (2) generates empirically testable hypotheses
6. User-friendliness	Useful in the field, practitioners can follow the logic, can be implemented in health education and public health, plausible and internally consistent

exercise behavior (adapted from Spruijt-Metz[38]). These are (1) correlation, (2) moderation, (3) mediation, (4) prescription, (5) elegance, and (6) user-friendliness (see Table 14.3 for an explanation of these criteria).

FOUR THEORIES FOR PROMOTING PHYSICAL ACTIVITY IN PEDIATRIC POPULATIONS

In a perfect world, intervention development would begin with a solid knowledge of the discrepancy between recommended levels of physical activity and current physical activity levels of the targeted population. Enough previous knowledge of the mediators of physical activity change in the target population would then be available to make an informed choice using these 6 criteria from the more than 50 theoretical frameworks that have been applied in health promotion research.[39] Often, however, knowledge of physical activity levels and correlates accrues as the research progresses. Furthermore, choosing a theory on the basis of one criteria might preclude another. This is particularly problematic given the current lack of solid mediational research.[48] There is, currently, no one theory or combination of theories that "works best" for pediatric populations.

To illustrate the progress in the field, we review pediatric physical activity promotion research that has employed four major theoretical backgrounds. Theories that attempt to understand motivation for physical activity have been categorized as belief–attitude theories, competence-based theories, control-based theories, or decision-making theories.[49] We focus on three of the most commonly used theoretical frameworks in physical activity interventions in youth and one theory that has recently been gathering more support in physical activity research. The commonly used theories are two belief–attitude theories, the health belief model and the theory of reasoned action, and one competence-based theory, the social cognitive theory. The more recently ascending theory, the self-determination theory, might be considered either a competence-based or a control-based theory.

THE HEALTH BELIEF MODEL AND PEDIATRIC PHYSICAL ACTIVITY

The health belief model (HBM) was originally developed around 1950 to explain widespread failure of the asymptomatic U.S. population to accept disease preventatives or to undergo screening tests for conditions such as lung cancer.[50] As one of the first psychosocial models of health-related behavior, several of its constructs have been incorporated in the study of pediatric physical activity. The main tenets of the HBM are that children and adolescents will not be physically active unless they (1) have minimal levels of motivation and knowledge about physical activity, (2) view themselves as potentially vulnerable to a relatively threatening condition (perceived threat) associated with not being physically active (like obesity or rejection by peers), (3) are convinced of relevant effectiveness of physical activity to prevent threatening condition (perceived benefits), and (4) anticipate few barriers to being physically active (perceived barriers). The HBM, as it might pertain to physical activity, is represented in Figure 14.1.

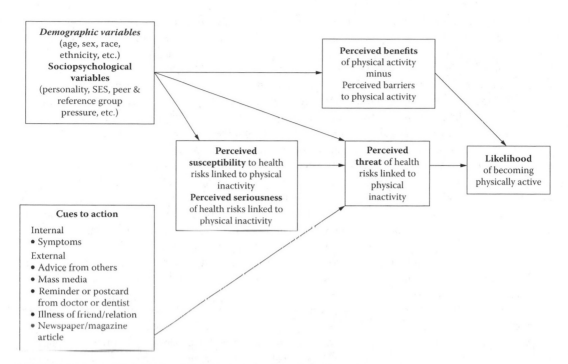

FIGURE 14.1 Health belief model (HBM) (From Janz NF, Champion VL, Strecher V. In Glanz K, Rimer BK, Lewis FM, Eds. *Health Behavior and Health Education: Theory, Research and Practice.* San Francisco: John Wiley & Sons. with permission.)

Few studies have examined the full model in relationship to physical activity, although one study did examine a full array of HBM constructs as potential predictors of fitness levels (using a modified version of the Harvard Step Test) in black and white adolescents.[51] HBM constructs accounted for 14% of the variance among black students in good and poor physical condition (severity 8%, susceptibility 3%, benefits 2%, social support 1%). Susceptibility accounted for 20% of the variance among white students in good and poor physical condition, barriers 5%, and benefits 2%.

Perceived benefits and perceived barriers, as part of the HBM, have received the most attention as correlates of child and adolescent physical activity. In their comprehensive review of correlates of physical activity in children and adolescents, Sallis and colleagues[29] found that perceived benefits of physical activity were related to physical activity in only 1 out of 7 studies in children and in 38% of 29 studies in adolescents. Perceived barriers were related to physical activity in 3 out of 3 studies in children (100%), but in only 33% of 15 studies in adolescents. A recent study examining relationships among perceived barriers, perceived benefits, and physical activity in 95 girls and boys (aged 9 to 16) and their parents (N = 171) found no relationship between perceived benefits and barriers and physical activity in boys, girls, children, or adolescents. Significant relationships between benefits and barriers and physical activity were found in parents. Children's perceptions of benefits of physical activity were weakly related to parents' perceptions, and child–parent perceptions of benefits were unrelated.[52] One study targeted perceived barriers and benefits in an intervention to increase physical activity in sedentary girls.[53] No relationship was found between these HBM variables and levels of physical activity at baseline. Baseline values of HBM variables did not predict physical activity levels postintervention, and changes in perceived barriers and benefits were not related to changes in physical activity over time. These findings suggest that these HBM constructs are not mediators of children's physical activity. However, HBM has not, to our knowledge, been evaluated or fully operationalized in its entirety in intervention studies.

The study of perceived benefits and barriers to physical activity offers a case in point for the importance of developmental, gender, and ethnic differences in correlates of physical activity. As children move into adolescence, determinants of physical activity change.[54–56] In a longitudinal study, Garcia et al. found that perceived barriers were significantly more likely to outweigh perceived benefits of physical activity after children transitioned into junior high school.[56]

The HBM has been modified and extended over the years to incorporate constructs from more recent theories. In the wake of the attitude theories that began to emerge decisively in the late 1960s, a measure of behavioral intentions is sometimes added to the HBM.[57] The publication of Bandura's seminal article on self-efficacy[58] also exerted some influence on the HBM. Concepts related to self-efficacy were originally considered to be incorporated in the perceived barriers construct of the HBM.[59] In 1988, Rosenstock et al. argued persuasively for the addition of self-efficacy to the model as an autonomous construct.[60] Recent research suggests that self-efficacy trumps barriers as a predictor of physical activity during school, but might contribute uniquely to variance in physical activity outside school in adolescent populations.[61] However, explained variance in physical activity by these variables remains low (usually around 6 to 10%).

The HBM has shown inconsistent correlations with physical activity in youth, and there is, to our knowledge, no available evidence of mediation effects. Critique of the model has included its lack of maturational constructs[42] and its emphasis on cognitive, belief-based constructs to the exclusion of more affective constructs.[38] A major problem with the HBM is that is was developed to predict isolated (often one-shot) illness-avoidance behaviors.[62] Physical activity is a complex behavior and, certainly where adherence and lifestyle adoption are concerned, an ongoing behavior. Isolated variables from the theory, such as perceived barriers to physical activity, have been somewhat more successful in predicting lower levels of physical activity than the entire model has been in predicting physical activity. As such, the HBM might actually be more useful for predicting nonparticipation in physical activity than uptake and lifestyle adoption of physical activity.

SOCIAL COGNITIVE THEORY AND PEDIATRIC PHYSICAL ACTIVITY

Social cognitive theory (SCT) posits that behavior is determined by the interaction among intrapersonal (e.g., cognitions), interpersonal (e.g., social), and environmental influences[63] (see Figure 14.2). This reciprocal determinism among factors, and particularly the inclusion of environmental influences, forms the basis of a growing interest in more comprehensive ecological models of behavior.[64] Although perhaps not originally intended, the empirical operationalization and evaluation of SCT within research regarding children's physical activity has been predominantly in the intrapersonal area. A specific focus has been on the relations between physical activity and the cognitive processes of self-efficacy and outcome expectancy. Self-efficacy refers to an individual's beliefs about their competency or confidence to perform a behavior, so general self-efficacy for physical activity would include an individuals' level of confidence for competently engaging in physical activity. Outcome expectancy involves the "judgment of the likely consequence [behaviors] will produce,"[65] with physical, social, and self-evaluative types of outcome expectancies. Examples of outcome expectancies for physical activity could include physical tiredness and discomfort, positive interaction with others on a sport's team, and feelings of self-satisfaction for attaining a physical activity goal.

There has been testing of whether and to what extent SCT constructs such as self-efficacy and outcome expectancies are correlates of children's physical activity. For example, Strauss and colleagues[66] found moderate correlations between various aspects of self-efficacy (including support seeking and ability to overcome barriers to being active) and vigorous physical activity among healthy 10 to 16 year olds, but such associations were not found for moderate intensity physical activity. Low self-efficacy has been shown to predict declines in physical activity across 1 year in elementary-aged children.[67] Collectively, approximately half of the cross-sectional studies examining

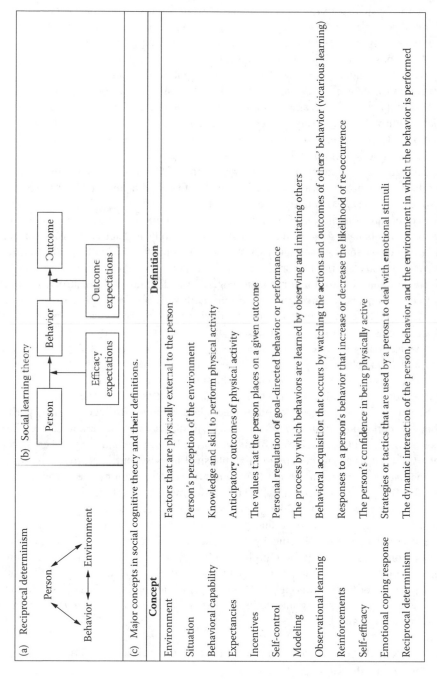

(a) Reciprocal determinism

Person

Behavior ← → Environment

(b) Social learning theory

Person → Behavior → Outcome

Efficacy expectations

Outcome expectations

(c) Major concepts in social cognitive theory and their definitions.

Concept	Definition
Environment	Factors that are physically external to the person
Situation	Person's perception of the environment
Behavioral capability	Knowledge and skill to perform physical activity
Expectancies	Anticipatory outcomes of physical activity
Incentives	The values that the person places on a given outcome
Self-control	Personal regulation of goal-directed behavior or performance
Modeling	The process by which behaviors are learned by observing and imitating others
Observational learning	Behavioral acquisition that occurs by watching the actions and outcomes of others' behavior (vicarious learning)
Reinforcements	Responses to a person's behavior that increase or decrease the likelihood of re-occurrence
Self-efficacy	The person's confidence in being physically active
Emotional coping response	Strategies or tactics that are used by a person to deal with emotional stimuli
Reciprocal determinism	The dynamic interaction of the person, behavior, and the environment in which the behavior is performed

FIGURE 14.2 Social cognitive theory (SCT) (formerly social learning theory) (From Baranowski T, Perry CL, Parcel GS. In Glanz K, Rimer BK, Lewis FM, Eds. *Health Behavior and Health Education: Theory, Research, and Practice.* San Francisco: John Wiley & Sons, 2002. With permission.)

self-efficacy and outcome expectations as correlates of children's physical activity have found significant positive associations.[68]

Social cognitive theory presents many constructs on which to attempt intervention to bring about increases in physical activity among children. Some school-based intervention trials have documented initial positive changes in physical activity self-efficacy resulting from intervention.[69,70] This suggests a prescriptive potential and relevance for modifying these constructs in children; although similar to physical activity itself, it appears difficult to sustain these higher initial levels of physical activity self-efficacy.[71] Few studies have investigated potential mediation within physical activity intervention for youth.[72] However, recently Dishman and colleagues[73] did find that an SCT-based physical activity intervention among adolescent girls increased their self-efficacy for physical activity, which in turn was positively related to their change in physical activity, suggesting, in part, a mediation role of self-efficacy. Other social–cognitive constructs of outcome expectancy, goal setting, and satisfaction did not show evidence of mediation in this study of adolescent girls. Other trials have failed to find significant increases in SCT constructs with physical activity intervention relative to control conditions, and/or failed to find significant relations between change in these constructs and physical activity (see, e.g., Wilson et al.[74]).

There are additional limitations of SCT to the study of children's physical activity. It is not clear whether individuals have general self-efficacy regarding physical activity across various types of physical activity or whether self-efficacy exists for engaging in specific physical activities (e.g., high self-efficacy for walking, but low self-efficacy for a specific sport) or within certain settings.[75] Further, self-efficacy may be a multicomponent cognitive and behavioral construct, including the ability to overcome barriers to physical activity, the ability to obtain support from others to be active, and to find and/or create environments conducive to being active, all of which may have different associations with children's physical activity.[76] For example, Trost and colleagues[77] found that children's self-efficacy for overcoming barriers to physical activity was a significant correlate of both boys' and girls' physical activity, while perceived self-efficacy for being active despite competing activities was essentially unrelated to children's physical activity.

Given the breadth of potential correlates and mediators that constitute the intrapersonal, interpersonal, and environmental factors that could affect children's physical activity, it is perhaps not surprising that the common evaluation of only a small subset of these potential correlates and mediators seems limited. Future research is likely best served not by replicating prior cross-sectional evaluation of SCT constructs in their relation to physical activity, but by further testing of SCT constructs as mediators. Further, the recent burgeoning of studies examining environmental correlates of physical activity (e.g., Saelens et al.[78,79]) allows for more complete testing of the SCT model and the reciprocal determination of children's physical activity between intrapersonal and environmental factors. For instance, it could be that playground availability (an environmental variable) moderates the relation between self-efficacy (an intrapersonal variable) and children's physical activity, such that only children with both high self-efficacy *and* playground availability are physically active, while children without either or both high self-efficacy and playground availability engage in less physical activity. Although SCT serves as a starting point, it is possible that more detailed theoretical models regarding interactions between intrapersonal and environmental factors will need to be generated and tested.

THEORY OF REASONED ACTION AND THEORY OF PLANNED BEHAVIOR, AND THEIR RELATION TO PEDIATRIC PHYSICAL ACTIVITY

The theory of reasoned action (TRA) would propose that the intention to engage in physical activity is the most proximal and strongest influence on children's physical activity. Intention is posited to be influenced by attitudes and subjective norms regarding physical activity, which are affected by perceived consequences and the influence of others, respectively. The theory of planned behavior (TPB) adds

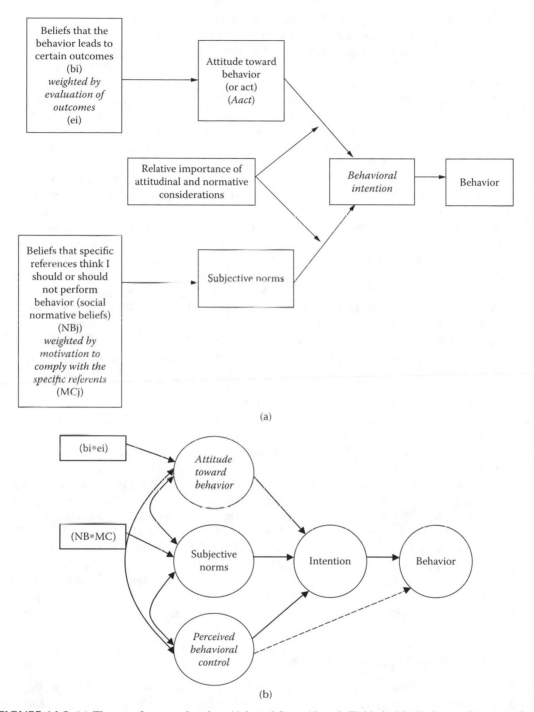

FIGURE 14.3 (a) Theory of reasoned action. (Adapted from Ajzen I, Fishbein M. *Understanding Attitudes and Predicting Social Behavior.* Englewood Cliffs, NJ: Prentice-Hall, 1980.) (b) The theory of planned behavior. (Adapted from Ajzen I, Madden JT. *J Exper Social Psychol* 1986;22: 453–74.)

perceived behavioral control as another factor influencing the intention to engage in a given behavior (Figure 14.3).

In cross-sectional evaluation of TRA/TPB factors of attitude, subjective norms and perceived behavioral control across a child's age and gender appear to be at least moderately related correlates (generally in the range of 0.1 to 0.4) of reported intention to be active (e.g., Hagger et al.[80]). There is some evidence of greater potency for the relation to children's physical activity intentions of subjective norms among younger elementary-aged children and perceived behavioral control among adolescents.[81–83] Indeed, some have found very low correlations between subjective norms and adolescents' intention to be active.[80]

Most studies of TRA/TPB among children have used the outcome of intentions to be active and thus failed to assess whether the TRA/TPB constructs are related to actual physical activity, although there are some exceptions. Trost and colleagues[84] found that attitudes, subjective norms, and perceived behavioral control around physical activity were independently related to adolescent girls' intentions to be active, but the intention to be active was only modestly associated with these girls' self-report of actual physical activity regardless of ethnicity and contrary to TRA or TPB. The authors conclude that "intentions and behaviors may not be closely aligned in adolescent girls" (p. 231). In this and a corresponding examination of TRA/TPB factors and the SCT construct of self-efficacy, perceived behavioral control and self-efficacy were found to be independently related to adolescent girls' physical activity, with self-efficacy positively associated with both moderate and vigorous intensity physical activity.[85] However, the limited explanatory power of TRA/TPB to explain variability in children's physical activity was further documented in a recent study that used more objective measures of children's physical activity (accelerometers). Attitudes and subjective norms were found to be associated with the intention to be physically active, intentions and perceived behavioral control were positively related to actual physical activity, but the variability in physical activity across children was not explained very well by these TRA/TPB factors.[86]

Perhaps to augment the explanatory power of the TRA/TPB model, recent investigations have combined this model with constructs from self-determination theory (detailed below), including extrinsic (e.g., active because others want me to be), intrinsic (e.g., active because I enjoy it), and introjective (e.g., active because otherwise I feel bad) motivators. The level of children's intrinsic motivation is highly related to the TRA/TPB constructs of attitudes, subjective norms, and perceived behavioral control around physical activity, with evidence that external or introjection factors are minimally related to these TRA/TPB constructs once the influence of intrinsic factors are taken into account.[82,87]

Whereas evidence documents cross-sectional relations between TRA/TPB constructs and children's physical activity, to our knowledge there has been no comprehensive evaluation of whether and how much TRA/TPB factors can be modified among children (e.g., increase positive attitudes) in order to increase physical activity. Such evaluation to test the mediation effects of the TRA/TPB for children's physical activity would need to assess whether these factors could be changed and whether such change is related to change in children's physical activity. It could be that it is difficult to conceive of ways to directly and rapidly change children's attitudes, subjective norms, and perceived behavioral control around physical activity. Self-determination models could provide avenues for such intervention (e.g., working to increase intrinsic motivation to change attitudes to change intentions to change physical activity levels).

SELF-DETERMINATION THEORY AND PEDIATRIC PHYSICAL ACTIVITY

The self-determination theory (SDT) was developed in part because the central focus of existing theories on cognition and efficacy appeared to limit the discussion of other important factors in human behavior.[45] SDT theorists, therefore, set out to integrate developmental theories, which conceptualize the person as an active organism, with behaviorist and cognitive theories, which view the person as predominantly reactive to social–environmental contexts. The SDT asserts that people have three *basic psychological needs: competence* (feeling effective), *relatedness* (feeling connected to others), and *autonomy* (perception of self as source of one's own behavior). These needs are considered innate and universal. They are therefore assumed to hold across age, gender, and culture, although the means to satisfy these needs may differ across various groups. Specific social–contextual

Type of motivation	Amotivation	Extrinsic motivation				Intrinsic motivation
Type of regulation	Non-regulation	External regulation	Introjected regulation	Identified regulation	Integrated regulation	Intrinsic regulation
Quality of behavior	Non-self-determined	⬛ ⬛ ⬛ ⬛ ⬛ ⬛ ⬛ ➤				Self-determined

FIGURE 14.4 The self-determination continuum. (Adapted from Ryan RM, Deci EL. Overview of self-determination theory: an organismic-dialectical perspective. In: Deci EL, Ryan RM, Eds. *Handbook of Self-Determination Research*. Rochester, NY: University of Rochester Press; 2002: 2–33.)

(or social–environmental) factors may be either supportive or antagonistic to these innate needs. Physical activity is related to needs in so as far as it fulfills them, and it is our job as exercise scientists to intervene in their world so that youth experience physical activity as fulfilling those needs. The SDT further postulates that behavior lives on a continuum of self-determination (from non-self-determined to self-determined). Levels of self-determination coincide with types of motivation (from amotivation to intrinsic motivation) and regulatory styles (Figure 14.4).

Intrinsic motivation is considered the optimal state of autonomy and challenge, and is associated with feelings of satisfaction, enjoyment, competence, and a desire to persist. According to this theory, people enjoy physical activity most if it is intrinsically motivated — conversely, one could say that the behaviors that people enjoy are most likely to be intrinsically motivated. Intrinsically motivated physical activity is therefore more likely to be undertaken and more likely to fulfill basic psychological needs. However, the SDT recognizes that some fairly important behaviors, such as regular physical activity, eating fruits and vegetables, and avoiding attractive energy dense foods, are going to be extrinsically motivated for many people. SDT suggests that participation in physical activity when it is extrinsically motivated can be enhanced by getting people to adopt regulatory styles that come closest to intrinsic regulation. At present, SDT is made up of four minitheories that build on these core theoretical concepts (see Box 1).

Research on SDT and physical activity in children and adolescents has mainly focused on measurement development, studies of interrelations between diverse constructs of the SDT and constructs from other theories such as the SCT, and relationships between SDT constructs and intentions to be physically active. Perceived competence has been related to sports enjoyment[88,89] and intrinsic motivation.[90] Intentions to be physically active or participate in leisure time physical activity have been related to many constructs in the SDT, including competence,[91] autonomy-supportive climates, and self-determined motivation.[92] Several studies have examined the relationship between SDT and physical activity. For instance, Wang and Biddle[93] studied the relations between constructs from the SDT and physical activity in 2500 12 to 15 year olds. They found that motivation and perceived competence was lower in older girls and that self-determination and motivation were related to recreational involvement and sports. In another study of 295 adolescents (mean age 14.5 years), Hagger and colleagues[94] showed that perceived autonomy support in physical education at week 1 was significantly related to self-reported leisure-time physical activity 5 weeks later.

The SDT has great promise because it offers a comprehensive view of human motivation but can be broken up into reasonably parsimonious minitheories. However, available research on the relationships between SDT variables and physical activity has generally employed fairly weak measures of physical activity, with a few notable exceptions.[95] Studies using objective measures of physical activity, such as accelerometry, are needed in order to understand SDT's possible contributions to the field of pediatric exercise science. To our knowledge, no published studies of SDT-based interventions on physical activity in pediatric populations are available to date, although several are ongoing. Hopefully, results from these studies will reveal whether constructs from the SDT actually mediate physical activity change.

BOX 1
Four Minitheories of Self-Determination Theory

---

1. Cognitive evaluation theory (CET) explains effects of contextual events (such as rewards, deadlines, praise) on intrinsic motivation, behavior, and experience. The influence of social contextual factors on intrinsic motivation is determined by two cognitive factors: perceived locus of causality (PLOC) and perceived competence.[133,134] *Perceived locus of causality* is related to autonomy needs: to what extent do external events shift PLOC away from intrinsic motivation? For instance, external rewards are hypothesized to shift perceived locus of causality to external motivation. This would lower intrinsic motivation, which would, in turn, lower physical activity. *Perceived competence* is related to the need for competence and the extent to which the social context is perceived as supporting competence (through, for instance, positive feedback). People actively attribute *functional significance* to social-contextual events: rewards, praise, or any other event can be *interpreted* either as *informational* (supports experience of competent engagement), *controlling* (pressures toward specific outcomes and undermines autonomy and intrinsic motivation), or *amotivating*.[62] The CET is most useful for studying behavior that people find interesting, challenging, or aesthetically pleasing, which is why it might be more useful for studying physical activity in athletes, but perhaps less useful for studying physical activity in adolescents who are not involved in competitive sports.

2. Organismic integration theory (OIT) examines how to transform externally regulated behaviors into self-regulated behaviors, and addresses the concept of *internalization,* especially with respect to the development of *extrinsic motivation*. The OIT was built to deal with the fact that socializing agents (schools, parents, public health advocates, doctors, etc.) often promote important — but for many uninteresting — behaviors that are not likely to be intrinsically motivated and are thus less likely to be performed. OIT addresses how we might prompt and promote self-regulation of these important behaviors. According to the OIT, extrinsically motivated behavior can become, to some extent, autonomous because people are naturally inclined to integrate ongoing experiences. The continuum of self-determination (Figure 14.4) represents constructs from the OIT. *Amotivation* is a lack of intention to act and results from feeling unable to achieve goals due to lack of competence or lack of value of activity or outcomes. In *external regulation* the motivation is to obtain rewards, avoid punishment, satisfy external demand or socially constructed contingency – this type of motivation is akin to operant conditioning. In *introjected regulation*, behavior is performed to avoid guild or shame or to enhance ego and feelings of self-worth. Behavior is ego-involved, controlling, and only partially integrated into self. In *identified regulation*, behavior (or the outcomes of that behavior) is accepted as personally important. The person identifies with the action or value to some extent. *Integrated regulation* is the most autonomous form of external regulation. Behavior (or its outcomes) is completely in line with personal values, goals, and needs. The difference between this form of external regulation and *intrinsic regulation* is that behavior under integrated regulation is still done to achieve personally important outcomes while behavior that is intrinsically regulated is done for inherent interest and enjoyment.

3. Causality orientations theory (COT) describes relatively stable individual differences in motivational orientations toward the social world. Motivation, behavior, and experience depend on social context and inner resources. The COT was developed to index aspects of personality integral to the regulation of behavior and experience. According the COT, there are three orientations to the social environment that differ in degree and promote self-determination.[135] Someone who is more *autonomously oriented* will regulate behavior based on interests and self-endorsed values. Autonomous orientation promotes intrinsic motivation and integrated regulation. *Controlled orientation* is related to behavior that is regulated and based on directives concerning how one "should" behave, and is related to external and introjected regulation. *Impersonal orientation* is related to amotivation and lack of intentional action.

4. Basic needs theory elaborates the concept of the three basic needs discussed in the main text, and their relation to life goals and daily behaviors. According to this minitheory, there will be a positive relationship between goal attainment and well-being only if it satisfies a basic psychological need. In other words, the pursuit of some goals that people may value highly (such as watching TV) may be negatively related to well-being if the goals take away from satisfaction of basic psychological needs (such as autonomy). *Intrinsic aspirations* (such as affiliation) provide direct satisfaction of basic needs, while *extrinsic aspirations* (such as looking like a model) do not.

HOT TOPICS IN PHYSICAL ACTIVITY RESEARCH: INDIVIDUAL DIFFERENCES AND CORRELATES OF PHYSICAL ACTIVITY

As various behavioral theories used to understand pediatric physical activity change, a major caveat about choice of theory must be noted. As mentioned above in the discussion of the health belief model, correlates of physical activity may differ according to demographics such as gender, ethnicity, and social and economic status, and according to age (usually used as a proxy for cognitive and physiological developmental status). Furthermore, new insights suggest that correlates of physical activity may differ for at-risk-for-overweight and overweight children. Beyond the scope of this chapter, but certainly important for consideration, is the possibility that correlates to physical activity will differ substantially for children with health problems, chronic illness, or disabilities.[96]

AGE, GENDER, AND ETHNIC DIFFERENCES IN CORRELATES OF PHYSICAL ACTIVITY

Similar to differences in physical activity prevalence across subpopulations of youth (e.g., gender, age, ethnicity), correlates of children's physical activity appear to differ by subpopulations. Gender differences in determinants of physical activity have repeatedly been found in adolescent populations.[97–99] Tappe et al.[100] reported that adolescent females considered "wanting to do other things with my time" to be a major barrier to physical activity, while adolescent males considered "having a girlfriend" and "use of alcohol and drugs" to be salient barriers to physical activity. Furthermore, mounting evidence points to pronounced ethnic and cultural differences in determinants of and barriers to physical activity.[54,101,102] For instance, African American girls differ from their Caucasian counterparts in their experience of availability of transportation, parental involvement, and boys' perception of girls who are physically active.[103] Latina girls report that major barriers to physical activity are self consciousness when they have to exercise with the boys, dissatisfaction with school PE programs, and feeling that the boys get all the attention.[104] Researchers have shown that perceived barriers to exercise differ substantially across cultural and ethnic groups in adult samples,[105] and they warn against a "color-blind" approach to perceived barriers of physical activity.[106] Perceived benefits and barriers may thus differ according to age, gender, and ethnicity. These considerations hold for most available constructs and theories that have been applied to children's physical activity, including those discussed in this chapter. The empirical literature has generally not advanced far enough to consider subpopulation differences when evaluating theoretical models to fit to children's physical activity. However, examination of whether the constructs in various models of health behavior are correlates, moderators, and/or mediators of children's physical activity begins the identification of influences on this behavior.

SOCIOECONOMIC STATUS AND CHILDREN'S PHYSICAL ACTIVITY

Relations are complicated between various child and family demographic factors, physical activity, and obesity. For example, obesity may be more prevalent among lower socioeconomic status (SES) children in comparison with children from higher SES families,[107–109] but one recent study finds higher rates of obesity among higher SES adolescents.[108] Further, relations between SES and obesity may not be consistent across ethnicity[107] or other factors (e.g., country). Although sparse, there is some evidence that socioeconomically disadvantaged children are less likely to be physically active during leisure time[110] and more likely than higher SES children to report no vigorous physical activity lasting 20 min or longer during any day of the prior week.[111] There are numerous potential mechanisms by which lower SES and corresponding environments in which lower SES families live may confer a disadvantage in children acquiring adequate amounts of physical activity. This includes among other things a lower perceived safety of the surrounding neighborhood in which children could play[112] and fewer physical activity facilities and resources.[113,114] Individual health beliefs may also make it less likely that lower SES children and families engage in physical activity and other healthy lifestyle behaviors.[115] Clearly, more comprehensive and theory-driven evaluations of environmental, individual, and demographic factors that contribute to children's physical activity and obesity are needed to understand the mechanisms and leverage points in order to intervene on these health issues.

CORRELATES OF PHYSICAL ACTIVITY IN OVERWEIGHT VERSUS NONOVERWEIGHT CHILDREN

Differences between obese and nonobese children in behavioral and other correlates and/or mediators of physical activity are confounded by a potential third variable and problems with causal directionality. However, the identification of correlates, moderators, and/or mediators that are specific to overweight children's physical activity could help focus interventions with this at-risk population. Overweight children, particularly girls, report higher barriers to physical activity than their nonoverweight peers, with body-related barriers to physical activity (e.g., self-consciousness about body when being active) among overweight girls in particular reported as being greater impediments than resource, social, and fitness barriers.[116] In one study, obese children reported lower adult support for physical activity,[116] but this weight status difference in social influences is not always observed.[117] Obese children indicate having lower physical activity self-efficacy than nonobese children, although their outcome expectancies or beliefs about physical activity appear similar.[117]

The direction of causality between childhood obesity and physical activity is not well specified, and it is possible it becomes a vicious cycle over time. For example, there are many aspects of being overweight in childhood that could preclude being more physically active. Stigmatization of overweight and obese children has been documented repeatedly,[118,119] and overweight children have less substantive peer networks.[120] Stigmatization of child overweight is evidenced by high rates of weight-related teasing directed toward overweight youth, with the frequency and negative effects of such teasing related to greater liking for isolative sedentary activities and loneliness.[121] Overweight has also been associated with increased experiences of anxiety, depression, suicidal thoughts, body dissatisfaction, and hopelessness,[122] particularly in Western youth.[123] These issues may interfere with obese children being more active. Overweight children may also be more physically uncomfortable engaging in physical activity, perhaps due to lower levels of physical fitness than their nonoverweight counterparts, thus precluding physical activity. It is not clear from the empirical literature whether unique factors correlate with, moderate, and/or mediate physical activity among obese vs. nonobese children because no studies have comprehensively examined these differences. Theory-based longitudinal and intervention studies are warranted to better understand the behavioral correlates, mediators, and moderators unique to obese children's physical activity.

CONCLUSION

Even using the more optimistic self-report estimates of children's overall physical activity, older children especially are not uniformly meeting the more rigorous recommendations for daily physical activity that lasts at least 60 min. Based on the more objective assessments of children's physical activity indicating lower overall physical activity (in comparison with self-report assessments) and minimal if any vigorous physical activity, efficacious interventions are needed to increase physical activity across the childhood population. Further, some subpopulations of children (e.g., overweight children) may require even more physical activity than currently recommended for children in order to become more optimally healthful.

This chapter, in an attempt to organize and evaluate factors related to children's physical activity, details various health behavior theories that have been, in part, applied to the examination of children's physical activity. There has been increasing consensus in the field that to increase the effectiveness of physical activity interventions in youth, research must focus on a better understanding of the mechanisms of physical activity behavior change.[19,48] It is only from theory that such mechanisms can be clearly delineated and therefore tested. However, a recently released review of 47 interventions to promote physical activity found only one study that examined whether a hypothesized mediator affected physical activity outcomes.[124] The majority of the research has remained at the correlates level, including mostly cross-sectional examination of the factors related to children's physical activity. This is appropriate to build and initially test theories, but it is merely a starting point to inform theory-based intervention to actually increase children's physical activity. Existing significant problems in the research arena have been identified, including: (1) theories and therefore mediators fail to be specified and evaluated within intervention trials, (2) current theoretical models often fail to account for substantial variability in physical activity, and (3) interventions often fail to effect substantial changes in selected mediating variables.[19] There is an increasing realization in the field that the current, predominantly cognitive theories fall short empirically,[125] and that theories of child and adolescent health behaviors must include the influence of affect as well as environment.[38,126] The infusion of new models (e.g., SDT, ecological models) and their adequate testing have the potential to explain more of the variance in children's physical activity and, thus, identify specific targets for intervention. Although we are not especially close to completely understanding why Jane runs, we can and must obtain a better understanding in order to help Jane run more often — and more importantly — to help all children engage in more physical activity in order to achieve and maintain health across their lifespan.

REFERENCES

1. Goran MI, Reynolds KD, Lindquist CH. Role of physical activity in the prevention of obesity in children. *Intl J Obes Related Metabol Disord: J Int Assoc Study Obes.* 1999;23(Suppl 3): S18–S33.
2. Hill JO, Wyatt HR, Reed GW, Peters JC. Obesity and the environment: where do we go from here? *Science.* 2003;299(5608): 853–855.
3. Kimm SY, Glynn NW, Kriska AM, et al. Decline in physical activity in black girls and white girls during adolescence [comment]. *New Engl J Med.* 2002;347(10): 709–715.
4. Luepker RV. How physically active are American children and what can we do about it? *Int J Obes Relat Metab Disord.* 1999;23 Suppl (2): S12–S17.
5. Micucci S, Thomas H, Vohra J. *The Effectiveness of School-Based Strategies for the Primary Prevention of Obesity and for Promoting Physical Activity and/or Nutrition, the Major Modifiable Risk Factors for Type 2 Diabetes: A Review of Reviews.* Ontario, Canada: The Ontario Public Health Association; 2002.
6. Resnicow K, Robinson T. School-based cardiovascular disease prevention studies: Review and synthesis. *Ann Epidemiol.* 1997;S7: S14–31.
7. Pate RR, Pratt M, Blair SN, et al. Physical activity and public health: A recommendation from the Centers for Disease Control and Prevention and the American College of Sports Medicine. *JAMA.* 1995;273: 402–7.
8. U.S. Department of Health and Human Services. *Healthy People 2010.* Washington, DC; 2000. Report No.: 017-001-00547-9.
9. Riddoch CJ, Bo Andersen L, Wedderkopp N, et al. Physical activity levels and patterns of 9- and 15-yr-old European children. *Med Sci Sports Exerc.* 2004;36 (1): 86–92.
10. Pratt M, Macera CA, Blanton C. Levels of physical activity and inactivity in children and adults in the United States: current evidence and research issues. *Med Sci Sports Exerc.* 1999;31(11 Suppl): S526–33.
11. Irving HM, Adlaf EM, Allison KR, Paglia A, Dwyer JJ, Goodman J. Trends in vigorous physical activity participation among Ontario adolescents, 1997–2001. *Can J Public Health.* 2003;94 (4): 272–4.
12. Centers for Disease Control and Prevention. Youth Risk Behavior Surveillance — United States, 2003. *Morbid Mortal Wkly Rept.* 2004;53(SS-2).
13. Epstein LH, Paluch RA, Kalakanis LE, Goldfield GS, Cerny FJ, Roemmich JN. How much activity do youth get? A quantitative review of heart-rate measured activity. *Pediatrics.* 2001;108(3): E44.

14. Pate RR, Freedson PS, Sallis JF, et al. Compliance with physical activity guidelines: prevalence in a population of children and youth. *Ann Epidemiol*. 2002;12(5): 303–8.

15. Patrick K, Norman GJ, Calfas KJ, et al. Diet, physical activity, and sedentary behaviors as risk factors for overweight in adolescence. *Arch Pediatr Adolesc Med*. 2004;158: 385–90.

16. Centers for Disease Control and Prevention. Physical activity levels among children aged 9–13 years — United States, 2002. *Morbid Mortal Wkly Rept*. 2003;52(33): 785–8.

17. Gordon-Larsen P, McMurray RG, Popkin BM. Adolescent physical activity and inactivity vary by ethnicity: The National Longitudinal Study of Adolescent Health. *J Pediatr*. 1999;135 (3): 301–6.

18. King AC, Stokols D, Talen E, Brassington GS, Killingsworth R. Theoretical approaches to the promotion of physical activity: forging a transdisciplinary paradigm. *Am J Prev Med*. 2002;23(2 Suppl): 15–25.

19. Baranowski T, Anderson C, Carmack C. Mediating variable framework in physical activity interventions. How are we doing? How might we do better? [erratum appears in *Am J Prev Med*. 1999 Jul. 17 (1): 98.]. *Am J Prev Med*. 1998;15(4): 266–97.

20. Stokols D. Establishing and maintaining healthy environments. Toward a social ecology of health promotion. *Am Psychol*. 1992;47(1): 6–22.

21. Corburn J. Confronting the Challenges in Reconnecting Urban Planning and Public Health. *Am J Public Health*. 2004;94 (4): 541–6.

22. Sallis JF, Kraft K, Linton LS. How the environment shapes physical activity: A transdisciplinary research agenda 1. *Am J Prev Med*. 2002;22 (3): 208.

23. Brownson RC, Baker EA, Housemann RA, Brennan LK, Bacak SJ. Environmental and policy determinants of physical activity in the United States. *Am J Public Health*. 2001;91(12): 1995–2003.

24. Sallis JF. Reflections on the physical activity interventions conference. *Am J Prev Med*. 1998;15 (4): 431–2.

25. Giles-Corti B, Donovan RJ. The relative influence of individual, social and physical environment determinants of physical activity. *Social Sci Med*. 2002;54(12): 1793–812.

26. Giles-Corti B, Donovan RJ. Relative influences of individual, social environmental, and physical environmental correlates of walking. *Am J Public Health*. 2003;93 (9): 1583–9.

27. DiClemente RJ, Crosby RA, Kegler MC. *Emerging Theories in Health Promotion Practice and Research Strategies for Improving Public Health*. 1st ed. San Francisco: Jossey-Bass; 2002.

28. Perry CL. *Creating Health Behavior Change*. Thousand Oaks, London: Sage Publications; 1999.

29. Sallis JF, Prochaska JJ, Taylor WC. A review of correlates of physical activity of children and adolescents. *Med Sci Sports Exercise*. 2000;32(5): 963–75.

30. Dishman RK, Motl RW, Saunders R, et al. Self-efficacy partially mediates the effect of a school-based physical-activity intervention among adolescent girls. *Prev Med*. 2004;38(5): 628–36.

31. Bauman AE, Sallis JF, Dzewaltowski DA, Owen N. Toward a better understanding of the influences on physical activity: the role of determinants, correlates, causal variables, mediators, moderators, and confounders. *Am J Prev Med*. 2002;23(2 Suppl): 5–14.

32. Motl RW, Dishman RK, Ward DS, et al. Examining social-cognitive determinants of intention and physical activity among black and white adolescent girls using structural equation modeling. *Health Psychol*. 2002;215: 459–67.

33. MacKinnon D. Analysis of mediating variables in prevention and intervention research. *NIDA Res Monograp.h* 1994;139:127–53.

34. Reynolds KD, Bishop DB, Chou C-P, Xie B, Nebeling L, Perry CL. Contrasting mediating variables in two 5–a-day nutrition intervention programs. *Prev Med*. 2004;39:882–93.

35. Chou C-P, Spruijt-Metz D, Azen SP. How Can Statistical Approaches Enhance Transdisciplinary Study of Drug Misuse Prevention? Substance Use and Misuse. 2004;39(10–12): 1867–1906.

36. McLean N, Griffin S, Toney K, Hardeman W. Family involvement in weight control, weight maintenance and weight-loss interventions: a systematic review of randomised trials. *Intl J Obes Related Metabolic Disorders: J Int Assoc Study Obes*. 2003;27(9): 987–1005.

37. Hansen WB, McNeal RB, Jr. The law of maximum expected potential effect: Constraints placed on program effectiveness by mediator relationships. *Health Edu. Res.* 1996;11(4): 501–7.

38. Spruijt-Metz D. *Adolescence, Affect and Health*. London: Psychology Press; 1999.

39. Glanz K, Rimer BK, Lewis FM. *Health Behavior and Health Education: Theory, Research, and Practice*. 3rd ed. San Francisco: Jossey-Bass; 2002.

40. Rothman AJ. "Is there nothing more practical than a good theory?" Why innovations and advances in health behavior change will arise if interventions are used to test and refine theory. *Int J Behav Nutrition Physical Activity*. 2004;1(11): 1–11.
41. Dishman RK, Buckworth J. Adherence to physical activity. In: Morgan WP, ed. *Physical Activity and Mental Health*. Philadelphia, PA: Taylor & Francis; 1997: 63–80.
42. Brown L, DiClemente R, Reynolds L. HIV prevention for adolescents: Utility of the Health Belief Model. *AIDS Ed Prev*. 1991;3:50–9.
43. Brodkin P, Weiss MR. Developmental differences in motivation for participating in competitive swimming. *J Sport Exercise Psychol* 1990;12(3): 248–63.
44. Kohl HW, 3rd, Hobbs KE. Development of physical activity behaviors among children and adolescents. *Pediatrics*. 1998;101(3 Pt 2): 549–54.
45. Frederick-Recascino CM. Self-determination theory and participation: motivation research in the sport and exercise domain. In: Deci EL, Ryan RM, Eds. *Handbook of Self-Determination Research*. Rochester, NY: University of Rochester Press; 2002:277–94.
46. Pate RR. Physical activity in young people. *Topics Nutrition*. 2000;1(8): 1–18.
47. Glanz K, Lewis FM, Rimer BK, eds. *Health Behavior and Health Education: Theory, Research, and Practice*. 2nd ed. San Francisco: Jossey-Bass Publishers; 1997.
48. Lewis BA, Marcus BH, Pate RR, Dunn AL. Psychosocial mediators of physical activity behavior among adults and children. *Am J Prev Med*. 2002;23(1): 26–35.
49. Biddle SJH, Nigg CR. Theories of exercise behavior. *Int J Sport Psychol Special Issue: Exercise Psychology*. 2000;31(2): 290–304.
50. Godin G, Shepard RJ. Use of attitude-behavior models in exercise promotion. *Sports Med*. 1990;10:103–21.
51. Desmond SM, Price JH, Lock RS, Smith D, Stewart PW. Urban black and white adolescents' physical fitness status and perceptions of exercise. *J School Health*. 1990;60(5): 220–6
52. Deflandre A, Antonini PR, Lorant J. Perceived benefits and barriers to physical activity among children, adolescents and adults. *Int J Sport Psychol*. 2004;35(1): 23–36.
53. Jamner MS, Spruijt-Metz D, Bassin S, Cooper DM. A controlled evaluation of a school-based intervention to promote physical activity among sedentary adolescent females: Project FAB. *J Adolescent Health*. 2004;344: 279–89.
54. Bungum TJ, Vincent ML. Determinants of physical activity among female adolescents. *Am J Prev Med* 1997;13(2): 115–22.
55. DiLorenzo TM, Stucky-Ropp RC, Vander Wal JS, Gotham HJ. Determinants of exercise among children. II. A longitudinal analysis. *Prev Med*. 1998;27(3): 470–7.
56. Garcia AW, Pender NJ, Antonakos CL, Ronis DL. Changes in physical activity beliefs and behaviors of boys and girls across the transition to junior high school. *J Adolescent Health*. 1998;22(5): 394–402.
57. Haefner D, Kirscht J. Motivational and behavioral effects of modifying health beliefs. *HSMHA Health Rept*.1970;85:478–84.
58. Bandura A. Self-efficacy: Toward a unifying theory of behavioral change. *Psychol Rev*. 1977;84:191–215.
59. Janz NK, Becker MH. The health belief model: A decade later. *Health Ed Quart*. 1984;2 (1): 1–47.
60. Rosenstock R, Strecher V, Becker M. Social learning theory and the health belief model. *Health Ed Quart*. 1988;15:175–83.
61. Allison KR, Dwyer JJ, Makin S. Self-efficacy and participation in vigorous physical activity by high school students. *Health Ed Behav*. 1999;26 (1): 12–24.
62. Biddle SJH, Mutrie N. *Psychology of Physical Activity: Determinants, Well-Being and Interventions*. New York: Routledge; 2001.
63. Bandura A. *Social Foundations of Thought and Action: A Social Cognitive Theory*. Englewood Cliffs, NJ: Prentice-Hall; 1986.
64. Sallis JF, Owen N. Ecological models. In: Glanz K, Lewis FM, Rimer BK, eds. *Health Behavior and Health Education: Theory, Research, and Practice* (2nd ed). San Francisco, CA: Jossey-Bass Publishers; 1996:403–24.
65. Bandura A. *Self-Efficacy: The Exercise of Control*. New York: W.H. Freeman and Company; 1997.

66. Strauss RS, Rodzilsky D, Burack G, Colin M. Psychosocial correlates of physical activity in healthy children. *Arch Pediatr Adolesc Med*. 2001;155 (8): 897–902.

67. Barnett TA, O'Loughlin J, Paradis G. One- and two-year predictors of decline in physical activity among inner-city schoolchildren. *Am J Prev Med*. 2002;23 (2): 121–8.

68. Sallis JF, Prochaska JJ, Taylor WC. A review of correlates of physical activity of children and adolescents. *Med Sci Sports Exerc*. 2000;32(5): 963–75.

69. Edmundson E, Parcel GS, Perry CL, et al. The effects of the Child and Adolescent Trial for Cardio-vascular Health Intervention on psychosocial determinants of cardiovascular disease risk behavior among third-grade students. *Am J Health Promot*. 1996;10(3): 217–25.

70. Stevens J, Story M, Ring K, et al. The impact of the Pathways intervention on psychosocial variables related to diet and physical activity in American Indian schoolchildren. *Prev Med*. 2003;37(70)–(79).

71. Edmundson E, Parcel GS, Feldman HA, et al. The effects of the Child and Adolescent Trial for Cardiovascular Health upon psychosocial determinants of diet and physical activity behavior. *Prev Med*. 1996;25:442–54.

72. Lewis BA, Marcus BH, Pate RR, Dunn AL. Psychosocial mediators of physical activity behavior among adults and children. *Am J Prev Med*. 2002;23(2 Suppl): 26–35.

73. Dishman RK, Motl RW, Saunders R, et al. Self-efficacy partially mediates the effect of a school-based physical-activity intervention among adolescent girls. *Prev Med*. 2004;38:628–36.

74. Wilson DK, Friend R, Teasley N, Green S, Lee Reaves I, Sica DA. Motivational versus social cognitive interventions for promoting fruit and vegetable intake and physical activity in African American adolescents. *Ann Behav Med*. 2002;244: 310–9.

75. Dzewaltowski DA. Physical activity determinants: a social cognitive approach. *Med Sci Sports Exerc*. 1994;26 (11): 1395–9.

76. Ryan GJ, Dzewaltowski DA. Comparing the relationships between different types of self-efficacy and physical activity in youth. *Health Educ Behav*. 2002;29 (4): 491–504.

77. Trost SG, Pate RR, Saunders R, Ward DS, Dowda M, Felton G. A prospective study of the determinants of physical activity in rural fifth-grade children. *Prev Med*. 1997;26 (2): 257–63.

78. Saelens BE, Sallis JF, Frank LD. Environmental correlates of walking and cycling: findings from the transportation, urban design, and planning literatures. *Ann Behav Med*. 2003;25 (2): 80–91.

79. Saelens BE, Sallis JF, Black JB, Chen D. Neighborhood-based differences in physical activity: an environment scale evaluation. *Am J Public Health*. 2003;93 (9): 1552–8.

80. Hagger MS, Chatzisarantis NL, Biddle SJH, Orbell S. Antecedents of children's physical activity intentions and behaviour: predictive validity and longitudinal effects. *Psychol Health*. 2001;16:391–407.

81. Craig S, Goldberg J, Dietz WH. Psychosocial correlates of physical activity among fifth and eighth graders. *Prev Med*. 1996;25 (5): 506–13.

82. Hagger MS, Chatzisarantis NL, Biddle SJ. The influence of autonomous and controlling motives on physical activity intentions within the theory of planned behaviour. *Br J Health Psychol*. 2002;7(Part 3): 283–97.

83. Mummery WK, Spence JC, Hudec JC. Understanding physical activity intention in Canadian school children and youth: an application of the theory of planned behavior. *Res Q Exerc Sport*.2000;71(2): 116–24.

84. Trost SG, Pate RR, Dowda M, Ward DS, Felton G, Saunders R. Psychosocial correlates of physical activity in white and African-American girls. *J Adolesc Health*. 2002;31(3): 226–33.

85. Motl RW, Dishman RK, Ward DS, et al. Examining social-cognitive determinants of intention and physical activity among black and white adolescent girls using structural equation modeling. *Health Psychol*. 2002;21 (5): 459–67.

86. Trost SG, Saunders R, Ward DS. Determinants of physical activity in middle school children. *Am J Health Behav*. 2002;26(2): 95–102.

87. Hagger MS, Armitage CJ. The influence of perceived loci of control and causality in the theory of planned behavior in a leisure-time exercise context. *J Appl Biobehav Res*. 2004;9 (1): 45.

88. Boyd MP, Weinmann C, Yin Z. The relationship of physical self-perceptions and goal orientations to intrinsic motivation for exercise. *J Sport Behav*. 2002;25(1): 1–18.

89. Boyd MP, Yin Z. Cognitive-affective sources of sport enjoyment in adolescent sport participants. *Adolescence*. 1996;31(122): 383–95.

90. Ferrer-Caja E, Weiss MR. Predictors of intrinsic motivation among adolescent students in physical education. *Res Q Exercise Sport*. 2000;71(3): 267–79.

91. Lintunen T, Valkonen A, Leskinen E, Biddle SJ. Predicting physical activity intentions using a goal perspectives approach: a study of Finnish youth. *Scand J Med Sci Sports*. 1999;9 (6): 344–52.

92. Standage M, Duda JL, Ntoumanis N. A model of contextual motivation in physical education: Using constructs from self-determination and achievement goal theories to predict physical activity intentions. *J Ed Psychol*. 2003;95(1): 97–110.

93. Wang JKC, Biddle SJH. Young people's motivational profiles in physical activity: a cluster analysis. *J Sport Exercise Psychol*. 2001;23:1–22.

94. Hagger MS, Chatzisarantis NLD, Culverhouse T, Biddle SJH. The processes by which perceived autonomy support in physical education promotes leisure-time physical activity intentions and behavior: A trans-contextual model. *J Ed Psychol*. 2003;95(4): 784–95.

95. Biddle S, Armstrong N. Children's physical activity: an exploratory study of psychological correlates. *Social Sci Med*. 1992;34(3): 325–32.

96. Wallander J, Siegel L, J., Eds. *Adolescent Health Problems*. New York, London: The Guilford Press; 1995.

97. Sallis JF, McKenzie TL, Elder JP, et al. Sex and ethnic differences in children's physical activity: discrepancies between self-report and objective measures. *Pediatr Exercise Sci*. 1998;10 (3): 277–84.

98. Stucky-Ropp RC, DiLorenzo TM. Determinants of exercise in children. *Prev Med*. 1993;22 (6): 880–9.

99. Trost SG, Pate RR, Dowda M, Saunders R, Ward DS, Felton G. Gender differences in physical activity and determinants of physical activity in rural fifth grade children. *J School Health*. 1996;66 (4): 145–50.

100. Tappe MK, Duda JL, Ehrnwald PM. Perceived barriers to exercise among adolescents. *J School Health*. 1989;59 (4): 153–5.

101. Bungum T, Pate R, Dowdu M, Vincent M. Correlates of physical activity among African-American and Caucasian female adolescents. *Am J Health Behavior*. 1999;23 (1): 25–31.

102. Gordon-Larsen P, McMurray RG, Popkin BM. Determinants of adolescent physical activity and inactivity patterns. *Pediatrics*. 2000;105 (6): E83.

103. Taylor WC, Yancey AK, Leslie J, et al. Physical activity among African American and Latino middle school girls: consistent beliefs, expectations, and experiences across two sites. *Women & Health*. 1999;302: 67–82.

104. Leslie J, Yancy A, McCarthy W, et al. Development and implementation of a school-based nutrition and fitness promotion program for ethnically diverse middle-school girls. *J Am Diet Assoc*. 1999;99 (8): 967–70.

105. Heesch KC, Brown DR, Blanton CJ. Perceived barriers to exercise and stage of exercise adoption in older women of different racial/ethnic groups. *Women Health*. 2000;30(4): 61–76.

106. Johnson MRD. Perceptions of barriers to healthy physical activity among Asian communities. *Sport, Ed Soc*. 2000;5(1): 51–70.

107. Goodman E, Slap GB, Huang B. The public health impact of socioeconomic status on adolescent depression and obesity. *Am J Public Health*. 2003;93(11): 1844–50.

108. Haas JS, Lee LB, Kaplan CP, Sonneborn D, Phillips KA, Liang SY. The association of race, socioeconomic status, and health insurance status with the prevalence of overweight among children and adolescents. *Am J Public Health*. 2003;93(12): 2105–10.

109. Wardle J, Jarvis MJ, Steggles N, et al. Socioeconomic disparities in cancer-risk behaviors in adolescence: baseline results from the Health and Behaviour in Teenagers Study (HABITS). *Prev Med*. 2003;36:721–30.

110. Kristjansdottir G, Vilhjalmsson R. Sociodemographic differences in patterns of sedentary and physically active behavior in older children and adolescents. *Acta Paediatr*. 2001;90:429–35.

111. Lee RE, Cubbin C. Neighborhood context and youth cardiovascular health behaviors. *Am J Public Health*. 2002;92(3): 428–36.

112. Molnar BE, Gortmaker SL, Bull FC, Buka SL. Unsafe to play? Neighborhood disorder and lack of safety predict reduced physical activity among urban children and adolescents. *Am J Health Promot*. 2004;18(5): 378–86.

113. Estabrooks PA, Lee RE, Gyurcsik NC. Resources for physical activity participation: does availability and accessibility differ by neighborhood socioeconomic status? *Ann Behav Med*. 2003;25(2): 100–4.

114. Wilson DK, Kirtland KA, Ainsworth BE, Addy CL. Socioeconomic status and perceptions of access and safety for physical activity. *Ann Behav Med.* 2004;28(1): 20–8.

115. Wardle J, Steptoe A. Socioeconomic differences in attitudes and beliefs about healthy lifestyles. *J Epidemiol Community Health* 2003;57(6): 440–3.

116. Zabinski MF, Saelens BE, Stein RI, Hayden-Wade HA, Wilfley DE. Overweight children's barriers to and support for physical activity. *Obes Res.* 2003;11(2): 238–46.

117. Trost SG, Kerr LM, Ward DS, Pate RR. Physical activity and determinants of physical activity in obese and non-obese children. *Int J Obes.* 2001;25:822–9.

118. Kimm SY, Barton BA, Berhane K, Ross JW, Payne GH, Schreiber GB. Self-esteem and adiposity in black and white girls: the NHLBI Growth and Health Study. *Ann Epidemiol.* 1997;7(8): 550–60.

119. Tiggemann M, Anesbury T. Negative stereotyping of obesity in children: The role of controllability beliefs. *J Appl Social Psychol* 2000;30(9): 1977–93.

120. Strauss RS, Pollack HA. Social marginalization of overweight children. *Arch Pediatr Adolesc Med.* 2003;157(8): 746–52.

121. Hayden-Wade H, Stein RI, Ghaderi A, Saelens BE, Zabinski MF, Wilfley DE. Prevalence, characteristics, and correlates of teasing experiences among overweight children versus non-overweight peers, in press.

122. Lobstein T, Baur L, Uauy R. *Obesity in Children and Young People: A Crisis in Public Health.* London, England: IASO International Obesity Task Force; 2004.

123. Ge X, Elder CH, Jr, Regnerus M, Cox C. Pubertal transitions, perceptions of being overweight, and adolescents' psychological maladjustment: Gender and ethnic differences. *Social Psychol Q.* 2001;64 (4): 363–75.

124. Holtzman J, Schmitz K, Babes G, et al. *Effectiveness of Behavioral Interventions to Modify Physical Activity Behaviors in General Populations and Cancer Patients and Survivors.* Rockville, MD: Prepared by the University of Minnesota Evidence-based Practice Center, under Contract No. 290–02–0009; 2004 June 2004. Report No.: AHRQ Publication No. 04–E027–1.

125. Jeffery RW. How can health behavior theory be made more useful for intervention research? *Int J Behav Nutrition Physical Activity.* 2004;1(11).

126. Bauer KW, Yang YW, Austin SB. "How can we stay healthy when you're throwing all of this in front of us?" Findings from focus groups and interviews in middle schools on environmental influences on nutrition and physical activity. *Health Ed Behav.* 2004;31(1): 34–46.

127. Sallis JF, Patrick K, Long BJ. Overview of the International Consensus Conference on physical activity guidelines for adolescents. *Ped Exerc Sci.* 1994;6:229–301.

128. Cavill N, Biddle SJ, Sallis JF. Health enhancing physical activity for young people: Statement of the United Kingdom Expert Consensus Conference. *Ped Exerc Sci.* 2001;13:12–25.

129. U.S. Department of Agriculture, U.S. Department of Health and Human Services. *Dietary Guidelines for Americans,* 2000 (5th ed.). U.S. Department of Agriculture, U.S. Department of Health and Human Services Washington, DC; 2000.

130. Corbin CB, Pangrazi RP. *Physical Activity for Children: A Statement of Guidelines for Children Ages 5–12.* 2nd ed: National Association for Sport & Physical Education; 2004.

131. Trost SG, Pate RR, Sallis JF, et al. Age and gender differences in objectively measured physical activity in youth. *Med Sci Sports Exerc.* 2002;34(2): 350–5.

132. Tudor-Locke C, Ainsworth BE, Adair LS, Du S, Popkin BM. Physical activity and inactivity in Chinese school-aged youth: the China Health and Nutrition Survey. *Int J Obes.* 2003;27(9): 1093–9.

133. Ryan RM, Connell JP. Perceived locus of causality and internalization: examining reasons for acting in two domains. *J Personality Social Psychol.* 1989;57(5): 749–61.

134. Hagger MS, Chatzisarantis NLD, Biddle SJH. The influence of autonomous and controlling motives on physical activity intentions within the theory of planned behaviour. *Br J Health Psychol.* 2002;7(3): 283–97.

135. Deci EL, Ryan RM. The general causality orientations scale: self-determination in personality. *J Res Personality.* 1985;19(2): 109–34.

15 Influence of the Built Environment on Physical Activity and Obesity in Children and Adolescents

Penny Gordon-Larsen and Kim D. Reynolds

CONTENTS

INTRODUCTION

As reviewed in earlier chapters, childhood obesity has rapidly increased among children and adolescents,[1] with no indication of abatement.[2] The obesity epidemic has been closely linked to an obesogenic environment[3] in which labor saving technologies and leisure options promote an inactive lifestyle and obesity.[4] For children, several societal trends have served to promote sedentary lifestyles: active transportation has decreased in favor of automobile transportation, in-school activity has declined, and a wide variety of sedentary activities is available to children compared with active leisure time activities. Three recent review articles conclude that environmental factors, either objectively or subjectively measured, are consistently related to physical activity.[5-7] In this chapter, we discuss the relationship between built environment factors and physical activity as it relates to obesity in children and adolescents.

In public health, the macro and built environment can be broadly conceived as the physical, legal, and policy environment, which presents barriers and facilitators to health-related behaviors, such as physical activity. In the planning and transportation fields, the built environment is defined as a multidimensional concept, broadly including patterns of human activity at various scales of geography within the physical environment.[8] Handy et al.[8] state that the built environment includes

(1) "urban design," the design of a city and its physical elements; (2) "land use," location and density of residential, commercial, industrial, forest, and other areas; and (3) "transportation system," physical infrastructure of roads, sidewalks, bike paths, and others.

Environments may influence physical activity behaviors by promoting or discouraging activity through built environment factors (e.g., availability of safe and affordable recreation facilities or walkable neighborhood design). Whereas the physical activity literature has not dealt extensively with quantification of built environment variables, the urban planning literature has traditionally focused on quantifying and characterizing the built environment, but without direct attention to physical activity. These two fields are now being blended to develop appropriate tools and measures, to advance our use of theory, and to better explain and predict physical activity and transportation behavior.[9–11]

Strategies to confront the obesity and inactivity epidemic that include built environment factors have substantial potential to affect an entire population,[6,12] rather than select individuals.[12,13] Supportive environments can provide a setting within which individual-level efforts may be optimized. Individual-level interventions have not had much success in long-term behavior change because of the lack of predictive power of behavior theories and lack of attention to change in mediating variables.[14] Furthermore, environmental barriers may limit the impact of these programs; for example, behavior change may be difficult without supportive environmental resources. Environmental and policy interventions have had enormous success in tobacco control through programs such as taxation and bans on indoor smoking,[15] although taxation strategies may be less well accepted in the built environment domain.[16] In addition, environmental and policy approaches can continue to influence behavior over time without requiring continued and active intervention by public health professionals.

The vast majority of the built environment and health literature has focused on adults. Few empirical studies have been conducted to examine the relationship of the built environment with physical activity among children. In a recent review of correlates of physical activity in youth, Sallis et al.[17] found that although built environment factors were understudied, there were consistent associations between childhood and adolescent activity patterns and factors such as access to programs, facilities, and opportunities for physical activity.

In this chapter, we focus on built environment correlates that present barriers and facilitators to physical activity. In addition, we present a short discussion on built environment factors and diet outcomes. Given the lack of research in youth, we present evidence for environment–activity relationships in adults and in youth where possible. Our focus is on environmental correlates research, as opposed to environmental intervention research, because there has been more correlate-oriented research. In addition, we focus on public health–oriented research, where there has been some examination of the linkage between environmental factors and health behaviors.

MEASURING THE BUILT ENVIRONMENT

Quantifying the built environment generally entails linkage to multiple resources and databases across geographic space and time. For example, population density is often measured using census data. Land use and diversity are often measured using land cover data or data describing the types of land use (e.g., commercial, residential, forest, urban). The built environment can be examined at various spatial scale levels, such as by census groupings (e.g., census block group), neighborhood, county, or region.

A central objective tool for characterizing the built environment is a geographic information system (GIS), a powerful tool to integrate these various dimensions of the built environment into a database that can then be linked to individual-level attribute data. A GIS is essentially a computerized map that allows the plotting of resource layers onto a coordinate system, which can then be used to spatially analyze the density and proximity of resources, environmental factors, and population characteristics, further allowing the evaluation of the impact of such facilities and

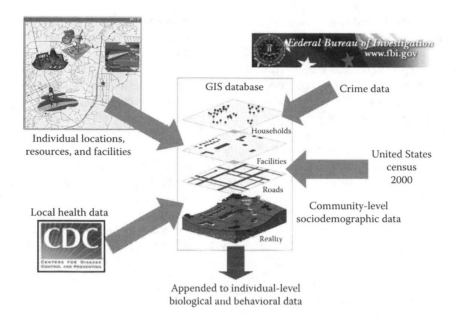

FIGURE 15.1 This example of the development of a geographic information system (GIS) database demonstrates the merging of respondent locations and facilities; location-specific community-level data such us crime data, sociodemographic data from the U.S census; and local health data, which are then merged to the individual-level biological and behavioral data to assess the relationship between community-level influences on individual-level health outcomes

environment characteristics on behavior. Using GIS, locations can be geocoded, or assigned a geographic reference such as latitude and longitude. Once geocoded, locations of individuals and resources, as well as built and social environment characteristics derived from public, federal, and commercial sources can be merged into a data set that is then joined to individual biological or social data (Figure 15.1). GIS methods have gained acceptance in the public health and medicine fields as a powerful tool to map, link, and integrate data related to physical location and time.[18-20]

THEORETICAL FRAMEWORK

Several theories have been used to characterize the influence of the built environment on health and social behavior. These models include social ecology, social cognitive theory, and the precede–proceed model.[21-25] In general these models address multiple levels of influence, including the individual, social, and environmental levels. The application of ecological models to the built environment includes attention to the physical environment (e.g., barriers and facilitators to physical activity, urban design, and transportation infrastructure) as well as policies and incentives (e.g., costs of physical activity, incentives for behavior, and regulation of environments). Health behavior theories are being developed and refined to accommodate the unique issues and concerns of the built environment on health behavior, particularly physical activity.[26,27] Once refined these theories will guide policy development to increase environmental supports for physical activity. Importantly, these theories will benefit from bridging research in geography, urban planning, and psychology, and the development of new theories that integrate multiple levels of influence.

The theory most commonly used to provide a framework for the effects of the built environment is ecological theory, or social ecology. Various models of social ecology have been proposed to characterize the complex personal and environmental influences on health and behavior.[3,23-25,28-33] Although ecological models differ in their classification of the ecosystem, they share many characteristics. In ecological models, health is determined by (1) individual actions and characteristics,

(2) factors outside the individual, and (3) an interaction between the two.[29] In ecological models, health behavior is determined by multiple levels of influence. The various levels of influence differ by the models proposed and typically include the interpersonal environment, the social environment, the cultural environment, and the physical environment.[23,30–32] A more recent formulation of the model by Swinburn et al.[3] adapted concepts of social ecology to obesity and classified environments by size and by type, including the micro level (e.g., churches, schools) and the macro level, which include larger units of aggregation such as the transportation system.

There is a clear need for new theoretical formulations and the adaptation of existing theoretical models for use in this area of research. These new theories can be drawn from several sources. King et al. recommend a number of alternative theories that should receive attention, including expanding the list of mediators and moderators beyond traditional psychosocial domains and particularly to explore meso and macro environments as described in theories of social ecology (see King et al.[26] for a comprehensive list). Further, research suggests that features of the built environment may trigger automatic evaluations, emotions, goals, and ultimately behaviors.[34,35] A rich literature on the built environment has been developed in the fields of environmental psychology and behavioral geography.[34–36]

SETTINGS AND KEY EXAMPLES

WALKING TO SCHOOL

Within the larger domain of physical activity, it is important to distinguish between leisure-time physical activity and nonleisure physical activity, such as walking and biking for transportation. Active transport to school through walking or bicycling, while understudied, is an important potential source of physical activity in children and adolescents.[37] Short of transportation to school, children may be less likely to use active transportation than adults, and they are more likely to be influenced by different neighborhood environment factors than adults.[5] Qualitative research indicates that walking for transportation has substantial appeal as a potential intervention target for increasing physical activity among mother–daughter pairs.[38]

Expanding the number of children who walk to school is one strategy advocated to increase physical activity[37] and has been listed as a health objective for the year 2010 (objective 22-14b).[39] Active commuting by children and adolescents has been associated with higher levels of physical activity[40] although this has been disputed.[41,42] Several model programs in the United States, and in other countries, have been developed to promote walking to school among children and their parents.[43–46]

Relatively few children walk to school in the United States. The Centers for Disease Control and Prevention report that only 31% of trips to school of 1 mile or less, among children 5 to 15 years of age, are made by walking.[39] Data from the statewide Georgia Asthma Study indicate that less than 19% of children living within 1 mile of school walked to school, and among all children, 4.2% walked to school most days of the week.[47] In addition to findings for walking to school, there has been a decline in the number of trips to any destination made by children by foot or by bicycle.[48] Studies conducted outside of the United States also show suboptimal levels of walking to school in Australia, the United Kingdom, and the Philippines.[40,49–52] Little research has been conducted to identify and test factors associated with walking to school. Some prior research has focused on the injury related implications of walking by children.[49,53,54]

A small number of papers have directly examined determinants and barriers of walking to school. Data from studies conducted in England, the United States, and the Philippines identified car ownership, greater distance to school, attendance at an independent school, and parental concern about abduction or molestation as significant predictors of using car transport to school. Conversely, significant predictors of walking to school include long distances to school, dangerous motor-vehicle traffic, low socioeconomic status, and females dwelling in urban areas.[40,50,55] A number of excellent reviews have examined the predictors of physical activity in children and adolescents.[17,56] The studies presented in these reviews have used more comprehensive measures of physical activity (e.g., moderate to vigorous levels of physical activity) and have not examined walking to school as an independent outcome measure. A body of research has been developed by researchers in geography and urban planning examining determinants of walking; however, this research has been conducted almost exclusively on adult populations.[5,7] Greater knowledge of the predictors of walking to school might influence public policy and assist public health professionals in the development of programs to promote walking to school. Further research on factors that influence decisions about active commuting to school has been advocated by public health researchers.[37] Recent research suggests that walking to school is lower among overweight or obese adolescents; factors such as lower SES, closer proximity to school, and lower levels of family acculturation were related to increases in the proportion of youth who walked to school.[57]

RECREATIONAL SPACES

Proximity to resources is another important environmental factor with influence on physical activity. Proximity may be thought of simply as physical (i.e., Euclidean or straight-line) distance. However, elements of proximity might also include travel distance (e.g., along the road network), traffic patterns (e.g., barriers to walkability and transportation to and from resources), cost of access, and parental support. Elementary school children have been shown to have higher levels of physical activity if they live in close proximity to playgrounds and parks and if their parents transport them to activity facilities.[58] Older children are also shown to rely on parental transportation to get to physical activity facilities.[59,60] Proximity to playgrounds has been shown to positively affect childhood physical activity.[61] Outdoor time, in particular, is important for promotion of physical activity among children and adolescents[17] and among preschool aged children.[62]

School environments may also influence activity levels, particularly those with high supervision level and activity related improvements.[63] Even at the preschool level, children attending higher quality schools with better resources had higher levels of moderate to vigorous physical activity.[64] In a school-based intervention, environment and policy interventions were effective in increasing school-based physical activity for boys, but not girls.[65]

One example of population-based research on the influence of community resources and programs on adolescent physical activity and inactivity found important environmental impacts.[56] Figure 15.2 presents the likelihood of being in the highest tertile of moderate to vigorous physical activity given participation in physical education (PE) classes, use of facilities, and neighborhood crime. Adolescents who had at least 1 day a week of PE were substantially more likely to be highly active; those who had daily PE had an over twofold increase in likelihood of being active than those with no PE. Adolescents who used a recreation center were similarly more likely to be highly active, and those who lived in a high crime neighborhood were less likely to be active. Thus, this research suggests that these modifiable environment factors play a major role in the physical activity patterns of U.S. adolescents.

Access to facilities and opportunities to exercise are consistent predictors of physical activity in children and adolescents,[17] and the presence of places to exercise, sidewalks, and access to open space have been related to physical activity in adults.[66-68] Access to resources including walking trails varies by SES with lower and middle SES populations having fewer free resources.[69] Trails are one promising avenue to provide access to physical activity resources particularly among women and those at lower SES levels.[70] Trails may be a cost-effective way to increase physical activity, particularly if trail construction costs can be minimized and the number of trail users increased.[71] Substantive questions remain unanswered about urban trails, including the trail design features that facilitate use, how characteristics of the trailside neighborhoods influence trail use, the degree to which user characteristics interact with trail design features, and the degree to which urban trails might serve as a resource for children and adolescents. Concerns about crime and injury may limit

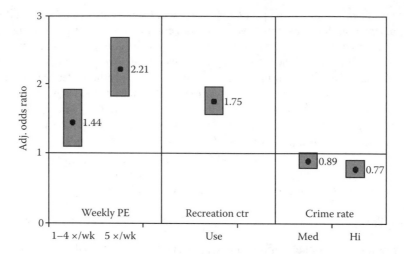

FIGURE 15.2 The relationship between modifiable environment factors and physical activity patterns of U.S. adolescents (Source: Data from Gordon-Larsen P, McMurray R, Popkin B, *Pediatrics*. 2000;105: 1–8). Figure shows odds ratios for likelihood of high levels of moderate to vigorous physical activity, adjusted for sex, age, SES, urban residence, in-school status, pregnancy, region, and month of interview. Reference categories are no weekly physical education, no community recreation center use, low neighborhood crime.

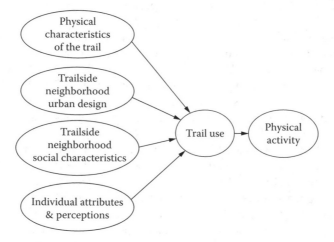

FIGURE 15.3 Conceptual model for understanding the impact of physical characteristics, neighborhood urban design, social characteristics, and individual attributes on trail use and physical activity.

use by children and adolescents.[61] Policy is also critical because it affects trail construction, trail maintenance, and connectivity between the trail, other transportation resources (bus lines), and neighborhoods.

Research on the levels of use and determinants of trail use has been initiated, with an emphasis on the exploration of built and social environmental predictors.[20,70,72–74] We present a conceptual model (Figure 15.3) and the data collection process (Figure 15.4) as one example of research involving the exploration of the built environmental determinants of urban trail use and physical activity.[75–77] Funded by the Robert Wood Johnson Foundation, this study is exploring determinants at multiple conceptual levels of influence as guided by models of social ecology and including (1) physical characteristics of the trails, (2) urban design of neighborhoods within 1 mile of the trails, (3) social characteristics of the neighborhoods, and (4) individual attributes and perceptions on trail use and physical activity for individuals sampled from the neighborhoods (see Figure 15.3). Using

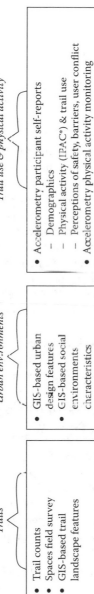
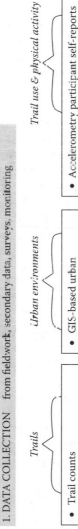
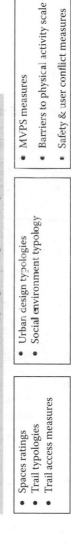

1. DATA COLLECTION from fieldwork, secondary data, surveys, monitoring

Trails

- Trail counts
- Spaces field survey
- GIS-based trail landscape features

Urban environments

- GIS-based urban design features
- GIS-based social environments characteristics

Trail use & physical activity

- Accelerometry participant self-reports
  - Demographics
  - Physical activity (IPAC*) & trail use
  - Perceptions of safety, barriers, user conflict
- Accelerometry physical activity monitoring

2. MEASURE GENERATION to create typologies, ratings, summary measures, scales

- Spaces ratings
- Trail typologies
- Trail access measures

- Urban design typologies
- Social environment typology

- MVPS measures
- Barriers to physical activity scale
- Safety & user conflict measures

3. MAPPING & MODELS to visualize/explain urban environmental relationships, trail use patterns, physical activity levels

Geographic visualization models
- 3-D trail & trailside neighborhood visualizations
- Origins–destinations of trail users
- Trail use & social difference mapping

Multi-level multiple & logistic regressions
- Determinants of trail use
- Physical activity & trail use
- Trail proximity, trail use, & physical activity
- Social difference & trail use

FIGURE 15.4 Levels of conceptualization and measurement for research on urban trails, an example of data collection, generation of measures, mapping, and models to understand the relationship among trail use, environmental factors, and physical activity. *The International Physical Activity Questionnaire.

the conceptual model to guide measurement, these relationships are tested using a series of GIS, accelerometry, and self-report measures (Figure 15.4). Findings from this work will answer questions related to neighborhood predictors of urban trail use at the built environmental, social environmental, and intrapersonal levels of influence. Research examining the determinants of physical activity at multiple levels has been called for in a recent review of environmental influences on walking.[27]

COMMUNITY DESIGN

The vast majority of the built environment and health literature is focused on adults. There is very little empirical support for these relationships among children. Furthermore, there is little work on the relationship of built environmental features to overall physical activity, especially objectively measured activity. Findings from research on community design are presented with the caveat that the adult findings are presented, given the lack of child and adolescent research in this area.

A review of 14 studies consistently shows an association between built environment factors (i.e., higher residential density, land mix, and connectivity) and walking or cycling.[5] Furthermore, that there was considerable consistency of results indicating associations between environmental factors (i.e., density, connectivity, land use) and walking or cycling.[5] Factors believed to be associated with walkability include neighborhood design and land use (e.g., distance and directness of route), which influences active- versus auto-oriented transportation choices,[78] and population density.[79–82] Residential land use diversity has been shown to be a very important predictor of walking, while bicycling is associated with density, diversity, and design, particularly of the origin, or residence, destination.[83] Individuals living in highly walkable neighborhoods report approximately two times the number of walking trips per week in contrast to low walkable neighborhood residents.[5]

Urban planners looking at environment and transportation find extremely low rates of walking for transport[84] and few pedestrian-favorable land-use policies.[78] Walking and biking increase with proximity, density, and interconnectedness of the road network and community.[82,85,86] Similarly walking and biking are also positively associated with higher population density,[79,80] greater land-use mix, pedestrian support such as sidewalks and interconnected road network,[82,87,88] and decreased air pollution.[78] In the public health literature, walking has been associated with age of home.[89] Other objectively measured environmental factors such as distance and density of resources, proximity to coast, sloped terrain, and composite measures have been shown to be associated with physical activity levels.[20,68,90,91]

The urban planning literature tends to control for only a limited range of SES factors; there is no concerted effort to look at relationships between individual factors and physical activity within different built environments.[88,92–94] Only recently has work become more focused in this area. For example, relative to dense urban form, urban sprawl has been shown to be associated with lower rates of walking and higher body mass index (BMI).[85] In addition, car ownership has been associated with increased obesity.[95] How these factors are mediated by sociodemographic factors and the impact of these transportation factors on physical activity levels is not known. Further the complex relationship between urban form, physical activity, and obesity across multiple environmental and sociodemographic settings is also unknown.

Over 75% of all trips less than 1 mile were made by automobile in 1995.[96] Walking trips made by adults dropped from 9.3% in 1977 to 7.2% in 1990 and again to 5.4% in 1995, with an even sharper decline among children.[96] One major issue influencing walking patterns among youth is the risk associated with walking. Pedestrian fatalities contribute to 12% of all traffic deaths, with higher risk among minorities and children.[97] Higher sprawl (widely dispersed population in low density development, poorly connected streets, limited market activity centers, low mixed land use) is a significant risk factor for pedestrian fatalities. The sprawling metro areas of the southern and western regions of the United States are the most dangerous for pedestrians.[97] This is of particular concern for children, particularly given that pedestrian injury is the second leading cause of unintentional injury–related death for children,[98] with highest risk among minority children[99] and in minority neighborhoods.[100] Among children, most of these pedestrian fatalities occur in residential neighborhoods, near the home of the child,[101] and specifically in driveways, parking lots, and sidewalks.[98]

NEIGHBORHOOD

While a majority of built environment research is focused on adults, empirical research suggests that there is important demographic variation in the relationship between environment factors and physical activity patterns. For example, research has shown sex differentials in the relationship between environment factors and patterns of walking; a positive association has been found between aesthetics, facilities convenience, and access to services and neighborhood walking for men, while convenience has been shown to be associated with neighborhood walking for women.[102] A cross-sectional analysis of land use patterns, travel time, and obesity in adults found that the relationship between the built environment and weight may vary across gender and ethnicity.[103] Further, research has shown small increases in pedestrian transport when adults moved from more to less car-dependent neighborhoods and small decreases associated with moves to more car-dependent neighborhoods.[104]

Spatial dimensions, such as the effects of clustering of the poor at the local and state level, and broader social class factors including access to resources, prestige, and stressors (e.g., racism) may play an important role. Large ethnic-specific spatial factors may contribute to inequality.[105–107] Societal inequality beyond individual SES may be related to health.[108–110] Even after adjusting for SES factors, physical activity is still lower in blacks than whites,[111] implicating other factors such as environmental context. Understanding how built environment factors may moderate or mediate social inequality is critically important in reducing health inequalities by race, ethnicity, and socioeconomic status.

Neighborhood environment is related to obesity, physical activity, and other health-related behaviors[85,86,112–115] and may have independent effects on disease risk.[116–119] Living in a disadvantaged neighborhood, independent of individual SES, is associated with increased coronary heart disease incidence,[120] providing a strong argument for inclusion of individual and area-level factors in research.[121–124] Others argue for population-wide physical activity–focused environmental interventions,[6] even though environmental influences are understudied.[24,125–127] While clearly there is not yet the empirical base to assert that widespread changes in the built environment will lead to population-wide increases in physical activity, early research is promising.[5,17,102,103] Furthermore, future work must seek to understand which specific types of environmental changes are likely to affect physical activity, which is at present unknown.[7]

Perceived neighborhood characteristics, such as aesthetics, convenience, and accessibility of activity resources have been shown to be associated with physical activity.[127–130] Greater perceived distance and street barriers to physical activity resources have also been found to be associated with decreased physical activity.[20] Perceived social and built environmental factors were positively associated with physical activity and walking, particularly at a neighborhood level.[131] A North Carolina study found that *perceived* presence of neighborhood trails and general access to places for physical activity were positively associated with activity.[86] Both perceived[132] and objective[56] crime have been shown to be associated with lower physical activity and higher inactivity. In addition, neighborhood disorder is associated with reduced outdoor physical activity.[133]

Perceived environmental factors have shown mixed results in their impact on physical activity; overall there was no (or minimal) impact of self-reported environmental characteristics on the likelihood of being physically active.[6,127,134,135] These studies might also be complicated by the use of self-reports of physical activity. However, more recent work indicates that both perceived and objective factors show good association with physical activity; it is unclear which has the greater impact on physical activity.[5,7]

PUBLIC POLICY

Laws and policies enacted by federal, state, and local authorities can directly influence the creation and maintenance of the built environment (e.g., ordinances on the segregation of residential and commercial land uses, funding and design of roads) and influence factors that facilitate or inhibit the use of the built environment (e.g., funding of after school programs at recreation centers). Laws and policies affect physical activity of children and adolescents through the wider built environment (e.g., roads, bike paths, land use mix) and also through specific built environments that are used more frequently by these age groups (e.g., school policy, parks, and recreation centers).

Several papers have reviewed the use of policy and noted its promise for fostering change in physical activity.[6,12,13,136] Pollard recently identified legal and policy barriers including federal, state, and local zoning laws that foster (1) the segregation of commercial and residential users into discrete geographic areas thereby limiting land use mix; (2) parking regulations that create greater distances between locations and discourage walking and bicycling; (3) street design standards that emphasize the fast flow of traffic to the detriment of safety, comfort, and accessibility for pedestrians and bicyclists; and (4) disparities in public expenditures that promote road development and sprawl.[136] Modifications in laws and policies have been recommended to promote the reuse of buildings and land in the urban core; to promote efficient development of new land, especially to encourage a mix of jobs, stores, and residences; to foster greater transportation choices (e.g., safe pedestrian paths) as well as connectivity between these and other transportation options; to support walk-to-school programs; to increase the use of traffic calming devices; and to facilitate accessible parks and open space.[136] The law can be used as a tool to configure the built environment to facilitate healthy behaviors.[137] Five main legal avenues are available that affect the built environment: environmental regulation to reduce toxic emissions, zoning ordinances and related developmental requirements, building and housing codes, taxation, and spending.[137] The public health community can also be a positive voice for improvements in the built environment by getting involved in the planning process early, by providing public health data, and by serving as advocates for the needs of special populations (e.g., children and adolescents, underserved populations).[137]

In schools, many policies focus on the health and safety of students through injury prevention, the removal of environmental hazards, and the limitation of tobacco and other substances.[138,139] Weschler et al. noted elements of policy that can be used to improve diet and physical activity in schools.[140] School policies can demonstrate commitment from school leadership, provide guidance for school staff, establish accountability for action, and help establish norms for healthy behavior. Targets of policy change might include mandated time for recess, enhanced funding and implementation of intramural programs, and the elimination of the use of physical activity as a punishment.[140] Policy regarding physical education has been carefully explored through the School Health Policies and Programs Study 2000,[141] is closely aligned with curriculum approaches, and is not reviewed here.

ZONING

The impetus for examining environmental correlates of physical activity is to focus on modifiable factors that can be altered through changes in public policy, in turn producing positive changes in health behaviors and disease risk. Policies may be grouped into legislation or regulations (e.g., formal policies written into law) and organizational policy (e.g., policies instituted within organizations), with environmental interventions being those that alter or control the physical or social environment.[13] A major area of importance in relation to policy impact is zoning, which is essentially the public regulation of the use of land. Zoning has generally favored automobile-oriented vs. pedestrian-oriented design.[26] Further, zoning has traditionally served to protect public health, safety, and welfare through regulation of land use.[142] However, zoning now prohibits health-promoting community design.[142] Hirschhorn urges public health officials to work with zoning commissions to protect health through the promotion of an activity friendly built environment.[142]

DIET ENVIRONMENT

In addition to important environmental influences on physical activity, environment also plays an important role in diet behaviors and practices. Though the present chapter focuses on environmental effects on physical activity and obesity, it is important to note the potentially critical role of the built environment as a determinant and a moderator of dietary behavior and to guide the reader toward some recent and essential research in this area. Our ability to address energy balance and to affect levels of obesity through environmental approaches will require us to better understand the impact of the built environment on both physical activity and dietary behavior and to address environmental factors that affect both behaviors. Finally, a deeper understanding of the shared and divergent environmental determinants of physical activity and dietary behavior is needed to guide intervention activities and policy decisions.

The literature in this area focuses largely on adults. Supermarkets are more likely located in wealthier and nonminority neighborhoods, and are associated with fruit and vegetable intake, even after controlling for socioeconomic factors.[143,144] Consistent positive associations are found between proximity to supermarkets and health food stores, and diet patterns and weight status,[145–147] though there is debate as to whether this is true for lower income populations as well.[148]

The number of fast food establishments and expenditure on away-from-home eating is growing at an exponential rate.[149–151] "Fast foods" and restaurant meals typically have higher energy densities and larger portion sizes than meals prepared at home,[152–155] which may affect total energy intake,[156–160] and consequently weight status.[156] Away-from-home eating, including restaurant and fast food consumption, is associated with a decrease in macro- and micronutrient intake and diet quality; weight gain; and increased BMI, energy density, and total energy intake.[161–167] Among children, away-from-home soda consumption is an important source of caloric intake.[168]

In the school setting, "competitive foods" or those that are sold in vending machines are an influential component of the dietary environment. These competitive foods, which are sold outside of the National School Lunch Program (which is federally regulated), are not subject to any federal nutrition guidelines.[169,170] Very few schools have nutrition policies, and most of fund-raising activities include sales of candy, fruit, and cookies.[171] Competitive foods have been shown to be higher in fat than those that are part of the school lunch program,[140,172,173] and include high-fat, energy-dense foods with a high prevalence of soda.[168] In fact, 98% of U.S. high schools have soft drink vending machines.[140] Much can be done to increase healthfulness of school lunch programs. For example, in a study of secondary school students, French et al.[174] found that reducing relative prices of low-fat snacks was successful in increasing low-fat purchases from vending machines.

FUTURE RESEARCH

A call for a greater focus on built environmental factors is common to most recent examinations of the obesity and inactivity epidemic, and includes factors such as urban design, transport, and policy to promote physical activity.[175,176] Several research agendas for work on the built environment and health have been proposed in recent years.[27,177,178] A wealth of research questions and methodological issues have been elucidated by these research agendas with a shared emphasis on the need to foster transdisciplinary approaches (i.e., methods and theories from multiple disciplines) and a need to better understand the factors that mediate and moderate the association between the built environment, physical activity, and health outcomes. The degree to which multiple levels of influence moderate the relationship between the built environment and physical activity is particularly interesting and has been strongly advocated in recent reviews.[27] This is a young area of research with a need for expansion in several areas as summarized in Table 15.1.

TABLE 15.1
Future Research Directions for Assessing the Relationship between Built Environment and Physical Activity

Interdisciplinary and transdisciplinary approaches to built environment and health outcomes research

Explore factors that mediate and moderate the relationships between the built environment, physical activity, and health outcomes

Develop innovative and sophisticated methods to assess the built environment

Expand research to target diverse environmental settings and diverse populations including youth, particularly minority youth

Use multiple research methods to assess change in the built environment and its impact on health behavior and health outcomes to establish causation

Confirm the association between the built environment and overall physical activity using objective measures

Assess the relationship between built environmental variables and indicators of obesity

Use longitudinal data to examine built environment factors and health outcomes over time

Expansion of research to include environment intervention studies

While we clearly do not have the empirical base to assert that widespread changes in the built environment will lead to populationwide increases in physical activity, there is building evidence of the important relationship between environmental correlates and physical activity behavior. Transportation, city and regional planning, and the physical activity literatures are all making headway in understanding environment–health relationships albeit from different perspectives. Innovative work across fields is essential in understanding the environment–health relationships. The formation of transdisciplinary research teams and transdisciplinary approaches is likely to speed progress in research on environment–health relationships.

There are three major areas in which transdisciplinary research on the built environment can push the field further. First, development of innovative and sophisticated methodologies to assess the built environment and health outcomes of interest is needed. Second, research on the built environment and health effects must expand to include diverse populations and environmental settings, including youth. Third, multiple research methodologies to assess change in environments and their impact on health outcomes is needed.

Given that the assessment of the built environment and the assessment of physical activity have largely developed in separate disciplines, there are relatively few studies to date that have integrated research using cutting edge measurement strategies for both physical activity and built environment. As a result, traditionally most studies having strong measures of the built environment focus on limited measures of physical activity, usually transportation behavior. Conversely, traditionally researchers using comprehensive and detailed physical activity measures have seldom addressed hypotheses involving the built environment. There is a major need to confirm predicted associations between the built environment and overall physical activity, particularly using objective measures of physical activity and objective and GIS-derived measures of the built environment. Similarly, there is a need to expand built environment–health relationships to include obesity as an outcome measure. Current research is emerging that is responsive to the call for trandisciplinary research that blends the best assessment strategies for the built environment with the best assessment strategies available for physical activity.

There is a great need to expand current research to investigate the relationship between built environment factors and health outcomes in diverse populations and in diverse environmental settings. Of critical importance is understanding these relationships in populations at highest risk, including ethnic minority, low income, and inner-city subpopulations. Given the predominance of literature on built environment and health in adults, and the dramatic increase in obesity in children and adolescence, there is a major need for research in youth that will confirm the associations between built environment factors and health outcomes seen in adults. Further research must explore the ways in which accepted features of the built environment (e.g., connectivity, density) differ in their effects on youth. As noted in a research article, there is a major need to use a life course, or developmental perspective to assess changes over time using longitudinal data.[26] Clearly, determining effective environmental supports and appropriate intervention strategies to overcome environmental barriers in understudied and underserved populations is needed.

Finally, multiple research methodologies to assess change in environments and their impact on health outcomes are needed. Studies of environmental change include longitudinal and intervention studies. Longitudinal data are crucial to understanding causality for posited environment and physical activity relationships. Most prior studies of the built environment have involved cross-sectional comparisons. Longitudinal studies are clearly needed to examine relations of environmental factors to particular physical activity behaviors and to understand causal relations between environmental factors and physical activity behaviors.[179] Thus, researchers must develop strong methods of collecting prospective and retrospective built environment data.

Intervention studies provide another method for producing change in the environment and are critically needed to understand fully the causal environment–behavior relationship.[7] Environment intervention studies must employ rigorous, standardized research methods and valid and reliable measures.[6,180] Intervention studies are most feasible when the focus is placed on changes in policy or on small scale elements of the built environment (e.g., equipment changes in schools) where a reasonable degree of control within a reasonable time frame can be achieved. Changes in relatively fixed elements of the built environment of our cities (e.g., land use mix, connectivity) are more complex and involve close collaborations between urban planers, community leaders, developers, and public health professionals. The use of quasi-experimental methods is perhaps a more fruitful way to approach this field of research as has been noted by prior authors.[27] The development of interventions in this area should be done in a transdisciplinary fashion, and as a result, hold promise for their potential novelty in the use of theory, design of intervention components, and effectiveness. To further maximize effectiveness of interventions, it is critical to develop a more extensive understanding of specific factors of the built environment that affect specific types of physical activity in subpopulations (e.g., male vs. female, children vs. adolescents, minority vs. nonminority, high vs. low income, urban vs. suburban).

Given the dramatic increase in obesity, particularly among youth, teasing apart the multiple levels of influence on youth health behaviors is critical. Understanding the relative contribution of built environment factors, public policy, and social environment factors as well as the interrelationships between these factors are necessary steps. Transdisciplinary approaches and methodological advances in measures of the built environment and physical activity can help the design of communities that encourage active living with the potential to positively affect physical activity and obesity at a population level.

REFERENCES

1. Ogden C, Flegal K, Carroll M, Johnson C. Prevalence and trends in overweight among US children and adolescents, 1999–2000. *JAMA*. 2002;288: 1728–1732.
2. Hedley A, Ogden L, Johnson C, Carrol M, Curtin L, Flegal K. Prevalence of overweight and obesity among US children, adolescents, and adults, 1999–2002. *JAMA*. 2002;291: 2847–2850.
3. Swinburn B, Egger G, Raza F. Dissecting obesogenic environments: the development and application of a framework for identifying and prioritizing environmental interventions for obesity. *Prev Med*. 1999;29: 563–570.
4. Hill J, Peters J. Environmental contributions to the obesity epidemic. *Science*. 1998;280: 1371–1374.
5. Saelens B, Sallis J, Frank L. Environmental correlates of walking and cycling: findings from the transportation, urban design, and planning literatures. *Ann Behav Med*. 2003;25: 80–91.

6. Sallis J, Bauman A, Pratt M. Environmental and policy interventions to promote physical activity. *Am J Prev Med.* 1998;15: 379–397.

7. Humpel N. Environmental factors associated with adults' participation in physical activity: A review. *Am J Prev Med.* 2002;22: 188–199.

8. Handy SL, Boarnet MG, Ewing R, Killingsworth RE. How the built environment affects physical activity: Views from urban planning. *Am J Prev Med.* 2002;23: 64–73.

9. Pikora T, Bull F, Jamrozik K, Knuiman M, Giles-Corti B, Donovan R. Developing a reliable audit instrument to measure the physical environment for physical activity. *Am J Prev Med.* 2002;23: 187–194.

10. Baker E, Brennan L, Brownson R, Houseman R. Measuring the determinants of physical activity in the community: current and future directions. *Res Q Exerc Sport.* 2000;71: 146–158.

11. Moudon A, Lee C. Walking and bicycling: an evaluation of environmental audit instruments. *Am J Health Promo.* 2003;18: 21–37.

12. King A, Jeffery R, Fridinger F, Dusenbury L, Provence S, Hedlund S. Environmental and policy approaches to cardiovascular disease prevention through physical activity: issues and opportunities. *Health Ed Q.* 1995;22: 499–511.

13. Schmid T, Pratt M, Howze E. Policy as intervention: environmental and policy approaches to the prevention of cardiovascular disease. *Am J Public Health.* 1995;85: 1207–1211.

14. Baranowski T, Anderson C, Carmack C. Mediating variable framework in physical activity interventions. How are we doing? How might we do better? *Am J Prev Med.* 1998;15: 266–297.

15. Buchner D. Physical activity to prevent or reverse disability in sedentary older adults. *Am J Prev Med.* 2003;23: 214–215.

16. Buzbee W. Urban form, health, and the law's limits. *Am J Public Health.* 2003;93: 1395–1398.

17. Sallis J, Prochaska J, Taylor W. A review of correlates of physical activity of children and adolescents. *Med Sci Sports Exercise.* 2000;32: 963–975.

18. Moore D, Carpenter T. Spatial analytic methods and geographic information systems: Use in health research and epidemiology. *Epidemiol Rev.* 1999;21: 143–161.

19. Croner CM. Public health, GIS, and the internet. *Annu Rev Public Health.* 2003;24: 57–82.

20. Troped P, Saunders R, Pate R. Associations between self-reported and objective physical environmental factors and use of a community rail-trail. *Prev Med.* 2001;32: 191–200.

21. Bandura A. *Social Foundations of Thought and Action: A Social Cognitive Theory.* Engelwood Cliffs, NJ: Prentice Hall, 1986.

22. Bandura A. Social cognitive theory: an agentic perspective. *Annu Rev Psychol.* 2001;52: 1–26.

23. Green L, Kreuter M. Health promotion planning. An educational and environmental approach. Mountain View, CA: Mayfield Publishing Company, 1991.

24. Sallis J, Owen N. *Physical Activity and Behavioral Medicine.* Thousand Oaks, CA: Sage, 1999.

25. Stokols D. Translating social ecological theory into guidelines for community health promotion. *Am J Health Promo.* 1996;10: 282–298.

26. King AC, Bauman A, Abrams DB. Forging trandisciplinary bridges to meet the physical inactivity challenge in the 21st century. *Am J Prev Med.* 2002;23: 104–106.

27. Owen N, Humpel N, Leslie E, Bauman A, Sallis J. Understanding environmental influences on walking: review and research agenda. *Am J Prev Med.* 2004;27: 67–76.

28. Cohen D, Scribner R, Farley T. A Structural model of health behavior: a pragmatic approach to explain and influence health behaviors at the population level. *Prev Med.* 2000;30: 146–154.

29. Green L, Richard L, Potvin L. Ecological foundations of health promotion. *Am J Health Promo.* 1996;10: 270–281.

30. McLeroy K, Bibeau D, Steckler A, Glanz K. An ecological perspective on health promotion programs. *Health Ed Q.* 1988;15: 351–377.

31. Richard L, Potvin L, Kishchuk N, Prlic H, Green L. Assessment of the integration of the ecological approach in health promotion programs. *Am J Health Promo.* 1996;10: 318–328.

32. Sallis J, Owen N. Ecological models of health behavior. In: Glanz K, Rimer B, Marcus Lewis F, Eds. *Health Behavior and Health Education: Theory, Research, and Practice.* San Francisco, CA: Jossey-Bass, 2002: 462–484.

33. Stokols D. Establishing and maintaining healthy environments: toward a social ecology of health promotion. *Am Psychologist.* 1992;47: 6–22.

34. Bargh J, Chartrand T. The unbearable automaticity of being. *Am Psychologist*. 1999;54:462–479.

35. Bargh J, Ferguson M. Beyond behaviorism: On the automaticity of higher mental processes. *Psychol Bull*. 2000;126: 925–945.

36. Amedeo D, Golledge R. Environmental perception and behavioral geography. In: Gaile G, Willmott C, eds. *Geography in America at the Dawn of the 21st Century*. New York: Oxford University Press, 2003: 133–148.

37. Tudor-Locke C, Ainsworth B, Popkin B. Active commuting to school: An overlooked source of childrens' physical activity? *Sports Med*. 2001;31: 309–313.

38. Gordon-Larsen P, Griffiths P. Barrers to physical activity: qualitative data on caregiver-daughter perceptions and practices. *Am J Prev Med*. 2004;27: 218–223.

39. Centers for Disease Control and Prevention and President's Council on Physical Fitness and Sports. *Healthy People 2010: Physical Activity and Fitness*. Washington, DC: U.S. Department of Health and Human Services, 2000. Retrieved July 19, 2005 from http://www.healthypeople.gov/Document/HTML/Volume2/22Physical.htm.

40. Tudor-Locke C, Ainsworth B, Adair L, Popkin B. Objective physical activity of Filipino youth stratified for commuting mode to school. *Med Sci Sports Exercise*. 2003;35: 465–471.

41. Metcalf B, Voss L, Jeffery A, Perkins J, Wilkin T. Physical activity cost of the school run: Impact on schoolchildren of being driven to school (EarlyBird 22). *BMJ*. 2004;329(7470): 1–2.

42. Tudor-Locke C, Neff L, Ainsworth BE, Addy C, Popkin B. Omission of active commuting to school and the prevalence of children's health-related physical activity levels: the Russian Longitudinal Monitoring Study. *Child Care Health Dev*. 2002;28: 507–512.

43. Division of Nutrition and Physical Activity, and National Center for Chronic Disease Prevention and Health Promotion. *Kids Walk-to-School*. Atlanta, GA: Centers for Disease Control. Retrieved July 18, 2005 from http://www.cdc.gov/nnccdphp/dnpa/kidswalk/.

44. U S Department of Transportation, and Pedestrian and Bicycle Information Center. *IWalk: International Walk to School*. Chapel Hill, NC: Highway Safety Research Center. Retrieved July 18, 2005 from http://www.iwalktoschool.org/.

45. U S Department of Transportation, and Pedestrian and Bicycle Information Center. *Walk and Bike to School*. Chapel Hill, NC: Highway Safety Research Center. Retrieved July 18, 2005 from http://www.walktoschool-usa.org/.

46. Sustrans. *Safe Routes to School*. United Kingdom: Department for Transport. Retrieved July 19, 2005 from http://www.saferoutestoschools.org.uk/index.php.

47. Bricker S, Kanny D, Mellinger-Birdsong A, Powell K, Shisler I. School transportation modes — Georgia, 2000. *Morbid Mortal Wkly Rept*. 2002;51: 704–705.

48. McCann B, DeLille B. Mean streets 2000: pedestrian safety, health and federal transportation spending, Columbia, South Carolina, 2000. Centers for Disease Control and Prevention.

49. Carlin J, Stevenson M, Roberts I, Bennett C, Gelman A, Nolan T. Walking to school and traffic exposure in Australian children. *Aust N Z J Public Health*. 1997;21: 286–292.

50. DiGuiseppi C, Roberts I, Li L, Allen D. Determinants of car travel on daily journeys to school: cross sectional survey of primary school children. *BMJ*. 1998;316: 1426–1428.

51. Hillman M. *Children, Transport, and the Quality of Life*. London: Policy Studies Institute, 1993.

52. Sleap M, Warburton P. Are primary school children gaining heart health benefits from their journeys to school? *Child Care Health Dev*. 1993;19: 99–108.

53. Roberts I. Why have child pedestrian death rates fallen? *BMJ*. 1993;306: 1737–1739.

54. Roberts I. Adult accompaniment and the risk of pedestrian injury on the school-home journey. *Injury Prev*. 1995;1: 242–244.

55. Dellinger A. Barriers to children walking and biking to school: United States, 1999. *Morbid Mortal Wkly Rept*. 2002;51: 701–704.

56. Gordon-Larsen P, McMurray R, Popkin B. Determinants of adolescent physical activity and inactivity patterns. *Pediatrics*. 2000;105: 1–8.

57. Reynolds K, Xie B, McConnell R, Wu J, Peters J. Predictors of walking to school. *Obes Res*. In review.

58. Sallis J, Nader P, Broyles S, Berry C, Elder J, McKenzie T, Nelson J. Correlates of physical activity at home in Mexican-American and Anglo-American preschool children. *Health Psychol*. 1993;12: 390–398.

59. Sallis J, Hovell M, Hofstetter C. Predictors of adoption and maintenance of vigorous physical activity in men and women. *Prev Med.* 1992;21: 237–251.

60. Hoefer W, McKenzie T, Sallis J, Marshall S, Conway T. Parental provision of transportation for adolescent physical activity. *Am J Prev Med.* 2001;21: 48–51.

61. Sallis J, McKenzie T, Elder J, Broyles S, Nader P. Factors parents use in selecting play spaces for young children. *Arch Ped Adolesc Med.* 1997;151: 414–417.

62. Burdetter H, Whitaker R, Daniels S. Parental report of outdoor playtime as a measure of physical activity of preschool children. *Arch Pediatr Adolesc Med.* 2004;158: 353–357.

63. Sallis J, Conway T, Prochaska J, McKenzie T, Marshall S, Brown M. The association of school environments with youth physical activity. *Am J Public Health.* 2001;91: 618–620.

64. Dowda M, Pate R, Trost S, Almeida M, Sirard J. Influences of preschool policies and practices on children's physical activity. *J Commun Health.* 2004;29: 183–196.

65. Sallis J, McKenzie T, Conway T, Elder J, Prochaska J, Brown M, et al. Environmental interventions for eating and physical activity: a randomized controlled trial in middle schools. *Am J Prev Med.* 2003;24: 209–217.

66. Evenson KR, Sarmiento OL, Tawney KW, Macon ML, Ammerman AS. Personal, social, and environmental correlates of physical activity in North Carolina Latina immigrants. *Am J Prev Med.* 2003;25: 77–85.

67. Ainsworth B, Wilcox S, Thompson W, Richter D, Henderson K. Personal, social, and physical environmental correlates of physical activity in African-American women in South Carolina. *Am J Prev Med.* 2003;25: 23–29.

68. Giles-Corti B, Donovan R. Socioeconomic status differences in recreational physical activity levels and real and perceived access to a supportive physical environment. *Prev Med.* 2002;35: 601–611.

69. Estrabrooks P, Lee R, Gyurcsik N. Resources for physical activity participation: does availability and accessibility differ by neighborhood socioeconomic status? *Ann Behav Med.* 2003;25: 100–104.

70. Brownson R, Housemann R, Brown D, Jackson-Thompson J, King A, Malone B, Sallis J. Promoting physical activity in rural communities: walking trail access, use, and effects. *Am J Prev Med.* 2000;18: 235–241.

71. Wang G, Macera C, Scudder-Soucie B, Schmid T, Pratt M, Buchner D, Heath G. Cost analysis of the built environment: the case of bike and pedestrian trails in Lincoln Neb. *Am J Public Health.* 2004;94: 549–553.

72. Lindsey G, Maraj M, Kuan S. Access, equity, and urban greenways: an exploratory investigation. *Profess Geographer* 2001;53: 332–346.

73. Lindsey G, Przybylski M. *Economic Considerations in Planning Urban Greenways: A Brief Review.* Indianapolis, IN: Center for Urban Policy and the Environment, 1998:19.

74. Lindsey G. Sustainability and urban greenways: indicators in Indianapolis. *J Am Planning Assoc.* 2003;69: 165–180.

75. Reynolds K, Wolch J, Fulton W, Weaver S, Spruijt-Metz D, Chou C, Williamson C. *Neighborhood Predictors of Class I Urban Trail Use.* Del Mar, CA: Active Living Research, 2004.

76. Reynolds K, Wolch J, Fulton W, Byrne J, Weaver S, Jerrett M, et al. *Urban Trails as an Environmental Resource to Increase Physical Activity.* Las Vegas, NV: North American Association of Obesity Research, 2004.

77. Reynolds K, Wolch J, Fulton W, Byrne J, Weaver S, Jerrett M, et al. *Research on Urban Trail Environments: Preliminary Findings.* San Diego, CA: Active Living Research, 2005.

78. Frank L. Land use and transportation interaction: implications of public health and quality of life. *J Planning Ed Res.* 2000;20: 6–22.

79. Ross C, Dunning A. *Land Use Transportation Interaction: An Examination of the 1995 NPTS Data.* Atlanta, GA: U.S. Department of Transportation: Federal Highway Administration, 1997.

80. Cervero R. Mixed land-uses and commuting: evidence from the American Housing Survey. *Transport Res-A* 1996;30: 361–377.

81. Parsons Q, Douglas I. *The Pedestrian Environment.* Vol. 4A. Portland, OR: 1,000 Friends of Oregon, 1993.

82. Frank L, Pivo G. Impacts of mixed use and density of utilization of three modes of travel: single-occupant vehicle, transit, and walking. *Transport Res Rec.* 1994;1466: 44–52.

83. Cervero R, Duncan M. Walking, bicycling, and urban landscapes: evidence from the San Francisco Bay area. *Am J Public Health.* 2003;93: 1478–1483.

84. Newman P, Kenworthy J. Transport and urban form in thirty-two of the world's principal cities. *Transport Rev.* 1991;11: 249–272.

85. Ewing R, Schmid T, Killingsworth R, Zlot A, Raudenbush S. Relationship between urban sprawl and physical activity, obesity, and morbidity. *Am J Health Promo.* 2003;18: 47–57.

86. Huston S, Evenson K, Bors P, Gizlice Z. Neighborhood environment, access to places for activity, and leisure-time physical activity in a diverse North Carolina population. *Am J Health Promo.* 2003;18: 58–69.

87. Cervero R, Kockelman K. Travel demand and the 3Ds: density, diversity, and design. *Transport Res-D.* 1997;2: 199–219.

88. Cervero R, Radisch C. Travel choices in pedestrian versus automobile oriented neighborhoods. *Transport Policy.* 1996;3: 127–141.

89. Berrigan D, Troiano RP. The association between urban form and physical activity in U.S. adults. *Am J Prev Med.* 2002;23: 74–79.

90. Sallis J, Hovell M, Hoffstetter C, Elder J, Hackley M, Caspersen C, Powell K. Distance between homes and exercise facilities related to frequency of exercise among San Diego residents. *Public Health Rept.* 1990;105: 179–186.

91. Bauman A, Smith B, Stoker L, Bellow B, Booth M. Geographical influences upon physical activity participation: evidence of a coastal effect. *Austral NZ J Public Health.* 1999;23: 322–324.

92. Cervero R, Gorham R. Commuting in transit versus automobile neighborhoods. *J Am Planning Assoc.* 1995: 210–225.

93. Handy S. Regional versus local accessibility: neo-traditional development and its implications for non-work travel. *Built Environment* 1992;18: 253–267.

94. Handy S. Urban form and pedestrian choices: study of Austin neighborhoods *Transport Res Rec.* 1996;1552: 135–144.

95. Bell A, Ge K, Popkin B. The road to obesity or the path to prevention: motorized transportation and obesity in China. *Obes Res.* 2002;10: 277–283.

96. U.S. Department of Transportation. *The Final Report: The National Bicycling and Walking Study.* Washington, DC: Federal Highway Administration, 1994.

97. Ernst M, McCann B. *Mean Streets 2002.* Washington, DC: Surface Transportation Policy Project, 2002. Retrieved July 19, 2005 from http://www.transact.org/PDFs/ms2002/MeanStreets2002.pdf.

98. SAFE KIDS Worldwide. *Report to the Nation on Child Pedestrian Safety.* Washington, DC: SAFE KIDS Worldwide, 2002.

99. Kim W, Palmisano P. Racial differences in childhood hospitalized pedestrian injuries. *Ped Emergency Care.* 1992;8: 221–224.

100. Braddock M, Lapidus G, Gregorino D, Kapp M, Banco L. Population, income, and ecological correlates of child pedestrian injury. *Pediatrics.* 1991;88: 1242–1247.

101. Sharples P, Storey A, Anynsley-Green A, Eyre J. Causes of fatal childhood accidents involving head injury in Northern region, 1979–86. *BMJ.* 1990;301: 1193–1197.

102. Humpel N, Owen N, Leslie E, Marshall AL, Bauman A, Sallis J. Associations of location and perceived environmental attributes with walking in neighborhoods. *Am J Health Promo.* 2004;18: 239–242.

103. Frank L, Andresen M, Schmid T. Obesity relationships with community design, physical activity and time spent in cars. *Am J Prev Med.* 2004;27: 87–96.

104. Massey D. The age of extremes: concentrated affluence and poverty in the twenty-first century. *Demography.* 1996;33: 395–412.

105. Wilson W. *The Truly Disadvantaged: The Inner City, The Underclass and Public Policy.* Chicago: University of Chicago Press, 1987.

106. Pebley A, Sastry N. Neighborhoods, poverty, and children's well-being: a review. In: Neckerman K, Ed. *Social Inequality.* New York: Russell Sage Foundation, 2004; 119–146.

107. Steckel R. Stature and the standard of living. *J Econ Lit.* 1995;33: 1903–1940.

108. Wilkinson R. Income distribution and life expectancy. *Am J Prev Med.* 1992;30: 165–168.

109. Wilkinson R. *Unhealthy Societies: The Afflictions of Inequality.* New York: Routledge, 1996.

110. Crespo C, Smit E, Andersen R, Carter-Pokras O, Ainsworth B. Race/ethnicity, social class and their relation to physical inactivity during leisure time: results from the Third National Health and Nutrition Examination Survey, 1988–1994. *Am J Prev Med*. 2000;18: 46–53.

111. Krizek K. A pre-test/post-test strategy for researching neighborhood-scale urban form and travel behavior. *Transport Res Rec*. 2000;1722: 48–55.

112. Sundquist J, Malmstrom M, Johansson S. Cardiovascular risk factors and the neighbourhood environment: a multilevel analysis. *Int J Epidemiol* 1999;28: 841–845.

113. Yen I, Kaplan G. Poverty area residence and changes in physical activity level: evidence from the Alameda County Study. *Am J Public Health*. 1998;88: 1709–1712.

114. Lee R, Cubbin C. Neighborhood context and youth cardiovascular health behaviors. *Am J Public Health*. 2002;92: 428–436.

115. Diez-Roux A, Nieto F, Muntaner C, Tyroler H, Comstock G, Shahar E, et al. Neighborhood environment and coronary heart disease: a multilevel analysis. *Am J Epidemiol*. 1997;146: 48–63.

116. Haan M, Kaplan G, Camacho T. Poverty and health: prospective evidence from the Alameda County study. *Am J Epidemiol*. 1987;125: 989–998.

117. MacIntyre S, Maciver S, Soorman A. Area, class and health: should we be focusing on places or people. *J Soc Pol*. 1993; 22.

118. Kaplan G. People and places: contrasting perspectives on the association between social class and health. *Int J Health Service*. 1996;26: 507–519.

119. Cohen DL, Spear S, Scribner R, Kissinger P, Mason K, Wildgen J. "Broken windows" and the risk of gonorrhea. *Am J Public Health*. 2000;90: 230–236.

120. Diez-Roux A. Investigating area and neighborhood effects on health. *Am J Public Health*. 2001;92: 1783–1789.

121. Krieger N, Williams D, Moss N. Measuring social class in US public health research: concepts, methodologies, and guidelines. *Ann Rev Pub Health*. 1997;18: 341–378.

122. O'Campo P, Gielen A, Faden R, Xzue X, Kass N, Wang M. Violence by male partners against women during the childbearing year: a contextual analysis. *Am J Public Health*. 1995;85: 1092–1097.

123. Diez-Roux A. Bringing context back into epidemiology: variables and fallacies in multi-level analysis. *Am J Public Health*. 1998;88: 216–222.

124. Diez-Roux A, Link B, Northridge M. A multilevel analysis of income inequality and cardiovascular risk factors. *Soc Sci Med*. 2000;50: 673–687.

125. Owen N, Leslie E, Salmon J, Fotheringham M. Environmental determinants of physical activity and sedentary behavior. *Exerc Sport Sci Rev*. 2000;28: 153–158.

126. Clark D. Physical activity and its correlates among urban primary care patients aged 55 years or older. *J Gerontol: Psych Sci Soc Sci*. 1999;54: 41–48.

127. King A, Castro C, Wilcox S, Eyler A, Sallis J, Brownson R. Personal and environmental factors associated with physical inactivity among different racial-ethnic groups of U.S. middle-aged and older-aged women. *Health Psychol*. 2000;19: 354–364.

128. Ball K, Bauman A, Leslie E, Owen N. Perceived environmental and social influences on walking for exercise in Australian adults. *Prev Med*. 2001;33: 434–440.

129. Booth M, Owen N, Bauman A, Clavisi O, Leslie E. Social-cognitive and perceived enviornmental influences associated with physical activity in older Australians. *Prev Med*. 2000;31: 15–22.

130. Wilcox S, Castro C, King A, Houseman R, Brownson R. Determinants of leisure time physical activity in rural compared with urban older and ethnically diverse women in the United States. *J Epidemiol Community Health*. 2000;54: 667–672.

131. Addy C, Wilson D, Kirtland K, Ainsworth B, Sharpe P, Kimsey D. Associations of perceived social and physical environmental supports with physical activity and walking behavior. *Am J Public Health*. 2004;94: 440–443.

132. Centers for Disease Control. Barriers to children walking and biking to school — US, 1999. *Morbid Mortal Wkly Rept*. 2002;51: 701–704.

133. Ross C, Mirowsky J. Neighborhood disadvantage, disorder, and health. *J Health Social Behav*. 2001;42: 258–276.

134. Sallis JF, Johnson MF, Calfas KJ, Caparosa S, Nichols JF. Assessing perceived physical environmental variables that may influence physical activity. *Res Q Exercise Sport*. 1997;68: 345–351.

135. Hovell M, Sallis J, Hofstetter C. Identifying correlates of walking for exercise: an epidemiologic prerequisite for physical activity promotion. *Prev Med.* 1989;18: 856–866.

136. Pollard T. Policy prescriptions for healthier communities. *Am J Health Promo.* 2003;18: 109–113.

137. Perdue W, Stone L, Gostin L. The built environment and its relationship to the public's health: the legal framework. *Am J Public Health.* 2003;93: 1390–1394.

138. Everett-Jones S, Brener N, McManus T. Prevalence of school policies, programs, and facilities that promote a health physical school environment. *Am J Public Health.* 2003;93: 1570–1575.

139. Small M, Jones S, Barrios L, Crossett L, Dahlberg L, Albuquerque M, et al. School policy and environment: Results from the School Health Policies and Programs Study 2000. *J School Health.* 2001;71: 325–334.

140. Wechsler H, Devereaux R, Davis M, Collins J. Using the school environment to promote physical activity and healthy eating. *Prev Med.* 2000;31: S121–S137.

141. Burgeson C, Wechsler H, Brener N, Young J, Spain C. Physical education and activity: results from the School Health Policies and Programs Study 2000. *J School Health.* 2001;71: 279–293.

142. Hirschhorn J. Zoning should promote public health. *Am J Health Promo.* 2004;18: 258–260.

143. Morland K, Wing S, Diez-Roux A, Poole C. Neighborhood characteristics associated with the location of food stores and food service places. *Am J Prev Med.* 2002;22: 23–29.

144. Morland K, Wing S, Roux A. The contextual effect of the local food environment on residents' diets: the athereosclerosis risk in communities study. *Am J Public Health.* 2002;92 :1761–1768.

145. Ransley J, Donnelly J, Botham H, Khara T, Greenwood D, Cade J. Use of supermarket receipts to estimate energy and fat content of food purchased by lean and overweight families. *Appetite.* 2003;41: 141–148.

146. Laraia B, Siega-Riz A, Kaufman J, Jones S. Proximity of supermarkets is positively associated with diet quality index for pregnancy. *Prev Med.* 2004;39: 869–875.

147. Cheadle A, Psaty B, Curry S. Community-level comparisons between the grocery store environment and individual dietary practices. *Prev Med.* 1991,20. 250 261.

148. Dibsdall L, Lambert N, Bobbin R, Frewer J, Preville M, Hebert R, Boyer R. Low-income consumers' attitudes and behavior towards access, availabilty and motivation to eat fruits and vegetables. *Public Health Nutrition.* 2003;6: 159–168.

149. USDA ARS Food Surveys Research Group. Data and documentation for the 1994–1996, and 1998 Continuing Surveys of Food Intake by Individuals (CSFII). Diet and Health Knowledge Survey. Washington, DC: National Technical Information Service.

150. Jekanowski M, Binkley J, Eales J. Convenience, accessibility and demand for fast food. *J Agricul Resour Econ.* 2001;26: 58–74.

151. Putnam J, Allshouse J. *Food Consumption, Prices and Expenditures, 1996,* SB-928. Washington DC: Department of Agriculture, 1996.

152. Prentice A, Jebb S. Fast food, energy density and obesity: a possible mechanistic link. *Obes Rev.* 2003;4: 187–194.

153. Young L, Nestle M. The contribution of expanding portions sizes to the US obesity epidemic. *Am J Public Health.* 2002;92: 246–249.

154. Young L, Nestle M. Expanding portion sizes in the US marketplace: implications for nutrition counseling. *J Am Diet Assoc.* 2003;103: 231–234.

155. Neilsen S, Popkin B. Patterns and trends in portion size, 1977–1998. *JAMA.* 2003;289: 450–453.

156. Poppitt S, Prentice A. Energy density and its role in the control of food intake: evidence from metabolic and community studies. *Appetite.* 1996;26: 153–174.

157. Diliberti N, Bordi P, Conklin M, Roe L, Rolls B. Increased portion size leads to increased energy intake in a restaurant meal. *Obes Res.* 2004;12: 562–568.

158. Rolls B, Bell E, Castellanos V, Chow M, Pelkman C, Thorwart M. Energy density but not fat content of foods affected energy intake in lean and obese women. *Am J Clin Nutr.* 1999;69: 863–871.

159. Rolls B, Morris E, Roe L. Portion size of food affects energy intake in normal-weight and overweight men and women. *Am J Clin Nutr.* 2002;76: 1207–1213.

160. Rolls B, Roe L, Kral T, Meengs J, Wall D. Increasing the portion size of a packaged snack increases energy intake of men and women. *Appetite.* 2004;42: 63–69.

161. Thompson O, Ballew C, Resnicow K, Must A, Bandini L, Cyr H, Dietz W. Food purchased away from home as a predictor of BMI z-score among girls. *Int J Obes.* 2004;28: 282–289.

162. Zoumas-Morse C, Rock C, Sobo E, Neuhouser ML. Children's patterns of macronutrient intake and associations with restaurant and home eating. *J Am College Nutrition*. 2004;101: 923–925.

163. Bowman S, Vinyard B. Fast food consumption of US adults: impact on energy and nutrition intake and overweight status. *J Am College Nutrition*. 2004;23: 163–168.

164. Ebbeling C, Sinclair K, Pereira MA, Garcia-Lago E, Feldman H, Ludwig D. Compensation for energy intake from fast food among overwieght and lean adolescents. *JAMA*. 2004;291: 2828–233.

165. French S, Story M. Fast food restaurant use among adolescents: associations with nutrient intake, food choices and behavioral and psychosocial variables. *Int J Obes*. 2001;25: 1823–1833.

166. Lin B, Guthrie J, Frazao E. *Nutrient Contribution of Food Away from Home, America's Eating Habits: Changes and Consequences*. Washington DC: U.S. Department of Agriculture: 1999: 213–242.

167. McCrory M, Fuss P, Hays N, Vinken A, Greenberg A, Roberts S. Overeating in America: association between restaurant food consumption and body fatness in healthy men and women ages 19–80. *Obes Res*. 1999;7: 564–571.

168. French S, Lin B, Guthrie J. National trends in soft drink consumption among children and adolescents age 6 to 17 years: prevalence, amounts, and sources, 1977/1978 to 1994/1998. *J Am Dietetic Assoc*. 2003;103: 1326–1331.

169. USDA. *National School Lunch Program and School Breakfast Program Nutrition Objectives for School Meals*. Washington DC: U.S. Department of Agriculture; 1994: 30218–30233.

170. USDA. *Competitive Food Service*. Washington DC: U.S. Department of Agriculture; 2002:105–106.

171. French S, Story M, Fulkerson J. School food policies and practices: a state-wide survey of secondary school principals. *J Am Diet Assoc*. 2002;102: 1785–179.

172. Story M, Hayes M, Kalina B. Availability of foods in high schools: Is there a cause for concern? *J Am Diet Assoc*. 1996;96: 123–126.

173. Harnack L, Snyder P, Story M, Holliday R, Lytle L, Neumark-Sztainer D. Availability of a la carte food items in junior and senior high schools: a needs assessment *J Am Dietetic Assoc*. 2000;100: 701–703.

174. French S, Jeffery R, Story M, Hannan P, Snyder M. A pricing strategy to promote low-fat snack choice through vending machines. *Am J Public Health*. 1997–87(5): 849–851

175. Kahn E, Heath G, Powell K, Stone E, Brownson R. Increasing physical activity: a report on recommendations of the Task Force on Community Preventive Services. *Morbid Mortal Wkly Rept*. 2001;50: 1–14.

176. Wilkinson R, Marmot M. *Solid Facts: Social Determinants of Health*. Denmark: World Health Organization, 2003.

177. Dannenberg A, Jackson R, Frumkin H, Schieber R, Pratt M, Kochtitzky C, Tilson H. The impact of community design and land-use choices on public health. A scientific research agenda. *Am J Public Health*. 2003;93: 1500–1508.

178. Srinivasan S, O'Fallon L, Dearry A. Creating healthy communities, healthy homes, health people: Initiating a research agenda on the built environment and public health. *Am J Public Health*. 2003;93: 1446–1450.

179. Humpel N, Marshall A, Leslie E, Bauman A, Owen N. Changes in neighborhood walking are related to changes in perceptions of environmental attributes. *Ann Behav Med*. 2004;27: 60–67.

180. Milat A, Stubbs J, Engelhard S, Weston P, Giles-Corti B, Fitzgerald S. Measuring physical activity in public open space — an electronic device versus direct observation. *Austral NZ J Public Health*. 2002;26: 50–51.

16 Community-Level Influences and Interventions for Pediatric Obesity

Leslie A. Lytle and Kathryn Schmitz

CONTENTS

OVERVIEW OF CHAPTER

The etiology and prevention of childhood obesity is complex and multifaceted. The epidemiology of this important public health problem implicates a wide range of factors including: genetics, family history and environment, early feeding practices, eating, physical activity (PA) and sedentary behaviors, the physical and social environment of schools and other community agencies where youth interact and make choices, and finally, the larger community and its related social and physical environments, including the built environment. Many of these aspects have been discussed in other chapters in this book. The focus of this chapter is on community-level preventive influences, not including the influence of the built environment or schools.

Community-level obesity programs focus on physical activity and healthful diet interventions. There are several prior reviews that have included discussion of community-based physical activity interventions in youth.[1-3] One of these[3] outlined why we need community-based physical activity interventions among youth, including the large amount of time youth spend in community settings that are conducive to activity; the capacity to involve adult role models in supporting and influencing youth activity; the potential for influencing community norms around physical activity; the informal, nongraded atmosphere (in contrast to school); and the provision of a place to put into practice what is learned in school. Many of these reasons also support community-based dietary interventions for youth.[4] Our discussion of the role of community in physical activity, diet, and pediatric obesity prevention starts with several premises. The first premise is that there is a link between both energy expenditure and energy intake with the subsequent development of pediatric obesity. The second premise is that increasing daily energy expenditure in youth may be approached by reducing sedentary behaviors and/or increasing physical activity. There is a lack of correlation between sedentary leisure habits in youth and physical activity levels in youth,[5] so it important to recognize that changing each of these two behaviors is a separate issue, though both may be addressed in a single intervention (e.g., replacing TV time with physical activity). The third premise is that a community intervention with a goal to improve dietary intake or eating behaviors, increase activity and/or fitness, and/or decrease sedentary behavior in youth is an obesity prevention intervention. We recognize, with regard to this final premise, that dietary recommendations will have a positive effect on obesity rates only if improvement of dietary intake occurs in the context of a healthy energy balance. An intervention targeting increased consumption of fruits, vegetables, dairy, or whole grain has the potential to have an adverse effect on energy balance. It is acknowledged that messages about energy balance for a youth population are made even more complex because the messages need to account for energy needs for growth and development.

In this chapter, we define community, discuss ecological models as a theoretical perspective that includes community, and provide a review of the literature on community-level influences and approaches to positively affect activity levels and food choices of youth. We close with suggested future directions for community-level preventive approaches to affect the obesity epidemic in youth.

DEFINING COMMUNITY

Other chapters in this book address school and built environment aspects of preventing pediatric obesity, as well as the behavioral aspects of eating and activity. To avoid overlap, our definition of community will exclude school and the built environment. We define community on two planes: physical spaces and the social influences in those places. It is the interrelatedness of people and organizations within common spaces that creates a sense of community. The VERB physical activity promotion campaign included the following as spaces and organizations that define community: "backyards, youth-serving organizations, community-based organizations, churches, parks and recreation departments, public or private sports organizations, businesses, government agencies, or any other place that can provide facilities and year-round or periodic event-based opportunities for tweens to be physically active and have fun."[6] In addition to many of these spaces and organizations, fast food outlets, other restaurants, grocery stores, and convenience stores also influence the eating behavior of youth. Each of these places is then influenced by the social interactions found there and the connectedness of the spaces themselves. Places become communities or part of communities based on the shared interests and goals of inhabitants, as well as the relationships and interdependence of the people and/or organizations in a given place.[7] A shared set of values, norms, and attachments imbues place with community, creating a symbolic unit of collective identity.[7,8] With this in mind, a family can be a community, as can Indian reservations, primary care health clinics, residential developments, neighborhoods, towns, and cities.

INFLUENCE OF COMMUNITY AS EXAMINED WITH AN ECOLOGICAL APPROACH

For both physical activity and eating behaviors, there is a vast literature on correlates or predictors of overweight and obesity. A review of these associations is beyond the scope of this chapter; readers are referred to Parsons et al.,[9] French et al.,[10] and Swinburn et al.[11] Summarizing and organizing these associations is a challenge. A social ecological model provides a structure for examining multiple levels of influence on eating and activity among youth, including individual, interpersonal, institutional, and community factors.[12] A recent Institute of Medicine committee concluded that both research and intervention efforts for social and behavioral approaches for primary prevention should be based on an ecological model that addresses not only the behaviors of individuals and families, but also the environmental context within which people live because

TABLE 16.1
Potential Community Influences of Pediatric Obesity

	Proximal	Distal
Social	Role models (peers, family, and other community members) for healthful eating and activity behaviors	Societal role models (media, advertising) for healthful eating and activity behaviors
	Incentives for healthful choices in the home, school, community	Structure and pace of society and culture
	School-level policies and practices related to physical education, nutrition education, food use	National guidelines, information, and recommendations about activity and diet
	Parental control, parenting style	Societal and cultural norms
	Normative expectations regarding eating and activity	Media messages and educational campaigns for healthy activity and eating habits (e.g., VERB, 5-a-Day Campaign)
	Family support for activity and healthy foods	Product advertising (soft drinks, fast foods, sedentary activities)
	Low levels of television viewing in the home	
Physical	Food access and availability at home, school, and at community venues	Legislation affecting access and availability of foods, activity options
	Food outlets (grocery stores, convenience stores, fast food, restaurants)	Taxation, pricing policies of foods
	Walkability of neighborhood, access to parks, bike trails, gyms, and activity facilities	Portion sizes, packages, nutritional content of packaged foods
	Financial resources needed for a healthy diet and active leisure time	Urban planning
	Portion sizes offered in local restaurants	Transportation planning
		Agricultural policy

those environments shape and support behavior.[13] There is strong support for studying the obesity epidemic using an ecological approach.[14–16]

Booth et al.[17] describe an attempt by an expert panel to identify broader contextual, environmental, societal, and policy variables that may be implicated in the obesity epidemic using a knowledge-mapping technique. They developed a framework that includes elements of an ecological approach (including a psychobiological core, and cultural and social influences) and also discuss proximal and distal "leverage points" or potential points of change. As a heuristic for thinking about the community factors and issues related to the childhood obesity epidemic, we modify their framework and suggest a rubric that organizes issues along two continuums: the proximal and distal levels of influence, and the social and physical environment. Table 16.1 gives examples of activity and eating influences in each of the four cells based on research, theory, and "best guesses" suggested in the literature.

Proximal aspects of the community are those that represent behavioral settings within the community where youth make decisions about how to spend their leisure time (to be active or sedentary) and what to eat. Proximal behavioral settings include homes, schools, grocery stores, restaurants, and other food outlets, and other community venues such as places of worship, recreation centers, and parks. More distal community influences include broader societal and cultural aspects as they are played out in the community; while they may influence foods consumed and activity choices made, a community's ability to intervene on distal factors is limited, at least in the short term.

Likewise, the community environment influences activity and dietary behavior of youth from a social and a physical perspective. The social environment is an important source of influence for youth because it provides the context for what is normative behavior in the behavioral setting and provides role models, incentives, and support for behavior through the actions and words of other members of the community. The physical environment includes the numbers and types of structures that support or hinder healthful activity and food choices as well as access and availability of food choices and opportunities for youth to be active. We acknowledge that there are obvious points of overlap between the four cells and that the four cells interact and influence each other in a dynamic, reciprocal relationship. Still we believe the rubric may have heuristic value in the consideration of community-level obesity factors.

COMMUNITY INTERVENTIONS TO PROMOTE PHYSICAL ACTIVITY AND POSITIVELY AFFECT DIETARY BEHAVIOR IN YOUTH

Research on community-based physical activity and dietary interventions in youth is scant, particularly compared with the number of school-based interventions, despite the finding that most of childhood and adolescent physical activity and dietary intake occurs outside the school setting.[18,19] What follows is a review of research on community interventions to increase physical activity and positively affect dietary behaviors among youth, as well as an example of nonresearch-oriented community interventions for promoting healthy physical activity and dietary intake among youth.

A review of the available literature uncovered peer-reviewed publications relating to 14 community-based interventions that included efforts to increase physical activity and eating behaviors among youth. This literature review is limited to intervention studies focusing on primary prevention; obesity treatment studies were not included. The review includes quasi-experimental and pilot studies. Summaries of these studies are provided in Table 16.2. None of them reported significant improvement in any measure of body size or composition. Eight of these studies focused specifically on African American youth and two others focused on Hispanic or Native American youth. Eleven of the studies focused on parents with their children, and many of these evaluated changes in the parents as well as the children; the results summarized in Table 16.2 are limited to youth outcomes. Of the 14 studies included in Table 16.2, six intervened on eating as well as exercise habits. Only two of these showed some improvements in physical activity or fitness.[20–22] Of the eight studies that focused exclusively on changing physical activity, three demonstrated improvements in physical activity and/or fitness. Most of the dietary studies were pilot studies; some positive trends in dietary behavior were seen.

LITERATURE REVIEW: PHYSICAL ACTIVITY INTERVENTIONS

In this section we provide a description of the five studies included in Table 16.2 that showed any significant improvement in physical activity or fitness.

The Daughters and Mothers Exercising Together intervention[23,24] was tested in two versions. The first[23] recruited mothers and daughters (aged 11 to 17) into a 12-week intervention that included a weekly educational session, a weekly physical activity session (supervised), and a prescription to do one to two more exercise sessions on their own. This version of the intervention was not successful in increasing physical activity among the daughters. The second version of Daughters and Mothers Exercising Together[24] set out to compare the relative efficacy of a community-based exercise intervention compared with a home-based one in mother–daughter pairs. Both intervention arms were asked to exercise three times weekly for 12 weeks. Mother–daughter pairs in the community-based (CB) group came to a fitness facility twice weekly and participated in some recreational fitness activity (rock-climbing, mountain biking) the third session. Mother–daughter pairs in the home-based (HB) group, were taught exercises to do at home on their own and encouraged to exercise together, but it was not required that they exercise together. The HB group pairs reported exercising together 59% of the sessions, while the CB group pairs always exercised together, based on the structure of the intervention. Adherence to the two interventions was 70% for the CB and 77% for the HB programs, notably better than in other studies reviewed herein. The PA changes in the two interventions were similar among the daughters, with girls reporting 1 to 2 more weekly sessions of aerobic exercise, 1.5 to 2 more weekly sessions of muscular strength

TABLE 16.2
Community-Based Interventions to Increase Physical Activity or Reduce Sedentary Behavior and Enhance a Healthy Diet in Youth

Participants	Design and Evaluation Method	Duration of Intervention	Goal	Intervention Strategies	Outcomes	Statistical Significance	Ref.
Mothers and adolescent daughters (n = 20 pairs)	RCT PILOT	12 weeks	To compare the efficacy of a home- vs. community-based intervention to increase physical activity in mothers and daughters.	Three sessions per week either in home-based (HB) or in a community-based (CB) intervention, plus encouragement to increase lifestyle activities (taking the stairs vs. the elevator).	Pre-post: Aerobic activity Muscular strength activity Flexibility activity HB vs. CB: Exercise sessions attended Fitness % body fat	Increased, $p = 0.02$ Increased, $p = 0.001$ Increased, $p < 0.0001$ HB: 70% CB: 77% NS NS	24
Students in 5th grade at start of study in 2 rural South Carolina communities (n = 436)	Quasi-experimental (one town each condition, not randomized)	18 months	To test the effects of a community-based intervention to increase PA.	After-school, summer, home, school, and community physical activity programs.	PA	Not significant in intervention vs. comparison communities	51
African American girls and their parents (n = 19 in TX and n = 16 in control)	RCT PILOT	12 weeks	To prevent obesity among 8-year-old African American girls with the Fun, Food, and Fitness Project.	Four-week summer day camp for girls followed by an 8-week home Internet intervention for girls and parents.	BMI PA Variety of dietary outcomes	NS NS NS, some favorable trends	27

TABLE 16.1 (CONTINUED)
Community-Based Interventions to Increase Physical Activity or Reduce Sedentary Behavior and Enhance a Healthy Diet in Youth

Participants	Design and Evaluation Method	Duration of Intervention	Goal	Intervention Strategies	Outcomes	Statistical Significance	Ref.
African American girls and their parents (n = 60)	RCT PILOT	12 weeks	To assess the feasibility, acceptability, and outcomes of 2 versions of a culturally relevant, family-based intervention to prevent excess weight gain in preadolescent African American girls.	Weekly group sessions with either girls or their parents or caregivers to promote healthy eating and increased PA (Analysis combined TX groups)	BMI PA Variety of dietary outcomes	Trend toward reduced BMI in TX vs. control, NS 11.7% increase in minutes of moderate to vigorous PA, NS Significant ($p = 0.03$) difference in intake of sweetened beverages by condition	28
African American girls and their parents (n = 54)	RCT PILOT	12 weeks	To describe and develop an after-school obesity-prevention program for African American girls.	Twice weekly after school intervention focused on increasing physical activity and healthy eating. There was also a family component	BMI PA Variety of dietary outcomes	NS Increased in TX more than control, NS NS	29
African American girls and their parents or guardians (n = 61)	RCT PILOT	12 weeks	To test the feasibility, acceptability, and potential efficacy of after-school dance classes and a family-based intervention to reduce television viewing, thereby reducing weight gain, among African American girls.	After school dance classes 5 days a week at 3 community centers, 45–60 min of dancing per session. Also, 5 lessons delivered during home visits with families.	BMI PA TV viewing time	TX improved more than control, NS TX improved more than control, NS TX decreased more than control, NS	30

Sample	Design	Duration	Objective	Intervention	Outcome measure	Results	Ref.
Hispanic and non-Hispanic white (Anglo) families with a 5th or 6th grade child (n = 206)	RCT	1 year	To assess the effectiveness of a family-based cardiovascular disease risk reduction intervention in two ethnic groups (Hispanic and non-Hispanic whites "Anglos").	Educational intervention to decrease intake of salt and fat, as well as increasing PA	PA BMI Variety of dietary outcome	Significant increase in PA for Anglo boys only at 24- and 48-month postintervention ($p = 0.02$ at both times) NS Significant differences for Anglo families for fat and sodium, both ethnic groups food frequency index	20,21
Black American families with children in the 5th to 7th grades (n = 94)	RCT	14 weeks	To promote aerobic physical activity among healthy black-American families with children in the 5th to 7th grades	One education and 2 fitness sessions per week for 14 weeks	Fitness Fitness session attendance	NS 20%	31
Mother–daughter pairs or triads with daughters aged 11–17 (20 pairs)	Pre-post	12 weeks	To assess whether a twice weekly education and participatory intervention would increase physical activity in mothers and daughters.	Once weekly 2-h educational session, once weekly 2-h activity session. Participants asked to exercise 1–2 times weekly outside of sessions.	PA Fitness Body weight	Nonsignificant increase Nonsignificant increase Increased: $p = 0.03$	23

TABLE 16.1 (CONTINUED)
Community-Based Interventions to Increase Physical Activity or Reduce Sedentary Behavior and Enhance a Healthy Diet in Youth

Participants	Design and Evaluation Method	Duration of Intervention	Goal	Intervention Strategies	Outcomes	Statistical Significance	Ref.
Low income African American residents of 6 rental communities administered by the Housing Authority of Birmingham District (AL)	RCT	1 year	To assess whether a community intervention could increase physical activity among low socioeconomic status African American residents of 3 low-income housing communities compared with 3 similar comparison communities.	Community based exercise program coordinated by project staff and led by a member of the community (who had training from the project staff). Activities included walking, aerobic dance, low-impact aerobics, games and sports, and weight lifting. Written educational materials were distributed.	PA	No increase, NS	52
Overweight African American girls aged 11–17 (n = 57)	Pre–post with comparisons of high vs. low attenders	6 months	To assess the impact of a nutrition and physical activity intervention on overweight low-income African American adolescent women.	Twice weekly sessions for months 1–4, once weekly sessions for months 5–6. Each 2-h session included an interactive educational component, 30–60 min of PA, and meal preparation.	PA BMI % body fat Variety of dietary outcomes	NS NS NS Significant difference in calorie intake between high attenders and low attenders	53

Population	Study design	Aim	Intervention	Outcome	Results	Ref
Low-fit children aged 9–12 (n = 12)	Pre-post	To assess the efficacy of a home-based behavioral program utilizing contingency contracts and parent-determined rewards to modify children's PA levels and thereby fitness levels.	Parents received training, then observed physical activity for a baseline level, then increased the goal weekly to increase after-school activity levels.	PA Fitness	No statistical analysis: 100% increase 36% increase	25
Low-income families with 7- to 12-year-old African American children (28 families)	RCT PILOT Single counseling session, follow-up at 4 weeks	To assess the efficacy of a behavioral intervention to decrease television viewing and increase physical activity in 7- to 12-year-old low income African American children.	A 20–30 min counseling session in a primary care medical clinic, written educational materials, and an electronic television time manager.	TV viewing time Hours playing outside Hours organized PA	NS between groups, both groups decreased Improved, $p = 0.06$ Improved, $p = 0.004$	26
Zuni Indian adolescents (n = 173)	Multiple cross-sectional samples of population over project	To enhance knowledge of diabetes and to support increased PA, increased fruit and vegetable intake, and reduced soft drink consumption among Zuni Indian youth.	Communitywide intervention with 4 intervention strategies: Establish supportive social networks. Construct wellness facility for teens. Diabetes education in school. Modify food supply available to teens.	BMI Fitness	Decreased, but NS Improved, $p < 0.05$	22

4 years (results reported for midpoint so far)

activity, and 2 to 3 more weekly sessions of flexibility activity at posttesting compared with pretesting. The lack of a no-exercise control group limits the ability to conclude that the HB and/or CB intervention was effective in increasing activity compared with no intervention. Hypotheses presented by the authors to explain the success of this family-based physical activity intervention, while others have not succeeded, include the higher socioeconomic status (SES) level of participants in this study and the choice to focus on changing physical activity only, not diet or other behaviors concurrent with physical activity changes.

Taggart et al.[25] tested whether physical education homework, with parents as the helpers, would improve the fitness and activity levels of 12 low-fitness children aged 9 to 12 years. Though this noncontrolled intervention did not assess statistical significance of the impact on physical activity and fitness, the changes were large, so we feel it is worthy of providing further details. The intervention focused solely on physical activity and was intensive for both parents and children. The participating children were asked to accumulate activity points, which differed by activity according to intensity. A baseline number of weekly points was established; then the parents and child decided together on a goal number of points to be earned for the following week, as well as the reward for doing so. Parents reviewed the contract with their child at the end of each week and a new contract established for the following week, according to success or failure of the child to achieve the point goal in the prior week. Parents received support from trained interventionists to teach them how to establish the contracts, assess and record points, and fade extrinsic rewards. The intervention approach allowed for a systematic increase in physical activity over the course of the study, which would then support improvements in fitness. This intensive 9- to 12-week intervention succeeded in doubling "points earned" and time spent in physical activity. The lack of a control group is a severe limitation of this small study. Further, the intensive nature of the intervention assumed ample available time, equipment, play spaces, and other resources on the part of the families to put toward physical activity, limiting the generalizability of this approach.

Ford et al.[26] intervened on 28 African American low-income families with 7- to 12-year-old children to compare the effects of a 5- to 10-min counseling session regarding limiting television viewing (13 families) to a more intensive behavioral intervention that included a longer (20 to 30 min) counseling session, a more specific set of written materials, and provision of an electronic television time-management device (15 families). Both interventions were provided within a primary care clinic setting. At 4 weeks of follow-up, television viewing time decreased significantly in both groups by nearly 14 hours per week, with no between-group differences in these changes. Time spent playing outside and time spent in organized physical activity increased slightly among the children in the more intensive intervention group and decreased significantly among children in the group that received the less intensive intervention. Comparison of these changes showed statistical significance between group differences. All of the results were self-reported. These are promising preliminary findings; the authors indicated intent to follow-up with a larger intervention.

The last of the studies to show any significant effect on physical activity or fitness was the Zuni Diabetes Prevention Program, a noncontrolled community intervention to improve eating and activity habits of Zuni Indian adolescents.[22] Inclusion of this study could be questioned because some of the teens included were already obese, contrary to our restriction of including only primary prevention interventions. If we define obesity prevention to include preventing the worsening of obesity, this study can be included. Further, one of the four intervention components involved school classroom curriculum, while this chapter is focused on community- rather than school-based intervention. On the other hand, the majority of the physical activity curriculum came in the form of a teen wellness center built and developed by and for the teens in the community. The published report provides results at 2 years into this 4-year intervention and shows significant improvements in fitness levels compared with baseline levels. Because improvements in fitness are likely to result from increased physical activity, this outcome can be used as a proxy for physical activity increase. Though there were improvements in BMI, the changes were not significant.

Four of the studies included in Table 16.2 are from the first phase of an NIH funded project called GEMS: Girls Health-Enrichment Multi-site Studies.[27-30] These studies were all focused on African American girls aged 8 to 10 years and intervened for 12 weeks. The results of these pilot studies were then used to develop the full-scale interventions, though two of the sites chose not to continue on with the project after the pilot phase.[27,29] Because these studies were intended as pilot and feasibility efforts, it should not be surprising that none of them demonstrated significant increases in PA or decreases in measures of body size or composition. However, given the paucity of data on community-based PA interventions among youth, they represent a sizable contribution to the literature.

LITERATURE REVIEW: DIETARY INTERVENTIONS

Several of the studies presented in Table 16.2 also address eating-related behaviors, including the research from the pilot GEMS studies, the Go-Girls Study, and the San Diego Family Health Project. While the Zuni Diabetes Prevention Program[22] included a community component for physical activity behavior change, all of the nutrition elements occurred at school and are not discussed here. Diet and food behavior results from these studies are summarized below.

Three of the four GEMS studies included interventions targeting both diet and physical activity behaviors.[27-29] While Robinson et al.[30] included several dietary outcome measures, their intervention did not target dietary change and are not discussed here. As previously stated, these GEMS studies were pilot studies intended to evaluate the feasibility and the potential effectiveness of the intervention; small sample sizes precluded hypothesis testing of outcomes. Still, these three studies give some indication of potential community-based strategies to reduce the prevalence of obesity in one high-risk segment of the youth population, African American girls. The three GEMS studies that included a dietary intervention component had several commonalities, including: a 12-week intervention period, the use of social cognitive theory as a basis for the intervention, intervention efforts at both the girl and family levels, and many common impact measures.

Baranowski and colleagues[27] tested the feasibility of a 12-week intervention that included a 4-week summer day camp for youth, followed by an 8-week Internet-based intervention for both youth and their families. The dietary goals of their Food, Fun and Fitness Project included (1) increasing fruit and vegetable consumption as a way to displace dietary fat and related calories in the diet, (2) increasing dietary fiber and water as a means to increase satiety, and (3) increasing water consumption to displace soft drink and sweetened fruit drink consumption. The day camp included a wide range of interactive activities focusing on increasing healthful food preferences, skill building (both for simple food preparation and in asking parents to increase healthful food options in the home), self-control through goal setting, decision making, and problem-solving challenges to choosing healthful foods. In addition, they used incentives for achieving behavior change goals.

The Internet component included a weekly behavioral and environmental focus for both the girl and parent, delivered via separate Web sites. Similar interactive activities as used in day camp were reinforced on the Web site for children using a comic book theme and including a photo album from camp, links to other Web sites, and an "ask the experts" column. The Web site for parents also included a comic book focus, a parent poll question, goal setting, recipes, and links.

Trends toward dietary outcomes were all in the desired direction, although no differences between treatment conditions resulted in a p-value < 0.20. At the end of the 12-week intervention period, youth randomized to the intervention group were consuming, on average, approximately 232 fewer calories and 1.2 times more servings of fruits and vegetables as compared with girls in the control group. In addition, there was a favorable trend in the intervention group, as compared with the control group, for a decrease in the consumption of sweetened beverages and an increased intake of water.

Apart from considering impact evaluation, the process evaluation showed the challenges of engaging youth and family in this Internet-based program. Mean Internet log-on rates for girls and parents in the intervention group averaged 48% and 47%, respectively, across the 8 weeks. Log-on rates dipped as low as 37% during 3 weeks of the intervention for girls and to 26% during 1 week for parents. The authors recognize the challenge in using the Internet as an intervention strategy for youth and family, and suggest that future work in this area needs to pay special attention to the Web content (especially the attractiveness, fun, and cognitive appropriateness of the images and activities) and consider the use of incentives and reminders to promote use of the Web site. While attendance at the summer camp was very good (overall 91.5% participation over 4 weeks), this approach may have limited feasibility as a new community program because of the per-child cost of such a tailored camp experience. If existing summer day camps adopt similar activities with an emphasis on healthful snack and food-related activities, then a broader population impact may occur.

The Memphis-based GEMS project[28] also targeted both girls and parents via group sessions conducted for 90 min/week for 12 weeks with separate groups for girls and parents. The dietary goals of the intervention included (1) eating a balanced diet, reducing high fat food and fast food; (2) increasing water consumption and decreasing sweetened beverage intake; (3) increasing fruit and vegetable intake; and (4) promoting healthy eating behavior such as not skipping meals, snacking only when hungry, and not eating while watching television. The group sessions for the girls included a 30-min nutrition component that included taste testing and snack preparation of fruits, vegetables, low-fat and low-sugar foods, and beverages; discussions on healthy eating habits; and nutrition education including label reading. The parent sessions included a nutrition component that included tips for families, food preparation, modifying family favorite recipes, and kid-friendly, healthful recipes.

At the end of the 12-week intervention period, combining the parent and child targeted interventions, girls in the intervention conditions reported a 34.1% decrease in servings of sweetened beverages. This reduction in intake resulted in a statistically significant difference between treatment conditions ($p = 0.03$). This effect was driven by differences seen in the parent-targeted intervention group as compared with the control group; the child-targeted intervention proved to be less potent. No other statistically significant differences were seen although trends for most of the dietary variables were in the correct direction. For example, adjusted mean difference of caloric intake between treatment conditions was −85.2 kcal ($p = 0.37$) with the intervention group reporting fewer calories than the control group.

Process data show excellent attendance at the sessions. Overall, at least 88% of participants attended at least 80% of the sessions with better attendance at the parent-targeted sessions (94% of parents attended at least 80% of sessions; 83% of youth attended at least 80% of sessions.) This experience is contrary to other community-based research attempting to involve families in youth health promotion programs by asking them to attend out-of-school sessions.[21,31,32] The success of the Memphis GEMS program might reflect a change in family perceptions of the importance of healthy eating and activity patterns of youth over the past decade or something that is unique to this particular population and research.

Post pilot study interviews and observations during the pilot experience suggested that running separate sessions for parents and their children was not the preferred approach. Parents opined that they would prefer to participate with their child and thought that their presence at common sessions would help girls make positive behavior changes. Running two separate interventions was costly, and in a full scale community trial would require a larger sample size to power two separate intervention conditions, incurring even higher costs. The Phase 2 GEMS trial will include girl and family joint sessions.

Story et al.[29] report on the Minnesota GEMS pilot study that engaged girls in after school programs and families in other activities including weekly family packets (periodically including ingredients for a low fat snack to make at home), family night events, and phone calls to families.

The dietary change goals for Minnesota's intervention program included (1) decreased consumption of high-fat foods; (2) increased consumption of fruits and vegetables; (3) decreased consumption of sweetened beverages; and (4) adoption of healthy weight-related eating practices.

The after-school program was run in three elementary schools using a club format with club meetings twice a week for 12 weeks. The club meetings included a nutrition component that included interactive activities related to choosing healthful snacks, nutrition education–related activities such as label reading and determining the amount of sugar in beverages, goal setting, and preparing and tasting lower fat snacks. The family component included take home packets for the family that included tips sheets, "Fridge facts," and occasionally, foods to make a snack. Two family nights were held at the schools that included booths and games, a low-fat meal, and family goal setting. Family phone calls incorporated elements of motivational interviewing.

At the end of the pilot 12-week intervention, no statistically significant differences were found in the dietary variables assessed and the evidence for trends was mixed. While number of servings of water per day, total energy intake, and proportion of energy from fat was in the desired direction, showing a trend toward improvement in the intervention condition relative to the control condition, changes in the servings of fruits, vegetables, and juice and sweetened beverage servings favored the control condition. The parents of girls in the intervention condition reported less availability of higher-fat foods, more low-fat food practices, and lower energy intake from fat in their own diets as compared with parents in the control group, all at statistically significant levels.

Process data indicate that attendance at the after-school sessions was nearly 88%, and 95% of girls and 88% of parents attended at least one family night event. Nearly all of the girls (92%) reported that they liked the after-school program "a lot," and 83% of families said they liked the take home packs and the family nights. The authors conclude that the enrollment rates and satisfaction levels with the program are encouraging and might suggest community-based settings, such as after-school programs, might represent "… an untapped resource, and offer potential for interventions to help youth acquire, maintain or increase positive health behaviors related to eating and physical activity."[29] They acknowledge that the challenges to such nonschool-based programs include maintaining attendance, keeping the program fun and the participants engaged, and providing transportation.

Like the GEMS studies reviewed, Go Girls,[32] was also a feasibility and pilot intervention, and focused on older African American female adolescents. This pilot research recruited 47 high school age girls from four public housing units in Georgia to participate in a nutrition and physical activity intervention for overweight girls. (Girls self-identified as "overweight," and weight loss was not a stated objective of the study. Therefore, we include the study as primary prevention.) The intervention was delivered in community space or apartments at the four public housing developments over a period of 6 months. The groups met twice weekly after school for the first four months and weekly the last 2 months. Some activities were held out in the community as field trip events.

The primary nutrition-related target behaviors included (1) increasing fruits and vegetables, (2) decreasing fat intake, and (3) decreasing fast food intake. The intervention was based on social cognitive theory (SCT), and each of the group sessions included an interactive educational and/or behavioral activity, 30 to 60 min of physical activity, and preparation and tasting of a low-fat, portion-controlled meal. The educational and/or behavioral activities included applying substitution, moderation, or abstinence to positively influence eating behavior change, participating in satiety training (helping girls recognize when they are full), learning about fat and caloric content of foods, and exercises on shopping for healthful foods. Families were not directly involved with the intervention but were invited to attend at least two sessions.

This feasibility study did not include a control group. They compared levels of change on a variety of activity and food-related variables by examining results from high attenders versus low attenders, dichotomized by attendance at at least 50% of the sessions. To assess the girls' diets, 24-h recalls and food frequencies were used. Results show no statistically significant difference in any of the dietary intake variables (including calories, energy from fat, fiber, cholesterol, and sodium) between pre- and postmeasures. However, greater levels of change were seen in high attenders as compared with low attenders for total calories, percent calories from fat (24-h recalls only), fiber (24-h recalls only), cholesterol, and sodium (food frequency only).

The study design and small sample size severely limit what can be learned about the impact of the program on outcome variables. However, some things were learned with regard to conducting a nutrition and activity program for overweight youth in a community setting. While recruitment of girls into the program was not difficult, attendance and retention were problematic. On average, participants attended 43% of the sessions and the drop out rate was 45%. The authors suggest that having more African American lay health educators involved in the intervention might have helped retention rates and also recommend screening potential participants for their readiness to change.

As for intervention strategies, process and formative evaluation suggest that the girls preferred an experiential, rather than didactic, learning experience, enjoyed getting away for field trips, enjoyed the use of incentives for participation and behavior change, and enjoyed the social benefits and the meals served in the program. Homework assignments were not well received, even with incentives. Family participation was very low, with only one to two parents attending sessions when invited. The authors suggest that more intensive and creative strategies for engaging parents are needed.

Nader et al.[20,21] examined the effectiveness of a family-based intervention to reduce cardiovascular risk factors in Mexican American and Anglo American families. Families with children in fifth or sixth grade were invited to participate in the study; 206 families were successfully recruited and half of the families were randomized to a year-long educational intervention to decrease the family's intake of high salt, high fat foods and to increase their physical activity. Families randomized to the intervention condition received 3 months of intensive weekly intervention, followed by 9 months of monthly or bimonthly maintenance sessions. The intensive sessions lasted 90 min, were held in the early evening at the local school, and included learning activities designed to be experiential, be fun, and use a behavioral focus including goal setting. The intensive sessions ended with a social time that included a healthy snack. The dietary educational intervention used the stoplight approach, categorizing foods as red (whoa), yellow (slow), and green (go) with respect to their saturated fat and sodium content. Six maintenance sessions were held over 9 months and addressed specific problems such as breaking behavior chains and family grocery shopping. Process data showed some variance in attendance rates between the two ethnic groups represented and the intensive and maintenance phases. Average attendance during the intensive intervention was 71% and 58% for Anglo and Mexican American families, respectively. For the maintenance phase, the average attendance rates were 42% for Anglo families and 39% for Mexican American families.[20]

While no statistically significant differences were seen for physical activity[20] or BMI[21] posttreatment, Anglo families reported lower fat and sodium intake on both 24-h recalls and 3-day food records, and both ethnic groups experienced improved diets as measured using a food frequency index, as compared with control families.[20] Children also experienced a significant reduction in diastolic blood pressure posttreatment. Continued follow-up of the cohort at 24 and 48 months showed that changes in dietary fat persisted for Anglo girls and changes in the food frequency index persisted at 48 months for the Mexican American girls.[21]

NONRESEARCH COMMUNITY APPROACHES TO PROMOTING HEALTHY EATING AND PHYSICAL ACTIVITY

In addition to the research reviewed above, there are numerous community-based interventions ongoing that intend to promote physical activity and plans for potential community strategies for healthful diets for youth. In this section we review examples of these programs as indication of some of the important ongoing intervention work that could benefit from further efficacy evaluation.

VERB is one of the most broad ranging youth physical activity initiatives in the United States to date for "tweens" (youth aged 9 to 13). Part of this initiative was partnerships with state, territorial,

TABLE 16.3
Summary of VERB Community Partners Program Features
(n = 31 Programs Reporting)

VERB Activity	Proportion of Communities Using the Activity (%)
Professional development for teachers and/or community leaders	45
Media campaigns	26
Minigrants for variety of programs	26
Provision of equipment	23
Web site and resource guide development	23
After school PA program implementation	16
Surveillance to assess current state of programming	16
Provision of money for special trips and events related to PA	16
Walk or bike to school program development and implementation	13
After school PA program development	10
After school PA program professional development	6
Education and informing the public	6
Implementation of community programs	6
Peer leader training	3
Development of community programs	3
Development of community partnerships	3
Provision of spaces	3
Focus groups and educational forums	3
Walking program development and implementation	3

and local educational organizations, as well as national organizations, to promote physical activity. Funding from a specific CDC program announcement was divided among 43 state, 4 territorial, and 15 local education agencies, as well as 8 national agencies for initiatives to increase physical activity among youth. The use of this funding by state, local, and national agencies provides a snapshot of the available community-based physical activity promotion programming and associated challenges. Of these 70 programs, 31 provided a summary that is available on the VERB website (http://www.cdc.gov/HealthyYouth/physicalactivity/projects/pdf/complete_text.pdf). None of these reports includes any indication of whether the efforts resulted in increased physical activity among youth. Evaluation of programs is costly; the funds were put toward other uses. A summary table of the use of the grant funds is provided in Table 16.3. The majority of organizations used the money for one of three types of initiatives: professional development for those who will provide physical activity programming to youth, minigrants for a variety of programs, and media campaigns to promote physical activity. The most common challenge noted by programs that provided a summary was funding for sustaining the efforts started, gaps not covered by the CDC grant, or evaluation efforts. Other challenges reported included transportation of youth to sites where physical activity opportunities existed, need for further professional development, building multiorganization coalitions, availability of sites and equipment for physical activity, diversity of needs across the area served by the program, and insurance liability costs. Several of these challenges (transportation, availability of spaces, availability of equipment) are correlated with children's physical activity levels,[33] which speaks to the importance of addressing these issues in future interventions. Another interesting common thread through many of the summaries is that there may be more opportunities than the public is aware of, given that a sizable number of the programs chose to development Web sites and/or resource guides or take some other action to inform the public of the opportunities for youth physical activity. Many of these efforts targeted parents.

To our knowledge, there is not a similar, concerted national intervention to positively influence the eating habits of youth at the community level. There are national nutrition education and health promotion campaigns that focus on eating a healthy diet including efforts by the U.S. Department of Agriculture to provide sound nutritional advice to the populace through the Food Guide Pyramid, the U.S. Dietary Guidelines, and food labeling. The Food Guide Pyramid is the national nutrition education tool that is widely disseminated to youth through school health education. Other national campaigns that may influence youth in the community include National Cancer Institute's (NCI) 5-a-day campaign and community-level grocery store and restaurant campaigns that use signage to identify healthful items in stores or on menus. However, these efforts are not specifically directed toward youth.

The data on the influence of these national or communitywide campaigns on the eating behavior of youth are sparse but their impact is believed to be minimal.[34] Poor effects of public health–related messages about food disseminated broadly at the community level might reflect the imbalance in the number, intensity, and sophistication of marketing messages promoting eating healthful foods relative to the overwhelming messages to choose high energy foods and to overconsume calories, in general. As an example, the NCI's 5-a-day campaign spent just under $3 million dollars for advertising in 1 year while food and food service companies spend more than $11 billion annually on direct media advertising.[34] In addition, the content of the public health messages related to a healthful diet may need to switch from eating more of some foods (e.g., fruits, vegetables, grains, low fat milk) and begin to focus on energy balance in the diet. A national education campaign that includes information on how to determine one's caloric needs, the caloric content of foods, and how physical activity and other energy expenditures affect calorie balance and weight might be helpful; the challenge in communicating these complicated messages is acknowledged.

Potential communitywide intervention strategies might include a ban on advertising to children. It is estimated that in 1997, food companies spent $12.7 billion dollars marketing their products to children and their parents.[34] The children's television–advertising market accounted for $1 billion dollars in 1999.[34] Other communitywide strategies might include taxation of low-nutritive, energy-dense foods because research shows that youth are very sensitive to the cost of snacks[35] or regulation of the food industry with regard to packaging and portion sizes of foods that are popular with youth.[36] These strategies parallel those used to reduce youth smoking rates and will likely be met with similar resistance by the food industry, as was experienced with the tobacco industry.

SUMMARY AND FUTURE DIRECTIONS

Much has been written about how community may influence youth activity patterns and food intakes, but there is very little empirical research on community-based interventions to define best practices for creating community-level healthier environments for activity and eating behaviors. The literature summarized in Table 16.2 demonstrates the infancy of the field. Quasi-experimental study designs with small sample sizes are the norm; the generalizability of the findings is very limited because of study design and also because of the specificity of the populations on which intervention studies have focused. The changes observed in these early studies are modest at best.

The main trial of the GEMS study, which is currently underway, will add significantly to the field, but will have limited generalizability because it targets only 8- to 10-year-old African American girls. In addition, a large community trial, The Trial of Activity in Adolescent Girls (TAAG) is underway and is evaluating school- and community-linked intervention approaches to increase physical activity levels in adolescent girls.[37] However, the results from TAAG are not currently available, and no dietary component is included. The vast majority of the published obesity-prevention evaluation trials have occurred in schools. Family-based prevention approaches are rare. Other community-level venues have great potential for preventive efforts including primary health and dental care, churches, community centers, recreation facilities, grocery stores, convenience stores, restaurants, and fast-food chains.

Review of the literature shows that most of the work to date on community-level childhood obesity-prevention interventions focuses exclusively on proximal factors and primarily on social factors in the community. There is a great need to gain a better understanding of the influences of other proximal, distal, social, and physical influences of childhood obesity through etiologic research and then to begin to work on intervention strategies that tap the four cells depicted in Table 16.1. Working at the community level will require interventions that utilize newer approaches including "bottom-up" approaches such as community organizing[8] and forming community partnerships.[38] Obesity-prevention efforts may learn much from the successes experienced in changing community-level youth access to tobacco through mobilizing community members to change the norms and physical environments of their communities.[39,40] Work is needed to link community agencies in common goals of improving the physical activity and eating behaviors of youth. The TAAG study is pioneering efforts in this area because it links schools and community agencies in working toward increasing out-of-school activity options for adolescent girls.[41] Creating community partnerships is a difficult, but potentially powerful, way to institute community change.

Other lessons that might be learned from the tobacco-prevention research with youth are "top-down" approaches that may include policy, pricing, and legislative actions that can help promote healthful behaviors and provide disincentives for less healthful choices. School-based research suggests that pricing affects youth choice of lower and higher fat foods from vending machines.[35] It is possible that similar pricing manipulations could occur in community settings (i.e., vending machines at community centers, churches, and recreation facilities) and have a positive influence on youth eating behavior in the community. More distal approaches might include regulations on packaging and portion sizes that would affect not only youth, but also many members of the community. There is a great deal of interest in the role of the food industry and national food policy in the obesity epidemic.[34,36] These areas represent distal factors that while difficult to affect, could have broad-reaching impact.

The early work on interventions that are focused at the group or family level in the community (Table 16.2) suggest that we need to find ways to engage and maintain families and groups in obesity-prevention activities and that we need more powerful intervention strategies. A great deal of work is needed with families because their potential to affect the eating and activity behaviors of youth is great.

We need to expand our understanding of the influence of socioeconomic status and social capital[42] on obesity in youth. Demographic characteristics (including ethnicity and socioeconomic status) of the families wherein youth are raised influence their risk of becoming overweight,[43] and their eating and activity patterns. Recently published data from the National Longitudinal Study of Adolescent Health[44] show that lower household income and lower parental education were strongly related to adolescent obesity and depression. The National Health Interview Survey showed that the consumption of foods high in fat among adolescent girls was inversely related to parental education.[45] Activity differences among ethnic and socioeconomic subgroups have been attributed to differences in perceived benefits of being active, perceptions of desirable body shape, lack of time and financial resources for leisure time activities by lower income families, and differences in real or perceived safety of neighborhoods.[15,46–48] It is likely that reducing levels of poverty in our nation is an important step in reducing the youth obesity epidemic.

Finally, a great deal of methodological work is needed for us to assess and evaluate the effectiveness of community-level interventions. We need valid and reliable assessment tools to assess the physical and social food and activity environments of our communities. In addition, we need to employ more sophisticated study designs and analytic techniques if we want to intervene on multiple levels of influence and assess multilevel associations using an ecological approach.[49]

Children do not grow up solely in school or in any one institution or program; they grow up in a community. If the community makes clear to youth that obtaining the recommended amount of daily activity is important, provides adult role models who are active, and provides adequate spaces, programs, equipment, staff, transportation, reinforcement, and other support to do so, more children will succeed in being physically active. Likewise, communities that offer a predominance of healthy food choices served in reasonable portion sizes, reinforce healthy eating choice, and offer adult role models who eat reasonable amounts of healthful foods will be more likely to have children who eat a healthful diet, rich in nutrients and of appropriate caloric content. One assumed positive outcome from such community support would be a reduced rate of childhood obesity and related metabolic disorders. Another positive outcome could be the development of a lifelong pattern of regular physical activity and healthy eating patterns,[50] resulting in lower risk for chronic disease.

References

1. Centers for Disease Control and Prevention. Guidelines for school and community programs to promote lifelong physical activity among young people. *Morb Mortal Wkly Rep.* 1997;46: 1–36.
2. Campbell K, Waters E, O'Meara S, Kelly S, Summerbell C. *Interventions for Preventing Obesity in Children* (Cohrane Review). The Cochrane Library, Issue 3. Chicester, UK: John Wiley & Sons, Ltd, 2004.
3. Pate RR, Trost SG, Mullis R, Sallis JF. Community interventions to promote proper nutrition and physical activity among youth. *Prev Med.* 2000;31: S138–S149.
4. French SA, Story M, Jeffery RW. Environmental influences on eating and physical activity. *Annu Rev Public Health.* 2001;22: 309–335.
5. Schmitz KH, Lytle LA, Phillips GA, Murray DM, Birnbaum AS, Kubik MY. Psychosocial correlates of physical activity and sedentary leisure habits in young adolescents: the Teens Eating for Energy and Nutrition at School study. *Prev Med.* 2002;34: 266–278.
6. Wong F, Huhman M, Heitzler C, Asbury L, Bretthauer-Mueller R, McCarthy S, et al. VERB — A social marketing campaign to increase physical activity among youth. *Prev Chronic Dis.* 2004;1: 1–7.
7. Green LW, Kreuter MW. CDC's planned approach to community health as an application of the PROCEED and an inspiration for PROCEED. *J Health Ed.* 1992;23: 140–147.
8. Minkler M, Wallerstein N. Improving health through community organization and community building. In: Glanz K, Rimer BK, Lewis FM, Eds. *Health Behavior and Health Education: Theory, Research, and Practice*, 3rd ed. San Francisco: Jossey-Bass, 2002: 279–311.
9. Parsons TJ, Power C, Logan S, Summerbell CD. Childhood predictors of adult obesity: a systematic review. *Int J Obes Relat Metab Disord.* 1999;23(Suppl 8): S1–S107.
10. French SA, Story M, Neumark-Sztainer D, Fulkerson JA, Hannan P. Fast food restaurant use among adolescents: associations with nutrient intake, food choices and behavioral and psychosocial variables. *Int J Obes Relat Metab Disord.* 2001;25: 1823–1833.
11. Swinburn BA, Caterson I, Seidell JC, James WP. Diet, nutrition and the prevention of excess weight gain and obesity. *Public Health Nutr.* 2004;7: 123–146.
12. Sallis JF, Owen N. Ecological models of health behavior. In: Glanz K, Rimer BK, Lewis FM, Eds. *Health Behavior and Health Education: Theory, Research, and Practice*, 3rd ed. San Francisco: Jossey-Bass, 2002: 461–484.
13. Smedley BD, Syme SL. *Promoting Health: Intervention Strategies from Social and Behavioral Research.* Washington, DC: National Academy Press, 2000.
14. Poston WS, 2nd, Foreyt JP. Obesity is an environmental issue. *Atherosclerosis.* 1999;146: 201–209.
15. Davison KK, Birch LL. Childhood overweight: a contextual model and recommendations for future research. *Obes Rev.* 2001;2: 159–171.
16. Stettler N. Environmental factors in the etiology of obesity in adolescents. *Ethn Dis.* 2002;12: S1–S5.
17. Booth SL, Sallis JF, Ritenbaugh C, Hill JO, Birch LL, Frank LD, et al. Environmental and societal factors affect food choice and physical activity: rationale, influences, and leverage points. *Nutr Rev.* 2001;59: S21–S39;discussion: S57–S65.
18. Ross JG, Dotson CO, Gilbert GG, Katz SJ. After physical education ... Physical activity outside of school physical education programs. *J Phys Ed, Recreation Dance.* 1985;56: 77–81.
19. Simons-Morton BG, O'Hara NM, Parcel GS, Huang IW, Baranowski T, Wilson B. Children's frequency of participation in moderate to vigorous physical activities. *Res Q Exerc Sport.* 1990;61: 307–314.

20. Nader PR, Sallis JF, Patterson TL, Abramson IS, Rupp JW, Senn KL, et al. A family approach to cardiovascular risk reduction: results from the San Diego Family Health Project. *Health Educ Q.* 1989;16: 229–244.
21. Nader PR, Sallis JF, Patterson TL, Abramson IS, Rupp JW, Senn KL, et al. Family-based cardiovascular risk reduction education among Mexican- and Anglo-Americans. *Family Commun Health.* 1992;15: 57–74.
22. Teufel NI, Ritenbaugh CK. Development of a primary prevention program: insight gained in the Zuni Diabetes Prevention Program. *Clin Pediatr* (Phila). 1998;37: 131–141.
23. Ransdell LB, Dratt J, Kennedy C, O'Neill S, DeVoe D. Daughters and mothers exercising together (DAMET): a 12–week pilot project designed to improve physical self-perception and increase recreational physical activity. *Women Health.* 2001;33: 101–116.
24. Ransdell LB, Taylor A, Oakland D, Schmidt J, Moyer-Mileur L, Shultz B. Daughters and mothers exercising together: effects of home- and community-based programs. *Med Sci Sports Exercise.* 2003;35: 286–296.
25. Taggart AC, Taggart J, Siedentop D. Effects of a home-based activity program. A study with low fitness elementary school children. *Behav Modif.* 1986;10: 487–507.
26. Ford BS, McDonald TE, Owens AS, Robinson TN. Primary care interventions to reduce television viewing in African-American children. *Am J Prev Med.* 2002;22: 106–109.
27. Baranowski T, Baranowski JC, Cullen KW, Thompson DI, Nicklas T, Zakeri IF, Rochon J. The Fun, Food, and Fitness Project (FFFP): the Baylor GEMS pilot study. *Ethn Dis.* 2003;13: S30–S39.
28. Beech BM, Klesges RC, Kumanyika SK, Murray DM, Klesges L, McClanahan B, et al. Child- and parent-targeted interventions: the Memphis GEMS pilot study. *Ethn Dis.* 2003;13: S40–S53.
29. Story M, Sherwood NE, Himes JH, Davis M, Jacobs DR, Jr., Cartwright Y, et al. An after-school obesity prevention program for African-American girls: the Minnesota GEMS pilot study. *Ethn Dis.* 2003;13: S54–64.
30. Robinson TN, Killen JD, Kraemer HC, Wilson DM, Matheson DM, Haskell WL, et al. Dance and reducing television viewing to prevent weight gain in African-American girls: the Stanford GEMS pilot study. *Ethn Dis.* 2003;13: S65–S77.
31. Baranowski T, Simons-Morton B, Hooks P, Henske J, Tiernan K, Dunn JK, et al. A center-based program for exercise change among black-American families. *Health Educ Q.* 1990;17: 179–196.
32. Resnicow K, Yaroch AL, Davis A, Wang DT, Carter S, Slaughter L, et al. GO GIRLS!: results from a nutrition and physical activity program for low-income, overweight African American adolescent females. *Health Educ Behav.* 2000;27: 616–631.
33. Sallis JF, Prochaska JJ, Taylor WC. A review of correlates of physical activity of children and adolescents. *Med Sci Sports Exerc.* 2000;32: 963–975.
34. Nestle M. *Food Politics.* Berkley, CA: University of California Press, 2002.
35. French SA. Pricing effects on food choices. *J Nutr.* 2003;133: 841S–843S.
36. Brownell KD, Horgen KB. *Food Fight: The Inside Story of the Food Industry.* New York: McGraw-Hill, 2004.
37. Stevens J, Murray DM, Catellier DJ, Lytle LA, Elder JP, Young DR, et al. Design of the Trial of Activity in Adolescent Girls (TAAG). *Contemp Clin Trials.* 2005;26: 223–233.
38. Israel BA, Schulz AJ, Parker EA, Becker AB. Review of community-based research: assessing partnership approaches to improve public health. *Annu Rev Public Health.* 1998;19: 173–202.
39. Perry CL, Williams CL, Komro KA, Veblen-Mortenson S, Forster JL, Bernstein-Lachter R, et al. Project Northland High School interventions: community action to reduce adolescent alcohol use. *Health Educ Behav.* 2000;27: 29–49.
40. Forster JL, Murray DM, Wolfson M, Blaine TM, Wagenaar AC, Hennrikus DJ. The effects of community policies to reduce youth access to tobacco. *Am J Public Health.* 1998;88: 1193–1198.
41. Lytle LA, Alexander CS, Moody J, Parra-Medinia D, Perry CL, Saksvig BI, et al. The Trial of Activity in Adolescent Girls (TAAG): Developing a school and community-linked intervention. Submitted.
42. Sampson RJ, Morenoff JD. Public health and safety in context: lessons from community-level theory on social capital. In: Smedly BD, Syme SL, Eds. *Promoting Health: Intervention Strategies from Social and Behavioral Research.* Washington, DC: National Academy Press, 2000: 366–389.

43. Gnavi R, Spagnoli TD, Galotto C, Pugliese E, Carta A, Cesari L. Socioeconomic status, overweight and obesity in prepuberal children: a study in an area of Northern Italy. *Eur J Epidemiol.* 2000;16: 797–803.

44. Goodman E, Slap GB, Huang B. The public health impact of socioeconomic status on adolescent depression and obesity. *Am J Public Health.* 2003;93: 1844–1850.

45. Lowry R, Kann L, Collins JL, Kolbe LJ. The effect of socioeconomic status on chronic disease risk behaviors among US adolescents. *JAMA* 1996;276: 792–797.

46. Harris MB, Koehler KM. Eating and exercise behaviors and attitudes of Southwestern Anglos and Hispanics. *Psychol Health.* 1992;7: 165–174.

47. Sobal J, Strunkard AJ. Socioeconomic status and obesity: a review of the literature. *Psychol Bull.* 1989;105: 260–275.

48. Wolf AM, Gortmaker SL, Cheung L, Gray HM, Herzog DB, Colditz GA. Activity, inactivity, and obesity: racial, ethnic, and age differences among schoolgirls. *Am J Public Health.* 1993;83: 1625–1627.

49. Lytle LA, Fulkerson JA. Assessing the dietary environment: examples from school-based nutrition interventions. *Public Health Nutr.* 2002;5: 893–899.

50. Kelder SH, Perry CL, Klepp KI, Lytle LA. Longitudinal tracking of adolescent smoking, physical activity, and food choice behaviors. *Am J Public Health.* 1994;84: 1121–1126.

51. Pate RR, Saunders RP, Ward DS, Felton G, Trost SG, Dowda M. Evaluation of a community-based intervention to promote physical activity in youth: lessons from Active Winners. *Amer J Health Promotion.* 2003;17: 171–182.

52. Lewis CE, Raczynski JM, Heath GW, Levinson R, Hilyer JC, Jr., Cutter GR. Promoting physical activity in low-income African-American communities; the PARR project. *Ethnic Dis,* 1993;3: 106–118.

53. Resnicow K, Yaroch AL, Davis A, Wang DT, Slaughter L, Coleman D, et al. Go Girls!: Results from a nutrition and physical activity program for low-income, overweight African-american adolescent females. *Health Educ Behav.* 2000;27: 616–631.

17 Obesity Prevention in Schools

Simone A. French and Mary Story

CONTENTS

INTRODUCTION

Schools are an optimal setting in which to reach child and adolescent populations with interventions to promote a healthy body weight through physical activity and eating behaviors that maintain energy balance. Over 95% of American youth ages 5 to 17 years from diverse socioeconomic and racial and ethnic backgrounds attend school.[1] Over half of the children and adolescents in the United States eat at least one meal from the school meals program,[2] and many consume foods and beverages purchased in school from school snack bars, vending machines, or a la carte areas.[3–6] Physical activity opportunities are provided in the school setting through physical education classes, recess breaks, and organized school sports programs such as intramural sports or interscholastic teams.[7] Schools also provide an environment in which students observe social norms and role models for food choices and physical activity behaviors. In addition to these environmental influences on food choices and physical activity behaviors, schools can promote and support healthful eating and physical activity behaviors through behaviorally oriented classroom curricula.

Several theoretical frameworks have been used to conceptualize the school environment with respect to health behaviors and obesity prevention. School health promotion frameworks have included healthy eating and physical activity promotion within a comprehensive school health promotion framework.[7,8] School-based behavioral intervention studies to prevent obesity and promote healthful eating and physical activity behaviors have commonly used social ecological theory or social cognitive theory as an organizational framework.[9–11]

Many school-based intervention studies have been conducted to promote healthful eating and physical activity behaviors among children and adolescents. However, few school-based obesity prevention interventions have been conducted. Several comprehensive reviews are available on childhood obesity prevention interventions and behavioral interventions that have targeted nutrition and physical activity behaviors in child and adolescent populations.[12–21] The findings of these comprehensive reviews are not repeated here. Overall, the results of school-based studies that targeted eating and physical activity behaviors have been positive. Consistent with these studies, school-based obesity-prevention interventions have shown some success in changing eating and physical activity behaviors but have been less successful in changing body weight or body fatness. The most recent review of the effectiveness of the childhood obesity-prevention interventions concluded that limited quality data are available and no generalizable conclusions can be drawn.[19]

The purpose of the present chapter is to highlight the most promising and innovative research directions to date in school-based obesity prevention. Exemplary school-based nutrition and physical activity intervention studies also are included. Emerging innovative intervention and policy approaches that have yet to be evaluated are described. Research recommendations are presented.

OBESITY PREVENTION INTERVENTIONS

Few well-designed and evaluated school-based obesity-prevention interventions have been conducted, although recently this area has received greater research attention and funding priority. The interventions conducted to date have built upon successful school-based interventions to promote healthful eating and physical activity behaviors. The latter studies are described in further detail later in the chapter. School-based obesity prevention interventions to date have included one or more components, such as behaviorally oriented classroom curricula, physical education class structure modifications, and changes in the content of the school meals. The following obesity prevention studies were selected based on their methodological quality and their specific targeting of obesity as the primary outcome. All four studies were school-based, randomized trials with schools as the unit of randomization.

PATHWAYS: SCHOOL-BASED INTERVENTION FOR AMERICAN INDIAN ELEMENTARY SCHOOL CHILDREN

Pathways[22] was one of the first randomized controlled trial primary prevention obesity interventions to target children. Pathways aimed to prevent obesity among third-, fourth- and fifth-grade American Indian schoolchildren (average age 7.6 ± .06 years), a population subgroup at high risk for the development of overweight and obesity. Forty-one schools serving American Indian communities in Arizona, New Mexico, and South Dakota were randomized to a 3-year intervention or to a no-treatment control group. The multicomponent intervention package was similar in the basic content areas to the CATCH intervention (Child and Adolescent Trial for Cardiovascular Health, described below)[23] and included a behavioral curriculum component as well as environmental changes that targeted food service and PE classes. Intervention components included a classroom curriculum during third, fourth and fifth grades that focused on promoting healthful eating behaviors and increasing physical activity; physical activity breaks of 2- to 10-min duration during class; food service changes to reduce the fat content of the school meals; changes in the physical education classes to increase both the frequency of PE classes and the amount of PE class time spent in moderate to vigorous physical activity; and a family involvement component that consisted of take-home activities and family events held at the school. The primary outcome was change in body fatness, estimated using equations developed specifically for the Pathways study, from measures of triceps and subscapular skinfold thickness, bioelectrical impedence measures, and height and weight. Secondary outcomes were changes in dietary intake (measured using standardized lunch-room observations and 24-h recalls) and physical activity (measured using Tri-Trac accelerometers and self-reported physical activity recalls).

Results were not significant for the primary outcome, change in body fatness (intervention–control difference: +0.2%) or body mass index (BMI) (intervention–control difference: –0.2 kg/m²). However, significant reductions in favor of students in the intervention schools were observed for the secondary behavioral change outcome, percent dietary fat intake, which was measured using standardized observations of students' intake during lunch (intervention–control difference: –4.2% kcal fat) and using 24-h dietary recalls (post-intervention only; intervention–control difference: 2.5% kcal fat). Energy intake was significantly lower among students in intervention schools only based on the 24-h recalls (intervention–control difference: –265 kcal), but not based on observed lunch intake. Physical activity was not significantly different between students in intervention and control schools based on objective data collected with physical activity monitors (Tri-Trac). However, self-reported physical activity significantly increased among students in intervention schools compared with those in control schools. These findings show that a multicomponent, 3-year, school-based intervention that includes both a classroom educational component and environmental changes in the structure of the PE classes and the school meals program can produce positive, significant effects on change in behaviors related to energy balance such as dietary intake, and perhaps physical activity levels, among elementary school children. Although effects on body fatness were not significant, the results are nevertheless promising because of the positive changes in behaviors related to long-term energy balance. A stronger intervention program that produces larger behavioral change effects might have a significant detectable impact on change in body fatness during the time window in which the intervention and evaluation activities are completed. Smaller behavioral changes that are achievable during a short time frame represented by the research time window potentially might be effective in preventing excess weight and fat gains during a longer time frame.

Pathways was also successful from a perspective of developing and implementing an obesity prevention program that involved a genuine collaboration between the American Indian community and the academic institutions. The program was culturally tailored using a collaborative process and was implemented in challenging social and physical settings in American Indian reservation schools in seven widely dispersed geographic locations. Its success in involving the tribal community, individual families, and school staff provides a model for future intervention efforts in this community as well as in other economically challenged communities that are at high risk for obesity.

Hip Hop to Health, Jr.: Preschool Intervention for African American Children in Head Start

A second school-based obesity prevention intervention targeted African American preschool children (average age 4 years) enrolled in the Head Start program. Hip Hop to Health, Jr.[24] randomized

12 Head Start centers either to an obesity prevention intervention or to a general health program control group. Children in the intervention program received 14 weeks of intervention; 40-min sessions 3 days per week. Parents received newsletters and home activities and were invited to attend an aerobics class 2 days per week. The intervention messages focused on increasing the choice of healthful foods such as fruits and vegetables, decreasing the choice of less healthful foods high in fat and sugar, and increasing physical activity levels. Children's weight and height were measured, and children's food intake and physical activity were reported by parents. In contrast to the results of Pathways (described above), significant intervention effects were observed for change in BMI at both follow-ups: year 1 (intervention–control difference: –0.066 kg/m^2; p <.01) and year 2 (intervention–control difference: –0.59 kg/m^2; p < .01). By contrast, changes in parent reports of their child's dietary intake (percent dietary fat) and physical activity behaviors were not significantly different between treatment and control groups. Interestingly, Pathways was successful in changing behaviors related to energy balance, but not body fatness, while Hip Hop to Health was successful in changing BMI but not eating and physical activity behaviors. The results of these two multi-component interventions are clearly promising, but strong conclusions, positive or negative, are not warranted based on the results of only two studies.

PLANET HEALTH: CLASSROOM CURRICULA FOR MIDDLE SCHOOL CHILDREN

A third obesity-prevention study, Planet Health,[25] randomized 10 schools to a classroom-based obesity prevention intervention program or to a no-treatment control group for a 2-year period. In each of the 2 years, students in grades 6 and 7 (average age 11.7 years) in intervention schools received 16 lessons delivered by trained classroom teachers in an integrated curriculum format (i.e., delivered as part of the curriculum across several different subject areas). Activities and messages focused on increasing physical activity and fruit and vegetable intake, and decreasing television viewing time and intake of high-fat food. Evaluation consisted of a classroom administered behavioral survey and measured body weight, height, and skinfold thickness. Unfortunately, only 65% of the students participated in the evaluation measures. Change in obesity prevalence, defined as a composite of the BMI and triceps skinfold measure, was the primary outcome. A significant intervention effect for change in obesity prevalence was observed among girls only (obesity prevalence odds ratio: 0.47; 95% confidence interval CI 0.24–0.93; p < .03). Mean BMI change was not reported. For behavior changes related to energy balance, the intervention was associated with a significant reduction in the number of hours of reported television viewing among girls and boys (treatmentcontrol difference: girls: –0.58 h/day; boys: –0.40 h/day; p < .001 for both). Among girls only, a significant intervention effect was observed for a decrease in energy intake and a significant increase in fruit and vegetable intake. The results of the Planet Health study are intriguing and suggest that a school-based obesity-prevention program can be effective using only a classroom-based intervention without school environmental intervention components such as changes in the cafeteria and food service or changes in the physical education classroom environment.

TELEVISION REDUCTION INTERVENTION: CLASSROOM CURRICULA FOR ELEMENTARY SCHOOL CHILDREN

A fourth school-based obesity-prevention intervention also primarily focused on a classroom curriculum approach and targeted a single behavior: television viewing.[26] Two schools were randomized either to a 1-year intervention program or to a no-treatment control group. Third and fourth graders in intervention schools received 18 lessons that were each of 30- to 50-min duration and were delivered by trained teachers as part of the usual classroom curriculum. A home-environmental intervention component was included by providing free television timing devices to parents. Parents could program their home televisions to operate a limited number of hours per week using these devices. Forty-two percent of the parents reported installing the television timing device on their household television set. Evaluation consisted of a classroom-administered survey, and measured height and weight. Children self-reported their physical activity and dietary intake via recall measures. Results showed a significant intervention effect for change in BMI (intervention–control difference 0.45 kg/m^2; $p < 0.002$). Television viewing hours per day was also significantly lower at follow up among intervention compared with control students (intervention–control difference: 5.5 h/week; $p < 0.001$). The results of this study are intriguing because they show that an intervention that focuses on a single behavioral target (reduced time spent TV viewing) can significantly have an effect on BMI in children over a 1-year period. The classroom intervention, combined with the home television time limiting device, significantly reduced television viewing hours per week and BMI.

To summarize, it is clear that there are few school-based primary obesity prevention trials from which to draw conclusions about effectiveness. The available studies are difficult to directly compare due to differences in the age group targeted, intervention content and format, and evaluation measures. Three of the four interventions reported significant intervention effects on change in BMI[24,26] or obesity prevalence[25] (among girls only). However, the differences among the studies' design, methods, and results are more notable than are the similarities. For example, the 1-year intervention–control difference for change in BMI was –0.66 kg/m^2 ($p < 0.01$) in 4-year-old preschoolers after a 14-week multibehavioral program that included a parental intervention component.[24] intervention–control difference in change in BMI at 1 year was –0.45 kg/m^2 ($p < 0.002$) among third and fourth graders 8.9 years old after an 18-lesson program that targeted only television viewing reduction through a classroom curriculum with an optional home television time monitor device.[26] By contrast, a 3-year intervention that targeted multiple behaviors among third-, fourth-, and fifth-grade students, and included both classroom curricula, school environmental changes, and a home and parent component[22] did not significantly change BMI. Intervention–control difference in change in BMI after 3 years was –0.20 kg/m^2 (NS), about half the size of the television reduction intervention effect[26] and about one-third the size of the preschool intervention effect.[24] An intriguing question is why a longer, more intensive intervention such as Pathways produced only a one-third to one-half size change in BMI compared with the shorter, less intensive, and less comprehensive interventions described in Fitzgibbon et al.[24] and in Robinson.[26]

SUMMARY

The main conclusion that can be drawn from the few school-based obesity-prevention interventions is that each of these interventions appears to hold promise, but further studies are needed. Future studies need to strengthen the intervention components and to include others that target different levels, such as school environment, home environment, and individual student and parent behaviors. Strengthening the intervention components might include expanding the home and parent component from the typical newsletter and home activity component to include a parent behavioral intervention and home environmental modifications such as installation of television time monitoring devices or the provision of key healthful foods such as fruits and vegetables. Strengthening the school environmental component might include more frequent, required physical education classes, more interesting and diverse physical education choices (e.g., dance, kick-boxing, intramural soccer), and schoolwide guidelines about food and beverage availability and sales.[7]

Research is needed to examine whether certain types of interventions may be more successful with children of different age, gender, or ethnic groups. For example, interventions that target preschool and elementary school age children might focus more on parents as agents of change; particular behaviors might be a greater focus among different age groups (e.g., greater television reduction emphasis among younger aged children, greater emphasis on more structured and diverse PE opportunities among high school aged children). School environmental changes may provide greater impact in high school vs. elementary school (e.g., changes in a la carte and vending machine food and beverage availability, emphasis on active transport to school, increases in the availability of gym and fitness facilities, and equipment after school hours). In addition to strengthening intervention components, additional research is needed to further clarify the behavioral targets of obesity-prevention interventions in children. For example, the most potent behavioral contributors to energy balance need to be identified (e.g., television viewing, leisure time physical activity, sugar-sweetened beverages, large portion sizes).

Clearly, a wealth of research questions are available and in need of data to draw conclusions about the most effective and promising school-based obesity-prevention intervention strategies and programs. Although currently few studies are available, a plethora of data are available on school-based interventions for eating and physical activity behavior change. These data, discussed in detail below, provide insights into fruitful directions to pursue in the design and evaluation of the next generation of school-based obesity-prevention interventions.

SCHOOL-BASED NUTRITION AND PHYSICAL ACTIVITY BEHAVIOR CHANGE INTERVENTIONS

Multicomponent school-based nutrition and physical activity intervention studies have demonstrated positive effects on student dietary intake and physical activity behaviors. The multicomponent nutrition intervention studies have included both individual and environmental change components. A substantial body of research also has examined environmental changes that influence food choices without including a classroom educational component. Physical activity behavior change interventions have focused more on environmental approaches, most often by targeting changes within the PE class structure. The multicomponent intervention studies are first reviewed, followed by the environmental change interventions for food and physical activity.

CHILD AND ADOLESCENT TRIAL FOR CARDIOVASCULAR HEALTH: CATCH

The largest, most comprehensive school-based intervention conducted to date was CATCH.[23] The aim of the CATCH intervention was to lower serum cholesterol among third- through fifth-grade students through a multicomponent intervention composed of a behaviorally based classroom curriculum based on social cognitive theory[11] and school environmental changes, including the school food service meals and the structure of the PE classes. Ninety-six schools in four states were randomized to the intervention or to a no-intervention control group for a 3-year period. The school food environmental intervention component included training the food service staff in specific food preparation behaviors designed to lower the fat and sodium content of the school meals. The intervention targeted a broad range of changes in food preparation methods and availability, including choosing lower fat foods, preparing foods to lower the fat content, and increasing intake of foods such as fruits and vegetables. Food service staff were encouraged to promote healthful foods to students and to place point-of-choice promotional signage in the school cafeteria.[27]

The goal of the CATCH PE program was to increase the time spent in moderate-to-vigorous physical activity to 40% of class time during regularly scheduled PE classes. Three 30-min PE classes per week was the minimum frequency and duration desired. This targeted increase in percent of class time spent in moderate-to-vigorous activity was accomplished through comprehensive teacher training and on-site research staff consultations with teachers who were responsible for teaching PE class.[28]

Results for CATCH's primary outcome, serum cholesterol, showed no significant intervention effects. Although not a primary outcome, no significant treatment-related differences were observed for BMI. However, significant intervention-related effects were observed for changes in the dietary and physical activity environmental and behavioral change targets. Significant reductions in the percent energy from fat were observed in the school meals (school-level food environment). Student-level dietary recalls showed significant intervention-related decreases in energy and percent fat intake. Significant intervention-related increases were observed in the percent of school PE class time spent in moderate-to-vigorous physical activity (school-level physical activity environment). Both intervention and control schools increased the percent of PE class time spent in moderate-to-vigorous PA, but the increase was larger among intervention schools compared with control schools (intervention–control difference: +7%; $p < 0.002$). No differences were observed in PE lesson length. At the individual level, intervention students reported greater increases in vigorous PA minutes per day compared with students in control schools. However, no significant differences were observed in change in fitness level, measured by the 9-min distance run.

The findings from CATCH show that a multicomponent intervention that includes an individual-level behavioral classroom curriculum in tandem with environmental changes in the cafeteria and the school meal nutritional content can produce positive significant effects both on students' dietary intake and physical activity behaviors and on the school food and physical activity environment. CATCH provides a model for intervention design and evaluation from which to develop obesity-prevention interventions. Elements of the environmental and individual behavioral intervention components can be strengthened to produce larger behavioral changes of a magnitude that will affect significant change in BMI. Greater involvement of parents and greater targeting of the home environment and of school policies related to food and physical activity opportunities are also potential methods to strengthen the intervention effects on BMI outcomes.

Five A Day for Better Health: School-Based Multicomponent Interventions to Increase Fruit and Vegetable Consumption among Children

A second major program of school-based nutrition intervention studies was initiated and funded by the U.S. National Cancer Institute to examine strategies to increase fruit and vegetable intake among youth.[17,29,30] Five school-based studies were evaluated: three randomized trials targeted fourth and fifth graders;[31–33] one quasi-experimental study targeted fourth and fifth graders;[34] and one randomized study targeted high school students.[35] Social cognitive theory[11] was the predominant theoretical framework guiding the interventions. Intervention programs were 2 to 3 years in duration. All studies included a classroom curriculum component of some type. Three studies included a food service intervention component,[31,32,35] and four studies included a parent–home component.[31–33,35] Overall, four of the five studies reported significant intervention effects for increasing fruit and vegetable intake.[31–34] Significant intervention effects were more often observed for fruit intake compared with vegetable intake.

Several innovative intervention components were implemented, and some unique results were observed in each of these studies. Reynolds et al.[31] observed significant intervention-related changes among parents' fruit and vegetable intake. Although the mechanism is not clear, if school-based nutrition interventions could produce changes in parent food choices and eating behaviors, they might considerably strengthen their effects on the targeted children. Parents serve as role models for healthful food choices, influence home food availability through purchases, and are responsible for home policies and practices that affect their children's food choices. In another approach, Foerster et al.[34] evaluated a school-based fruit and vegetable intervention with and without a community intervention component. The intervention provides a model for the types of study designs called for to intervene at multiple levels and through multiple channels in the community and is currently a rare example of such an approach that also includes a separate evaluation of the community component. Although the school-only and the school-plus-community intervention conditions did not differ in their effects on fruit and vegetable intake, both produced significantly greater increases in fruit and vegetable intake compared with the control schools. Finally, the only study to examine an intervention among high school students did not find significant changes in fruit and vegetable intake.[35] The pattern of change observed was a significant increase in the intervention schools during the first intervention year, followed by a "catch-up" among the control schools. The authors attribute the increase in fruit and vegetable intake in the control schools to a districtwide change in the school food service aimed at meeting the national guidelines for school meals. No documentation is provided to show that the observed changes are attributable to school district policy changes. However, if this were the case, the study results show the powerful effects that policy changes can produce on dietary outcomes such as students' fruit and vegetable consumption. These policy-related changes in behavior could far surpass the effects of school-based behavioral curricula and/or cafeteria-based interventions, and warrant further research using research designs and methods that enable a strong evaluation of the effects of such policy changes on food choices.

To summarize, the results of CATCH[23] and the Five A Day school-based interventions[17] show that multicomponent interventions can produce positive effects on food choices and dietary intake. A limitation of these studies is that the individual intervention components cannot be evaluated separately. Therefore, it is not known whether educational behavioral curricula targeting individual knowledge and behavior or changes in the school food environment are each independently effective in changing behavior, or whether both are necessary. Additional studies that are designed to directly evaluate the separate and combined effects of individual-level and environmental interventions are clearly needed and would provide useful information about the size of the effects on behavior associated with intervention strategies that target different levels of influence.

Environmental Interventions: Food and Physical Activity

The multicomponent interventions reviewed above clearly show promise for promoting desired eating and physical activity behaviors among youth in school settings. However, such interventions are expensive, time-consuming, and logistically challenging to implement. Emphasis on using available classroom time to learn academic content related to national testing requirements has created an added barrier to securing teacher and classroom time for implementing nutrition and physical activity curricula. Interest in school-based interventions that focus on environmental change to promote healthful eating and physical activity behaviors has increased in recent years in the hope of providing logistically feasible, low-cost interventions that will produce comparable impact on eating behavior change.

The school environment can be conceptualized as including any factor that influences students' eating and physical activity behaviors.[7] Environmental influences can include social, physical, and institutional variables (e.g., school policies). The multicomponent studies reviewed above have focused on certain school environmental variables, such as the school food service and school meals, and school physical education classes. Several recent reviews have described a wider set of school environmental opportunities for intervention strategies.[7,16,17] For example, physical activity environmental interventions have not yet evaluated changes in availability of school recess, intramural sports, sports equipment and facilities, physical activity breaks during regular school hours, active travel to school, after school activities, and summer day camps. Nutrition environmental interventions are only just beginning to evaluate changes in availability of competitive foods and beverages, including cafeteria a la carte, school stores, vending machines, school fundraising activities, classroom incentives, and rewards. Little research has been done on the effects of school, district, or state-level policy changes regarding the school food and physical activity environment, the role of school policies, or school faculty and administrative staff as role models in influencing student behavior and the school normative environment for healthful eating and physical activity behaviors.

ENVIRONMENTAL INTERVENTIONS: FOOD PRICING, AVAILABILITY, AND PROMOTION

Empirical data are available from a series of several well-designed school-based interventions that targeted only environmental factors to change students' food choices. These interventions have changed the pricing, availability, and promotion of targeted foods and evaluated their effects on food choices and dietary intake.

FOOD PRICING

Changes in food prices have been examined in several school-based studies for their effect on food purchases. CHIPS (Changing Individuals' Purchase of Snacks) is the methodologically strongest study to date to examine the effects of pricing strategies on food choices.[36] The aim of CHIPS was to increase the purchase of lower fat snacks from vending machines in 12 high schools and 12 work sites by lowering prices on the targeted snacks. In addition to price changes, the independent effect of point-of-purchase promotion was evaluated. Four pricing levels (low fat and high fat snacks at equal price, 10, 25, and 50% low fat snack price reduction) and three promotional signage levels (no sign, low fat label only, low fat label plus a promotional sign) were crossed in a Latin square design, with each of the 12 experimental conditions implemented in a random order in each school or work site for a 1-month period. Results showed that sales of the lower fat snacks significantly increased in direct proportion to the magnitude of the price reduction. Price reductions of 10, 25, and 50% were associated with 9, 39, and 93% increases in the proportion of lower fat snacks sold. Under equal prices, low fat snacks made up about 11% of all vending snacks sold. Under the 50% price reduction condition, lower fat snacks made up about 21% of all snacks sold. Promotional signage in combination with low fat labels had small but independent significant effects on sales of lower fat snacks.

In one of several pilot studies for CHIPS, prices on fresh fruit and vegetables were reduced by 50% for a 3-week period in two high school cafeterias.[37] Minimal promotional activity was implemented (small signs near the fruit and vegetable area). Results showed a fourfold increase in sales of fresh fruit and a twofold increase in sales of baby carrots during the price reduction period. Sales returned to baseline levels when prices were returned to usual. These results show the generalizability of the price reduction strategy to healthful foods such as fruits and vegetables.

One issue to consider in food pricing studies is the effects of price reductions on sales volume. In the CHIPS study,[36] aggregate sales data were tracked. Data on individual purchases were not collected. While a price reduction of 10% did not increase the total volume of lower fat snacks sold, price reductions of 25 and 50% did. This pattern of findings suggests that with smaller price reductions, customers may change their snack choice to a more healthful snack. With larger price reductions, however, it is possible that customers may purchase additional snack items at the reduced price. This may result in increasing their total energy intake, an unintended and undesirable effect, given that limiting total energy intake is a concern. Depending on the food type (e.g., fresh fruit or vegetables vs. vending machine snack foods), the amount of the price reduction needs to be considered in terms of its potential effect on food choice and amount or number of foods purchased. Another strategy that warrants evaluation is concurrent increases in the prices of less healthful foods and decreases in prices of healthful foods. Small price increases on less healthful foods might increase revenues enough to subsidize price reductions on more healthful foods. Larger price increases on less healthful foods could curb demand for less healthful foods and perhaps increase sales of lower priced, more healthful foods. Effects of price increases and decreases implemented in tandem on food purchases and revenues need to be examined.[38] In addition, research is needed to examine whether these pricing strategies are effective only in settings that have a constrained array of food choices, such as a school or work site cafeteria, or whether pricing strategies also are effective in less constrained food purchase settings, such as grocery stores.

FOOD AVAILABILITY

A second environmental intervention that has been evaluated with positive results is increasing the availability of healthful food choices in the school cafeteria.[39–42] Four studies (three in elementary schools and one in high schools) found increases in student choice of targeted foods when availability of the targeted foods was increased. In TACOS (Trying Alternative Cafeteria Options in Schools),[39] 20 high schools were randomized to an intervention or control group for a 2-year period. In intervention schools, the availability of lower fat foods in school cafeteria a la carte areas was increased, and school-wide promotional activities were implemented by student groups to promote the lower fat a la carte foods. Sales of lower fat a la carte foods were measured continuously using the computerized point of sales data collected from the school food service. After 2 years, the availability of lower fat foods in a la carte areas increased 51% in intervention school cafeterias, and decreased 5% in control school cafeterias. Sales of lower fat foods significantly increased by 10% over 2 years in intervention schools, compared with a decrease of 2.8% in control schools ($p < 0.002$).

Whitaker et al[40] increased the availability of lower fat entreés in the school lunch meal in 16 elementary schools during 14 consecutive school months. During a baseline period of 6 months, a lower fat entrée was available on 23% of school lunch days. During the subsequent 8 months, the lower fat entrée was available on 71% of the school lunch days. No educational signage or promotional activities were implemented. Results showed that during the baseline period, 39% of the students selected the lower fat entrée. During the increased availability period, 29% of the students selected the lower fat entrée. However, the fat content of the average student meal decreased from 36 to 30% calories from fat. In a follow-up study,[41] a promotional newsletter targeting students' parents was evaluated for its incremental effect on student entrée choice. Sixteen elementary schools were randomized to an "availability only" or to an "availability plus parent newsletter" condition. Low fat entreés were available as one of two entrée choices daily in all schools. After a 5-month baseline period, intervention schools received a promotional program. School lunch menus that children carried home highlighted the lower fat entreés, and parents received a mailed copy of the school menu, plus nutrition information and a letter requesting them to encourage their child to select the lower fat entrée at school. Results showed a significant increase in the proportion of students who selected the lower fat entrée in schools assigned to the availability plus promotion condition (35.5%) compared with the availability only condition (32.2%)

Perry et al.[42] randomized 26 elementary schools to a no-treatment control group or to an intervention in which the availability of fruits and vegetables in the school lunch meal was increased and food service staff verbally encouraged students to choose and consume fruits and vegetables from the lunch line. Taste tests and contests were held in the lunchroom periodically during the 2-year intervention. Based on observations of lunchtime food intake, the intervention significantly increased students' intake of fruit and vegetable servings (not including potatoes).

The results of these school-based randomized trials provide strong evidence that increasing the availability of healthful foods, such as lower fat entreés, fruit and vegetables, and lower fat a la carte foods, is effective in increasing students' choices of the targeted foods. All four studies were methodologically strong in design, implementation, and evaluation, and were consistent in the pattern of results obtained across studies. The results were consistent across a variety of food types, in both the school meal and the a la carte food settings, and among both elementary school and high school age groups. In most of the studies, a promotional component was implemented in tandem with the availability component.[39,41,42] However, similar results were observed when no promotion was present.[40] A further intriguing finding observed in several cross-sectional school-based studies suggests that the availability of high fat foods is associated with lower intake of more healthful foods.[43,44] These findings suggest that the effects of simultaneous increases in the availability of healthful foods and decreases in the availability of less healthful foods warrant further evaluation in school-based studies that intervene by changing food availability.

FOOD PROMOTION

Most of the school-based nutrition interventions reviewed above, both the environmental interventions alone and the multicomponent interventions that included a school cafeteria component, included a food promotion component. Promotional activities most often consist of promotional or informational signage at the point-of-purchase or elsewhere in the cafeteria, posters, table tents, taste tests, contests, coupons, or fliers. Promotional activities have been implemented in tandem with the food pricing and the availability strategies described previously, and the effects of each strategy are impossible to evaluate separately. However, the studies that were designed to evaluate the independent effects of promotional activities and pricing[36] or promotional activities and availability[40] did find small but independent and significant effects for promotion on student food choices. Promotional activities typically are easy and inexpensive to implement, consistently show positive effects on food choices, and therefore should be implemented broadly to support healthful food choices in school settings.

The results of the environmental interventions described above provide consistent empirical support for the effectiveness of food pricing, availability, and promotion strategies to promote healthful food choices in school settings. Additional research is needed to further develop these promising intervention strategies. Simultaneous increases and decreases in food prices or food availability, and identification of the most effective promotional strategies warrant further careful evaluation.

ENVIRONMENTAL INTERVENTIONS FOR PHYSICAL ACTIVITY

Fewer school-based studies are available that have evaluated the effects on physical activity levels of environmental interventions to increase physical activity opportunities. The results of two well-designed and evaluated school-based physical activity interventions are described below.

MSPAN: MIDDLE SCHOOL PHYSICAL ACTIVITY AND NUTRITION STUDY

Sallis et al.[45] conducted an environmental intervention that targeted both the school physical activity and food environment. MSPAN randomized 24 middle schools to a 2-year physical activity and nutrition intervention in which school environment and policy changes were targeted. No classroom component was included in the intervention. Physical activity interventions included targeting the amount of PE class time spent in moderate-to-vigorous physical activity and increasing the time spent in physical activity during leisure periods, such as recess, and organized school-based physical activities. These changes were implemented by increasing the amount of school-based supervision available to students for physical activity, increasing the number of organized physical activities available at school, and increasing access to sports equipment at school. Schools received financial incentives to purchase sports and physical activity equipment. The nutrition intervention targeted increases in the availability and marketing of lower fat foods from all food sources in school (e.g., school meals, a la carte, school stores, bag lunch from home). School policy changes were targeted through the formation of school health policy councils, student health committees, and parent education.

Evaluation measures consisted of student self-reported energy expenditure from moderate-to-vigorous physical activity; body weight and height, based on mailed student surveys; and observed physical activity during PE classes and during leisure time at school, measured by trained research staff observers. Results showed significant intervention increases in physical activity only among boys. Increases in physical activity among boys were observed both in PE classes and in non-PE school settings, before and after school and during lunch period. A significant decrease in self-reported BMI was observed among boys in intervention schools compared with boys in control schools. No significant intervention effects were observed among girls for change in physical activity or BMI. No significant effects were observed for dietary fat or eating behaviors. Although the results appear somewhat promising for increasing physical activity levels among boys, the lack of process data makes the results difficult to interpret. It is not clear why the physical activity intervention was effective among boys but not among girls. The lack of significant intervention effects for food choices may be due to the greater complexity of intervening with food availability in multiple food venues. Contamination may also have worked differentially against finding a significant intervention effect for food choices versus physical activity. Schools within districts were randomized. School food service is typically organized at the central district level, so any changes in food availability or in foods ordered centrally would presumably affect all schools in the district, including those assigned to the control group. At any rate, in the absence of process data, no firm interpretations of the results are possible.

SPARK: Sports, Play, and Active Recreation for Kids in Elementary Schools

The SPARK study examined the effects of training elementary school physical education teachers to implement a PE curricula and classroom management program to increase the amount of PE class time that children spent in moderate to vigorous activity and to increase cardiorespiratory fitness among children.[46] Seven elementary schools were randomly assigned to one of two experimental conditions or to a no-treatment control group. In one experimental group, trained PE specialists implemented the SPARK PE curricula and classroom management program. In the second experimental group, trained classroom teachers implemented the SPARK PE curricula and classroom management program. In the control group, the usual PE programs were continued.

The SPARK lessons lasted 30 min and included health-fitness activities and skill-fitness activities. Health-fitness activities included aerobic dance, aerobic games, walking or jogging, and jump rope. Skill-fitness activities included basketball and soccer. Students were also taught behavior change skills, such as goal setting, self-monitoring, self-reinforcement, and problem solving. Measures of physical activity included accelerometer data and self-reported physical activity. Classroom PE physical activity levels were measured using in-person observation by trained research staff following a standardized measurement protocol. Fitness measures were collected using standardized protocols and included a 1-mile run, and timed sit-ups, pull-ups, and sit-and-reach tests. Results showed that compared with students in the control group, students in the two intervention groups spent significantly more time in PE classes, and spent significantly more time in moderate to vigorous physical activity during PE class time. There were no significant intervention-related changes in physical activity levels outside of school. Among boys, there were no significant intervention effects for any fitness measure. Among girls, significant differences in favor of the PE specialist-led group compared with the control group were observed for the mile run time and for the sit-ups measure. No significant differences were found among girls for the pull-up and sit-and-reach measure. No significant intervention effects were found for change in skinfolds among boys or girls. Results of the SPARK study showed that classroom teachers can be trained to implement PE classes that result in greater time spent in physical activity among students.

Summary

The results of both MSPAN and SPARK are consistent in demonstrating that school PE classes can be structured to increase the amount of classroom time students spend engaged in physical activity. In addition, increases in physical activity outside of PE class during the school day were observed among boys in the MSPAN study. In MSPAN, a significant decrease in BMI (based on student self-reported height and weight) was observed among boys in the intervention schools compared with the control schools. However, mediating analyses that examine changes in physical activity in relation to changes in BMI were not reported. Overall, these results suggest that changes in PE class structure through teacher training programs is a worthwhile means to increase children's physical activity during PE class. Additional physical activity opportunities during the school day may further increase physical activity levels among students. These increases in physical activity potentially may be effective in promoting energy balance and preventing excess weight gain among students.

EMERGING POLICY INITIATIVES FOR SCHOOL-BASED OBESITY PREVENTION

In recognition of the importance of the school food environment and physical activity opportunities for the prevention of excess weight gain among children and adolescents, policy initiatives are emerging in several areas of school-based nutrition, physical activity, and obesity prevention.[47–50] Policy initiatives at the district and state level and, most recently, at the federal level have led to the adoption of new guidelines for school food availability and physical activity requirements.[48,49] At the national level, legislators are developing initiatives to address issues related to the school food environment and physical activity opportunities. Issues are being explored such as the funding of school meals, revenues generated from the sales of competitive foods, and revenues generated from corporate contracts for in-school sales of soft drinks from vending machines and other in-school marketing and advertising activities. In addition, some districts and states have incorporated BMI surveillance and monitoring into their health reporting and feedback to parents.[51–53] The issue of in-school food and beverage advertising has gained national attention and active calls for the implementation of guidelines to limit in-school food and beverage marketing.[54]

FEDERAL POLICY INITIATIVES

The most recent U.S. federal level policy initiatives for childhood obesity prevention efforts have emerged from the reauthorization of the Child Nutrition Bill (S2507, July 2004) and new initiatives in 2003 to 2004 from the Senate Committee on Agriculture, Nutrition, and Forestry, led by Senators Tom Harkin and Patrick Leahy. The Child Nutrition Bill addresses legislation concerning the school meals program and nutrition education. Notable new features of the bill include reauthorization of the fruit and vegetable snacks program and addressing "junk" food in schools. The fruit and vegetable snack program was initially pilot tested by the USDA in 2002 to 2003 in 100 schools in four states and on one American Indian reservation.[55] The program provided fruit and vegetables to schools to provide as free snacks to students on a daily basis throughout the school year. The new child nutrition bill specifies $9 million in mandatory funding to expand the fruit and vegetable school snack program to add four additional states and two additional American Indian reservations to the program. A second feature of the bill is a new focus on addressing junk food in schools. The bill calls for each local education agency that participates in the school meals program to develop a local school wellness policy by 2006. The policy must include goals for nutrition education and physical activity, and include nutrition guidelines for all foods and beverages sold in school. It also authorizes $4 million for USDA to work with local education agencies to establish healthy school nutrition environments, promote efforts to reduce childhood obesity, and prevent diet-related chronic diseases.

Additional efforts in the United States at the federal level to address the issue of childhood obesity include those of the Senate Committee on Agriculture, Nutrition, and Forestry. Two General Accounting Office (GAO) reports have been commissioned by the Senate Agriculture Committee as background research on the school meals program and on the school food environment. In April 2004, the GAO issued their report to congressional requesters on "School Meal Programs: Competitive Foods Are Available in Many Schools; Actions Taken to Restrict Them Differ by State and Locality."[49] The findings from this report are described in detail in the section entitled "State and District Policy Initiatives." A second GAO report was commissioned (July 2004) to be published in the fall of 2005. The report describes revenue sources and amounts generated from school sales of competitive foods and beverages.

The Democratic staff of the U.S. Senate Committee on Agriculture, Nutrition, and Forestry generated a white paper in May 2004 entitled "Food Choices at School: Risks to Child Nutrition and Health. Call for Action."[56] This paper describes the foods available in schools and focuses on competitive foods and their potential impact on children's choice of school meals and on dietary quality.

Overall, these federal level efforts have been energized by both the increasing number of local and state actions in the area of school-based nutrition and physical activity policy, more frequent and intense advocacy from other federal nutrition related agencies such as the USDA and the Centers for Disease Control and Prevention, and the increasing media attention on the problem of childhood obesity and the school environment as a potential setting in which to reach children to promote healthful eating and physical activity behaviors and energy balance.

STATE POLICY INITIATIVES

Recently a flurry of legislative activity has occurred at the state level to address school policies regarding nutrition, physical activity, and obesity prevention. In 2003 through April 2004, 71 bills were introduced in 33 states for school-based nutrition and BMI policy; 64 bills in 27 states were introduced for school-based physical education policies.[49]

California has led the country in the number and scope of school-based nutrition and physical activity legislation introduced and passed in recent years. In 2002, a bill was passed that requires all foods and beverages sold in schools to meet specific nutrition criteria. The bill was never implemented because its implementation was contingent on increases in funding for the school meals program that did not occur. However, its passage established the political groundwork and grassroots support needed for further policy work in the area of school-based nutrition and obesity prevention. In April 2004, the California Senate passed another bill (SB1566) that established nutrition standards for all school foods and beverages without requiring the authorization of new funding. SB 1566 is now being considered by the State Assembly.[48]

Arkansas, another state on the forefront of obesity-prevention legislative initiatives, recently passed comprehensive, cutting-edge legislation (ARK ACT 1220) to address childhood obesity-prevention efforts in schools.[51] In April 2003, ARK ACT 1220 was passed and required the formation of a Child Health Advisory Committee to develop statewide nutrition and physical activity standards. The bill requires schools to report all sources and amounts of revenues from competitive food sales and soft drink contracts, prohibits access to vending machines in elementary schools, and requires student BMI to be measured and reported to parents, along with information about healthy BMI levels. In 2004 to 2005, the Department of Education will implement the nutrition and physical activity standards and annually monitor and evaluate their effectiveness. The Arkansas Center for Health Improvement is developing and implementing standardized statewide BMI assessments and reporting.

SCHOOL DISTRICT POLICY INITIATIVES

In addition to the state-level initiatives, several district-level policies have been passed recently to address school food availability. The Los Angeles Unified School District, the second largest district in the United States, recently passed legislation to prohibit the sale of soft drinks from vending machines in all schools starting in January 2004. In addition, the sale of fried chips, candy, and other snack foods from vending machines is prohibited starting June 1, 2004.[48,49]

The New York City Public School District is the largest district in the United States, and it eliminated the sale of candy, soft drinks and other snack foods from school vending machines in the fall of 2003. School vending machines are limited to selling only water, 100% fruit juice, and low fat snacks.[49]

The Philadelphia School District recently passed a comprehensive school nutrition policy that includes components to address the following areas: (1) nutrition education in schools, (2) school food service guidelines for all foods and beverages sold in school, (3) staff training, (4) family and community involvement, and (5) program evaluation. The Food Trust (www.thefoodtrust.org)

convenes the Philadelphia Nutrition Education Network and the School Nutrition Policy Task Force to guide the development, implementation, and evaluation of the school nutrition policy for the Philadelphia School District.

SCHOOL LINKS WITH COMMUNITY RESOURCES

In addition to policy initiatives, new efforts are underway at the district and school level to link with the community to enhance the schools' ability to provide healthful foods and greater physical activity opportunities for students.[47] Efforts to enhance the availability of fresh fruits and vegetables have resulted in school linkages with local farmers' markets and with efforts to develop school gardening programs.[57,58] Neighborhood programs to provide walking buses to school and to develop safe bike and walk paths to school are being initiated to encourage and support active commuting to schools. A walking bus is an adult-led walking program to collect children throughout the neighborhood to walk as a group to school.

In addition to the USDA-funded fruit and vegetable snack program described above,[55] local schools in several states have been able to increase the availability of fresh produce for their school meals program through the Department of Defense FRESH Program (www.feedsecurity.org/california/cfjc_dod_faq.pdf), the use of school-based gardens, and local farmers' markets. For example, the Edible Schoolyard is a nonprofit program being implemented at the Martin Luther King Junior Middle School in Berkeley, CA. Students participate in all phases of the cultivation of produce, including planting seeds, raising and tending plants, preparing meals with the food grown, and recycling waste back into the garden. Classroom lessons incorporate hands-on activities in the garden and kitchen.[59]

Schools can also be connected with communities to increase physical activity opportunities for youth by making their facilities available after school and during weekend hours. Organized after-school programs could specifically target physical activity and nutrition behaviors or incorporate them as components of existing programs whose primary focus involves other activities.[47] For example, the Girls Health Enrichment Multi-Site Studies (GEMS) aimed to prevent obesity among 8- to 10-year-old African American girls.[60-64] In a set of four pilot interventions, girls and their parents were recruited through school settings and other community channels to participate in after-school programs that targeted healthful eating and physical activity for obesity prevention. Intervention formats included summer camp programs, after-school programs, and family-based programs. Behaviors targeted included reducing television viewing, increasing physical activity, and increasing fruit and vegetable intake. The results of the GEMS pilot interventions were promising, and two of the GEMS full-scale trials are currently underway. The GEMS interventions demonstrate the feasibility and potential effectiveness of linking obesity prevention intervention efforts across school-, family-, and community-based settings.

The proliferation of new policy initiatives at the state and district level and of new school-based local programs offer an important opportunity to evaluate the effects of school-based policy, and environmental and programmatic changes, on children's eating and exercise behaviors and body weight. It is important that funding and support are provided to capitalize on the opportunities provided by these new initiatives to collect evaluation data. Such data can be used to guide new directions in school-based policy and program development to effectively address the childhood obesity epidemic and further school-based obesity prevention efforts. The Center for Disease Control and Prevention's School Health Index provides an assessment instrument to measure and evaluate school nutrition and physical activity environments and practices.[65] In addition, schools, districts, and states may monitor individual student behaviors related to nutrition, physical activity, and body weight.[51-53]

It is hoped that these legislative and policy initiatives at the national, state, and district levels will further highlight the important role that the school environment can play in promoting the development and support of healthful food and physical activity behaviors that will promote energy balance and maintain a healthful body weight. Funding is needed for further school-based research to evaluate the effects of policy and school-based environment changes on the prevention of obesity and the promotion of healthful eating and physical activity behaviors among children and adolescents.

RESEARCH RECOMMENDATIONS

Broadly speaking, research related to youth obesity prevention must address the question of defining the most appropriate outcome to target with interventions. Is it reasonable to evaluate the success of school-based interventions primarily on changes in body mass, or are changes in behaviors related to energy balance the most appropriate evaluation outcome? Which specific behavior or combination of behaviors are the most effective to target for intervention, and what magnitude of change is needed to prevent excess weight gain among children and adolescents?

Specific recommendations for research include the following:

1. Evaluate intervention components at different levels to determine the relative effectiveness of educational, environmental, and policy changes on students' BMI, eating and physical activity behaviors, and the school food and physical activity environment.
2. Evaluate specific behavioral targets to determine the relative effectiveness of changes in specific behaviors on changes in body mass (e.g., television viewing, changes in PE class frequency and/or structure, decreases in soft drink consumption).
3. Evaluate methods to increase parental involvement, parental behavior changes, and home environmental changes through school-based obesity prevention interventions.
4. Evaluate interventions that link school-based obesity prevention efforts with other community settings such as primary care, youth groups, community centers, sports leagues, and after school programs.
5. Evaluate policy interventions at the state, district, and school level for policies related to the school food environment and physical activity requirements and opportunities.

REFERENCES

1. U.S. Department of Education, National Center for Education Statistics, 1990. Retrieved from http://nces.ed.gov/pubsearch/pubsinfo.asp?pubid=91076.
2. Dwyer J. The School Nutrition Dietary Assessment Study. *Am J Clin Nutr.* 1995;61(Suppl): 173S–177S.
3. Wechsler H, Brener ND, Kuester S, Miller C. Food services and foods and beverages available at school: Results from the School Health Policies and Programs Study, 2000. *J School Health.* 2001;71: 313–324.
4. French SA, Story M, Fulkerson JA, Gerlach AF. Food environment in secondary schools: a la carte, vending machines, food policies and practices. *Am J Public Health.* 2003;93: 1161–1167.
5. Harnack L, Snyder P, Story M, Holliday R, Lytle L, Neumark-Sztainer D. Availability of a la carte food items in junior and senior high schools: a needs assessment. *J Am Diet Assoc.* 2000;100: 701–703.
6. Story M, Hayes M, Kalina B. Availability of foods in high schools: is there a cause for concern? *J Am Diet Assoc.* 1996;96: 123–126.
7. Wechsler H, Devereaux RS, Davis M, Collins J. Using the school environment to promote physical activity and healthy eating. *Prev Med.* 2000;31: S121–S137.
8. Allensworth DD, Kolbe LJ. The comprehensive school health program: exploring an expanded concept. *J School Health.* 1987;57: 409–412.
9. Stokols D. Establishing and maintaining health environments: toward a social ecology of health promotion. *Am Psychol* 1992;47: 6–22.

10. Glanz K, Rimer BF, Lewis FM. *Health Behavior and Health Education*, 3rd ed. San Francisco: Jossey-Bass, 2002.

11. Bandura A. *Social Foundations of Thought and Action*. Englewood Cliffs, NJ: Prentice-Hall; 1986

12. Lobstein T, Baur L, Uauy R. Obesity in children and young people: a crisis in public health. *Obes Rev.* 2004;5(Suppl 1): 4–85.

13. Schmitz MKH, Jeffery RW. Public health interventions for the prevention and treatment of obesity. *Med Clin N Am.* 2000;84(2): 491–512.

14. Resnicow K. School-based obesity prevention: population versus high-risk interventions. *Ann NY Acad Sci.* 1993;699: 154–166.

15. Resnicow K, Robinson TN. School-based cardiovascular disease prevention studies: review and synthesis. *Ann Epidemiol.* 1997;S7: S14–S31.

16. Jago R, Baranowski T. Non-curricular approaches for increasing physical activity in youth: a review. *Prev Med.* 2004;39: 157–163.

17. French SA, Stables G. Environmental interventions to promote vegetable and fruit consumption among youth in school settings. *Prev Med.* 2003;37: 593–610.

18. Lytle L, Achterberg C. Nutrition education for children: what works and why. *J Nutr Educ.* 1995;27: 250–260.

19. Campbell K, Waters E, O'Meara S, Kelly S, Summerbell C. Interventions for preventing obesity in childhood: a systematic review. *Obes Rev.* 2001;2: 149–157.

20. Fulton JE, McGuire MT, Caspersen CJ, Dietz WH. Interventions for weight loss and weight gain prevention among youth: current issues. *Sports Med.* 2001;31: 153–165.

21. Stone EJ, McKenzie TL, Welk GJ, Booth ML. Effects of physical activity interventions in youth: review and synthesis. *Am J Prev Med.* 1998;15: 298–315.

22. Caballero B, Clay T, Davis SM, Ethelbah B, Holy Rock B, Lohman T, et al. Pathways: a school-based, randomized controlled trial for the prevention of obesity in American Indian schoolchildren. *Am J Clin Nutr.* 2003;78: 1030–1038.

23. Luepker RV, Perry CL, McKinlay SM, Nader PR, Parcel GS, Stone EJ, et al. Outcomes of a field trial to improve children's dietary patterns and physical activity: the Child and Adolescent Trial for Cardiovascular Health (CATCH). *JAMA.* 1996;275: 768–776.

24. Fitzgibbon ML, Stolley MR, Schiffer L, Van Horn L, Kaufer Christoffel K, Dyer A. Two-year follow-up results for Hip-Hop to Health, Jr.: a randomized controlled trial for overweight prevention in preschool minority children. *J Pediatr.* 2005;146(5): 618–625.

25. Gortmaker SL, Peterson K, Wiecha J, Sobol AM, Dixit S, Fox MK, Laird N. Reducing obesity via a school-based interdisciplinary intervention among youth: Planet Health. *Arch Pediatr Adolesc Med.* 1999;153: 409–418.

26. Robinson TN. Reducing children's television viewing to prevent obesity: a randomized controlled trial. *JAMA.* 1999;282: 1561–1567.

27. Osganian SK, Ebzery MK, Montgomery DH, Nicklas TA, Evans MA, Mitchell PD, et al. Changes in the nutrient content of school lunches: results from the CATCH Eat Smart food service intervention. *Prev Med.* 1996;25: 400–412.

28. McKenzie TL, Nader, PR, Strikmiller PK, Yang M, Stone EJ, Perry CL, et al. School physical education: effect on the Child and Adolescent Trial for Cardiovascular Health. *Prev Med.* 1996: 25: 423–431.

29. Heimendinger J, Van Duyn M, Chapelsky D, Foerster S, Stables G. The National 5 a Day for Better Health Program: a large-scale nutrition intervention. *J Public Health Management Practice.* 1996;2: 27–35.

30. Stables G, Subar AF, Patterson BH, Dodd K, Heimendinger J, Van Duyn MA, et al. Changes in vegetable and fruit consumption and awareness among US adults: results of the 1991 and 1997 5 A Day for Better Health Program surveys. *J Am Diet Assoc.* 2002;102: 809–817.

31. Reynolds KD, Franklin FA, Binkley D, Raczynski JM, Harrington KF, Kirk KA, et al. Increasing the fruit and vegetable consumption of fourth graders: results from the High 5 Project. *Prev Med.* 2000;30: 309–319.

32. Perry CL, Bishop DB, Taylor G, Murray DM, Mays RW, Dudovitz BS, et al. Changing fruit and vegetable consumption among children: the 5–a-Day Power Plus Program in St. Paul, Minnesota. *Am J Public Health.* 1998;88: 603–609.

33. Baranowski T, Davis M, Resnicow K, Baranowski J, Doyle C, Lin LS, et al. Gimme 5 fruit, juice and vegetables for fun and health: Outcome evaluation. *Health Educ Behav.* 2000;27: 96–111.

34. Foerster SB, Gregson J, Beall DL, Hudes M, Magnuson H, Livingston S, et al. The California children's 5 A Day Power Play! campaign: evaluation of a large-scale social marketing initiative. *Family Commun Health.* 1998;21: 46–64.

35. Nicklas TA, Johnson CC, Myers L, Farris RP, Cunningham A. Outcomes of a high school program to increase fruit and vegetable consumption: gimme 5 — a fresh nutrition concept for students. *J School Health.* 1998;68: 248–253.

36. French SA, Jeffery RW, Story M, Breitlow KK, Baxter JS, Hannan P, Snyder MP. Pricing and promotion effects on low-fat vending snack purchases: the CHIPS Study. *Am J Public Health.* 2001;91: 112–117.

37. French SA, Story M, Jeffery RW, Snyder P, Eisenberg M, Sidebottom A, Murray D. Pricing strategy to promote fruit and vegetable purchase in high school cafeterias. *J Am Diet Assoc.* 1997;97: 1008–1010.

38. Hannan P, French SA, Story, M, Fulkerson JA. A pricing strategy to promote sales of lower fat foods in high school cafeterias: acceptability and sensitivity analysis. *Am J Health Promo.* 2002;17: 1–6.

39. French SA, Story M, Fulkerson JA, Hannan P. Environmental intervention to increase sales of lower fat foods in high school cafeterias: the TACOS study. *Am J Public Health.* 2004;94: 1507–1512.

40. Whitaker RC, Wright JA, Finch AJ, Psaty BM. An environmental intervention to reduce dietary fat in school lunches. *Pediatrics.* 1993;91: 1107–1111.

41. Whitaker RC, Wright JA, Koepsell TD, Finch AJ, Psaty BM. Randomized intervention to increase children's selection of low fat foods in school lunches. *J Pediatr.* 1994;125: 535–540.

42. Perry CL, Bishop, DB, Taylor GL, Davis M, Story M, Gray C, Bishop SC, Warren Mays RA, Lytle LA, Harnack L. A randomized school trial of environmental strategies to encourage fruit and vegetable consumption among children. *Health Educ Behav.* 2004;31(1): 65–76.

43. Kubik MY, Lytle LA, Hannan PJ, Perry CL, Story M. The association of the school food environment with dietary behaviors of young adolescents. *Am J Public Health.* 2003;93: 1168–1173.

44. Cullen KW, Eagan J, Baranowski T, Owens E, deMoor C. Effect of a la carte and snack bar foods at school on children's lunchtime intake of fruits and vegetables. *J Am Diet Assoc.* 2000;100: 1482–1486.

45. Sallis JF, McKenzie TL, Conway TL, Elder JP, Prochaska JJ, Brown M, Zive MM, Marshall SJ, Alcaraz JE. Environmental interventions for eating and physical activity: a randomized controlled trial in middle schools. *Am J Prev Med.* 2003: 24: 209–217.

46. Sallis JF, McKenzie TL, Alcaraz JE, Kolody B, Faucette N, Hovell MF. The effects of a 2-year physical education program (SPARK) on physical activity and fitness in elementary school students: Sports, Play and Active Recreation for Kids. *Am J Public Health.* 1997;87: 1328–1334.

47. Healthy Schools for Healthy Kids. Princeton, NJ: Robert Woods Johnson Foundation. *Healthy Schools for Healthy Kids.* 2004. Retrieved from www.rwjf.org/publications/publications/pdfs/healthy-Schools.pdf.

48. National Conference of State Legislatures. Nutrition, Obesity and Physical Education. Health Policy Tracking Service. NETSCAN iPublishing Inc. March, 2004. Contact: Lee Dixon, Director of NCSL HPTS at lee.Dixon@netscan.org.

49. US General Accounting Office. *School Meal Programs: Competitive Foods Are Available in Many Schools; Actions Taken to Restrict Them Differ by State and Locality.* Washington, DC: General Accounting Office. GAO-04-673. 2004.

50. Institute of Medicine of the National Academies. Committee on Prevention of Obesity in Children and Youth. *Preventing Childhood Obesity: Health in the Balance.* Koplan JP, Liverman CT, Krak VI Eds. Washington, DC: The National Academies Press, 2004.

51. General Assembly of the State of Arkansas. Act 1220 of 2003. An act to create a child health advisory committee. State of Arkansas, 84th General Assembly. Regular session, 2003. House Bill 1583.

52. Chomitz VR, Collins J, Kim J, Kramer E, McGowan R. Promoting healthy weight among elementary school children via a health report card approach. *Arch Pediatr Adolesc Med.* 2003;157: 765–772.

53. Scheier LM. School health report cards attempt to address the obesity epidemic. *J Am Diet Assoc.* 2004;104: 341–344.

54. Story M, French S. Food advertising and marketing directed at children and adolescents in the US. *Int J Behavior Nutr Phys Activity.* 1;2004. Retrieved July 12, 2005 from http://www.ijbnpa.org/content/1/1/3.

55. Buzby JC, Guthrie JF, Kantor LS. *Evaluation of the USDA Fruit and Vegetable Pilot program: report to Congress.* USDA Food Assistance and Nutrition Research Program. Washington DC: USDA Economic Research Service. May 2003.

56. Democratic Staff of the Senate Committee on Agriculture, Nutrition and Forestry. Food choices at school: risks to child nutrition and health. Call for action. May 18, 2004. Retrieved July 12, 2005 from http://www.harkin.senate.gov/wellness/Food_Choices_at_School.pdf.

57. Stone MK. A food revolution in Berkeley: the edible schoolyard: Berkeley's Martin Luther King Jr. Middle School planted a garden. www.edibleshoolyard.org.

58. Mascarenhas M, Gottlieb R. The farmer's market salad bar: assessing the first three years of the Santa Monica–Malibu Unified School District program. Report prepared by Occidental College Community Food Security Project for the Santa Monica–Malibu Unified School District Food and Nutrition Services. 1600 Campus Road. Los Angeles, CA. 90041.

59. Edible Schoolyard. 2004. *The Edible Schoolyard.* Available at http://www.edibleschoolyard.org. Accessed June 4, 2004.

60. Kumanyika SK, Story M, Beech BM, Sherwood NE, Baranowski JC, Powell TM, et al. Collaborative planning for formative assessment and cultural appropriateness in the Girls Health Enrichment Multi-Site Studies (GEMS): a retrospection. *Ethn Dis.* 2003;13: S1–S15.

61. Baranowski T, Baranowski JC, Cullen KW, Thompson DI, Nicklas T, Zakeri IF, et al. The Fun, Food and Fitness Project (FFFP): The Baylor GEMS pilot study. *Ethn Dis.* 2003;13: S1-30–S1-39.

62. Beech BM, Klesges RC, Kumanyika SK, Murray DM, Klesges L, McClanahan B, et al. Child- and parent-targeted interventions: the Memphis GEMS pilot study. *Ethn Dis.* 2003;13: S1-40–S1-53.

63. Story M, Sherwood NE, Himes JH, Davis M, Jacobs DR, Cartwright Y, et al. An after-school obesity prevention program for African American girls: the Minnesota GEMS pilot study. *Ethn Dis.* 2003;13: S1-54–S1-64.

64. Robinson TN, Killen JD, Kraemer HC, Wilson DM, Matheson DM, Haskell WL, et al. Dance and reducing television viewing to prevent weight gain in African American girls: the Stanford GEMS pilot study. *Ethn Dis.* 2003;13: S1-65–S1-77.

65. CDC. 2004. School Health Index. Available at http://www.cdc.gov/HealthyYouth/shi/index.htm. Accessed May 18, 2004.

18 Dietary Approaches for Obesity Treatment and Prevention in Children and Adolescents

Cara B. Ebbeling and David S. Ludwig

CONTENTS

INTRODUCTION

From a theoretical perspective, successful dietary prevention or treatment of obesity should be relatively simple: maintain energy intake equal to or less than energy expenditure. From a practical perspective, this prescription has become increasingly difficult for most adults, and many children, to follow. Though controversy exists as to how genetic and environmental factors interact to promote excessive weight gain, it is generally agreed that adverse changes in diet quality have played an important role in the epidemic of obesity among children. In this chapter, we first examine how children's diets have changed over the past few decades and then review studies that have examined conventional and popular diet approaches. Finally, we explore the possibility that a diet focused on reducing the postprandial rise in blood glucose may be more effective than either low-fat or low-carbohydrate diets.

Before beginning, one conceptual point merits consideration. Traditionally, management of epidemic disease has employed two very disparate strategies, prevention and treatment; the former is considered substantially less costly and more effective from a public health perspective. However, this paradigm, developed to combat infectious disease among high-risk populations,[1] does not apply well to obesity, a noncommunicable disease for which virtually the entire American population is at risk. In this case, the distinction between prevention and treatment becomes arbitrary because risks for cardiovascular disease and type 2 diabetes, among other obesity comorbidities, increase across a continuum ranging from normal weight to overweight and obesity. Thus, the aim of this chapter is to determine what dietary approaches best promote achievement and maintenance of a healthy body weight for all children, regardless of baseline body weight. For severe obesity requiring intensive intervention, the reader is directed elsewhere.[2]

SECULAR TRENDS IN CHILDREN'S DIETS

From 1971 to 2000, total daily energy consumption among adults increased by 335 kcal in women and 168 kcal in men,[3] an amount sufficient to explain all of the weight gain in the general population during this time. Among children, daily energy intake appears to have increased in some subpopulations, especially adolescents, and remained stable in others,[4,5] though methodology used to obtain these estimates can be problematic. Nevertheless, diet quality among children and adolescents has undergone radical changes in ways that would likely increase risk for obesity, as summarized below with regard to beverage consumption, fast food intake, portion sizes, and meal patterns. These changes could promote a positive energy balance by stimulating eating in the absence of hunger (e.g., ubiquity of high calorie snack foods), by effects on satiation (i.e., leading to overconsumption at a meal), or by effects on satiety (i.e., causing hunger to return relatively quickly).

BEVERAGE CONSUMPTION

In the 1970s, children drank approximately 1 cup of soft drink for every 2 cups of milk; today, that ratio is reversed.[6-8] Over the past 20 years, soft drink consumption by children ages 6 to 17 years has increased from a mean of 5 oz/day to 12.[7] Currently, soft drinks constitute the leading source of added sugars in the diets of adolescents,[9,10] amounting to 36.2 g/day for females and 57.7 g/day for males, figures that approach or exceed the limits for total added sugar consumption recommended by the U.S. Department of Agriculture (USDA).[11] Assuming an average sugar content of 11%,[12] these beverages contributed 100 kcal/day more to the diet of adolescent males in 1994 than in 1989, accounting for about 37% of the observed increase in total energy intake in this population according to one report.[5]

Soft drinks may cause weight gain, in part, because of the apparently poor satiating properties of sugar in liquid form. Calories from soft drinks appear to increase total energy intake, rather than displace energy from other sources.[13,14] In addition, children in particular may consume soft drinks for reasons other than to satisfy hunger, including thirst, hedonic reward, or social desirability. Among school-age children, those consuming an average of 9 oz/day or more had total energy intakes that were 188 kcal/day higher than nonconsumers.[15] Among adults, total energy consumption among 16 subjects was greater on the day that an energy-containing beverage was given at lunch, compared with the preceding day.[13]

Observational studies indicate an independent association between soft drink consumption and body weight. We studied 548 ethnically diverse middle school students over two academic years and observed that each additional serving of sugar-sweetened drink increased the risk of becoming obese by 60%, after controlling for potentially confounding factors.[16] Berkey et al.[17] examined 1-year changes in soft drink consumption and body weight among 10,000 participants in the Growing Up Today Study, reporting direct associations in both boys and girls that were largely explained by total energy intake. These findings are supported by a recent randomized controlled trial using a cluster design, based in six primary schools in southwestern England.[18] A targeted program to reduce soft drink consumption decreased the incidence of obesity in the intervention group by 7.7% compared with the control group.

FAST FOOD INTAKE

Perhaps no dietary pattern typifies children's eating habits today better than fast food. Once an occasional event, fast food has become regular fare for most American youth. On any given day, one in three children consume fast food;[19] three in four do so each week.[20] Fast food consumption has increased by a remarkable fivefold among children since the 1970s, now exceeding 10% of total energy intake.[21]

Fast food, as presently marketed, contains numerous unhealthful components, including extraordinarily large portion sizes, very high energy density, high content of refined carbohydrate and *trans* fatty acids, low content of fiber and micronutrients, and primordial palatability (appealing to innate preferences for sugar, fat, and salt). Each of these aspects has been linked to excessive weight gain or obesity-associated comorbidities.[22,23]

A nationally representative study by Bowman et al.[19] of approximately 6212 children ages 4 to 18 years found that energy consumption was 187 kcal/day greater on days when fast food was consumed, compared with days without fast food. Studies of adolescents by McNutt et al.[24] and French et al.[20] reached similar conclusions. Moreover, certain individuals may be especially susceptible to the adverse effects of fast food. We studied the diets of 54 lean and overweight adolescents who consumed fast food regularly.[25] Whereas lean individuals compensated perfectly for the large amount of energy in a habitual fast food meal by decreasing consumption of other foods commensurately, overweight subjects did not. On days when the overweight adolescents consumed fast food, total energy intake was 409 kcal greater than on days without fast food.

While there are no prospective studies of fast food and obesity in children, we recently examined data from 3031 young adults, ages 18 to 30 years, over a 15 year period.[26] Individuals in the highest compared with the lowest categories of fast food intake at baseline and follow-up gained an extra 10 lb and had a twofold greater increase in insulin resistance.

PORTION SIZES

In the 1950s, soft drinks were served in 6.5-oz sizes; today, servings of up to 64 oz (4 pounds!) can be readily obtained.[27] This trend toward increasingly large portion sizes seems to have affected virtually all foods prepared outside the home, from packaged snacks to meals at sit-down restaurants.[28]

When adults and children are served large compared with standard portions of food, they eat more food, and total energy intake tends to increase, at least over the short term. Diliberti et al.[29] covertly manipulated the size of a pasta entrée consumed by 180 adults in a cafeteria-style restaurant. Individuals who purchased the large size (377 vs. 248 g) increased their energy intake of the entrée by 43% (172 kcal) and of the entire meal by 25% (159 kcal). Similarly, Levitsky and Youn[30] found that energy intake increased at a buffet lunch among college students when portion size was covertly increased. McConahy et al.[31] examined dietary habits and body weight of approximately 5000 children, ages 2 to 5 years, participating in the Continuing Survey of Food Intake by Individuals. Portion size alone accounted for 17 to 19% of the variance in energy intake, whereas body weight explained only 4%. Fisher et al.[32] studied 30 children during two series of lunches in which either age-appropriate or excessively large entrée portion sizes were provided. They found that energy consumption from the entrée and meal increased by 25 and 15%, respectively, when portion size was doubled. Increased food intake was attributed to increases in average bite size.

MEAL PATTERNS

The dietary changes discussed above — involving beverages, fast food, and portion sizes — are inextricably related to fundamental changes in meal patterns of children. In the 1970s, most food was prepared at home and consumed primarily as regular meals. Today, the proportion of food prepared and eaten away from home has increased to 30% among adolescents,[33] and frequency of snacking has increased markedly among all age groups.[34] Not surprisingly, the quality of foods eaten away from home is consistently lower than foods eaten at home.[35,36] At the same time, the prevalence of skipping breakfast, a phenomenon associated with a 4.5-fold higher risk for obesity in adults,[37] has increased by 13 to 20% in adolescents.[38]

In light of the discussion above, a conceptually straightforward approach to the prevention and treatment of obesity in children would be to reduce consumption of soft drinks and fast food, decrease portion sizes of meals and snacks, and increase the proportion of foods consumed at home (though this approach has not been specifically studied).

CURRENT DIETARY APPROACHES

Most multicentered, school-based studies — such as DISC[39] and CATCH[40] — have compared an intervention group that received behavioral treatment designed to decrease dietary fat and reduce cardiovascular disease risk with a control group that received minimal or no intervention. Many of these treatments have achieved decreases in fat consumption. However, these studies do not demonstrate significant, long-term reductions in body weight in the intervention compared with control groups,[22,41] raising the possibility that other dietary approaches might be more efficacious for weight control. Regarding a family-based approach, the comprehensive behavioral intervention of Epstein et al.[42] that uses the "Traffic Light Diet" seems promising. With this diet, foods are categorized as green, yellow, or red based on energy density. Participants are instructed to restrict total caloric intake, particularly by limiting energy-dense "red foods." In perhaps the longest follow-up of any obesity treatment study in children, a decrease in percent overweight (7.5%) was observed after 10 years in the experimental group compared with an increase in the untreated control group (14.3%),[42] though less than half of the children in the experimental group maintained a 20% decrease in percent overweight.[43] Moreover, this study did not directly assess the effects of the diet *per se*, as the control group did not receive an intervention of equal intensity.

Indeed, there have been virtually no clinical trials examining the effects of any specific dietary prescription in children, controlling for the effects of potentially confounding factors such as treatment intensity, behavioral intervention strategies, and physical activity. While comprehensive approaches aiming to modify diet, physical activity, family behavior, and the social and physical environment will undoubtedly be needed, studies involving multiple modalities cannot assess the efficacy of any specific component (e.g., diet). Therefore, in the absence of data relating directly to the efficacy of varying diet prescriptions in children, it is necessary to refer to the adult literature.

SCOPE OF AVAILABLE DIETARY APPROACHES

Widespread debate regarding dietary recommendations for weight management has focused largely on optimal carbohydrate-to-fat ratios.[44,45] Low-fat, high-carbohydrate diets remain the cornerstone of public health guidelines.[46] Nevertheless, diets that impose extreme fat or carbohydrate restriction have become increasingly popular alternatives, with carbohydrate to fat ratios ranging from >5:1

TABLE 18.1
Available Dietary Approaches

Type of Diet	Carbohydrate/Fat (%)	Example(s)
Low fat	50–60/≤30	USDA Food Guide Pyramid (pre-2005)
	45–65/25–35	USDA MyPyramid
Very low fat	70–75/≤10	Eat More, Weigh Less (Ornish Diet)
Low carbohydrate	≤10/60	Atkins' Diet
Low energy density	Variable[a]	Volumetrics
Low glycemic load	Variable	South Beach Diet
		Glucose Revolution
		Sugar Busters

[a] Typically low in fat due to the high energy-density of this macronutrient.

to <1:5.[47] Recently, approaches focusing on other dietary factors, rather than a specific macronutrient composition, have been proposed, including low energy density and low glycemic load. Table 18.1 compares the nutrient profiles of these conventional and alternative diets.

From a practical perspective, the USDA Food Guide Pyramid (recently updated to MyPyramid) has been widely recommended for promoting healthful eating among children in the context of a low-fat diet.[46,48,49] The pyramids convey messages to eat a variety of grains, fruits, and vegetables, and to limit fat intake to approximately 30% or less of total calories. A more extreme very-low-fat, Ornish-type diet — with 10% or less of total calories from fat and 70 to 75% from carbohydrates is based on consumption of plant foods containing ample amounts of complex carbohydrates and dietary fiber.[50] At the opposite extreme, a very-low-carbohydrate, Atkins-type diet — with approximately 10% of calories from carbohydrates and 60% from fat — recommends unlimited consumption of animal foods (e.g., meat, fish, poultry, eggs) along with controlled portions of cheese and nonstarchy vegetables to promote weight loss.[51]

Divergent hypotheses linking macronutrient consumption with obesity are central to the debate regarding dietary guidelines. Proponents of low-fat and very-low-fat diets argue that people who eat less fat consume fewer calories because fat has a higher energy density and is less satiating than complex carbohydrates or protein.[52–55] They also contend that carbohydrate is preferentially oxidized during the postprandial period, enhancing energy expenditure, and that energy from fat is stored most efficiently.[54,55] In contrast, proponents of Atkins-type diets argue that carbohydrate restriction stabilizes blood sugar and prevents hyperinsulinemia, thereby limiting storage of metabolic fuels, controlling carbohydrate cravings, and promoting satiety.[51] They also argue that glucagon secretion in response to high protein intake may counteract the adverse effects of insulin on body weight. According to Ornish,[56] the high fiber content of very-low-fat diets has a similar beneficial effect in preventing hyperinsulinemia by slowing carbohydrate absorption, rather than restricting carbohydrate consumption, to avoid rapid increases in blood glucose following a meal.

Some proponents of low-fat diets have approached the debate regarding optimal macronutrient composition for weight management by noting that energy intake is the most critical variable, attributing greater weight loss on very-low-carbohydrate diets to lower energy intake due in part to limited food choices.[57,58] Perhaps a more fundamental issue pertains to optimal strategies for controlling energy intake. Behavioral interventions often focus on counting calories or following a comprehensive food exchange system to impose energy restriction,[42,59] although *ad libitum* diets have been evaluated in several studies.[60–67] An *ad libitum* approach, regardless of the carbohydrate-to-fat ratio, does not disregard the importance of energy intake but, rather, shifts the primary focus from external restriction to internal physiologic control of intake based on the satiety hypotheses presented above.

EFFICACY OF AVAILABLE DIETS

Prior systematic reviews are not mutually consistent, with some authors concluding that low-fat diets are efficacious for weight management[53,68] and others that dietary fat is not an important determinant of adiposity.[69,70] The inconsistency may be largely due to differences in study selection criteria. Many studies cited as a basis for recommending low-fat diets used short-term (i.e., less than 6 months) interventions, were not designed to specifically evaluate changes in body weight, or had a control condition in which patients did not receive any nutrition education or dietary counseling.[53,68] Clearly, the relevance of such studies for evaluating efficacy is problematic, underscoring the need for well-defined review criteria.

We systematically updated previous reviews of long-term randomized controlled trials (RCTs) designed to evaluate weight-control diets in adults,[69,70] directing attention to macronutrient composition and prescription strategies (i.e., energy-restricted vs. *ad libitum*). We focused largely on adult studies because of the paucity of pediatric and adolescent data, as discussed above. Studies were identified using a Medline search and referring to published reviews and commentaries. When multiple reports were generated from the same study, we reviewed each article and reported data based on the largest participant follow-up rate. Study selection criteria are listed below.

- Intervention was 6 months or more in duration.
- Body weight was a primary outcome.
- Study was designed to compare diets containing 1000 kcal/day or more.
- Nutrition education and behavioral counseling provided the basis for intervention (i.e., no provision of food by the investigators).
- Intensity of nutrition education and behavioral counseling was similar across diets.
- Participants were free-living.
- Results were published in a peer-reviewed journal.
- Follow-up rate could be calculated based on reported data.

As summarized in Table 18.2, several studies have shown that significant weight loss can be achieved over 3 to 6 months with energy-restricted or *ad libitum* diet prescriptions varying widely in macronutrient composition.[60,63,64,66,71–74] However, follow-up rates have been disappointing, and weight loss at 12 to 18 months of follow-up infrequently exceeds 5% of baseline weight.[60–62,64,65,67,75–77] While *ad libitum* very-low-carbohydrate diets seem to be more efficacious than energy-restricted low-fat diets over the short term,[63,64,66,67] Foster et al.[64] found no significant group difference in mean body weight at 12 months. Similar results were obtained in a study by Stern et al.[67] that included patients with type 2 diabetes. With regard to pediatric data from a short-term study, Sondike et al.[78] reported greater weight loss (9.9 vs. 4.1 kg) in adolescents who were instructed to follow an *ad libitum* very-low-carbohydrate diet vs. an *ad libitum* low-fat diet for 12 weeks. However, findings from this study must be interpreted cautiously in light of adult data indicating poor compliance and weight regain over the long term on an Atkins-type diet.[64,67] In addition, there is widespread concern regarding the safety of severe carbohydrate restriction, especially in children.[79,80] While very-low-carbohydrate diets may have some beneficial effects on risk factors for CVD and type 2 diabetes,[64,67] the overall effects of this approach on disease processes, growth, and development are not known.

Very-low-fat diets have been shown to promote weight loss in several adult studies.[81–84] However, these studies are not included in our systematic review for one or more of the following reasons: the design was not an RCT,[82,83] body weight was not a primary outcome,[84] the intensity of intervention varied (i.e., very-low-fat diets combined with other intensive lifestyle changes were compared with usual care),[84] or information about follow-up rate was not included in the report.[81]

Dietary interventions based on energy density (i.e., calories per mass of food) also have been considered as an approach for weight management. A series of short-term feeding studies, summarized by Rolls,[85] suggest that reducing energy density decreases energy intake independent of macronutrient ratio, possibly due to effects on satiation and satiety. Based on a preliminary report of *ad libitum* diets in obese women, greater weight loss was achieved at 6 months by reducing energy density — with emphasis on increasing consumption of water-rich foods and decreasing consumption of high-fat foods — in comparison with reducing fat intake only;[86] however, weight loss did not differ between dietary intervention groups at 12 months.

In summary, data regarding optimal dietary approaches for weight management in children are lacking, and long-term studies of available interventions in adults have not demonstrated efficacy. Therefore, research into the development and testing of novel dietary approaches to obesity prevention and treatment is warranted. An emerging body of literature suggests that a focus on macronutrient ratio is too simplistic and that the quality of dietary carbohydrate and fat is an important consideration.[47] From this perspective, a low-glycemic load diet may be an especially attractive alternative, in light of preliminary data from animal studies, feeding studies in children and adults, and small-scale clinical trials as reviewed below.

REDUCED GLYCEMIC LOAD DIET

CLASSIFICATION OF DIETARY CARBOHYDRATE

All carbohydrates can be digested or converted to glucose. The terms "complex carbohydrate" and "simple sugar" are based on the belief that rates of digestion and absorption are determined by saccharide chain length. Current public health guidelines reflect this perspective by advocating increased consumption of starchy foods and decreased consumption of sugar in the context of a low-fat diet.[46] However, this classification scheme based on chemical structure has limited physiological relevance given the well-documented overlap in biological responses to foods varying in saccharide chain length.[87,88] For example, Wahlqvist et al.[87] demonstrated similar changes in blood glucose, insulin, and fatty acid concentrations after consumption of glucose as a monosaccharide, disaccharide, oligosaccharide, or polysaccharide. Bantle et al.[88] found no differences in blood glucose responses to meals with sucrose compared with meals containing a similar amount of energy from either potato or wheat starch. Nevertheless, the physiological effects of carbohydrates do vary substantially, as demonstrated by marked differences in glycemic and insulinemic responses to ingestion of isoenergetic amounts of white bread vs. pasta.[89] For this reason, Jenkins et al.[90] proposed the glycemic index as an alternative system for classifying carbohydrate-containing foods.

The glycemic index (GI) is a term that describes the rise in blood glucose over a 2-h postprandial period following consumption of a food portion containing a standardized amount of carbohydrate.[90] It is calculated as the incremental area under the blood glucose–response curve after consuming 50 g of available carbohydrate from a test food, divided by the area under the curve after consuming 50 g of carbohydrate from a reference food (i.e., glucose or white bread).[91] Foods that are rapidly digested and absorbed, or metabolically transformed into glucose, have a high GI.[92,93] Examples of high-GI foods include white bread, prepared breakfast cereals, potato products, and sugar-sweetened beverages. Unprocessed grains, nonstarchy vegetables, fruits, and legumes tend to have a low GI. Regular consumption of high-GI meals, compared with isoenergetic and nutrient-controlled low-GI meals, causes higher average 24-h blood glucose and insulin levels.[94,95]

Because GI is derived from studies of foods containing a standard amount of carbohydrate, the term glycemic load (GL, defined as the arithmetic product of GI and carbohydrate amount) is used to characterize how actual portion sizes, meals, or diets affect postprandial glycemia.[96] Recently, this concept has received experimental validation, in that calculated GL accurately predicted the observed glycemic responses to test meals differing in carbohydrate source and amount.[97]

TABLE 18.2
Systematic Review of Studies Examining Efficacy of Available Dietary Approaches

Duration (months)	N[a]	Strategy	Energy Distribution[b]	Follow-up Rate[a]	Weight Change[c]	N[a]	Strategy	Energy Distribution[b]	Follow-up Rate[a]	Weight Change[c]	Ref.[d]
			Diet Prescription 1					**Diet Prescription 2**			
		Low-fat *Ad libitum*	(Prescription target)				Low-carbohydrate *Ad libitum*	(Prescription target)			60
3	66		≤25%F	96%	4.8%	63		≤18% C	95%	6.4%	
12	61			88%	2.1%	59			89%	2.9%	
		Low-fat *Ad libitum*					Energy-restricted				61,71,75
6	47		62%C, 21%F, 16%P	77%	5.5%	42		54%C, 30%F, 16%P	69%	4.8%	
12	39		58%C, 25%F, 17%P	64%	3.1%	36		52%C, 31%F, 17%P	59%	1.0%	
18	39		26%F	64%	0.5%	35		33%F	57%	+2.3%	
		Low-fat Energy-restricted					Energy-restricted				76
12	16		26%F	70%	3.2%	13		34%F	57%	3.7%	
		Low-fat Energy-restricted	(Prescription target)				Low-carbohydrate Energy-restricted	(Prescription target)			72
6	42		58%C, 21%F, 21%P	74%	(ITT) 5.0%	40		35%C, 35%F, 30% P	75%	(ITT) 6.4%	
		Low-fat *Ad libitum*					Energy-restricted				62,73
6	28		61%C, 21%F, 17%P	~70%	6.2%	29		54%C, 27%F, 16%P	~73%	13.6%	
18	26		59%C, 24%F, 16%P	~65%	2.2%	22		54%C, 28%F, 16%P	~55%	8.8%	
		Low-fat Energy-restricted					Moderate-fat Energy-restricted				77
18	10		50%C, 30%F, 19%P	20%	3.3%	25		47%C, 35%F, 19%P	50%	5.4%	

Months	Intervention (arm 1)	n	Energy distribution	Follow-up	Weight change	Intervention (arm 2)	n	Energy distribution	Follow-up	Weight change	Ref
6	Low-fat Energy-restricted	20	53%C, 29%F, 18%P	74%	4.2%	Low-carbohydrate Ad libitum	22	30%C, 46%F, 23%P	85%	9.3%	63
3	Low-fat Energy-restricted (Prescription target)	21	60%C, 25%F, 15%P	70% (ITT)	2.7%	Low-carbohydrate Ad libitum (Prescription Target)	28	10%C, 60%F, 30%P	85% (ITT)	6.8%	64
6		18		60%	3.2%		24		73%	7.0%	
12		17		57%	2.5%		20		61%	4.4%	
12	Low-fat Energy-restricted	7	55%C, 29%F, 18%P	88%	+1.9%[e]	Low glycemic load Ad libitum	7	52%C, 29%F, 20%P	88%	3.7%[e]	65
6	Low-fat Energy-restricted	34	52%C, 29%F, 19%P	57% (ITT)	6.7%	Low-carbohydrate Ad libitum	45	8%C, 68%F, 26%P	76%	12.9% (ITT)	66
6	Low-fat Energy-restricted	36	51%C, 33%F, 16%P	53% (ITT)	1.4%	Low-carbohydrate Ad libitum	43	37%C, 41%F, 22%P	67% (ITT)	4.4%	67,74
12		43	50%C, 34%F, 16%P	63%	2.3%		44	30%C, 52%F, 18%P	69%	3.9%	

[a] Sample sizes represent the number of active participants who completed follow-up measurements. Follow-up rates were calculated based on the number of participants who were randomly assigned to a dietary intervention group.

[b] Energy distribution data are based on self-report of dietary intake, if available: the prescription targets are otherwise listed (C, carbohydrate; F, fat; P, protein).

[c] Weight change data are derived from participants who were available for follow-up measurements except where indicated as intention to treat (ITT).

[d] When multiple reports were generated from the same study, the article containing the most long-term data is listed as the primary reference.

[e] Weight change data are based on BMI, rather than absolute body weight, given that subjects were adolescents.

PHYSIOLOGICAL MECHANISMS

Circulating blood glucose levels are tightly controlled by homeostatic regulatory mechanisms that normally ensure a smooth transition from the postprandial period to the postabsorptive state. However, rapid digestion and absorption of carbohydrate from high-GL meals seem to challenge these mechanisms.[98] During the early postprandial period (0 to 2 h after a meal), hyperglycemia resulting from consumption of a high-GL meal stimulates pancreatic beta cells to release insulin and inhibits alpha cells from releasing glucagon. This relative hyperinsulinemia and hypoglucagonemia directs metabolic fuels toward storage and away from oxidation by upregulating glycogenesis and lipogenesis and downregulating gluconeogenesis and lipolysis. During the middle postprandial period (2 to 4 h after a meal), persistent elevation of insulin levels and suppression of glucagon levels continue to stimulate uptake of glucose by insulin-sensitive tissues and may cause hypoglycemia. Free fatty acid concentrations are also suppressed. At this time, hunger increases in response to the relatively low circulating concentrations of metabolic fuels. The physiological significance of these metabolic changes is demonstrated by the counterregulatory hormone response that occurs during the late postprandial period (4 to 6 h after a meal).

EXPERIMENTAL EVIDENCE

Animal Studies

Animal studies provide evidence for a direct effect of GI on nutrient partitioning away from oxidation and toward storage. In two studies reported by Kabir et al.,[99,100] rats were fed a diet containing either high-GI or low-GI starch for 3 weeks. Insulin-stimulated glucose oxidation was lower and incorporation of glucose into lipid was higher in the rats fed the high-GI starch. Moreover, consumption of the high-GI starch caused greater fatty acid synthetase activity in adipose tissue and lower phosphoenolpyruvate carboxykinase mRNA in liver, indicating increased lipogenesis and decreased gluconeogenesis in these respective tissues. In a study by Pawlak et al.,[101] two groups of growing rats were treated with identical diets that differed only in the GI of the starch. Food was provided in variable amounts to maintain the same mean body weight between groups. After 2 months, rats fed the high-GI starch became more energy efficient, as demonstrated by a progressive decrease in food energy requirements compared with those fed the low-GI starch. At the end of the study, despite having the same mean body weight, animals in the high-GI group had 70 to 90% more body fat and a commensurate reduction in lean body mass compared with animals in the low-GI group.

Hunger and Energy Intake

Adult studies have consistently indicated less hunger and voluntary energy intake in response to decreases in GL achieved by dietary manipulations affecting carbohydrate quality (i.e., GI) or quantity (i.e., carbohydrate amount), as previously reviewed.[92] Three studies substantiate these findings in children. We compared the effects of three different breakfast meals that contained the same amount of energy but varied in GL (high, moderate, low) in obese adolescents under controlled conditions.[102] Two of the breakfasts had identical macronutrient composition (64% carbohydrate, 20% fat, and 16% protein) but varied in GI owing to different carbohydrate sources (i.e., high-GI instant oatmeal vs. moderate-GI steel-cut oats). The third breakfast, a vegetable omelet, achieved a low GL by reduction in both carbohydrate amount (40%) and GI. Hunger ratings and cumulative voluntary energy intake over the 5-h postprandial period were highest following the high-GL meal, intermediate following the moderate-GL meal, and lowest following the low-GL meal. Moreover, the interval between completion of the meal and initiation of voluntary energy intake from foods on a buffet platter was shortest following the high-GL breakfast. Using a similar study design, Ball et al.[103] also observed less prolonged satiety in obese adolescents following high- vs. low-GL meal replacements that were controlled for energy and macronutrient composition (43 to 45% carbohydrate, 29 to 32% fat, 25 to 27% protein) but varied in GI. In a study of preadolescent children ranging from normal weight to obese, Warren et al.[104] fed breakfasts matched for energy but differing in GI due to variations in types of cereal and bread. They subsequently observed food intake during lunch in the naturalistic setting of a school cafeteria. Hunger ratings and voluntary energy intake at lunchtime were higher following the high- vs. low-GI breakfasts. Taken together, these studies provide consistent evidence that GL has a significant effect on energy intake over the short term.

Energy Metabolism

We recently examined the effects of GL on energy metabolism in 39 overweight and obese young adults.[105] Subjects were randomly assigned to receive either low-fat or low-GL diets designed to reduce body weight by 10%. After approximately 10 weeks, both groups lost a similar amount of weight and showed similar changes in body composition. Subjects in the low-fat group showed the expected decrease in resting energy expenditure (REE) that has been previously demonstrated to occur with weight loss.[106] However, subjects in the low-GL group showed a significantly smaller decline in REE (a difference of 80 kcal/day). This group also reported less hunger.

Short-Term Weight Loss

Reducing GL seems to be a promising weight management strategy based on several short-term intervention studies that relied on outpatient counseling to foster changes in dietary intake. Bouche et al.[107] conducted a crossover study of 11 overweight men treated for 5 weeks on low- vs. high-GI diets that were controlled for energy and macronutrient composition (39 to 42% carbohydrate, 37 to 38% fat, 18 to 20% protein). Fat mass in the trunk region was approximately 500 g less after the low-GI diet. Slabber et al.[108] compared low- vs. high-GI diets (1000 to 1200 kcal, 50% carbohydrate, 30% fat, 20% protein) in 16 obese women for 12 weeks using a crossover design. Body weight decreased more with the low-GI diet (7.4 vs. 4.5 kg). In an outcomes assessment study of 107 patients attending a pediatric obesity clinic, Spieth et al.[109] prescribed either an *ad libitum* low-GL load diet (45 to 50% carbohydrate, 30 to 35% fat, 20 to 25% protein) emphasizing low-GI carbohydrate sources or an energy-restricted low-fat diet (55 to 60% carbohydrate, 25 to 30% fat, 15 to 20% protein). Patients on the low-GL diet lost more weight, resulting in a group difference of 1.5 kg/m^2 for change in body mass index (BMI) over a mean of 4 months. Clapp[110] treated 12 pregnant women with low- vs. high-GI diets (55 to 60% carbohydrate, 20 to 25% fat, 17 to 19% protein) and found less maternal weight gain (11.8 vs. 19.7 kg) and lower infant birth weight (3.27 vs. 4.25 kg) with the low-GI diet. This study may have particular relevance to the prevention of pediatric obesity, in light of evidence suggesting that body weight may be programmed by intrauterine events.[111] In contrast, Sloth et al.[112] reported no significant difference in weight loss among overweight subjects treated for 10 weeks with low- vs. high-GI diets. However, this study may have been underpowered because there appears to have been a progressive divergence in rates of weight loss over time favoring the low-GI group (1.9 vs. 1.3 kg) at 10 weeks. In any event, these short-term studies do not meet the criteria specified for our systematic review, underscoring the need for long-term clinical trials.

LONG-TERM EFFICACY AND FEASIBILITY

Long-term efficacy was examined by us in one small-scale study of 16 obese adolescents who were randomly assigned to a low-GL diet or a conventional low-fat diet.[65] The low-GL treatment encouraged consumption of low- to moderate-GL meals and snacks, with 45 to 50% of energy from carbohydrate and 30 to 35% of energy from fat (particularly healthful sources such as canola and olive oils); while the conventional treatment emphasized intake of low-fat products, with 55 to 60% of energy from "complex" carbohydrate and 25 to 30% from fat. At 12 months, BMI had decreased more in the low-GL group compared with the low-fat group (1.3 vs. +0.7 kg/m²). Based on these data, an *ad libitum* low-GL diet, focusing on GI and without strict limitation on carbohydrate intake, appears to be a promising alternative to a conventional energy-restricted diet. To our knowledge, this is the only study of diet composition in which differences between intervention groups persisted at 12 months of follow-up. Clearly, these findings require confirmation with a larger number of subjects and in other populations.

The feasibility and long-term efficacy of an *ad libitum* low-GL diet may be due, in part, to the flexibility of the approach. As noted above, *ad libitum* diet prescriptions rely on internal satiety mechanisms to control energy intake, hypothetically diminishing the need for reliance on laborious calorie-counting regimens or food exchange systems to externally impose energy restriction. This potential flexibility may be particularly beneficial for adolescents who have a strong desire for autonomy and often resist the attempts of well-meaning adults who make an effort to support dietary change by imposing external controls. Indeed, children with type 1 diabetes were more easily able to select their own foods, achieved better glycemic control, and experienced less family conflict when given a low-GI diet prescription compared with a regimented meal plan based on an exchange system.[113]

As noted above,[65] we typically reduce the GL of a conventional low-fat, high-carbohydrate diet by replacing high-GI carbohydrate-containing foods with low-GI alternatives and sources of healthful fat. Thus, we cannot dismiss the possibility that the quality of dietary fat may have contributed to long-term weight control in our adolescent efficacy study.[65] Indeed, data from a mouse model reported by Wang et al.[114] suggest that polyunsaturated fatty acids may protect against obesity via beneficial effects on hypothalamic neuropeptides regulating energy balance. Perhaps, individuals can succeed with weight management on *ad libitum* diets varying widely in macronutrient composition when adequate attention is directed toward dietary quality with respect to both carbohydrate and fat.[47] Further mechanistic research is warranted to address this topic.

POTENTIAL EFFECTS ON OBESITY-RELATED COMORBIDITIES

Pediatric obesity, while historically viewed as an aesthetic problem, confers increased risk for numerous medical complications.[22] Of particular concern, the clustering of CVD risk factors, referred to as the "insulin resistance syndrome," has been identified in children as young as 5 years of age,[115] and prevalence of the syndrome is high among obese children.[116] Optimal approaches to weight management, therefore, must take into account the effects of diet on risk for CVD and type 2 diabetes.

Although limited data exist on the relationship between dietary intake and disease processes in children, most epidemiologic studies of adults,[117–124] but not all,[125–127] provide evidence that the quality of dietary carbohydrate and fat influences risk. Dietary GI[117–119] and GL[118,120] are inversely associated with HDL-cholesterol concentrations, and GL has a stronger (direct) association with triglyceride levels than either GI or carbohydrate amount.[120] Moreover, individuals in the highest categories of GL appear to be at substantially increased risk for incident coronary heart disease[121] and type 2 diabetes.[96,122,124] Regarding the quality of dietary fat, partially hydrogenated (*trans*) fat — frequently contained in commercial bakery products and fast foods[128] — increases risk for CVD[129] and type 2 diabetes,[123] while unsaturated fats from vegetable and marine sources decrease risk.[123,129]

PRACTICAL CONSIDERATIONS FOR PRESCRIBING LOW GLYCEMIC LOAD DIETS

A low-GL food pyramid is presented in Figure 18.1, and corresponding food choice lists are presented in Table 18.3. These teaching tools were developed to assist families in reducing GL by replacing high-GI sources of carbohydrate with low-GI sources and healthful oils. Thus, the primary focus is on the quality of carbohydrate and fat, rather than the relative quantity of these macronutrients.

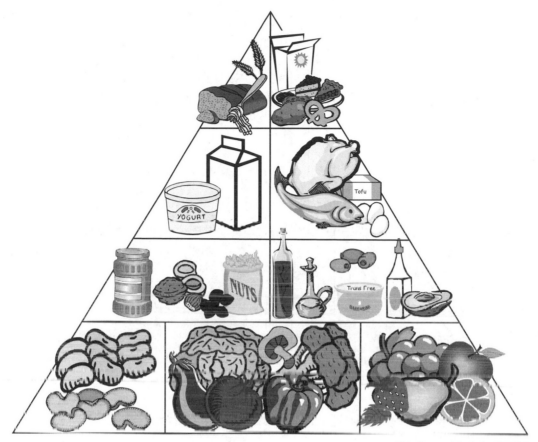

Ebbeling and Ludwig, © 2004

FIGURE 18.1 Low-glycemic load pyramid.

Intervention messages are inherently different from available low-fat and very-low-carbohydrate approaches in that there is no restriction on total dietary fat or carbohydrate.

Nonstarchy vegetables, legumes, and fruits have a low GL and, thus, are on Level 1 of the pyramid and form the foundation of the diet. Sources of healthful oils — including nuts and seeds — are on Level 2. Protein-rich foods — including milk and other recommended sources of protein — are on Level 3. Moderate- and high-GL foods are differentiated from one another on Level 4. Intervention messages encourage *ad libitum* consumption of foods on Levels 1 to 3 of the pyramid, along with a few servings of moderate-GL foods and limited intake of high-GL foods on Level 4.

An *ad libitum* approach to consuming foods on Levels 1 to 3 necessitates education regarding hunger and satiety, such that individuals recognize when to initiate and stop eating based on these feelings. Moreover, portion size information must be directed toward what it means to "eat plenty" of the foods on Level 1, to complement meals and snacks with foods on Levels 2 and 3, and to monitor intake of foods on Level 4. Interactive activities that utilize food models and cooking demonstrations with taste-testing are enjoyable educational strategies, when logistically feasible.

CONCLUSIONS

Hundreds of studies in recent years have aimed to prevent or treat obesity in children and adults by dietary modification. Most of these studies have not achieved significant long-term weight reduction. Moreover, very few of these studies were designed to examine the effects of any specific

TABLE 18.3
Food Choice Lists for a Low-Glycemic Load Diet

Carbohydrate					
Vegetables		Legumes	Fruit		Dairy	Grains

Low Glycemic Load

Nonstarchy

Vegetables		Legumes	Fruit		Dairy	Grains
Alfalfa sprouts	Mushrooms	Beans	Apples	Lemon	Milk, whole, 2%	
Artichoke	Okra	Black-eyed peas	Apricot	Lime	Yogurt plain, sugar-free	
Asparagus	Onions	Chickpeas	Berries	Nectarines		
Bamboo shoots	Peppers	Hummus	Cantaloupe	Oranges		
Beans (green, wax)	Radishes	Lentils	Cherries	Peaches		
Bok choy	Salsa	Split peas	Clementines	Pears		
Broccoli	Scallions		Grapefruit	Plums		
Brussels sprouts	Snow peas		Grapes	Tangelos		
Cabbage	Sauerkraut		Honeydew	Tangerines		
Carrots	Spinach		Kiwi			
Cauliflower	Summer squash					
Celery	Swiss chard					
Cucumber	Tomatoes					
Eggplant	Turnip					
Greens	Water chestnuts					
Kohlrabi	Zucchini					
Leeks						
Lettuce						

Moderate Glycemic Load

Starchy					Breads	Cereal	Grains
Acorn squash	Green peas	Pumpkin	Applesauce	Dried fruit	**Breads**	**Cereal**	**Grains**
Beets	Parsnips	Yam	Banana	Mango	Flourless	High fiber	Barley
Butternut	Plantain		Canned fruit	Papaya	Pumpernickel	Steel-cut oats	Basmati rice
squash				Pineapple	Stone ground	**Pasta**	Brown rice
				Watermelon	Whole grain	*al dente*	Bulgur
							Kasha
							Parboiled rice
							Quinoa
							Wheat berries
							Wild rice

High Glycemic Load

Starchy	Baked Beans	Fruit juices	Juice drinks	Yogurt sugar-sweetened	Breads	Cereal	Grains
Corn	Baked Beans	Fruit juices	Juice drinks	Yogurt sugar-sweetened	**Breads**	**Cereal**	**Grains**
French fries					Bagel	Most varieties	Couscous
Potato, boiled					Bread	**Pasta**	Millet
Potato, baked					Bread sticks	Canned	Rice
Sweet potato					Buns	**Snacks**	Rice cakes
					Cornbread	Crackers	**Sweet Desserts**
					Muffin	Pizza	Cake
					Pancakes	Popcorn	Cookies
					Pita	Pretzels	Danish
					Roll	Snack chips	Doughnuts
					Stuffing		Pie
					Taco shell		
					Tortilla		
					Waffle		

(continued)

TABLE 18.3 (CONTINUED)
Food Choice Lists for a Low-Glycemic Load Diet

Healthful Fat

Nuts		Seeds	Oils		Other
Almonds	Pecans	Flaxseed	Canola oil	Peanut oil	Avocado
Almond butter (natural)	Pine nuts	Pumpkin seeds	Mayonnaise	Salad dressing (Italian style)	Olives
Brazil nuts	Pistachios	Sesame seeds	Olive oil	Soybean oil	
Cashews	Soy nuts	Sunflower seeds		*Trans*-free spreads	
Hazelnuts	Walnuts				
Macadamia nuts					
Peanuts					
Peanut butter (natural)					

Protein

Cheese	Eggs	Fish and Shellfish, not breaded		Poultry, not breaded	Soy Products	Deli Meat
Cheddar	Egg substitutes	Bass	Clams	Chicken	Seitan	Chicken breast
Cottage	Egg whites	Catfish	Crab	Cornish hen	Tempeh	Turkey breast
Feta	Whole eggs	Cod	Lobster	Duck	Textured vegetable protein	Turkey ham
Monterey Jack		Flounder	Oysters	Turkey	Tofu	
Mozzarella		Grouper	Scallops			
Parmesan		Haddock	Shrimp			
Ricotta		Halibut				
Swiss		Herring				
		Mackerel				
		Mahi mahi				
		Salmon				
		Sardines				
		Snapper				
		Sole				
		Swordfish				
		Trout				
		Tuna				

dietary approaches *per se*, independent of potentially confounding factors. Thus, based on available data, no specific diet can be said to be efficacious, let alone effective, in the prevention or treatment of childhood obesity. Nevertheless, novel diets focused on nutrient quality (e.g., low GL) rather than macronutrient ratio, show considerable promise. Pending definitive RCTs, a practical approach to the prevention and treatment of childhood obesity would include reducing consumption of sugar-sweetened beverages and fast food, decreasing portion sizes, increasing intake of low energy dense foods such as vegetables and fruit, focusing on the quality of dietary carbohydrate and fat, and encouraging consumption of foods prepared at home.

REFERENCES

1. Awofeso N. What's new about the "new public health"? *Am J Public Health*. 2004;94: 705–709.
2. Styne DM, Ed. *Pediatr Clinics N Am*. 2001;48: 823–1069.
3. Wright JD, Kennedy-Stephenson J, Wang CY, McDowell MA, Johnson CL. Trends in intake of energy and macronutrients — United States, 1971–2000. *Morbid Mortal Wkly Rep*. 2004;53: 80–82.
4. Troiano RP, Briefel RR, Carroll MD, Bialostosky K. Energy and fat intakes of children and adolescents in the united states: data from the national health and nutrition examination surveys. *Am J Clin Nutr*. 2000;72: 1343S–1353S.
5. Morton JF, Guthrie JF. Changes in children's total fat intakes and their food group sources of fat, 1989–91 versus 1994–95: implications for diet quality. *Fam Econ Nutr Rev*. 1998;11: 44–57.
6. Nielsen SJ, Popkin BM. Changes in beverage intake between 1977 and 2001. *Am J Prev Med*. 2004;27: 205–210.
7. French SA, Lin B H, Guthrie JF. National trends in soft drink consumption among children and adolescents age 6 to 17 years: prevalence, amounts, and sources, 1977/1978 to 1994/1998. *J Am Diet Assoc*. 2003;103: 1326–1331.
8. Jacobson M. *Liquid Candy: How Soft Drinks are Harming Americans*. Washington, DC: Center for Science in the Public Interest. 2005.
9. Guthrie JF, Morton JF. Food sources of added sweeteners in the diets of Americans. *J Am Diet Assoc*. 2000;100: 43–51.
10. Bowman SA. Diets of individuals based on energy intakes from added sugars. *Fam Econ Nutr Rev*. 1999;12: 31–38.
11. Welsh S, Davis C, Shaw A. *USDA's Food Guide: Background and Development*. Hyattsville, MD: U.S. Department of Agriculture, 1993.
12. Matthews RH, Pehrsson PR, Farhat-Sabet M. *Sugar Content of Selected Foods: Individual and Total Sugars*. Washington, DC: U.S. Department of Agriculture, 1987.
13. Mattes RD. Dietary compensation by humans for supplemental energy provided as ethanol or carbohydrate in fluids. *Physiol Behav*. 1996;59: 179–187.
14. De Castro JM. The effects of the spontaneous ingestion of particular foods or beverages on the meal pattern and overall nutrient intake of humans. *Physiol Behav*. 1993;53: 1133–1144.
15. Harnack L, Stang J, Story M. Soft drink consumption among US children and adolescents: nutritional consequences. *J Am Diet Assoc*. 1999;99: 436–441.
16. Ludwig DS, Peterson KE, Gortmaker SL. Relation between consumption of sugar-sweetened drinks and childhood obesity: a prospective, observational analysis. *Lancet*. 2001;357: 505–508.
17. Berkey CS, Rockett HR, Field AE, Gillman MW, Colditz GA. Sugar-added beverages and adolescent weight change. *Obes Res*. 2004;12: 778–788.
18. James J, Thomas P, Cavan D, Kerr D. Preventing childhood obesity by reducing consumption of carbonated drinks: cluster randomised controlled trial. *BMJ*. 2004;328: 1237.
19. Bowman BA, Gortmaker SL, Ebbeling CB, Pereira MA, Ludwig DS. Effects of fast food consumption on energy intake and diet quality among children in a national household survey. *Pediatrics*. 2004;113: 112–118.
20. French SA, Story M, Neumark-Sztainer D, Fulkerson JA, Hannan P. Fast food restaurant use among adolescents: associations with nutrient intake, food choices and behavioral and psychosocial variables. *Int J Obes*. 2001;25: 1823–1833.

21. Guthrie JF, Lin B-H, Frazao E. Role of food prepared away from home in the American diet, 1977–78 versus 1994–96: changes and consequences. *Int J Obes*. 2002;34: 140–150.

22. Ebbeling CB, Pawlak DB, Ludwig DS. Childhood obesity: public-health crisis, common sense cure. *Lancet*. 2002;360: 473–482.

23. Prentice AM, Jebb SA. Fast foods, energy density and obesity: a possible mechanistic link. *Obes Rev*. 2003;4: 187–194.

24. McNutt SW, Hu Y, Schreiber GB, Crawford PB, Obarzanek E, Mellin L. A longitudinal study of the dietary practices of black and white girls 9 and 10 years old at enrollment: the NHLBI Growth and Health Study. *J Adolesc Health*. 1997;20: 27–37.

25. Ebbeling CB, Sinclair KB, Pereira MA, Garcia-Lago E, Feldman HA, Ludwig DS. Compensation for energy intake from fast food among overweight and lean adolescents. *JAMA*. 2004;291: 2828–2833.

26. Pereira MA, Kartashov AI, Ebbeling CB, Van Horn L, Slattery ML, Jacobs DR, Jr., Ludwig DS. Fast food habits, weight gain, and insulin resistance (the CARDIA study): 15-year prospective analysis. *Lancet*. 2005;365: 36–42.

27. Brownell KD, Horgen KB. *Food Fight: The Inside Story of the Food Industry, America's Obesity Crisis, and What We Can Do About It*. Chicago, IL: Contemporary Books, 2004.

28. Nielson SJ, Popkin BM. Patterns and trends in food portion sizes, 1977–1998. *JAMA*. 2003;289: 450–453.

29. Diliberti N, Bordi PL, Conklin MT, Roe LS, Rolls BJ. Increased portion size leads to increased energy intake in a restaurant meal. *Obes Res*. 2004;12: 562–568.

30. Levitsky DA, Youn T. The more food young adults are served, the more they overeat. *J Nutr*. 2004;134: 2546–2549.

31. McConahy KL, Smiciklas-Wright H, Mitchell DC, Picciano MF. Portion size of common foods predicts energy intake among preschool-aged children. *J Am Diet Assoc*. 2004;104: 975–979.

32. Fisher JO, Rolls BJ, Birch LL. Children's bite size and intake of an entree are greater with large portions than with age-appropriate or self-selected portions. *Am J Clin Nutr*. 2003;77: 1164–1170.

33. Nicklas TA, Baranowski T, Cullen KW, Berenson G. Eating patterns, dietary quality and obesity. *J Am Coll Nutr*. 2001;20: 599–608.

34. Jahns L, Siega-Riz AM, Popkin BM. The increasing prevalence of snacking among US children from 1977 to 1996. *J Pediatr*. 2001;138: 493–498.

35. Neumark-Sztainer D, Hannan PJ, Story M, Croll J, Perry C. Family meal patterns: associations with sociodemographic characteristics and improved dietary intake among adolescents. *J Am Diet Assoc*. 2003;103: 317–322.

36. Gillman MW, Rifas-Shiman SL, Frazier AL, Rockett HRH, Camargo CA, Field AE, et al. Family dinner and diet quality among older children and adolescents. *Arch Fam Med*. 2000;9: 235–240.

37. Ma Y, Bertone ER, Stanek EJ, 3rd, Reed GW, Hebert JR, Cohen NL, et al. Association between eating patterns and obesity in a free-living US adult population. *Am J Epidemiol*. 2003;158: 85–92.

38. Siega-Riz AM, Popkin BM, Carson T. Trends in breakfast consumption for children in the United States from 1965–1991. *Am J Clin Nutr*. 1998;67: 748S-756S.

39. Obarzanek E, Kimm SY, Barton BA, VanHorn LL, Kwiterovich PO, Simons-Morton DG, et al. Long-term safety and efficacy of a cholesterol-lowering diet in children with elevated low-density lipoprotein cholesterol: seven-year results of the Dietary Intervention Study in Children (DISC). *Pediatrics*. 2001;107: 256–264.

40. Luepker RV, Perry CL, McKinlay SM, Nader PR, Parcel GS, Stone EJ, et al. Outcomes of a field trial to improve children's dietary patterns and physical activity: the Child and Adolescent Trial for Cardiovascular Health (CATCH). *JAMA*. 1996;275: 768–776.

41. Epstein LH, Myers MD, Raynor HA, Saelens BE. Treatment of pediatric obesity. *Pediatrics*. 1998;101: 554–570.

42. Epstein LH, Valoski A, Wing RR, McCurley J. Ten-year follow-up of behavioral, family-based treatment for obese children. *JAMA*. 1990;264: 2519–2523.

43. Epstein LH, Valoski AM, Wing RR, McCurley J. Ten year outcomes of behavioral family-based treatment for childhood obesity. *Health Psychol*. 1994;13: 373–383.

44. Butler D. Science of dieting: slim pickings. *Nature*. 2004;428: 252–254.

45. Stephenson J. Low-carb, low-fat diet gurus face off. *JAMA*. 2003;289: 1767–1768, 1773.

46. http://www.mypyramid.gov (accessed July 2005).

47. Ludwig DS, Jenkins DJ. Carbohydrates and the postprandial state: have our cake and eat it too? *Am J Clin Nutr.* 2004;80: 797–798.

48. Barlow SE, Dietz WH. Obesity evaluation and treatment: expert committee recommendations. *Pediatrics.* 1998;102: E29.

49. Nicklas T, Johnson R. Position of the American Dietetic Association: dietary guidance for healthy children ages 2 to 11 years. *J Am Diet Assoc.* 2004;104: 660–677.

50. Ornish D. *Eat More, Weigh Less.* New York: Harper Collins Publishers, 2001.

51. Atkins RC. *Atkins for Life.* New York: St. Martin's Griffin, 2004.

52. Astrup A. The role of dietary fat in the prevention and treatment of obesity. Efficacy and safety of low-fat diets. *Int J Obes Relat Metab Disord.* 2001;25: S46–S50.

53. Bray GA, Popkin BM. Dietary fat does affect obesity! *Am J Clin Nutr.* 1998;68: 1157–1173.

54. Hill JO, Melanson EL, Wyatt HT. Dietary fat intake and regulation of energy balance: implications for obesity. *J Nutr.* 2000;130: 284S–288S.

55. Jequier E. Pathways to obesity. *Int J Obes.* 2002;26: S12–S17.

56. Ornish D. Was Dr Atkins right? *J Am Diet Assoc.* 2004;104: 537–542.

57. Astrup A, Meinert Larsen T, Harper A. Atkins and other low-carbohydrate diets: hoax or an effective tool for weight loss? *Lancet.* 2004;364: 897–899.

58. Bray GA. Low-carbohydrate diets and realities of weight loss. *JAMA.* 2003;289: 1853–1855.

59. Wylie-Rosett J, Swencionis C, Caban A, Friedler AJ, Schaffer N. *The Complete Weight Loss Workbook: Proven Techniques for Controlling Weight-Related Health Problems.* Alexandria, VA: American Diabetes Association, 1997.

60. Baron JA, Schori A, Crow B, Carter R, Mann JI. A randomized controlled trial of low carbohydrate and low fat/high fiber diets for weight loss. *J Public Health.* 1986;76: 1293–1296.

61. Jeffery RW, Hellerstedt WL, French SA, Baxter JE. A randomized trial of counseling for fat restriction versus calorie restriction in the treatment of obesity. *Int J Obes.* 1995;19: 132–137.

62. Harvey-Berino J. Calorie restriction is more effective for obesity treatment than dietary fat restriction. *Ann Behav Med.* 1999;21: 35–39.

63. Brehm BJ, Seeley RJ, Daniels SR, D'Alessio DA. A randomized trial comparing a very low carbohydrate diet and a calorie-restricted low fat diet on body weight and cardiovascular risk factors in healthy women. *J Clin Endocrinol Metab.* 2003;88: 1617–1623.

64. Foster GD, Wyatt HR, Hill JO, McGuckin BG, Brill C, Mohammed BS, et al. A randomized trial of a low-carbohydrate diet for obesity. *N Engl J Med.* 2003;348: 2082–2090.

65. Ebbeling CB, Leidig MM, Sinclair KB, Hangen JP, Ludwig DS. A reduced glycemic load diet in the treatment of adolescent obesity. *Arch Pediatr Adolesc Med.* 2003;157: 773–779.

66. Yancy WS, Olsen MK, Guyton JR, Bakst RP, Westman EC. A low-carbohydrate, ketogenic diet versus a low-fat diet to treat obesity and hyperlipidemia. *Ann Intern Med.* 2004;140: 769–777.

67. Stern L, Iqbal N, Seshadri P, Chicano KL, Daily DA, McGrory J, et al. The effects of low-carbohydrate versus conventional weight loss diets in severely obese adults: one-year follow-up of a randomized trial. *Ann Intern Med.* 2004;140: 778–785.

68. Astrup A, Grunwald GK, Melanson EL, Saris WHM, Hill JO. The role of low-fat diets in body weight control: a meta-analysis of *ad libitum* dietary intervention studies. *Int J Obes.* 2000;24: 1545–1552.

69. Pirozzo S, Summerbell C, Cameron C, Glasziou P. Should we recommend low-fat diets for obesity? *Obes Rev.* 2003;4: 83–90.

70. Willett WC. Is dietary fat a major determinant of body fat? *Am J Clin Nutr.* 1998;67: 556S–562S.

71. Shah M, McGovern P, French S, Baxter J. Comparison of a low-fat, ad libitum complex-carbohydrate diet with a low-energy diet in moderately obese women. *Am J Clin Nutr.* 1994;59: 980–984.

72. Lean MEJ, Han TS, Prvan T, Richmond PR, Avenell A. Weight loss with high and low carbohydrate 1200 kcal diets in free living women. *Eur J Clin Nutr.* 1997;51: 243–248.

73. Harvey-Berino J. The efficacy of dietary fat vs. total energy restriction for weight loss. *Obes Res.* 1998;6: 202–207.

74. Samaha FF, Iqbal N, Seshadri P, Chicano KL, Daily DA, McGrory J, et al. A low-carbohydrate as compared with a low-fat diet in severe obesity. *N Engl J Med.* 2003;348: 2074–2081.

75. Shah M, Baxter JE, McGovern PG, Garg A. Nutrient and food intake in obese women on a low-fat or low-calorie diet. *Am J Health Promot.* 1996;10: 179–182.

76. Pascale RW, Wing RR, Butler BA, Mullen M, Bononi P. Effects of behavioral weight loss program stressing calorie restriction versus calorie plus fat restriction in obese individuals with NIDDM or a family history of diabetes. *Diabetes Care*. 1995;18: 1241–1248.

77. McManus K, Antinoro L, Sacks F. A randomized controlled trial of a moderate-fat, low-energy diet cmpared with a low fat, low-energy diet for weight loss in overweight adults. *Int J Obes*. 2001;25: 1503–1511.

78. Sondike SB, Copperman N, Jacobson MS. Effects of a low-carbohydrate diet on weight loss and cardiovascular risk factors in overweight adolescents. *J Pediatr*. 2003;142: 253–258.

79. St. Jeor ST, Howard BV, Prewitt TE, Bovee V, Bazzarre T, Eckel RH. Dietary protein and weight reduction: a statement for healthcare professionals from the Nutrition Committee of the Council on Nutrition, Physical Activity, and Metabolism of the American Heart Association. *Circulation*. 2001;104: 1869–1874.

80. Bravata DM, Sanders L, Huang J, Krumholz HM, Olkin I, Gardner CD, Bravata DM. Efficacy and safety of low-carbohydrate diets: a systematic review. *JAMA*. 2003;289: 1837–1850.

81. Fleming RM. The effect of high-, moderate-, and low-fat diets on weight loss and cardiovascular disease risk factors. *Prev Cardiol*. 2002;5: 110–118.

82. Koertge J, Weidner G, Elliott-Eller M, Scherwitz L, Merritt-Worden TA, Marlin R, et al. Improvement in medical risk factors and quality of life in women and men with coronary artery disease in the multicenter lifestyle demonstration project. *Am J Cardiol*. 2003;91: 1316–1322.

83. Mueller-Cunningham WM, Quintana R, Kasim-Karakas SE. An ad libitum, very low-fat diet results in weight loss and changes in nutrient intakes in postmenopausal women. *J Am Diet Assoc*. 2003;103: 1600–1606.

84. Ornish D, Scherwitz LW, Billings JH, Gould L, Merritt TA, Sparler S, et al. Intensive lifestyle changes for reversal of coronary heart disease. *JAMA*. 1998;280: 2001–2007.

85. Rolls BJ. The role of energy density in the overconsumption of fat. *J Nutr*. 2000;130: 268S–271S.

86. Ello-Martin J, Roe L, Rolls B. A diet reduced in energy density results in greater weight loss than a diet reduced in fat. *Obes Res*. 2004;12: A23.

87. Wahlqvist ML, Wilmshurst EG, Richardson EN. The effect of chain length on glucose absorption and the related metabolic response. *Am J Clin Nutr*. 1978;31: 1998–2001.

88. Bantle JP, Laine DC, Castle GW, Thomas JW, Hoogwerf BJ, Goetz FC. Postprandial glucose and insulin responses to meals containing different carbohydrates in normal and diabetic subjects. *N Engl J Med*. 1983;309: 7–12.

89. Granfeldt Y, Bjorck I, Hagander B. On the importance of processing conditions, product thickness and egg addition for the glycaemic and hormonal responses to pasta: a comparison with bread made from "pasta ingredients". *Eur J Clin Nutr*. 1991;45: 489–499.

90. Jenkins DJA, Wolever TMS, Taylor RH, Barker H, Fielden H, Baldwin JM, et al. Glycemic index of foods: a physiological basis for carbohydrate exchange. *Am J Clin Nutr*. 1981;34: 362–366.

91. Wolever TMS, Jenkins DJA, Jenkins AL, Josse RG. The glycemic index: methodology and clinical implications. *Am J Clin Nutr*. 1991;54: 846–854.

92. Ebbeling CB, Ludwig LS. Treating obesity in youth: should dietary glycemic load be a consideration? *Adv Pediatr*. 2001;48: 179–212.

93. Foster-Powell K, Holt SHA, Brand-Miller JC. International table of glycemic index and glycemic load values: 2002. *Am J Clin Nutr*. 2002;76: 5–56.

94. Jenkins DJ, Wolever TM, Collier GR, Ocana A, Rao AV, Buckley G, et al. Metabolic effects of a low-glycemic-index diet. *Am J Clin Nutr*. 1987;46: 968–975.

95. Miller JC. Importance of glycemic index in diabetes. *Am J Clin Nutr*. 1994;59: 747S-752S.

96. Salmeron J, Manson JE, Stampfer MJ, Colditz GA, Wing AL, Willett WC. Dietary fiber, glycemic load, and risk of non-insulin-dependent diabetes mellitus in women. *JAMA*. 1997;277: 472–477.

97. Brand-Miller JC, Thomas M, Swan V, Ahmad ZI, Petocz P, Colagiuri S. Physiological validation of the concept of glycemic load in lean young adults. *J Nutr*. 2003;133: 2728–2732.

98. Ludwig DS. The glycemic index: physiological mechanisms relating to obesity, diabetes, and cardio-vascular disease. *JAMA*. 2002;287: 2414–2423.

99. Kabir M, Rizkalla SW, Quignard-Boulange A, Guerre-Millo M, Boillot J, Ardouin B, et al. A high glycemic index starch diet affects lipid storage-related enzymes in normal and to a lesser extent in diabetic rats. *J Nutr*. 1998;128: 1878–1883.

100. Kabir M, Rizkalla SW, Champ M, Luo J, Boillot J, Bruzzo F, Slama G. Dietary amylose-amylopectin starch content affects glucose and lipid metabolism in adipocytes of normal and diabetic rats. *J Nutr.* 1998;128: 35–43.

101. Pawlak DB, Kushner JA, Ludwig DS. Effects of dietary glycaemic index on adiposity, glucose homoeostasis, and plasma lipids in animals. *Lancet.* 2004;364: 778–785.

102. Ludwig DS, Majzoub JA, Al-Zahrani A, Dallal GE, Blanco I, Roberts SB. High glycemic index foods, overeating, and obesity. *Pediatrics.* 1999;103: E26.

103. Ball SD, Keller KR, Moyer-Mileur LJ, Ding YW, Donaldson D, Jackson WD. Prolongation of satiety after low versus moderately high glycemic index meals in obese adolescents. *Pediatrics.* 2003;111: 488–494.

104. Warren JM, Henry CJ, Simonite V. Low glycemic index breakfasts and reduced food intake in preadolescent children. *Pediatrics.* 2003;112: E414.

105. Pereira MA, Swain J, Goldfine AB, Rifai N, Ludwig DS. Effects of a low-glycemic load diet on resting energy expenditure and heart disease risk factors during weight loss. *JAMA.* 2004;292: 2482–2490.

106. Leibel RL, Rosenbaum M, Hirsch J. Changes in energy expenditure resulting from altered body weight. *N Engl J Med.* 1995;332: 621–628.

107. Bouche C, Rizkalla SW, Luo J, Vidal H, Veronese A, Pacher N, et al. Five-week, low-glycemic index diet decreases total fat mass and improves plasma lipid profile in moderately overweight nondiabetic men. *Diabetes Care.* 2002;25: 822–828.

108. Slabber M, Barnard HC, Kuyl JM, Dannhauser A, Schall R. Effects of a low-insulin-response, energy-restricted diet on weight loss and plasma insulin concentrations in hyperinsulinemic obese females. *Am J Clin Nutr.* 1994;60: 48–53.

109. Spieth LE, Harnish JD, Lenders CM, Raezer LB, Pereira MA, Hangen SJ, Ludwig DS. A low glycemic index diet in the treatment of pediatric obesity. *Arch Pediatr Adol Med.* 2000;154: 947–951.

110. Clapp JF. Diet, exercise, and feto-placental growth. *Arch Gynecol Obstet.* 1997;261: 101–108.

111. Whitaker RC, Dietz WH. Role of the prenatal environment in the development of obesity. *J Pediatr.* 1998;132: 768–776.

112. Sloth B, Krog-Mikkelsen I, Flint A, Tetens I, Bjorck I, Vinoy S, et al. No difference in body weight decrease between a low-glycemic-index and a high-glycemic-index diet but reduced LDL cholesterol after 10-wk ad libitum intake of the low-glycemic-index diet. *Am J Clin Nutr.* 2004;80: 337–347.

113. Gilbertson HR, Brand-Miller JC, Thorburn AW, Evans S, Chondros P, Werther GA. The effect of flexible low glycemic index dietary advice versus measured carbohydrate exchange diets on glycemic control in children with type 1 diabetes. *Diabetes Care.* 2001;24: 1137–1143.

114. Wang H, Storlien LH, Huang XF. Effects of dietary fat types on body fatness, leptin, and ARC leptin receptor, NPY, and AgRP mRNA expression. *Am J Physiol Endocrinol Metab.* 2002;282: E1352–1359.

115. Young-Hyman D, Schlundt DG, Herman L, DeLuca F, Counts D. Evaluation of the insulin resistance syndrome in 5- to 10-year-old overweight/obese African-American children. *Diabetes Care.* 2001;24: 1359–1364.

116. Weiss R, Dziura J, Burgert TS, Tamborlane WV, Taksali SE, Yeckel CW, et al. Obesity and the metabolic syndrome in children and adolescents. *N Engl J Med.* 2004;350: 2362–2374.

117. Buyken AE, Toeller M, Heitkamp G, Karamanos B, Rottiers R, Muggeo M, Fuller JH. Glycemic index in the diet of European outpatients with type 1 diabetes: relations to glycated hemoglobin and serum lipids. *Am J Clin Nutr.* 2001;73: 574–581.

118. Ford ES, Liu S. Glycemic index and serum high-density lipoprotein cholesterol concentration among US adults. *Arch Intern Med.* 2001;161: 572–576.

119. Frost G, Leeds AA, Dore CJ, Madeiros S, Brading S, Dornhorst A. Glycemic index as a determinant of serum HDL-cholesterol concentration. *Lancet.* 1999;353: 1045–1048.

120. Liu S, Manson JE, Stampfer MJ, Holmes MD, Hu FB, Hankinson SE, Willett WC. Dietary glycemic load assessed by food-frequency questionnaire in relation to plasma high-density-lipoprotein cholesterol and fasting plasma triacylglycerols in postmenopausal women. *Am J Clin Nutr.* 2001;73: 560–566.

121. Liu S, Willett WC, Stampfer MJ, Hu FB, Franz M, Sampson L, et al. A prospective study of dietary glycemic load, carbohydrate intake, and risk of coronary heart disease in women. *Am J Clin Nutr.* 2000;71: 1455–1461.

122. Salmeron J, Ascherio A, Rimm EB, Colditz GA, Spiegelman D, Jenkins DJ, et al. Dietary fiber, glycemic load, and risk of NIDDM in men. *Diabetes Care.* 1997;20: 545–550.

123. Salmeron J, Hu FB, Manson JE, Stampfer MJ, Colditz GA, Rimm EB, Willett WC. Dietary fat intake and risk of type 2 diabetes in women. *Am J Clin Nutr.* 2001;73: 1019–1026.

124. Schulze MB, Liu S, Rimm EB, Manson JE, Willett WC, Hu FB. Glycemic index, glycemic load, and dietary fiber intake and incidence of type 2 diabetes in younger and middle-aged women. *Am J Clin Nutr.* 2004;80: 348–356.

125. Meyer KA, Kushi LH, Jacobs DR, Slavin J, Sellers TA, Folsom AR. Carbohydrates, dietary fiber, and incident type 2 diabetes in older women. *Am J Clin Nutr.* 2000;71: 921–930.

126. Stevens J, Ahn K, Juhaeri, Houston D, Steffan L, Couper D. Dietary fiber intake and glycemic index and incidence of diabetes in African-American and white adults: the ARIC study. *Diabetes Care.* 2002;25: 1715–1721.

127. vanDam RM, Visscher AWJ, Feskens EJM, Verhoef P, Kromhout D. Dietary glycemic index in relation to metabolic risk factors and incidence of coronary heart disease: the Zutphen Elderly Study. *Eur J Clin Nutr.* 2000;54: 726–731.

128. Litin L, Sacks F. Trans-fatty-acid content of common foods. *N Engl J Med.* 1993;329: 1969–1970.

129. Hu FB, Stampfer MJ, Manson JE, Rimm E, Colditz GA, Rosner BA, et al. Dietary fat intake and the risk of coronary heart disease in women. *N Engl J Med.* 1997;337: 1491–1499.

19 Breastfeeding and Overweight

Elsie M. Taveras and Matthew W. Gillman

CONTENTS

INTRODUCTION

Over 75 years ago, the *Journal of the American Medical Association* published a study that reported a reduction in risk of obesity among children 7 to 13 years of age who had been breastfed during infancy compared with those who had been artificially fed.[1] In the decades since this report, the relationship between breastfeeding and later overweight has been examined in many epidemiological studies that now include outcomes of overweight and obesity from childhood into adulthood. In a review of studies published between 1976 through 1999, Butte[2] reported that most studies showed no association between breastfeeding and later overweight. Several of the studies published since 1999 have addressed the limitations of earlier studies and have included larger sample sizes and adjustment for potential confounders, most importantly parental obesity. Taken as a whole, these most recent studies suggest that breastfeeding is associated with reduced risk of childhood overweight.[3] Whether infant feeding is related to later overweight is especially important today given the high rates and profound consequences of childhood overweight.

This overview is organized into four sections. The first section cites current data on breastfeeding initiation, duration, and exclusivity in the United States. In the second section we review published literature on the association of breastfeeding and overweight by age group and highlight the strengths and limitations of studies published within the last 10 years. In the third section we explore potential mechanisms that may mediate the relationship between breastfeeding and overweight. Finally, in the last section we discuss clinical and public health implications.

PREVALENCE OF BREASTFEEDING INITIATION, EXCLUSIVITY, AND DURATION IN THE UNITED STATES

Prolonged and exclusive breastfeeding has multiple health benefits for infants and their mothers.[4–7] Both the American Academy of Pediatrics (AAP) and the World Health Organization (WHO) recommend exclusive breastfeeding for the first 6 months of life and continuation of any breast-feeding until 12 months.[8,9]

Although rates of breastfeeding initiation have increased in recent years from a low of 25% in the 1970s[10] to 65% in 2001,[11] breastfeeding continuation lags behind the national goals of 50% at 6 months and 25% at 12 months (short by 23 and 13 percentage points, respectively).[12] Initiation and maintenance of *exclusive* breastfeeding are also low in the United States. Between 1991 and 1994, 47% of mothers were exclusively breastfeeding at 7 days after birth, but exclusive breast-feeding rates were only 10% at 6 months.[13] In 2001, exclusive breastfeeding rates at 6 months were just 7.9% in a national study of 896 households.[11] Moreover, racial and ethnic minorities and women of lower socioeconomic position initiate and maintain breastfeeding rates at much lower lev-els,[10,13–16] and these groups have particularly high rates of obesity in childhood and beyond.[17,18]

ASSOCIATION OF BREASTFEEDING WITH OVERWEIGHT IN CHILDREN AND ADOLESCENTS

Despite differences in methodology, several recent studies are consistent in demonstrating a reduced risk of overweight among children and adolescents who were ever breastfed as infants.[19–27] Some of the studies also indicate that increased duration of breastfeeding predicts lower rates of child and adolescent overweight.[19,22–24,27]

We reviewed studies that examined the association of breastfeeding with overweight in child-hood, adolescence, and adulthood that were published in the last 10 years and had a minimum sample size of 100 per feeding group. We focused on studies published in the last decade because of the many limitations of earlier studies, which included inadequate sample sizes, varying defini-tions of breastfeeding, inconsistent measurement and definitions of "at risk of overweight" and overweight, and lack of adjustment for confounders.[3] Because breastfeeding could also potentially benefit failure to thrive, we further limited our review to studies that reported odds ratios (OR) of overweight rather than differences in mean body mass index. Table 19.1, Table 19.2, and Table 19.3 show the 15 studies that met our criteria. Seven studies focused on preschool children under 6 years of age (Table 19.1), seven reported outcomes of children and adolescents between the ages of 6 to 15 (Table 19.2), and four studies reported outcomes of older adolescents and adults (Table 19.3). We present the review by age group for ease of comparison of studies that have similar end points for measurement of overweight and because studies of younger children may be subject to less confounding and those of older adolescents may be more meaningful in predicting adult obesity and its related comorbidities.[28]

STUDIES OF PRESCHOOL-AGED CHILDREN

Of the seven studies of breastfeeding and overweight among preschool-aged children, two[19,20] considered breastfeeding both as a dichotomous variable (e.g., ever vs. never) and as breastfeeding duration (e.g., length of any or exclusive breastfeeding), one[21] used only a dichotomous definition, and four[22,27,29,30] had only duration data. The definitions of overweight included age–sex-specific body mass index (BMI) above the 90th, 95th, 97th, or 98th percentiles and one study[27] defined overweight as a BMI greater than 25 mg/kg[2]. To define the percentiles, four of the studies[19–22] used reference data from countries where the studies were conducted, and one[29] used study cohort–based reference data.

In the three studies using the dichotomous breastfeeding exposure, the odds ratios for over-weight (age–sex-specific BMI above the 95th, 97th, or 98th percentiles) in the breastfeeding group ranged from 0.70 to 0.84. Among 3-year-old children in Scotland, Armstrong et al.[21] reported an odds ratio of 0.72 (95% confidence interval [CI]: 0.65, 0.79) for having a BMI > 95th percentile and an odds ratio of 0.70 (95% CI: 0.61, 0.80) for having a BMI > 98th percentile. Von Kries et al.[19] reported an odds ratio of 0.75 (95% CI: 0.57, 0.98) for having a BMI > 97th percentile among

5- to 6-year-old children in Germany, and Hediger et al.[20] reported an odds ratio of 0.84 (95% CI: 0.62, 1.13) for having a BMI > 95th percentile among U.S. children ages 3 to 5. Hediger et al.[20] and von Kries et al.[19] also demonstrated a reduction in being "at risk of overweight" (age–sex-specific BMI above the 85th or 90th percentiles) with adjusted odds ratios of 0.63 (95% CI; 0.41, 0.96)[20] and 0.79 (95% CI; 0.68, 0.93).[9]

Of the six studies that examined breastfeeding duration, four observed an inverse association between breastfeeding and overweight and two did not. Von Kries et al. observed a protective "dose-response" effect, i.e., decreased odds of overweight with increasing duration.[19] In race-specific analyses of 12,587 4-year-old U.S. children, Grummer-Strawn and Mei[22] showed an inverse association between breastfeeding and overweight only among non-Hispanic whites, but not among non-Hispanic blacks or Hispanics. In comparison with children who were breastfed for more than 6 months, O'Callaghan et al.[29] observed an increase in odds of overweight in children who were never breastfed (OR 1.4, 95% CI: 0.8, 2.3), breastfed for less than 2 weeks and for 3 to 6 weeks (OR 1.1, 95% CI: 0.6, 2.0), and those who were breastfed for 7 weeks to 3 months (OR 1.6, 95% CI: 1.0, 2.7). Finally, Bogen et al.[30] found a reduction in overweight risk among 4-year-old low-income white children who were breastfed for at least 16 weeks (OR 0.71, 95% CI: 0.56, 0.92) and whose mothers had not smoked in pregnancy, compared with those who were never breastfed. Hediger et al.[20] and Poulton and Williams[27] did not show a clear inverse relationship between breastfeeding and overweight in this age group. Both studies, however, had wide confidence intervals for the breastfeeding categories of longest duration and may have been underpowered to detect an association.

The studies by von Kries et al.[19] and Grummer-Strawn and Mei[22] were unique in this age group for examining prolonged breastfeeding, that is, breastfeeding for over 1 year. Von Kreis et al. found a 57% reduction in the adjusted odds of being overweight at 5 to 6 years of age when contrasting those who were breastfed for at least 12 months with those who were never breastfed (Table 19.4). Grummer-Strawn and Mei found a 51% reduction for a similar comparison.

Two of the six studies[19,20] reported the association between *exclusive* breastfeeding and overweight. In both studies, exclusive breastfeeding was associated with decreased odds of overweight and "at risk of overweight," but the odds ratios included unity in the study by Hediger et al.[20]

Finally, all of the studies adjusted for potential confounders such as markers of socioeconomic status, but only four[22,27,29,31] included parental body mass index or overweight status. In most cases, adjustment for parental BMI resulted in modest attenuation (8% to 25%) of the effect estimates.

STUDIES OF CHILDREN AGES 6 TO 15

Of the seven studies of breastfeeding and overweight among children and young adolescents ages 6 to 15 years, two[23,24] considered breastfeeding both as a dichotomous variable and as breastfeeding duration, two[25,26] used only a dichotomous definition, and three[27,32,33] had only duration data. The studies used an age–sex-specific BMI between the 85th to 95th percentiles or BMI greater than 90th percentile to define "at risk of overweight," BMI over 95th or 97th percentiles to define overweight, and one study defined overweight as a BMI of greater than 25 mg/kg[2].

Among the four studies using the dichotomous breastfeeding exposure, as for the younger children, all showed a reduction in being "at risk of overweight" and overweight in the breastfeeding group with odds ratios ranging from 0.46 to 0.80. In a study of 2108 German children ages 9 to 10 years, Liese et al.[23] reported an OR of 0.66 (95% CI: 0.52, 0.87) for having a BMI greater than the 90th percentile. Gillman et al.[24] reported an OR of 0.95 (95% CI: 0.84, 1.07) for being "at risk of overweight" (age- and sex-specific BMI 85th to 94th percentiles) and 0.78 (95% CI: 0.66, 0.91) for being overweight (BMI > 95th percentile) among 15,341 U.S. adolescents. Toschke et al.[25] reported an OR of 0.80 (95% CI: 0.71, 0.90) for having a BMI over the 90th percentile and 0.80 (95% CI: 0.66, 0.96) for having a BMI over the 97th percentile among 33,768 children ages 6 to 14 in the Czech Republic. Finally, in a small study of 480 6-year-old German children, Bergmann

TABLE 19.1
Association of Breastfeeding with Overweight — Studies of Children under 6 Years of Age

Country	N	Age (yr)	BMI Cutpoints to Define Outcomes	Breastfeeding Exposure		Results (AOR, 95% CI)		Covariates	Ref.
				Dichotomous	Duration	Dichotomous	Duration		
Australia	3909	5	BMI 85th – 94th % BMI > 95th% From study cohort data	—	Never breastfed	—	1.2 (0.8, 1.7)	Birth weight, gender, gestational age, feeding problems, sleep problems, parental BMI, education, and income	29
					BF < 2 weeks		1.5 (1.0, 2.2)		
					BF 3–6 weeks		1.3 (0.8, 1.9)		
					BF 7 weeks–3 months		1.1 (0.7, 1.7)		
					BF 4–6 months		1.4 (0.9, 2.1)		
					BF > 6 months		1.0 (ref)		
					Never breastfed		1.4 (0.8, 2.3)		
					BF < 2 weeks		1.1 (0.6, 2.0)		
					BF 3–6 weeks		1.1 (0.6, 2.0)		
					BF 7 weeks–3 months		1.6 (1.0, 2.7)		
					BF 4–6 months		0.7 (0.3, 1.4)		
					BF > 6 months		1.0 (ref)		
Germany	9357	5–6	BMI > 90th% BMI > 97th% From German national data	Ever vs. never BF	Exclusive BF	0.79 (0.68, 0.93) 0.75 (0.57, 0.98)	0.89 (0.73, 1.07)	Parental education, maternal smoking during pregnancy, birth weight, child having his or her own bedroom, and frequent consumption of butter	19
					2 months		0.87 (0.72, 1.05)		
					3–5 months		0.67 (0.49, 0.91)		
					6–12 months		0.43 (0.17, 1.07)		
					> 12 months				
					Exclusive BF		0.90 (0.65, 1.24)		
					2 months		0.65 (0.44, 0.95)		
					3–5 months		0.57 (0.33, 0.99)		
					6–12 months		0.28 (0.04, 2.04)		
					> 12 months				

Country	Sample size	Age (years)	Overweight definition	Comparison	AOR (95% CI)	Breastfeeding category	AOR (95% CI)	Covariates	Ref
United States	2685	3–5	BMI 85th–94th%	Ever vs. never exclusively BF	0.63 (0.41, 0.96)	Never exclusively BF	1.0 (ref)	Maternal BMI, child's birth weight, race/ethnicity, gender, age, and timing of introduction of solid foods	20
			BMI > 95th%		0.84 (0.62, 1.13)	Exclusive BF 2 mon	0.57 (0.32, 1.02)		
			From U.S. national data			Exclusive BF 3–5 mon	0.69 (0.35, 1.33)		
						Exclusive BF 6–8 mon	0.55 (0.27, 1.12)		
						Exclusive BF 9 mon	0.76 (0.32, 1.80)		
						Never exclusively BF	1.0 (ref)		
						Exclusive BF 2 mon	0.98 (0.67, 1.43)		
						Exclusive BF 3–5 mon	0.70 (0.33, 1.48)		
						Exclusive BF 6–8 mon	0.65 (0.34, 1.24)		
						Exclusive BF 9 mon	0.75 (0.29, 1.95)		
Scotland	32,200	3	BMI > 95th%	BF vs. formula at 6–8 weeks	0.72 (0.65, 0.79)	—	—	Socioeconomic status, birth weight, and gender	21
			BMI > 98th%		0.70 (0.61, 0.80)				
			From U.K. national data						
United States	177,304	4	BMI > 95th%	—	—	Never breastfed	1.0 (ref)	Child's gender, race/ethnicity, and birth weight and mother's age, education, pre-pregnancy BMI, weight gain during pregnancy, and postpartum smoking	22
			From U.S. national data			BF < 1 month	0.98 (0.94, 1.03)		
						BF 1–2.9 months	0.88 (0.83, 0.93)		
						BF 3–5.9 months	0.81 (0.76, 0.87)		
						BF 6–11.9 months	0.73 (0.68, 0.79)		
						BF 12 months	0.72 (0.65, 0.80)		
United States	73,458	4	BMI > 95th%	—	—	Never breastfed	1.0 (ref)	Maternal age, education, parity, marital status, pregnancy conditions, delivery method, child sex, birth weight, birth order, and birth year	30
			From U.S. national data			BF < 8 weeks	0.97 (0.86, 1.09)		
						BF 8–15 weeks	0.80 (0.62, 1.03)		
						BF 16–26 weeks	0.71 (0.56, 0.92)		
						BF > 26 weeks	0.55 (0.42, 0.71)		
New Zealand	980	3–5	BMI > 25 kg/m²	—	—	Never BF	1.0 (ref)	Gender, birth weight, mother's education, and mother and father being overweight	27
						BF 6 months	0.75 (0.43, 1.32)		
						BF > 6 months	1.01 (0.48, 2.15)		
						At age 5 years			

Note: Inclusion criteria were studies published in the last 10 years, which had a minimum sample size of 100 per feeding group, and reported odds ratios for overweight.
AOR = adjusted odds ratio; (ref) = reference group.

TABLE 19.2
Association of Breastfeeding with Overweight — Studies of Children Ages 6–15 Years

Country	N	Age (yr)	BMI Cutpoints to Define Outcomes	Breastfeeding Exposure — Dichotomous	Breastfeeding Exposure — Duration	Results (AOR, 95% CI) — Dichotomous	Results (AOR, 95% CI) — Duration	Covariates	Ref.
United Kingdom	3550	6	BMI > 90th % BMI > 97th % From U.K reference data	—	Never BF BF 2 months BF 3–4 months BF 5–10 months BF > 10 months Never BF BF 2 months BF 3–4 months BF 5–10 months BF > 10 months	—	1.0 (ref) 0.72 (0.54, 0.95) 0.86 (0.61, 1.15) 0.98 (0.77, 1.24) 1.29 (0.84, 1.81) 1.0 (ref) 0.65 (0.41, 1.00) 0.83 (0.44, 1.21) 0.90 (0.58, 1.22) 1.05 (0.45, 1.69)	Social class, birth weight, household crowding, and fat intake	32
Germany	2108	9–10	BMI > 90th % From German national data	Ever vs. never BF	Never breastfed Any BF < 6 months Any BF > 6 months[a] Never breastfed Exclusive BF < 2 months Exclusive BF 2–4 months Exclusive BF > 5 months[b]	0.66 (0.52, 0.87)	1.0 (ref) 0.71 (0.51, 0.98) 0.56 (0.53, 0.90) 1.0 (ref) 0.70 (0.49, 0.99) 0.68 (0.48, 0.98) 0.51 (0.33, 0.80)	Child's age, gender, nationality, city of study, socioeconomic status, and environmental tobacco smoke	23
United States	15,341	9–14	BMI 85th–94th % BMI > 95th % From U.S. national data	Mostly/only breast milk vs. mostly/only formula for first 6 months of life	Any BF	0.95 (0.84, 1.07) 0.78 (0.66, 0.91)	0.93 (0.81, 1.05) 0.92 (0.87, 0.98) For every increment of 3 months of breastfeeding	Child's age, gender, Tanner stage, weekly hours of television and physical activity, daily energy intake, birth weight, birth order, household income, and mother's smoking, dietary restraint, BMI, weight cycling, and weight concerns	24

Country	N	Age (y)	Overweight definition	Breastfeeding category	AOR (95% CI)	Adjusted for	Ref
Czech Republic	33,768	6–14	BMI > 90th %; BMI >97th% From Czech Republic reference sample	Ever vs. never BF	0.80 (0.71, 0.90); 0.80 (0.66, 0.96)	Parental education, parental obesity, maternal smoking, birth weight, daily hours of television viewing, physical activity, and having siblings.	25
United Kingdom	1541	4–8	BMI > 95th% From U.K. national data	BF < 1 week; 1 wk to 1 month; 2–3 months; 4–6 months; 7–9 months; >9 months	1.0 (ref); 1.04 (0.57, 1.90); 0.68 (0.34, 1.35); 0.94 (0.50, 1.78); 1.14 (0.61, 2.16); 0.61 (0.28, 1.32)	Gender, parent's BMI, maternal smoking during pregnancy, birth weight, and social class	33
Germany	480	6	BMI 90th–97th%; BMI >97th% From French national data	BF 3 months vs. < 3 months	0.53 (0.31, 0.89); 0.46 (0.23, 0.92)	Mother's BMI, smoking in pregnancy, and social status	26
New Zealand	980	7–15	BMI > 25 kg/m² From international reference data	Never BF; BF 6 months; BF > 6 months	1.0 (ref); 0.85 (0.49, 1.46); 0.70 (0.30, 1.63) At age 15 years	Gender, birth weight, mother's education, and mother and father being overweight	27

Note: AOR = adjusted odds ratio; (ref) = reference group.

[a] Category includes breastfeeding 6 to 12 months and over 1 year.
[b] Category includes exclusively breastfeeding for 5 to 6 months and over 6 months.

TABLE 19.3
Association of Breastfeeding with Overweight — Studies of Older Adolescents and Adults

Country	N	Age (yr)	BMI Cutpoints to Define Outcomes	Breastfeeding Exposure Dichotomous	Breastfeeding Exposure Duration	Results (AOR, 95% CI) Dichotomous	Results (AOR, 95% CI) Duration	Covariates	Ref.
New Zealand	980	18–26	BMI > 25 kg/m²	—	Never BF BF 6 months BF > 6 months	—	1.0 (ref) 1.18 (0.83, 1.68) 0.97 (0.59, 1.60) At age 26 years	Gender, birth weight, mother's education, and mother and father being overweight	27
United Kingdom	9287	33	BMI 30 kg/m²	BF > 1 month vs. never	—	M: 0.93 (0.74, 1.17) F: 0.84 (0.67, 1.05)	—	Social class, mother's BMI, and mother's smoking	34
United Kingdom	1090	9–18	BMI > 95th% From U.K. national data	—	BF <1 week 1 week to 1 month 2–3 months 4–6 months 7–9 months > 9 months	—	1.0 (ref) 1.25 (0.65, 2.39) 0.69 (0.32, 1.52) 1.31 (0.62, 2.74) 2.02 (0.80, 5.10) 0.73 (0.23, 2.27)	Gender, parent's BMI, maternal smoking during pregnancy, birth weight, and social class	33

Brazil	2250	18	BMI 85th plus subscapular and triceps skinfolds 90th From World Health Organization data	—	Any BF
					  <1 month
					  1–2 months
					  3–5 months
					  6–8 months
					  9–11 months
					  12 months
					Predominant BF
					  <1 month
					  1–1.9 months
					  2–2.9 months
					  3–3.9 months
					  4 months
						—	
							1.08 (0.63, 1.84)
							1.09 (0.64, 1.84)
							0.38 (0.20, 0.72)
							1.20 (0.64, 2.24)
							1.05 (0.46, 2.42)
							1.0 (ref)
							
							1.42 (0.79, 2.56)
							1.14 (0.59, 2.22)
							1.02 (0.53, 1.94)
							0.80 (0.43, 1.48)
							1.0 (ref)
								Family income, maternal education at birth, maternal BMI, skin color, birth weight, gestational age, maternal smoking during pregnancy, and current behavioral variables (smoking, alcohol drinking, type of diet, and physical activity)	35

TABLE 19.4
Crude and Adjusted Odds Ratios (95% Confidence Intervals) of the Association between Having Been Breastfed and Breastfeeding Duration on Being Overweight (BMI > 90th Percentile) or Obese (BMI > 97th Percentile) in Children Aged 5 or 6 in Rural Bavaria

	Being Overweight		Being Obese	
	Crude Odds Ratio	Adjusted Odds Ratio[a]	Crude Odds Ratio	Adjusted Odds Ratio[a]
Ever breastfed (n = 5184)	0.70 (0.61 to 0.80)	0.79 (0.68 to 0.93)	0.61 (0.50 to 0.76)	0.75 (0.57 to 0.98)
Exclusively breastfed for:				
>2 months (n = 2084)	0.87 (0.74 to 1.02)	0.89 (0.73 to 1.02)	0.84 (0.64 to 1.10)	0.90 (0.65 to 1.24)
3–5 months (n = 2052)	0.64 (0.53 to 0.76)	0.87 (0.73 to 1.07)	0.50 (0.36 to 0.69)	0.65 (0.44 to 0.95)
6–12 months (n = 863)	0.51 (0.38 to 0.67)	0.67 (0.49 to 0.91)	0.38 (0.22 to 0.64)	0.57 (0.33 to 0.99)
>12 months (n = 5184)	0.36 (0.16 to 0.82)	0.43 (0.17 to 1.07)	0.61 (0.50 to 0.76)	0.28 (0.04 to 2.04)

Note: Ref = reference group.

[a] Odds ratios adjusted for level of parental education, maternal smoking during pregnancy, low birth weight, own bedroom, and frequent consumption of butter.

Adapted from von Kries R, Koletzko B, Sauerwald T, et al. *BMJ*. 1999;319: 147–50.

and Bergmann[26] reported an odds ratio of 0.53 (95% CI: 0.31, 0.89) for having a BMI between the 90th to 97th percentile and an OR of 0.46 (95% CI: 0.23, 0.92) for having a BMI over the 97th percentile).

Of the five studies that examined breastfeeding duration, Liese et al.,[23] Gillman et al.,[24] and Poulton and Williams[27] observed an inverse association between breastfeeding duration and overweight. Wadsworth et al.[32] found no relationship between breastfeeding duration and overweight and a suggestion that the lowest prevalence of overweight was associated with the shortest period of breastfeeding (OR 0.65, 95% CI: 0.41, 1.00, for children breastfed 2 months or less compared with those breastfed more than 10 months) among 3550 6-year-old children living in the United Kingdom. These children, however, were born in 1946, and the authors suggested that residual confounding by social factors associated with breastfeeding today (but not in the 1940s) might account for the inverse relationship observed in recent studies. Li et al.[33] also found no clear inverse relationship between breastfeeding and overweight in a study of 2631 offspring of a 1958 British cohort when they were between the ages of 4 to 8 and 9 to18 years. Compared with children who were breastfed for less than 1 week, the odds of being overweight were 0.94 (95% CI: 0.50, 1.78) for children who were breastfed for 4 to 6 months, 1.14 (95% CI: 0.61, 2.16) for children breastfed for 7 to 9 months, and 0.61 (95% CI: 0.28, 1.32) for those breastfed more than 9 months. This study, however, was limited by a small sample of 1541 children between the ages of 4 to 8 and 1090 children ages 9 to 18. In more than half of the breastfeeding duration categories, the sample size was less than 200.

Similar to the studies by von Kries et al.[19] and Grummer-Strawn and Mei,[22] Liese et al.[23] was also able to examine prolonged breastfeeding and its effect on overweight. Among a subset of 1754 children in their study who had been breastfed, the odds ratio was 0.41 (95% CI: 0.18, 0.90) for breastfeeding over 1 year compared with children who were breastfed less than 6 months.

Two of the studies reported the association between exclusive breastfeeding[23] or "mostly/only feeding breast milk"[24] and overweight. In both studies, exclusive breastfeeding and its duration were associated with decreased odds of overweight. Finally, five[24-27,33] of the seven studies included parental BMI as a potential confounder in their analyses. In all cases, adjustment for parental BMI resulted in modest attenuation of the effect estimates. In the study by Gillman et al.,[24] adjustment for maternal BMI attenuated the odds of overweight among adolescents who had been mostly or only fed breast milk by approximately 11%.

STUDIES OF OLDER ADOLESCENTS AND ADULTS

Four studies reported outcomes at ages greater than or equal to 18 years. Only one study[34] used a dichotomous breastfeeding exposure. The other three examined the association of breastfeeding duration with overweight. The outcomes differed in each study (Table 19.3).

In the study that used a dichotomous breastfeeding exposure, Parsons et al.[34] observed slightly decreased odds of overweight among men (OR 0.93, 95% CI: 0.74, 1.17) and women (OR 0.84, 95% CI: 0.67, 1.05) who had been breastfed for more than 1 month compared with those who had never been breastfed among 9287 33-year-old adult participants of the 1958 British birth cohort.

None of the three studies that examined duration of *any* breastfeeding[27,33,35] observed an inverse association between breastfeeding and overweight in this age group. However, all three had small sample sizes.

Victora et al.[35] also examined the relationship between duration of *predominant* breastfeeding and odds of overweight in a cohort of 2250 Brazilian men. Compared with men who had been breastfed for 4 months or more, the odds of overweight appeared to be higher for those who had never been breastfed (OR 1.42, 95% CI: 0.79, 2.56), breastfed for 1 to 1.9 months (OR 1.14, 95% CI: 0.59, 2.22), or breastfed for 2 to 2.9 months (OR 1.02, 95% CI: 0.53, 1.94), but wide confidence intervals prevent strong inferences.

All of the studies in this age group included parental BMI or overweight status in their analyses. Parsons et al.[34] observed a 5 to 7% attenuation in the odds for being obese among 33-year-old men and women who had been breastfed more than 1 month after adjusting for maternal BMI in separate multivariate models.

STRENGTHS AND LIMITATIONS OF STUDIES

Of the studies that met our review criteria, seven[19,21,22,24,25,30,34] deserve particular mention because of large sample sizes and adjustment for important potential confounders. Despite somewhat different exposure and outcome definitions, the five studies that examined a dichotomous breast-feeding exposure tend to agree on the magnitude of risk reduction for overweight, comparing children, adolescents, and adults who had been breastfed with those who were formula-fed: adjusted odds ratios ranged from 0.70 to 0.80 among children; in the one study of adults, the odds ratios were 0.84 for women and 0.93 for men. Four of the seven studies that had duration data[19,22,24,30] also showed that increased duration of breastfeeding predicted lower rates of later overweight.

Because of relatively large sample sizes and adjustment for numerous potential confounders, 3 of the 15 studies reviewed[22,24,30] provide the best evidence for a protective, dose-response relationship between breastfeeding duration and overweight. In a racially and ethnically diverse population of 12,587 4-year-old children in the United States, Grummer-Strawn and Mei[22] found that duration of breastfeeding was inversely associated with overweight (defined as a BMI-for-age at or above the 95th percentile based on the 2000 Centers for Disease Control growth charts) among non-Hispanic whites but not among non-Hispanic blacks or Hispanics. Among non-Hispanic whites, the adjusted odds ratio of overweight by breastfeeding for 6 to 12 months compared with never breastfeeding was 0.70 (95% CI: 0.50, 0.99) and for more than 12 months compared with never was 0.49 (95% CI: 0.25, 0.95). Similarly, Bogen et al.[30] studied 73,458 white and black low-income children and found that duration of breastfeeding was inversely associated with overweight only among white children whose mothers had not smoked during pregnancy. These two studies are the largest conducted among low-income populations and the only studies to date that stratified their analyses by race and ethnicity. The authors observed differential effects by racial and ethnic groups suggesting that the association between breastfeeding and overweight may be mediated by behavioral factors that differ across racial and ethnic groups (Table 19.5). Gillman et al.[74] also found an association of increased breastfeeding duration with decreased overweight among 15,341 older children and adolescents in the United States. In their study, the adjusted odds ratio for overweight declined with duration of breastfeeding, with the lowest odds ratio associated with more than 9 months of breastfeeding (Figure 19.1).

Three cohort studies[26,27,34] have provided information about the possible preventive influence of breastfeeding at multiple ages. These studies allow us to identify the time course of BMI differences and the development of overweight. Bergmann and Bergmann[26] studied 480 German children from birth to 6 years of age. The authors collected nutritional data at birth; when the children were 3, 6, 12, 18 months; and yearly thereafter until the children were 6 years old, as well as anthropometric data including triceps and subscapular skinfolds. They also obtained parental BMI, socioeconomic status, and smoking history at each visit. Breastfeeding was considered a dichotomous exposure: breastfeeding 3 months or more compared with less than 3 months. Breast-fed children in the study began to diverge from formula-fed children in BMI and adiposity between 3 to 4 years of age (Figure 19.2). In another cohort of 1037 children born in Dunedin, New Zealand, and followed from birth to 26 years of age, Poulton and Williams[26] found that the association of breastfeeding with decreased overweight was largely confined to late childhood (ages 7 and 11 years) and adolescence. Among those breastfed for more than 6 months compared with those who were never breastfed, a relatively weak relationship (odds ratios ranged from 0.86 to 1.01) was observed before the age of 7 years, which strengthened in late childhood from 7 to 11 years (odds ratios ranged from 0.25 to 0.67), and stabilized during adolescence (ORs approximately 0.70 in

TABLE 19.5
Adjusted Odds Ratios of the Association between Breastfeeding and Overweight in Children Aged 4 Years, by Race and Ethnicity.

Race/Ethnicity and Breastfeeding Duration	N	Overweight (%)	Odds Ratio	95% Confidence Interval
White, non-Hispanic				
Never breastfed	3174	14.5	1.00 (ref)	—
<1 month	643	14.3	0.99	0.77–1.27
1–2.9 months	510	14.9	1.14	0.87–1.50
3–5.9 months	377	10.6	0.73	0.51–1.05
6–11.9 months	448	9.8	0.7	0.50–0.99
≥12 months	150	6.7	0.49	0.25–0.95
Black, non-Hispanic				
Never breastfed	1659	13.3	1.00 (ref)	—
<1 month	456	18	1.32	0.98–1.76
1–2.9 months	332	16.6	1.31	0.93–1.83
3–5.9 months	261	17.2	1.27	0.88–1.83
6–11.9 months	203	19.2	1.36	0.91–2.01
≥12 months	56	14.3	0.87	0.40–1.89
Hispanic				
Never breastfed	1478	22.5	1.00 (ref)	—
<1 month	520	24.6	1.12	0.88–1.43
1–2.9 months	536	21.5	0.9	0.70–1.16
3–5.9 months	394	21.6	0.89	0.67–1.18
6–11.9 months	315	22.9	0.98	0.72–1.32
≥12 months	70	28.6	1.11	0.64–1.92
Other				
Never breastfed	773	16.2	1.00 (ref)	—
<1 month	87	17.2	1.01	0.55–1.87
1–2.9 months	73	17.8	1.03	0.53–1.98
3–5.9 months	32	3.4	0.46	0.13–1.58
6–11.9 months	23	8.7	0.52	0.12–2.31
≥12 months	17	11.8	0.46	0.10–2.18

Note: Odds ratio adjusted for child's gender, race/ethnicity, and birth weight and mother's age, education, prepregnancy BMI, weight gain during pregnancy, and postpartum smoking. Ref = reference group.

Source: Modified from Grummer-Strawn LM, Mei Z. *Pediatrics.* 2004;113(2):e81–86. Data from 12,587 participants in the Centers for Disease Control and Prevention Pediatric Nutrition Surveillance System.

ages 13 to 15 years) before somewhat weakening again in adulthood (ORs 0.79 at age 21 and 0.97 at age 26). In the study by Parsons et al.[34] of the 1958 British cohort of 9287 children, BMI data were collected at 7, 11, 16, and 33 years. The authors observed that breastfeeding and BMI were unrelated in childhood but an inverse relationship of BMI with duration of breastfeeding was evident at ages 16 and 33 years in females, and at 33 years in males. The results of these studies are consistent with the suggestion by Dietz[36] that the association between breastfeeding and overweight may remain latent in early childhood and appear at a later point in development.

One of the main limitations of the studies published before 1999 was the inability to adjust for potential confounders and thus, to know whether residual confounding by shared cultural determinants of both breastfeeding and obesity could explain the observed results. All of the studies summarized in Table 19.1, Table 19.2, and Table 19.3 involved adjustment for a number of traditional social and economic factors, but 4 of the 14 studies did not adjust for parental BMI or

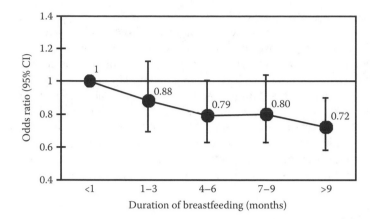

FIGURE 19.1 Risk of overweight in adolescence by duration of breastfeeding in infancy. Data from 15,341 9- to 14-year-old participants of the Growing Up Today study. (*Source:* Adapted from Gillman MW, Rifas-Shiman SL, Camargo CA, Jr., et al. *JAMA.* 2001;285: 2461–2467.)

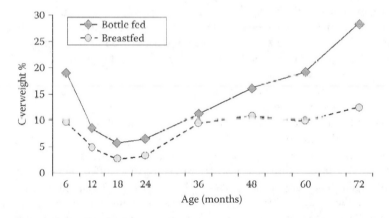

FIGURE 19.2 Prevalence of overweight (BMI > 90th percentile) among 480 children followed from birth to 6 years of age. (Adapted from Bergmann KE, Bergmann RL. *Int J Obes Relat Metab Disord.* 2003;27:162–72.)

overweight status.[19,21,23,32] Because parental obesity is generally related to both offspring overweight[28] and breastfeeding initiation and duration,[37,38] failure to adjust for it in analyses may lead to an overestimation of the effect of breastfeeding on overweight. Adjustment for parental BMI in most studies attenuated the effects of breastfeeding by as little as 5% in one study[34] to as much as 25% in another study.[33] Finally, few of the studies adjusted for nutrition and physical activity behaviors of children and adolescents, leaving open the possibility of residual confounding.

Future observational studies would be stronger if they directly measured why women choose to either breast- or formula-feed their infants and carefully measured other potential confounders that minimize the effects of differences between breastfeeding and formula-feeding. Additional data from a time when breastfeeding was more common in lower socioeconomic strata and overweight more common in higher socioeconomic strata might also help. Finally, it is possible that now-planned follow-up of participants in a Belarussian randomized trial to increase breast-feeding rates will address the limitations of residual confounding.[39] Crossovers could introduce noise, however, and generalizability to countries with higher rates of obesity would be an issue.

Another approach to minimizing confounding is within-family (most often sibling-pair) analyses. Because siblings usually share many genetic and environmental factors, this approach allows for a better understanding of the true effect of early life exposures on health outcomes over time, independent of numerous confounding factors that are not satisfactorily controlled using traditional cohort methods. Siblings may, however, differ on several factors that could be confounders, such as age (or birth order), sex, and Tanner stage. These factors should also be considered as covariates in sibling-pair analyses. Preliminary data from the Growing Up Today Study of 1542 sibling pairs with discordant overweight status (Gillman MW, unpublished data) have shown that the within-family adjusted odds ratios for breastfeeding duration appears similar to the overall (not within-family) estimate. With a smaller sample size, however, the within-family estimate is associated with a much wider confidence interval. In contrast, Nelson et al.[40] did not find that discordant breastfeeding of sibling pairs predicted BMI z-scores or discordant overweight status among 850 sibling pairs. Larger studies of siblings are needed to examine this relationship.

POTENTIAL MECHANISMS

If having been breastfed does indeed protect against future overweight, at least two types of mechanisms could be at play: behavioral and metabolic. Children naturally regulate their energy intake, but parents' behavior may override the appetite signals. Birch and Fisher[41] have reported that preschool children of parents who used highly controlling feeding practices had lower self-regulation of energy intake and, among the girls, increased adiposity. In infancy, it is possible that compared with parents who bottle-feed, mothers who breast-feed may be more responsive to the infant's signals for frequency and volume of feedings. Breastfed infants would thus learn better self-regulation of their energy intake and gain less excess weight over time even in the face of the energy surfeit that characterizes our society.

In a recent systematic review of parental feeding styles and later child eating and weight status,[42] the authors found that increased parental feeding restriction (i.e., restricting children's access to preferred foods), but not other feeding domains, was associated with later increased eating and weight status among children. Thus, one underlying pathway by which breastfeeding may be related to child and adolescent overweight is through its influence on maternal feeding restriction.

Only a few studies have addressed how breastfeeding may affect maternal control of infant feeding. Infants appear to be able to adjust the volume of milk consumed to maintain a constant energy intake.[43] Fomon et al.[43] suggested that because breastfeeding mothers are less able than bottle-feeding mothers to monitor how much milk their infants consume, the quantity of milk consumed is primarily under the infants' control. Thus, breastfeeding may promote maternal feeding styles that are less controlling.[43] It is also likely that feeding duration and intake in bottle-fed infants may be influenced by visual cues. Parents who bottle-feed their infants may be more responsive to visible milk remaining in the bottle and, consequently, more likely to have their infants finish the bottle even when the infants are satiated. This hypothesis is supported by one study that found that breastfed infants at 6 to 9 months consumed less nonmilk food offered to them than bottle-fed infants did.[44]

Two longitudinal studies have examined the relationship between breastfeeding and maternal feeding control. Fisher et al.[45] found that mothers who breastfed their infants for at least 12 months used lower levels of control in feeding, including less restriction and pressure to eat, than mothers who did not breast-feed their infants for at least 12 months, suggesting that breastfeeding may promote parenting feeding styles that are more responsive to infant cues of hunger and satiety and, thus, promote shared mother–infant regulation of food intake.[45]

Data from 1160 mother–infant pairs participating in Project Viva, a prospective observational cohort study of gestational diet, pregnancy outcomes, and offspring health, have also shown that longer breastfeeding duration is related to less maternal restriction of infant feeding but not pressure to eat at 12 months of age, even after controlling for preexisting maternal attitudes toward control of infant feeding[46] (Figure 19.3). No studies to date, however, report prospective data linking infant feeding type and duration with maternal control over infant feeding with adiposity in childhood.

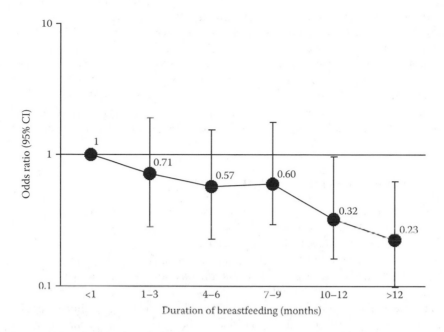

FIGURE 19.3 Relationship of breastfeeding duration with maternal restriction of child's intake at age 1 year, odds ratios, and 95% confidence intervals for each category compared with the reference group of never breastfed or breastfed less than 1 month. Estimates are adjusted for gender only. Data from 1160 mother–infant pairs participating in Project Viva. (Adapted from Taveras EM, Scanlon KS, Birch L, Rifas-Shiman SL, Rich-Edwards JW, Gillman MW. *Pediatrics.* 2004;114(5): e577–583.)

A second mechanism could be related to the metabolic influences of ingested breast milk. A few studies suggest that breast milk feeding could alter the adipoinsular axis. Lucas et al.[47,48] found higher plasma insulin concentrations in formula-fed infants and a prolonged insulin response at 6 days of age compared with breastfed infants. Higher insulin levels would be expected to stimulate fat deposition and thus affect early development of adipocytes. A study of Pima Indian children ages 5 to 9 years found that fasting plasma insulin concentration correlated with the rate of weight gain per year in both boys ($r = 0.42$; $P < 0.0001$) and girls ($r = 0.20$; $P < 0.01$) and was associated with change in relative weight and in triceps skinfold thickness, thus supporting the hypothesis that fasting hyperinsulinemia may promote rapid deposition of fat and adiposity.[49] Some studies of children and adults have shown a link between breastfeeding and plasma insulin, obesity, type II diabetes, and glucose tolerance.[50–52] Singhal et al.[53] conducted two randomized trials among preterm infants: in one, the infants received either preterm (energy-enriched) or standard formula, and in the other they received either preterm formula or banked donated breast milk. The authors found that infants that were randomly assigned human milk instead of formula, for just 4 weeks, had substantial benefits 13 to 16 years later in lipid profile,[54] blood pressure,[55] and insulin resistance.[53]

Another hormone that may mediate the protective effect of breastfeeding on overweight is leptin. Leptin is secreted by adipose and other tissues, and serves to regulate energy intake in response to satiety. Breast milk contains leptin, whereas commercial infant formulas do not.[56] The presence of leptin in breast milk may have a positive effect on satiety and regulation of energy intake.[56] Studies are inconclusive, however, as to whether infants receiving breast milk have higher or lower blood leptin concentrations than those receiving formula.[57–59] Part of the discrepancy may be related to the fact that leptin is derived from adipocytes, so that one must take into account the body composition at the time of leptin measurement, which is not straightforward in infants. Laboratory measurement issues may also play a role because one must account for the fat in breast milk.[56] Only one epidemiologic follow-up study has examined the long-term effects of breastfeeding on leptin. Among almost 1000 initial subjects, Singhal et al.[53] measured leptin concentrations in 197 at ages 13 to 16 years. The participants who had received preterm formula had higher leptin (adjusted for fat mass) levels than the other two groups. In analyses without randomization, the highest percentage of breast milk intake was related to the lowest leptin–fat mass concentrations. This study suggests a long-lasting effect of breast milk on leptin metabolism. On the other hand, it is limited because it included no term infants, who constitute the large majority of individuals who will grow up to have problems with obesity, and had low follow-up rates. Future studies should prospectively examine the link between infant feeding type and duration, and leptin status later in childhood.

CLINICAL AND PUBLIC HEALTH IMPLICATIONS

The role of breastfeeding in obesity prevention has taken on new urgency in the twenty-first century. While some point out that breastfeeding *initiation* rates have risen close to the Healthy People 2010 goals in the United States in recent decades, rates of breastfeeding (and exclusive breastfeeding) *maintenance* until at least 6 months of age lag far behind national goals.[12] In addition, racial and ethnic minorities and women of lower socioeconomic position initiate and maintain breastfeeding rates at much lower levels,[10,16,60,61] and these groups have particularly high rates of obesity in childhood and beyond.[18] Such disparities make it essential to address the validity of epidemiologic associations between breastfeeding and later obesity, both by carefully controlling for potential confounding by sociocultural factors and by evaluating plausible mechanisms, including behavioral and metabolic effects.

For a variety of reasons, breastfeeding remains the best choice for infant feeding; thus, there is little risk to cautiously promoting breastfeeding for overweight prevention. New approaches for counseling, however, are needed for women who choose to bottle-feed. Strategies to assist bottle-feeding parents in promoting infant self-regulation of energy intake may decrease their children's risk of later overweight.

In summary, the evidence to date suggests that having been breastfed, as opposed to bottle fed, is associated with lower prevalence of overweight. While these relationships might be confounded by sociocultural determinants of both the decision to breast-feed and obesity, plausible but under-studied mechanisms have emerged. One posits that the act of breastfeeding itself promotes lifelong self-regulation of energy intake, while another raises the possibility that breast milk may affect the adipoinsular axis. The growing evidence that having been breastfed may lower one's risk of excess weight gain later in life may support efforts of health professionals and public health researchers in formulating policies to increase breastfeeding initiation and promote prolonged breastfeeding across the country. Continued promotion and support of breastfeeding could help to attenuate the dramatically rising prevalence of obesity in the United States and elsewhere.

ACKNOWLEDGMENTS

Dr. Taveras is supported in part by the Minority Medical Faculty Development Program of the Robert Wood Johnson Foundation and a grant from the U.S. National Institutes of Health (HL 64925 – S1). Dr. Gillman is supported in part by grants from the U.S. National Institutes of Health (HD 34568, HL 64925, HL 68041).

REFERENCES

1. Hoefer C, Hardy MC. Later development of breast fed and artificially fed infants. *JAMA*. 1929;92: 615–619.
2. Butte NF. The evidence for breastfeeding. *Ped Clin N Am*. 2001;48: 189–198.

3. Dewey KG. Is breastfeeding protective against child obesity? *J Hum Lact.* 2003;191(1): 9–18.
4. Scariati PD, Grummer-Strawn LM, Fein SB. A longitudinal analysis of infant morbidity and the extent of breastfeeding in the United States. *Pediatrics.* 1997;99(6): E5.
5. Dewey KG, Heinig MJ, Nommsen-Rivers LA. Differences in morbidity between breastfed and formula-fed infants. *J Pediatr.* 1995;126(5 Pt 1): 696–702.
6. Howie PW. Protective effect of breastfeeding against infection in the first and second six months of life. *Adv Exper Med Biol.* 2002;503: 141–147.
7. Dermer A. Breastfeeding and women's health. *J Women Health.* 1998;7(4): 427–433.
8. American Academy of Pediatrics. Breastfeeding and the use of human milk. Work Group on Breastfeeding [comment]. *Pediatrics.* 1997;100(6): 1035–1039.
9. Kramer MS, Kakuma R. *The Optimal Duration of Exclusive Breastfeeding.* Geneva: Department of Nutrition for Health and Development, Department of Child and Adolescent Health and Development, World Health Organizatio, 2001.
10. Ryan AS, Wenjun Z, Acosta A. Breastfeeding continues to increase into the new millennium. *Pediatrics.* 2002;11(6): 1103–1109.
11. Li R, Zhao Z, Mokdad A, Barker L, Grummer Strawn L. Prevalence of breastfeeding in the United States: the 2001 National Immunization Survey. *Pediatrics.* 2003;111(5 Part 2): 1198–1201.
12. U. S. Department of Health and Human Services. *Healthy People 2010:* Conference ed. Vols I and II. Washington, DC: U. S. Department of Health and Human Services, Office of the Assistant Secretary for Health January 2000.
13. Li R, Ogden C, Ballew C, Gillespie C, Grummer-Strawn L. Prevalence of exclusive breastfeeding among US infants: the Third National Health and Nutrition Examination Survey (Phase II, 1991–1994). *Am J Public Health.* 2002;92(7): 1107–1110.
14. Li R, Grummer-Strawn L. Racial and ethnic disparities in breastfeeding among United States infants: Third National Health and Nutrition Examination Survey, 1988–1994. *Birth.* 2002;29(4): 251–257.
15. U. S. Department of Health and Human Services. *Healthy People 2010:* Conference ed. Vols I and II. Washington, DC: U. S. Department of Health and Human Services, Office of the Assistant Secretary for Health January 2000.
16. Forste R, Weiss J. The decision to breastfeed in the United States: Does race matter? *Pediatrics.* 2001;108: 291–296.
17. Strauss RS, Pollack HA. Epidemic increase in childhood overweight, 1986–1998. *JAMA.* 2001;286(22): 2845–2848.
18. Hedley AA, Ogden CL, Johnson CL, Carroll MD, Curtin LR, Flegal KM. Prevalence of overweight and obesity among US children, adolescents, and adults, 1999–2002. *JAMA.* 2004;291(23): 2847–2850.
19. von Kries R, Koletzko B, Sauerwald T, et al. Breast feeding and obesity: cross sectional study. *BMJ.* 1999;319: 147–150.
20. Hediger ML, Overpeck MD, Kuczmarski RJ, Ruan WJ. Association between infant breastfeeding and overweight in young children. *JAMA.* 2001;285(19): 2453–2460.
21. Armstrong J, Reilly JJ, Team CHI. Breastfeeding and lowering the risk of childhood obesity. *Lancet.* 2002;359: 2003–2004.
22. Grummer-Strawn LM, Mei Z. Does breastfeeding protect against pediatric overweight? Analysis of longitudinal data from the Centers for Disease Control and Prevention Pediatric Nutrition Surveillance System. *Pediatrics.* 2004;113(2): E81–86.
23. Liese AD, Hirsch T, von Mutius E, Keil U, Leupold W, Weiland SK. Inverse association of overweight and breastfeeding in 9- to 10-y-old children in Germany. *Int J Obes Relat Metab Disord.* 2001;25(11): 1644–1650.
24. Gillman MW, Rifas-Shiman SL, Camargo CA, Jr., et al. Risk of overweight among adolescents who had been breast fed as infants. *JAMA.* 2001;285: 2461–2467.
25. Toschke AM, Vignerova J, Lhotska L, Osancova K, Koletzko B, von Kries R. Overweight and obesity in 6- to 14-year-old Czech children in 1991: protective effect of breastfeeding. *J Pediatr.* 2002;141: 764–769.
26. Bergmann KE, Bergmann RL. Early determinants of childhood overweight and adiposity in a birth cohort study: role of breastfeeding. *Int J Obes Relat Metab Disord.* 2003;27: 162–172.
27. Poulton R, Williams S. Breastfeeding and risk of overweight. *JAMA.* 2001;286(12): 1449–50.

28. Whitaker RC, Wright JA, Pepe MS, Seidel KD, Dietz WH, Jr. Predicting obesity in young adulthood from childhood and parental obesity. *N Engl J Med.* 1997;337: 869–873.

29. O'Callaghan MJ, Williams GM, Anderson MJ, Bor W, Najman JM. Prediction of obesity in children at 5 years: a cohort study. *J Paediatr Child Health.* 1997;33: 311–316.

30. Bogen DL, Hanusa BH, Whitaker RC. The effect of breastfeeding with and without formula use on the risk of obesity at 4 years of age. *Obes Res.* 2004;12(9): 1527–1535.

31. Hediger ML, Overpeck MD, Ruan WJ, Troendle JF. Early infant feeding and growth status of US-born infants and children aged 4–71 mo: analyses from the third National Health and Nutrition Examination Survey, 1988–1994. *Am J Clin Nutr.* 2000;72(1): 159–167.

32. Wadsworth M, Marshall S, Hardy R, Paul A. Breast feeding and obesity. Relation may be accounted for by social factors. *BMJ.* 1999;319(7224): 1576.

33. Li L, Parsons TJ, Power C. Breast feeding and obesity in childhood: cross sectional study. *BMJ.* 2003;327(7420): 904–905.

34. Parsons TJ, Power C, Manor O. Infant feeding and obesity through the lifecourse. *Arch Dis Child.* 2003;88(9): 793–794.

35. Victora CG, Barros F, Lima RC, Horta BL, Wells J. Anthropometry and body composition of 18 year old men according to duration of breastfeeding: birth cohort study from Brazil. *BMJ.* 2003;327: 901.

36. Dietz WH. Breastfeeding may help prevent childhood overweight. *JAMA.* 2001;285(19): 2506–2507.

37. Li R, Jewell S, Grummer-Strawn L. Maternal obesity and breastfeeding practices. *Am J Clin Nutrition* 2003;77(4): 931–936.

38. Donath SM, Amir LH. Does maternal obesity adversely affect breastfeeding initiation and duration? *Breastfeed Rev.* 2000;8(3): 29–33.

39. Kramer MS, Guo T, Platt RW, et al. Breastfeeding and infant growth: biology or bias? *Pediatrics.* 2002;110(2): 343–347.

40. Nelson MC, Gordon-Larsen P, Adair LS. Are adolescents who were breastfed less likely to be overweight? Reducing the effect of confounding through the use of sibling pair analyses. *Proc Soc Epidemiol Res.* 2004;S55: 218–S.

41. Birch LL, Fisher JO. Development of eating behaviors among children and adolescents. *Pediatrics.* 1998;101: 539–548.

42. Faith MS, Francis L, Sherry B, Scanlon KS, Birch LL. Relationship between maternal feeding style and child energy intake and body composition: findings from a quantitative and qualitative literature review [abstract]. *Obes Res.* 2001;9: 123S.

43. Fomon SJ, Filmer LJ, Jr., Thomas LN, Anderson TA, Nelson SE. Influence of formula concentration on caloric intake and growth of normal infants. *Acta Paediatr Scand.* 1975;64(2): 172–181.

44. Dewey KG, Heinig MJ, Nommsen LA, Lonnerdal B. Adequacy of energy intake among breastfed infants in the DARLING study: relationships to growth velocity, morbidity, and activity levels. Davis Area Research on Lactation, Infant Nutrition and Growth. *J Pediatr.* 1991;119(4): 538–547.

45. Fisher JO, Birch LL, Smiciklas-Wright H, Picciano MF. Breastfeeding through the first year predicts maternal control in feeding and subsequent toddler energy intakes. *J Am Diet Assoc.* 2000;100(6): 641–646.

46. Taveras EM, Scanlon KS, Birch L, Rifas-Shiman SL, Rich-Edwards JW, Gillman MW. Association of breastfeeding with maternal control of infant feeding at age 1 year. *Pediatrics.* 2004;114(5): e577–583.

47. Lucas A, Sarson DL, Blackburn AM, Adrian TE, Aynsley-Green A, Bloom SR. Breast vs. bottle: endocrine responses are different with formula feeding. *Lancet.* 1980;1: 1267–1269.

48. Lucas A, Boyes S, Bloom SR, Aynsley-Green A. Metabolic and endocrine responses to milk fed in six-day-old term infants: differences between breast and cow's milk formula feeding. *Acta Paediatr Scand.* 1981;70: 195–200.

49. Odeleye OE, de Courten M, Pettitt DJ, Ravussin E. Fasting hyperinsulinemia is a predictor of increased body weight gain and obesity in Pima Indian children. *Diabetes.* 1997;46(8): 1341–1345.

50. Young TK, Martens PJ, Taback SP, et al. Type 2 diabetes mellitus in children: prenatal and early infancy risk factors among native Canadians. *Arch Pediatr Adolesc Med.* 2002;156(7): 651–655.

51. Ravelli AC, van der Meulen JH, Osmond C, Barker DJ, Bleker OP. Infant feeding and adult glucose tolerance, lipid profile, blood pressure, and obesity. *Arch Dis Child.* 2000;82(3): 248–252.

52. Pettitt DJ, Forman MR, Hanson RL, Knowler WC, Bennet PH. Breastfeeding and incidence of non-insulin-dependent diabetes mellitus in Pima Indians. *Lancet.* 1997;350: 166–168.

53. Singhal A, Fewtrell M, Cole TJ, Lucas A. Low nutrient intake and early growth for later insulin resistance in adolescents born preterm. *Lancet.* 2003;361: 1089–1097.

54. Singhal A, Cole TJ, Fewtrell M, Lucas A. Breastmilk feeding and lipoprotein profile in adolescents born preterm: follow-up of a prospective randomised study. *Lancet.* 2004;363(9421): 1571–1578.

55. Singhal A, Cole TJ, Lucas A. Early nutrition in preterm infants and later blood pressure: two cohorts after randomised trials. *Lancet.* 2001;357(9254): 413–419.

56. Locke R. Preventing obesity: the breast milk-leptin connection. *Acta Paediatr.* 2002;91: 891–896.

57. Soumerai SB, McLaughlin TJ, Spiegelman D, Hertzmark E, Thibault G, Goldman L. Adverse outcomes of underuse of beta blockers in elderly survivors of acute myocardial infarction. *JAMA.* 1997;277: 115–121.

58. Lonnerdal B, Havel PJ. Serum leptin concentrations in infants: effects of diet, sex, and adiposity. *Am J Clin Nutr.* 2000;72: 484–489.

59. Shimizu T, Satoh Y, Shoji H, et al. Lack of plasma leptin response to feeding in newborn infants. *J Paediatr Child Health.* 2004;40(1–2): 42–43.

60. Li R, Ogden C, Ballew C, Gillespie C, Grummer-Strawn L. Prevalence of exclusive breastfeeding among US infants: the Third National Health and Nutrition Examination Survey (Phase II, 1991–1994). *Am J Public Health.* 2002;92: 1107–1110.

61. Li R, Grummer-Strawn L. Racial and ethnic disparities in breastfeeding among United States infants: Third National Health and Nutrition Examination Survey (1988–1994). *Birth.* 2002;29: 251–257.

Index